Key Concepts in Nutrition and Metabolism

Key Concepts in Nutrition and Metabolism

Edited by Vivian Belt

Syrawood Publishing House
New York

Published by Syrawood Publishing House,
750 Third Avenue, 9th Floor,
New York, NY 10017, USA
www.syrawoodpublishinghouse.com

Key Concepts in Nutrition and Metabolism
Edited by Vivian Belt

International Standard Book Number: 978-1-68286-495-1 (Hardback)

Cataloging-in-Publication Data

Key concepts in nutrition and metabolism / edited by Vivian Belt.
p. cm.
Includes bibliographical references and index.
ISBN 978-1-68286-495-1
1. Nutrition. 2. Metabolism. 3. Physiology. I. Belt, Vivian.
QP141.K49 2017
613.2--dc23

Printed in China.

TABLE OF CONTENTS

PREFACE

Metabolism is the process whereby food is converted into energy by living organisms. This book on nutrition and metabolism deals with topics related to physical activity and metabolism as well as the chemical reactions that occur during the metabolic process. Metabolic activity changes according to the requirement of energy by cells. This book is a valuable compilation of topics, ranging from the basic to the most complex advancements in the field of nutrition and metabolism. For all readers who are interested in these fields, the research included in this book will serve as an excellent guide to develop a comprehensive understanding. It will serve as a reference to a broad spectrum of readers.

The information contained in this book is the result of intensive hard work done by researchers in this field. All due efforts have been made to make this book serve as a complete guiding source for students and researchers. The topics in this book have been comprehensively explained to help readers understand the growing trends in the field.

I would like to thank the entire group of writers who made sincere efforts in this book and my family who supported me in my efforts of working on this book. I take this opportunity to thank all those who have been a guiding force throughout my life.

Editor

Associations among the plasma amino acid profile, obesity, and glucose metabolism in Japanese adults with normal glucose tolerance

Chisa Takashina[1], Ichizo Tsujino[1*], Taku Watanabe[1], Shinji Sakaue[2], Daisuke Ikeda[1], Asuka Yamada[1], Takahiro Sato[1], Hiroshi Ohira[2], Yoshinori Otsuka[3], Noriko Oyama-Manabe[4], Yoichi M. Ito[5] and Masaharu Nishimura[2]

Abstract

Background: Amino acids (AAs) are emerging as a new class of effective molecules in the etiology of obesity and diabetes mellitus. However, most investigations have focused on subjects with obesity and/or impaired glucose regulation; the possible involvement of AAs in the initial phase of glucose dysregulation remains poorly understood. Furthermore, little attention has been given to possible associations between the pattern/degree of fat deposition and the plasma AA profile. Our objective was therefore to determine the relationships between plasma AA concentrations and the type/degree of obesity and glucose regulation in Japanese adults with normal glucose tolerance.

Methods: Eighty-three subjects with normal glucose tolerance were classified as obese or nonobese and as visceral obesity or nonvisceral obesity. Correlations between the plasma levels of 23 AAs and somatometric measurements, visceral fat area (VFA), subcutaneous fat area (SFA), and 75-g oral glucose tolerance test results were analyzed.

Results: Obesity or visceral obesity was associated with higher levels of branched-chain AAs (isoleucine, leucine, and valine), lysine, tryptophan, cystine, and glutamate but lower levels of asparagine, citrulline, glutamine, glycine, and serine ($p < 0.04$). Age- and gender-adjusted analyses indicated that VFA was positively correlated with tryptophan and glutamate levels, whereas VFA and SFA were negatively correlated with citrulline, glutamine, and glycine levels ($p < 0.05$). The fasting and 2-h plasma glucose levels or the homeostasis model assessment of insulin resistance were positively correlated with valine, glutamate, and tyrosine levels but negatively correlated with citrulline, glutamine, and glycine levels. The homeostasis model assessment for the β-cell function index was positively correlated with leucine, tryptophan, valine, and glutamate levels but negatively correlated with citrulline, glutamine, glycine, and serine levels ($p < 0.05$).

Conclusions: The present study identified specific associations between 10 AAs and the type/degree of obesity, and indices of glucose/insulin regulation, in Japanese adults with preserved glucose metabolism. With the growing concern about the increasing prevalence of obesity and diabetes, the possible roles of these AAs as early markers and/or precursors warrant further investigation.

Keywords: Visceral obesity, Oral glucose tolerance test, Insulin secretion, Insulin resistance, Branched-chain amino acid, Glycine, Glutamate, Glutamine

* Correspondence: itsujino@med.hokudai.ac.jp
[1]First Department of Medicine, Hokkaido University Hospital, North 14, West 5, Kita-ku, Sapporo 060-8648, Japan
Full list of author information is available at the end of the article

Background

Globally, the prevalence of diabetes mellitus (DM), impaired glucose tolerance (IGT), and metabolic syndrome is increasing; these disorders are becoming a major economic and social burden [1]. Insulin resistance plays a central role in the pathogenesis of these disorders, through defects in insulin-mediated glucose uptake and/or glucose release by the liver, muscles, and other peripheral tissues. There is a well-established epidemiological relationship between obesity and insulin resistance. However, this relationship has been investigated less thoroughly in nondiabetic subjects with normal glucose metabolism than in subjects with DM or IGT.

Amino acids (AAs) are emerging as a new class of effective molecules in the etiology of obesity and DM. During a 12-year follow-up study, plasma levels of branched-chain AAs (BCAAs; isoleucine, leucine, and valine), tyrosine, and phenylalanine were reported to predict the development of DM in nondiabetic subjects [2]. Prior clinical studies have also identified significant associations between the plasma levels of specific AAs and body mass index (BMI) [3, 4] or glucose regulation [5]. However, most investigations involved subjects with obesity and/or impaired glucose regulation [6–8]. Thus, the possible involvement of AAs in the initial phase of glucose dysregulation remains poorly understood. Furthermore, little attention has been given to possible associations between the pattern and degree of fat deposition and the plasma AA profile. This is of clinical interest because visceral adipose tissue demonstrates a stronger association with metabolic disturbances and cardiovascular risks than subcutaneous adipose tissue [9, 10]. Finally, most related studies involved mainly non-Asian subjects [4, 5, 11], who differ physically and metabolically from the Asian population [12, 13]. Indeed, a community-based observational study documented that Asians have a lower BMI but a higher percentage of body fat than Caucasians [14]. Based on these and other publications from around the world [15, 16], a definition for obesity specific to the Japanese population was proposed as BMI ≥ 25 kg/m^2 [17], which differed from that for Europeans (BMI ≥ 30 kg/m^2).

The aim of the present study was to investigate the relationships between the plasma AA profile and the type/degree of obesity as well as glucose and insulin regulation, in normoglycemic Japanese adults. Using a detailed analysis of the indices of insulin resistance, sensitivity, and secretion derived from the 75-g oral glucose tolerance test (75-g OGTT), this study identified significant associations between AAs and the development of aberrant glucose regulation in nondiabetic Japanese adults.

Methods

Subjects

Ninety-four healthy Japanese volunteers aged 20–60 years were recruited between March 2009 and March 2010 from the medical students, interns, employees, and paramedical staff of Hokkaido University Hospital. We excluded subjects with a history of DM, chronic kidney disease, or liver disease, and those taking medications that could affect glucose metabolism, such as angiotensin-converting enzyme inhibitors, angiotensin II receptor inhibitors, statins, quinolones, antimicrobial agents, and any drug that presents hormonal effects. Finally, those unable to undergo magnetic resonance imaging (MRI) for any reason were excluded. This study was approved by the Ethical Committee on Human Experiments of Hokkaido University Graduate School of Medicine (MED08-003), and written informed consent was obtained from all subjects.

All subjects underwent somatometry, blood sampling, 75-g OGTT, and MRI within a week of their enrollment, during which there was no significant change in their lifestyle, including their dietary intake, or their physical condition.

Somatometry

Height and body weight (BW) were measured using standard methods on the same day as the blood sampling for plasma AA measurements and the 75-g OGTT. Waist circumference (WC) was measured in the standing position, at the umbilical level, after expiration during natural breathing. BMI was calculated using the following formula: BW (kg)/(height (m))^2. The subjects were divided into two groups based on the BMI cutoff value for obesity determined for the Japanese population (BMI ≥ 25 kg/m^2) [17].

The 75-g OGTT

The subjects were tested using the standard 75-g OGTT procedure [18]. Briefly, the subjects were fasted from 11 pm on the previous day until 9 am, when they were given 300 ml of aqueous solution containing 75 g of glucose to drink within 5 min. Blood samples were collected from an antecubital vein immediately before ingestion of the solution (fasting plasma glucose [FPG]) and 30, 60, 90, and 120 min after ingestion. The samples were collected in tubes containing fluoride and maintained at 4 °C until they were centrifuged, within 2 h, to measure the plasma glucose (PG) and plasma insulin levels. The results were interpreted according to the World Health Organization definitions: normal glucose tolerance (NGT; FPG < 110 mg/dl and 2-h PG < 140 mg/dl), impaired fasting glucose (FPG 110–125 mg/dl and 2-h PG < 140 mg/dl), IGT (FPG < 126 mg/dl and 2-h PG 140–199 mg/dl), and DM (FPG ≥ 126 mg/dl or 2-h PG ≥

200 mg/dl) [19]. Insulin resistance was determined using the homeostasis model assessment of insulin resistance (HOMA-IR) index, calculated as follows: FPG (mg/dl) × fasting plasma insulin (μU/ml) / 405 [20]. Insulin sensitivity was assessed by calculating the oral glucose insulin sensitivity (OGIS) index using a spreadsheet downloaded from the OGIS website [21, 22]. Insulin secretion was measured using the homeostasis model assessment of β-cell function index (HOMA-β), calculated as follows: (fasting plasma insulin (μU/ml) × 360)/(FPG (mg/dl) – 63) [20]. Insulin secretion was also expressed in terms of the insulinogenic index (II): 0–30 min insulin increment (μU/ml)/0–30 min PG increment (mg/dl) [23].

Measurement of plasma AA concentrations

Separate blood specimens were collected from the antecubital vein into heparinized tubes at the time the fasting blood specimens were obtained for the 75-g OGTT. The plasma was separated at 4 °C and stored at −80 °C until the measurements were made. The plasma was deproteinized in a final concentration of 80 % acetonitrile, and the plasma AAs were identified and quantified using high-performance liquid chromatography (L-8500; Hitachi, Ltd., Tokyo) after derivatization (SRL, Inc., Tokyo) [24, 25].

Twenty-three compounds were analyzed in each plasma sample to cover the main essential AAs acquired from the diet (histidine, isoleucine, leucine, lysine, methionine, phenylalanine, threonine, tryptophan, and valine) as well as the nonessential AAs (alanine, arginine, asparagine, α-aminobutyric acid, citrulline, cystine, glutamate, glutamine, glycine, ornithine, proline, serine, taurine, and tyrosine). Of these, the BCAAs are isoleucine, leucine, and valine.

Evaluation of visceral and subcutaneous fat by MRI

The MRIs were performed with an Achieva 1.5 T (Philips Medical System, Best, The Netherlands) equipped with a gantry coil. Coronal, sagittal, and long-axis scout images were obtained, covering the whole body from the cervix to the pelvis. Transverse axial fat imaging was then performed during repeated breath-holds, using a T1-turbo field echo (TFE) sequence with spectral attenuated inversion recovery (SPAIR) for water suppression. The acquisition parameters were as follows: field of view, 450 × 310 mm; (repetition time)/(echo time), 3.6/1.7 ms; acquisition matrix, 128 × 100; slice thickness, 6 mm; flip angle, 10°; and TFE factor, 30. For SPAIR, the repetition time was 206 ms, and the inversion time was 80 ms.

The areas of visceral and subcutaneous fat were measured using commercially available software (FatChecker, VOX-BASE; J-MAC system, Sapporo, Japan). In brief, a transaxial image at the level of the umbilicus was selected from the stack of abdominal short-axis images. In this image, fat tissue was distinguished from the other tissues (muscles and bones) based on the minimum and maximum signal intensities of each tissue, calculated using an approximation of the Gaussian distribution of the overall histogram. The boundaries between the subcutaneous fat and visceral fat were automatically traced using the software's tracking operation. The subcutaneous fat and visceral fat were identified as the regions outside and inside of these boundaries, respectively. Each fat region identified with this method was visually confirmed, and the border manually corrected as needed. The subcutaneous fat area (SFA) and visceral fat area (VFA) were calculated from the number of pixels in the histograms and the pixel size. The subjects were divided into two groups based on the widely used VFA cutoff value of 100 cm^2: the visceral obesity group (VFA ≥ 100 cm^2) and the nonvisceral obesity group (VFA < 100 cm^2) [17].

Data analysis

All values are presented as mean ± SD. The obese and nonobese groups, and the visceral obesity group and nonvisceral obesity groups, were compared in terms of demographic parameters, somatometric indices, 75-g OGTT results, SFA, VFA, and plasma AA concentrations using chi-square tests or unpaired *t*-tests, as appropriate.

Plasma AA concentrations were also compared between men and women using an unpaired *t*-test.

Associations between plasma AA concentrations and other variables (age, BW, BMI, WC, VFA, SFA, FPG, 2-h PG, HOMA-IR, OGIS, HOMA-β, and II) were assessed by Pearson's correlation analysis and also by multivariate logistic regression analysis adjusted for age and gender.

The reproducibility of the SFA and VFA measurements was determined using randomly selected MRI images from 10 subjects, measured by two investigators (AY and CT) separated by an interval of at least 2 weeks. The reproducibility analysis was conducted using Bland–Altman plots and intraclass correlation coefficients. The investigators were unaware of the somatometric data or the blood test results.

All statistical analyses were conducted using JMP software version 10, and p values <0.05 were considered statistically significant.

Results

Among the 94 adult volunteers, 11 subjects were excluded from the analysis because the 75-g OGTT test indicated that they had DM ($n = 3$) or IGT ($n = 8$). The remaining 83 subjects, 66 men and 17 women all with NGT, were divided into two groups based on their BMI: obese ($n = 10$) or nonobese ($n = 73$). These subjects were also divided into two groups based on their VFA: visceral obesity ($n = 18$) or nonvisceral obesity ($n = 65$). The two pairs of groups were compared in terms of demographic, somatometric, 75-g OGTT, and MRI data (Table 1). The obese group presented significantly higher somatometric parameters (BW, BMI, and WC), FPG, insulin resistance (HOMA-IR), insulin secretion (II), and SFA, but a lower insulin sensitivity (OGIS) than the nonobese group (all $p < 0.001$). The visceral obesity group included significantly more men than the nonvisceral obesity group, as well as significantly higher age, somatometric parameters (BW, BMI, and WC), and II (all $p \leq 0.017$).

Table 2 shows that, for the essential AAs, obesity and visceral obesity were both associated with higher plasma concentrations of the three BCAAs (isoleucine, leucine, and valine; all $p \leq 0.033$). Lysine levels were higher in the obese group ($p = 0.006$), and tryptophan levels were higher in the visceral obesity group ($p = 0.004$). In contrast, the analysis revealed remarkably different impacts of obesity and visceral obesity on the nonessential AA profile. Obesity was associated with higher levels of cystine and glutamate but lower levels of glycine. Visceral obesity was associated with higher levels of glutamate but lower levels of asparagine, citrulline, glutamine, glycine, and serine.

Comparison of the AA concentrations between men and women showed that those of 11 AAs were higher in men than in women, but serine levels were lower in men than in women (Additional file 1: Table S1). There were significant correlations between age and the plasma concentrations of four AAs (Additional file 2: Table S2). In a subgroup analysis involving only the 66 men, 7 of the 10 AAs that exhibited significantly different concentrations in the overall analysis on 83 subjects still showed different plasma concentrations between visceral and nonvisceral obesity groups (Additional file 3: Table S3). The men were further divided into two subsets (each $n = 33$) according to whether they were aged above or below the median age of 35. A comparison of AA concentrations showed that significant differences existed for two AAs (glutamate and glutamine) in the older subset (>35 years) and for eight AAs in the younger subset (Additional file 4: Table S4). Overall, these results suggested significant impacts of gender and age on the AA concentrations. At the same time, they also indicated the associations between AA concentrations and visceral obesity because significant differences of the concentrations of some AAs remained between the subjects with or without visceral obesity in the age- and gender-adjusted analyses.

The associations between AAs and the glucose regulation of the NGT subjects was investigated by Pearson's correlation analysis (Table 3, Additional file 5: Table S5) and by age- and gender-adjusted logistic regression analysis (Table 4, Additional file 6: Table S6) of the plasma AA concentrations of all 83 subjects and the

Table 1 Somatometric measurements and the results of 75-g oral glucose tolerance test and magnetic resonance imaging

	Overall ($n = 83$)	Obese ($n = 10$)	Nonobese ($n = 73$)	p values [a]	Visceral obesity ($n = 18$)	Nonvisceral obesity ($n = 65$)	p values[b]
Gender (male/female)	66/17	10/0	56/17	0.114	18/0	48/17	**0.017**
Age (years)	34.0 ± 5.7	35.2 ± 3.8	33.8 ± 5.9	0.487	37.1 ± 7.0	33.2 ± 5.0	**0.009**
Somatometric measurements							
Body weight (kg)	65.5 ± 9.9	79.5 ± 8.5	63.5 ± 8.5	**<0.001**	72.0 ± 8.2	63.7 ± 9.6	**0.001**
Body mass index (kg/m^2)	22.5 ± 2.4	26.7 ± 2.3	21.9 ± 1.8	**<0.001**	24.1 ± 2.6	22.0 ± 2.2	**0.001**
Waist circumference (cm)	78.8 ± 7.2	88.9 ± 5.8	77.4 ± 6.2	**<0.001**	84.8 ± 6.7	77.2 ± 6.4	**<0.001**
75 g-oral glucose tolerance test							
Fasting plasma glucose (mg/dl)	91.7 ± 8.1	100.7 ± 5.2	90.4 ± 7.6	**<0.001**	91.9 ± 9.4	91.6 ± 7.7	0.868
2-h plasma glucose (mg/dl)	104.3 ± 16.1	110.3 ± 17.2	103.4 ± 15.9	0.209	108.1 ± 19.2	103.2 ± 15.1	0.255
Insulin resistance (HOMA-IR)	1.2 ± 0.8	2.1 ± 1.6	1.1 ± 0.5	**<0.001**	1.5 ± 1.3	1.2 ± 0.6	0.067
Insulin sensitivity (OGIS)	446.6 ± 47.1	394.0 ± 52.0	453.8 ± 41.8	**<0.001**	436.6 ± 65.4	449.4 ± 40.9	0.312
Insulin secretion (HOMA-β)	71.3 ± 37.8	78.8 ± 53.6	70.3 ± 35.4	0.507	82.4 ± 45.7	68.2 ± 35.0	0.159
Insulin secretion (II)[c]	0.3 ± 0.2	0.5 ± 0.4	0.3 ± 0.1	**<0.001**	0.4 ± 0.4	0.3 ± 0.1	**0.004**
Magnetic resonance imaging-derived fat area							
Visceral fat area (cm^2)	77.1 ± 34.3	88.0 ± 39.2	75.6 ± 33.6	0.285	127.6 ± 27.1	63.1 ± 19.8	**<0.001**
Subcutaneous fat area (cm^2)	122.9 ± 42.5	176.8 ± 51.2	115.5 ± 35.6	**<0.001**	136.4 ± 43.5	119.2 ± 41.8	0.129

Data are mean ± SD. obese: BMI ≥ 25, nonobese: BMI < 25; visceral obesity: visceral fat area ≥ 100 cm^2, nonvisceral obesity: visceral fat area < 100 cm^2
HOMA-β, homeostasis model assessment for β-cell function index; HOMA-IR, homeostasis model assessment for insulin resistance; II, insulinogenic index; OGIS, oral glucose insulin sensitivity. [a]obese vs nonobese, [b]Visceral obesity vs Nonvisceral obesity, [c]$n = 81$ (Data set from 2 subjects were excluded due to unphysiological glucose/insulin levels. Bold numbers indicate significant differences between the two groups with p <0.05

Table 2 Plasma amino acid concentrations in the obese, nonobese, visceral obese, and nonvisceral obese groups

(nmol/ml)	Overall ($n = 83$)	Obese ($n = 10$)	Nonobese ($n = 73$)	p values[a]	Visceral obesity ($n = 18$)	Nonvisceral obesity ($n = 75$)	p^b values[a]
Essential AAs							
Histidine	85.42 ± 9.71	88.02 ± 9.95	85.06 ± 9.69	0.370	84.83 ± 7.94	85.58 ± 10.19	0.774
Isoleucine	64.07 ± 12.09	72.94 ± 12.74	62.86 ± 11.57	**0.013**	70.99 ± 10.59	62.16 ± 11.85	**0.005**
Leucine	125.07 ± 20.71	139.34 ± 15.73	123.12 ± 20.62	**0.019**	136.51 ± 15.93	121.90 ± 20.85	**0.007**
Lysine	187.46 ± 26.41	208.75 ± 23.59	184.55 ± 25.56	**0.006**	186.83 ± 21.20	187.64 ± 27.82	0.909
Methionine	26.51 ± 3.71	26.69 ± 3.89	26.48 ± 3.71	0.871	25.81 ± 3.97	26.70 ± 3.65	0.370
Phenylalanine	57.67 ± 6.79	59.54 ± 4.86	57.41 ± 7.00	0.356	59.13 ± 8.34	57.26 ± 6.31	0.305
Threonine	129.23 ± 26.66	126.43 ± 19.06	129.61 ± 27.62	0.726	122.77 ± 23.68	131.02 ± 27.33	0.248
Tryptophan	56.04 ± 10.08	53.93 ± 6.27	56.33 ± 10.49	0.484	61.94 ± 15.43	54.40 ± 7.38	**0.004**
Valine	231.17 ± 30.90	261.89 ± 27.62	226.96 ± 29.03	**<0.001**	244.87 ± 25.78	227.38 ± 31.30	**0.033**
Nonessential AAs							
Alanine	342.61 ± 79.73	359.03 ± 99.02	340.36 ± 77.28	0.491	349.52 ± 83.12	340.70 ± 79.33	0.681
Arginine	66.10 ± 16.33	70.04 ± 17.12	65.56 ± 16.27	0.420	64.26 ± 10.86	66.62 ± 17.58	0.591
Asparagine	46.49 ± 6.19	46.17 ± 7.03	46.53 ± 6.12	0.865	42.73 ± 5.92	47.53 ± 5.89	**0.003**
α-ABA	20.11 ± 5.50	22.01 ± 5.98	19.85 ± 5.42	0.247	20.17 ± 6.39	20.10 ± 5.28	0.963
Citrulline	28.34 ± 6.20	26.23 ± 6.23	28.63 ± 6.19	0.254	25.57 ± 4.99	29.11 ± 6.32	**0.031**
Cystine	36.67 ± 6.41	41.47 ± 7.06	36.02 ± 6.08	**0.011**	37.59 ± 7.53	36.42 ± 6.11	0.497
Glutamate	57.93 ± 19.19	70.06 ± 17.04	56.27 ± 18.97	**0.032**	71.88 ± 24.25	54.07 ± 15.68	**<0.001**
Glutamine	524.27 ± 55.46	514.17 ± 80.48	525.66 ± 51.75	0.542	495.84 ± 60.17	532.15 ± 51.86	**0.013**
Glycine	220.56 ± 34.87	197.88 ± 41.43	223.67 ± 33.00	**0.027**	193.69 ± 30.16	228.00 ± 32.51	**<0.001**
Ornithine	80.34 ± 16.80	86.87 ± 14.91	79.44 ± 16.94	0.192	81.85 ± 15.20	79.92 ± 17.30	0.669
Proline	147.67 ± 39.39	141.67 ± 32.09	148.50 ± 40.40	0.610	151.29 ± 33.02	146.67 ± 41.15	0.662
Serine	116.31 ± 19.30	112.34 ± 15.82	116.86 ± 19.76	0.491	104.54 ± 16.36	119.57 ± 18.87	**0.003**
Taurine	74.99 ± 18.72	69.79 ± 15.03	75.70 ± 19.15	0.352	71.52 ± 15.75	75.95 ± 19.47	0.377
Tyrosine	61.26 ± 9.71	66.44 ± 13.47	60.55 ± 8.97	0.072	62.76 ± 9.47	60.84 ± 9.80	0.461

Data are mean ± SD. obese: BMI ≥ 25, nonobese: BMI < 25; visceral obesity: visceral fat area ≥ 100 cm^2, nonvisceral obesity: visceral fat area < 100 cm^2
AA amino acid, *α-ABA* α-aminobutyric acid, *BMI* body mass index
[a]Obese vs Nonobese, [b]Visceral obesity vs Nonvisceral obesity. Bold numbers indicate significant differences between the two groups with p <0.05

somatometric parameters (BW, BMI, and WC), body fat areas (VFA and SFA), and the indices derived from the 75-g OGTT (HOMA-IR, OGIS, HOMA-β, and II).

Regarding the essential AAs, the age- and gender-adjusted analysis showed that the levels of tryptophan and valine correlated positively with the somatometric parameters (BW, BMI, and WC), VFA, and/or SFA. Leucine, tryptophan, and valine levels exhibited positive correlations with insulin resistance (HOMA-IR) or insulin secretion (HOMA-β and II). Notably, none of the 75 g-OGTT parameters were associated with the concentrations of the remaining six essential AAs.

The plasma concentrations of nonessential AAs exhibited positive or negative correlations with the other parameters. The most widespread associations were identified for glutamate and glutamine. Plasma glutamate levels positively correlated with all the somatometric parameters, BW, BMI, WC, VFA and SFA, glucose levels (FPG and 2 h-PG), insulin resistance (HOMA-IR), and insulin secretion (HOMA-β and II) but negatively correlated with insulin sensitivity (OGIS). Interestingly, plasma glutamine levels negatively correlated with all the somatometric parameters and the 75 g-OGTT parameters (except FPG, 2 h-PG, and OGIS). Plasma glycine levels negatively correlated with the somatometric parameters (BW, BMI, and WC), VFA and SFA but correlated positively with insulin sensitivity (OGIS) and negatively with insulin resistance (HOMA-IR) and insulin secretion (HOMA-β and II). Citrulline levels negatively correlated with BW, BMI, WC, VFA and SFA, insulin resistance (HOMA-IR), and insulin secretion (HOMA-β and II). Conversely, tyrosine levels positively correlated with BW and HOMA-IR but negatively correlated with insulin sensitivity (OGIS). Finally, alanine levels correlated positively with WC and serine levels correlated negatively with HOMA-β.

Table 3 Correlations of plasma amino acid concentrations with indices of obesity and glucose metabolism

	Body weight	BMI	WC	VFA	SFA	FPG	2-h PG	HOMA-IR	OGIS	HOMA-β	II
Essential AAs											
Histidine	—	—	—	—	—	—	—	—	—	—	—
Isoleucine	0.413	0.305	0.345	0.332	—	—	—	—	—	—	—
Leucine	0.488	0.300	0.361	0.413	—	—	—	—	—	—	—
Lysine	0.307	—	0.290	—	—	0.236	—	—	−0.257	—	—
Methionine	—	—	—	—	—	—	—	—	—	—	—
Phenylalanine	0.276	—	—	—	—	—	—	—	—	—	—
Threonine	—	—	—	—	—	—	—	—	—	—	—
Tryptophan	—	—	—	0.289	—	—	—	—	—	—	—
Valine	0.539	0.387	0.482	0.397	—	0.254	—	0.219	−0.297	—	—
Nonessential AAs											—
Alanine	—	—	—	—	—	—	—	—	—	—	—
Arginine	—	—	—	—	—	—	—	—	—	—	—
Asparagine	—	—	—	—	—	—	—	—	—	—	—
α-ABA	—	—	—	—	—	—	—	—	—	—	—
Citrulline	—	—	−0.242	—	−0.395	—	—	−0.291	—	−0.375	—
Cystine	0.276	—	0.285	—	—	0.236	—	—	—	—	—
Glutamate	0.548	0.443	0.528	0.568	—	0.439	0.302	0.292	−0.458	—	—
Glutamine	−0.241	−0.289	−0.326	−0.272	−0.396	—	−0.220	−0.398	—	−0.311	—
Glycine	−0.333	−0.418	−0.426	−0.426	−0.294	—	−0.247	−0.317	0.303	−0.231	—
Ornithine	—	—	—	—	—	—	—	—	—	—	—
Proline	—	—	—	—	—	—	—	—	—	—	—
Serine	−0.368	−0.273	−0.351	−0.379	—	—	—	—	0.258	—	—
Taurine	—	—	—	—	—	−0.240	—	—	—	—	—
Tyrosine	0.335	—	0.314	0.252	—	0.269	—	—	−0.327	—	—

Each number indicates a correlation coefficient for two variables that showed statistically significant correlation by Pearson's analysis. *AA* amino acid, *α-ABA* α-aminobutyric acid, *BMI* body mass index, *FPG* fasting plasma glucose, *HOMA-β* homeostasis model assessment for β-cell function index, *HOMA-IR* homeostasis model assessment of insulin resistance, *II* insulinogenic index, *OGIS* oral glucose insulin sensitivity, *SFA* subcutaneous fat area, *VFA* visceral fat area, *WC* waist circumference, *2-h PG* 2-h plasma glucose

The reproducibility of the fat area measurements performed by two independent observers was validated by using Bland–Altman plots. Only small intraobserver (VFA: −0.4 ± 5.9 (2SD), SFA: −0.1 ± 1.9) and interobserver (VFA: −1.5 ± 8.4, SFA: 0.0 ± 2.0) differences were detected. The intraclass correlation coefficients for intraobserver reproducibility were 1.000 for VFA and SFA, and for interobserver reproducibility, these were 0.9995 for VFA and 1.000 for SFA.

Discussion

The present study, exclusively involving Japanese adults with NGT, demonstrated that the plasma levels of specific AAs were associated with parameters of obesity, and/or indices of insulin resistance, sensitivity, and secretion derived from the 75-g OGTT. These findings support possible associations of AAs with the type and degree of obesity and glucose regulation in the Asian population with preserved glucose metabolism.

An important result of the present study was the establishment of a link between plasma AA levels and type of obesity: visceral or subcutaneous. We demonstrated that tryptophan is positively associated only with VFA, whereas valine, one of the three BCAAs, is positively associated only with SFA. These data suggest that the known associations between obesity and certain AAs may be derived from a distinct link with visceral fat and/or subcutaneous fat. A previous study on Japanese adults reported similar results; however, the participants did not undergo 75-g OGTT, and those with DM or IGT were not excluded [26]. Conversely, citrulline, glutamine, and glycine negatively correlated with both VFA and SFA, and glutamate positively correlated with both VFA and SFA. These AAs may have broad associations with the overall deposition of fat, rather than with the pattern of fat deposition. Importantly, 88 % of the subjects were considered nonobese (BMI < 25 kg/m^2), and 78 % of them were considered not to have significant visceral

Table 4 Age- and gender-adjusted correlations of plasma amino acid concentrations with obesity and glucose metabolism indices

	Body weight	BMI	WC	VFA	SFA	FPG	2-h PG	HOMA-IR	OGIS	HOMA-β	II
Essential AAs											
Histidine	—	—	—	—	—	—	—	—	—	—	—
Isoleucine	—	—	—	—	—	—	—	—	—	—	—
Leucine	—	—	—	—	—	—	—	—	—	0.288	—
Lysine	—	—	—	—	—	—	—	—	—	—	—
Methionine	—	—	—	—	—	—	—	—	—	—	—
Phenylalanine	—	—	—	—	—	—	—	—	—	—	—
Threonine	—	—	—	—	—	—	—	—	—	—	—
Tryptophan	—	—	—	0.206	—	—	—	—	—	0.259	—
Valine	0.202	0.247	0.296	—	0.348	—	—	0.380	-	0.272	0.419
Nonessential AAs											
Alanine	—	—	0.184	—	—	—	—	—	—	—	—
Arginine	—	—	—	—	—	—	—	—	—	—	—
Asparagine	—	—	—	—	—	—	—	—	—	—	—
α-ABA	—	—	—	—	—	—	—	—	—	—	—
Citrulline	−0.183	−0.286	−0.358	−0.285	−0.382	—	—	−0.296	-	−0.323	−0.307
Cystine	—	—	—	—	—	—	—	—	—	—	—
Glutamate	0.247	0.327	0.352	0.362	0.401	0.395	0.310	0.436	−0.377	0.243	0.403
Glutamine	−0.265	−0.308	−0.282	−0.233	−0362	—	—	−0395	—	−0.341	−0.434
Glycine	−0.221	−0.364	−0.316	−0.311	−0.311	—	—	−0.325	0.226	−0.309	−0.380
Ornithine	—	—	—	—	—	—	—	—	—	—	—
Proline	—	—	—	—	—	—	—	—	—	—	—
Serine	—	—	—	—	—	—	—	—	—	−0.280	—
Taurine	—	—	—	—	—	—	—	—	—	—	—
Tyrosine	0.164	—	—	—	—	—	—	0.226	−0.238	—	—

Each number indicates a standardized coefficient for two variables that showed significant association in the age- and gender-adjusted multiple logistic regression analysis. *AA* amino acid, *α-ABA* α-aminobutyric acid, *BMI* body mass index, *FPG* fasting plasma glucose, *HOMA-β* homeostasis model assessment for β-cell function index, *HOMA-IR* homeostasis model assessment of insulin resistance, *II* insulinogenic index, *OGIS* oral glucose insulin sensitivity, *SFA* subcutaneous fat area, *VFA* visceral fat area, *WC* waist circumference, *2-h PG* 2-h plasma glucose

obesity (VFA < 100 cm^2). Thus, this study demonstrated a significant link between AAs in the blood and body fat in nonobese and nonviscerally obese adult Asians.

Three possibilities could contribute to an explanation of the association between plasma AA levels and the type/degree of obesity identified in the present study: 1. plasma AA levels affect the type/degree of obesity; 2. different obesity types affect plasma AA levels; and 3. there are confounding factors that affect both plasma AA levels and obesity.

The first possibility relates to the appetite-regulating effects of certain AAs. Glutamate is a substrate in the formation of gamma aminobutyric acid, a known appetite enhancer [27]. In contrast, glutamine increases the secretion of glucagon-like peptide (GLP)-1, which is an appetite suppressor [28]. Therefore, the positive correlation of glutamate and the negative associations of glutamine with the obesity-related indices may be related to the regulation of food intake. In addition, an animal study showed that glycine reduces visceral fat through the oxidization of free fatty acids in adipose tissue [29]. This function is consistent with the negative correlation between high plasma glycine levels and BMI, VFA, and SFA.

The second possibility is that the two types of obesity could affect the AA levels. For instance, a study on rats and human specimens revealed that BCAAs including valine are catabolized in visceral and subcutaneous adipose tissue [30]. Also, a rat model of obesity exhibited enhanced protein degradation and reduced catabolic activities toward BCAAs, which could increase their plasma levels [31]. However, a different catabolism of AAs in visceral and subcutaneous fat tissue has not been clearly demonstrated, indicating the need for further research to support this speculation.

The third possibility is that confounding factors, such as dietary intake or exercise, may affect AA levels and obesity. For example, glutamate is abundant in wheat protein, which is the second highest dietary carbohydrate in Japan. In some subjects, excess wheat intake may have caused both an increase in the levels of glutamate and an increase in BMI, VFA, and SFA. Conversely, prolonged submaximal exercise has been reported to reduce plasma leucine concentration and BMI [32]. This finding may be consistent with the significantly lower concentration of leucine in the nonobese group compared with the obese group.

With regard to the link between AAs and the indices of glucose regulation, the present study identified positive correlations of glutamate concentration with FPG and 2-h PG in the Japanese NGT subjects. This finding is partially supported by prior studies in which plasma glutamate, valine, and tyrosine levels were elevated in patients with metabolic syndrome [6] or type 2 DM [33, 34]. These data support the presence of a mechanistic link between an altered plasma AA profile and aberrant glucose regulation, even in subjects with a preserved glucose metabolism. A recent prospective study on 2,422 normoglycemic individuals demonstrated that the plasma levels of five AAs (isoleucine, leucine, valine, tyrosine, and phenylalanine) predicted the development of diabetes during a 12-year follow-up [2]. These results and ours support a possible role for AA metabolism early in the development of DM.

In the present study, the plasma levels of six AAs exhibited relationships with the index of insulin resistance (HOMA-IR) and/or the index of insulin sensitivity (OGIS). Glutamate and tyrosine levels were positively correlated with HOMA-IR and negatively correlated with OGIS, whereas the opposite was the case for glycine. Single associations were also identified for valine, citrulline, and glutamine (with HOMA-IR). This complex network of interactions between AAs and insulin regulation is partially supported by a recent study conducted on Japanese type 2 DM patients, in which the levels of the BCAAs (isoleucine, leucine, and valine), alanine, glutamate, proline, and tyrosine positively correlated with HOMA-IR [8]. The fact that a positive correlation of valine, glutamate, and tyrosine with HOMA-IR was already present in our NGT subjects allows a speculation that these AAs may be associated with the initial phase of the development of glucose dysregulation. Oral glutamate supplements have been reported to impair insulin sensitivity and to induce the development of diabetes in animal studies [35]. In addition, feeding animals with BCAAs induced insulin resistance, along with the chronic phosphorylation of mTOR, JNK, and $IRS1_{Ser307}$ [3]. Also, valine is a glycogenic AA and, in a rat study, its oral administration increased the PG level [36]. These data support an incremental effect of glutamate and valine on blood glucose levels. Finally, as tyrosine is a precursor of catecholamines, the accumulation of this AA could promote an increase in blood glucose level through the anti-insulin action of catecholamines. Collectively, prior studies and ours suggest that specific AAs may indirectly induce an increase in blood glucose level through the stimulation of insulin resistance.

Glutamine has been reported to induce the secretion of GLP-1 in healthy and diabetic subjects [28], suggesting that this AA reduces PG levels through the stimulatory effect of GLP-1 on insulin secretion. Also, leucine synergistically stimulates insulin secretion and lowers blood glucose when ingested with glucose in healthy humans [37]. In addition, in healthy first-degree relatives of type 2 DM patients, oral glycine has been reported to increase insulin secretion without affecting insulin sensitivity [11]. Also, in another human study, single oral administration of glycine significantly stimulated insulin secretion whereas, when given together with glucose, it augmented insulin action and attenuated the increase of blood glucose levels [38]. Thus, further studies are required to clarify the mechanisms by which AAs affect glucose/insulin regulation.

WC is a basic and widely used somatometric index of visceral fat adiposity. In Japan, the cutoff levels for visceral fat obesity are 85 cm for men and 90 cm for women, because these cutoff levels correlate well with a VFA of 100 cm^2 [12]. Indeed, in our NGT subjects, WC was greater in the visceral obesity group than in the nonvisceral obesity group. The correlation analysis indicated that WC was correlated with the plasma levels of six AAs, which is a greater number than for BMI (five AAs) and VFA (five AAs). These suggest that WC is not only a marker of visceral obesity but also a noninvasive parameter that could be used in future studies on possible associations between AAs and obesity and/or glucose regulation.

Our study had some limitations. First, we did not collect lifestyle data for subjects; thus, we could not exclude the possibility that factors related to lifestyle, such as dietary intake and/or physical activity, affected the subjects' plasma AA profiles, obesity, and glucose metabolism [39]. Second, only one participant had a BMI $\geq$ 30 kg/m^2, and so the findings cannot be extrapolated to a population with higher BMI. Similarly, due to the racial variation in the relation between AAs and insulin resistance/sensitivity, the results need to be interpreted cautiously when extrapolated to other races [40]. Finally, the observational nature of the present study did not allow a direct investigation of the causal relationships between the parameters. However, only Japanese adults with preserved glucose metabolism were included in the study following careful selection using the 75-g OGTT. Thus, the results obtained are meaningful for future basic and clinical research on the potential role of AAs in the pathogenesis and/or prevention of obesity and DM.

Conclusions

The present study identified specific associations between 10 AAs and the type and degree of obesity, or indices of glucose/insulin regulation, in Japanese adults with preserved glucose metabolism. With the growing concern about the increasing prevalence of obesity and DM, the possible roles of these AAs as early markers and/or precursors of these conditions warrant further investigation.

Ethics approval and consent to participate

The present study was approved by the Ethical Committee on Human Experiments of Hokkaido University Graduate School of Medicine (MED08-003), and written informed consent was obtained from all subjects.

Consent for publication

Not applicable.

Additional files

Additional file 1: Table S1. Comparison of plasma amino acid concentrations between men and women. (DOC 45 kb)

Additional file 2: Table S2. Correlations between plasma amino acid concentrations and age. (DOC 42 kb)

Additional file 3: Table S3. Plasma amino acid concentrations in visceral obesity and nonvisceral obesity groups in 66 men. (DOC 46 kb)

Additional file 4: Table S4. Plasma amino acid concentrations in visceral obesity and nonvisceral obesity groups in two age groups. (DOC 56 kb)

Additional file 5: Table S5. Correlations between plasma amino acid concentration and indices of obesity and glucose metabolism. (XLS 19 kb)

Additional file 6: Age- and gender-adjusted correlations between plasma amino acid concentration and indices of obesity and glucose metabolism. (XLS 20 kb)

Abbreviations

AA: Amino acid; VFA: Visceral fat area; SFA: Subcutaneous fat area; BCAA: Branched-chain amino acid; DM: Diabetes mellitus; IGT: Impaired glucose tolerance; BMI: Body mass index; OGTT: Oral glucose tolerance test; MRI: Magnetic resonance imaging; BW: Body weight; WC: Waist circumference; PG: Plasma glucose; NGT: Normal glucose tolerance; IFG: Impaired fasting glucose; FPG: Fasting plasma glucose; HOMA-IR: Homeostasis model assessment for insulin resistance; OGIS: Oral glucose insulin sensitivity; HOMA-β: Homeostasis model assessment of β-cell function; II: Insulinogenic index; HPLC: High-performance liquid chromatography; SPAIR: Spectral attenuated inversion recovery; GLP-1: Glucagon-like peptide-1.

Competing interests

There were no potential conflicts of interest relevant to this article to report.

Authors' contributions

SS and DI designed the experiments; CT, DI, and AY conducted the experiments; CT, TS, DI, and IT analyzed the data; NOM conducted and analyzed the MRI; CT, TW, and IT wrote the original manuscript; YMI provided advice with and reviewed the statistical analysis; HO and YO provided academic suggestions, reviewed, and edited the manuscript; and MN was responsible for the final content. All authors read and approved the final manuscript.

Acknowledgments

The authors thank J-MAC (Sapporo, JAPAN) for its support in the evaluation of visceral and subcutaneous fat area using MRI, and also thank Crimson Interactive Pvt. Ltd. (Tokyo, JAPAN) for scientific English editing throughout the revised manuscript.

Funding

There was no financial support for this study.

Author details

[1]First Department of Medicine, Hokkaido University Hospital, North 14, West 5, Kita-ku, Sapporo 060-8648, Japan. [2]First Department of Medicine, Hokkaido University Graduate School of Medicine, Sapporo, Japan. [3]Department of Human Developmental Science, Faculty of Education, Hokkaido University, Sapporo, Japan. [4]Department of Diagnostic and Interventional Radiology, Hokkaido University Hospital, Sapporo, Japan. [5]Department of Biostatistics, Hokkaido University Graduate School of Medicine, Sapporo, Japan.

References

1. Wild S, Roglic G, Green A, Sicree R, King H. Global prevalence of diabetes: estimates for the year 2000 and projections for 2030. Diabetes Care. 2004; 27:1047–53.
2. Wang TJ, Larson MG, Vasan RS, Cheng S, Rhee EP, McCabe E, et al. Metabolite profiles and the risk of developing diabetes. Nat Med. 2011;17: 448–53.
3. Newgard CB, An J, Bain JR, Muehlbauer MJ, Stevens RD, Lien LF, et al. A branched-chain amino acid-related metabolic signature that differentiates obese and lean humans and contributes to insulin resistance. Cell Metab. 2009;9:311–26.
4. Chevalier S, Marliss EB, Morais JA, Lamarche M, Gougeon R. Whole-body protein anabolic response is resistant to the action of insulin in obese women. Am J Clin Nutr. 2005;82:355–65.
5. Schwenk WF, Haymond MW. Decreased uptake of glucose by human forearm during infusion of leucine, isoleucine, or threonine. Diabetes. 1987; 36:199–204.
6. Kamaura M, Nishijima K, Takahashi M, Ando T, Mizushima S, Tochikubo O. Lifestyle modification in metabolic syndrome and associated changes in plasma amino acid profiles. Circ J. 2010;74:2434–40.
7. Mansour A, Mohajeri-Tehrani MR, Qorbani M, Heshmat R, Larijani B, Hosseini S. Effect of glutamine supplementation on cardiovascular risk factors in patients with type 2 diabetes. Nutrition. 2015;31:119–26.
8. Nakamura H, Jinzu H, Nagao K, Noguchi Y, Shimba N, Miyano H, et al. Plasma amino acid profiles are associated with insulin, C-peptide and adiponectin levels in type 2 diabetic patients. Nutr Diabetes. 2014;4:e133.
9. Liu J, Fox CS, Hickson DA, May WD, Hairston KG, Carr JJ, et al. Impact of abdominal visceral and subcutaneous adipose tissue on cardiometabolic risk factors: the Jackson Heart Study. J Clin Endocrinol Metab. 2010;95:5419–26.
10. Yamashita S, Nakamura T, Shimomura I, Nishida M, Yoshida S, Kotani K, et al. Insulin resistance and body fat distribution. Diabetes Care. 1996;19:287–91.
11. Gonzalez-Ortiz M, Medina-Santillan R, Martinez-Abundis E, von Drateln CR. Effect of glycine on insulin secretion and action in healthy first-degree relatives of type 2 diabetes mellitus patients. Horm Metab Res. 2001;33:358–60.
12. Kadowaki T, Sekikawa A, Murata K, Maegawa H, Takamiya T, Okamura T, et al. Japanese men have larger areas of visceral adipose tissue than Caucasian men in the same levels of waist circumference in a population-based study. Int J Obes (Lond). 2006;30:1163–5.
13. Chiu KC, Chuang LM, Yoon C. Comparison of measured and estimated indices of insulin sensitivity and beta cell function: impact of ethnicity on insulin sensitivity and beta cell function in glucose-tolerant and normotensive subjects. J Clin Endocrinol Metab. 2001;86:1620–5.
14. Wang J, Thornton JC, Russell M, Burastero S, Heymsfield S, Pierson Jr RN. Asians have lower body mass index (BMI) but higher percent body fat than do whites: comparisons of anthropometric measurements. Am J Clin Nutr. 1994;60:23–8.

15. Hsu WC, Araneta MR, Kanaya AM, Chiang JL, Fujimoto W. BMI cut points to identify at-risk Asian Americans for type 2 diabetes screening. Diabetes Care. 2015;38:150–8.
16. Consultation WHOE. Appropriate body-mass index for Asian populations and its implications for policy and intervention strategies. Lancet. 2004;363: 157–63.
17. Examination Committee of Criteria for 'Obesity Disease' in J, Japan Society for the Study of O. New criteria for 'obesity disease' in Japan. Circ J. 2002;66: 987–92.
18. WHO Expert Committee on Diabetes Mellitus: Diabetes Mellitus. Tech. Rep. Ser., no. 727. Geneva: WHO; 1985.
19. WHO. Definition, diagnosis and classification of diabetes mellitus and its complications. Part 1: diagnosis and classification of diabetes mellitus. Geneva: WHO; 1999.
20. Matthews DR, Hosker JP, Rudenski AS, Naylor BA, Treacher DF, Turner RC. Homeostasis model assessment: insulin resistance and beta-cell function from fasting plasma glucose and insulin concentrations in man. Diabetologia. 1985;28:412–9.
21. OGIS (Oral Glucose Insulin Sensitivity) [http://webmet.pd.cnr.it/ogis/, Accessed 1 Dec 2015]
22. Mari A, Pacini G, Murphy E, Ludvik B, Nolan JJ. A model-based method for assessing insulin sensitivity from the oral glucose tolerance test. Diabetes Care. 2001;24:539–48.
23. Seltzer HS, Allen EW, Herron Jr AL, Brennan MT. Insulin secretion in response to glycemic stimulus: relation of delayed initial release to carbohydrate intolerance in mild diabetes mellitus. J Clin Invest. 1967;46:323–35.
24. Deyl Z, Hyanek J, Horakova M. Profiling of amino acids in body fluids and tissues by means of liquid chromatography. J Chromatogr. 1986; 379:177–250.
25. Sugino T, Shirai T, Kajimoto Y, Kajimoto O. L-ornithine supplementation attenuates physical fatigue in healthy volunteers by modulating lipid and amino acid metabolism. Nutr Res. 2008;28:738–43.
26. Yamakado M, Tanaka T, Nagao K, Ishizaka Y, Mitushima T, Tani M, et al. Plasma amino acid profile is associated with visceral fat accumulation in obese Japanese subjects. Clin Obes. 2012;2:29–40.
27. Wu Q, Clark MS, Palmiter RD. Deciphering a neuronal circuit that mediates appetite. Nature. 2012;483:594–7.
28. Greenfield JR, Farooqi IS, Keogh JM, Henning E, Habib AM, Blackwood A, et al. Oral glutamine increases circulating glucagon-like peptide 1, glucagon, and insulin concentrations in lean, obese, and type 2 diabetic subjects. Am J Clin Nutr. 2009;89:106–13.
29. El Hafidi M, Perez I, Zamora J, Soto V, Carvajal-Sandoval G, Banos G. Glycine intake decreases plasma free fatty acids, adipose cell size, and blood pressure in sucrose-fed rats. Am J Physiol Regul Integr Comp Physiol. 2004; 287:R1387–1393.
30. Lackey DE, Lynch CJ, Olson KC, Mostaedi R, Ali M, Smith WH, et al. Regulation of adipose branched-chain amino acid catabolism enzyme expression and cross-adipose amino acid flux in human obesity. Am J Physiol Endocrinol Metab. 2013;304:E1175–1187.
31. She P, Olson KC, Kadota Y, Inukai A, Shimomura Y, Hoppel CL, et al. Leucine and protein metabolism in obese Zucker rats. PLoS One. 2013;8:e59443.
32. Blomstrand E, Ek S, Newsholme EA. Influence of ingesting a solution of branched-chain amino acids on plasma and muscle concentrations of amino acids during prolonged submaximal exercise. Nutrition. 1996;12:485–90.
33. Fiehn O, Garvey WT, Newman JW, Lok KH, Hoppel CL, Adams SH. Plasma metabolomic profiles reflective of glucose homeostasis in non-diabetic and type 2 diabetic obese African-American women. PLoS One. 2010;5:e15234.
34. Lips MA, Van Klinken JB, van Harmelen V, Dharuri HK, t Hoen PA, Laros JF, et al. Roux-en-Y gastric bypass surgery, but not calorie restriction, reduces plasma branched-chain amino acids in obese women independent of weight loss or the presence of type 2 diabetes. Diabetes Care. 2014;37: 3150–6.
35. Collison KS, Zaidi MZ, Saleh SM, Inglis A, Mondreal R, Makhoul NJ, et al. Effect of trans-fat, fructose and monosodium glutamate feeding on feline weight gain, adiposity, insulin sensitivity, adipokine and lipid profile. Br J Nutr. 2011;106:218–26.
36. Doi M, Yamaoka I, Fukunaga T, Nakayama M. Isoleucine, a potent plasma glucose-lowering amino acid, stimulates glucose uptake in C2C12 myotubes. Biochem Biophys Res Commun. 2003;312:1111–7.
37. Kalogeropoulou D, Lafave L, Schweim K, Gannon MC, Nuttall FQ. Leucine, when ingested with glucose, synergistically stimulates insulin secretion and lowers blood glucose. Metabolism. 2008;57:1747–52.
38. Gannon MC, Nuttall JA, Nuttall FQ. The metabolic response to ingested glycine. Am J Clin Nutr. 2002;76:1302–7.
39. Sekhar RV, Patel SG, Guthikonda AP, Reid M, Balasubramanyam A, Taffet GE, et al. Deficient synthesis of glutathione underlies oxidative stress in aging and can be corrected by dietary cysteine and glycine supplementation. Am J Clin Nutr. 2011;94:847–53.
40. Tillin T, Hughes AD, Wang Q, Wurtz P, Ala-Korpela M, Sattar N, et al. Diabetes risk and amino acid profiles: cross-sectional and prospective analyses of ethnicity, amino acids and diabetes in a South Asian and European cohort from the SABRE (Southall And Brent REvisited) Study. Diabetologia. 2015;58:968–79.

2

Evaluation of markers of beige adipocytes in white adipose tissue of the mouse

Rolando A. Garcia*, James N. Roemmich and Kate J. Claycombe

Abstract

Background: There is a growing interest in exploiting the induction of beige or "brite" (brown in white) adipocytes (beigeing) to combat obesity and its comorbidities. However, there is some uncertainty regarding the best markers to evaluate the occurrence or magnitude of beigeing in white adipose tissue in the mouse model.

Methods: We evaluated the transcript expression of several thermoregulatory genes and proposed beige markers employing cell culture, whole white adipose tissue, and the adipocyte and stromal vascular fractions.

Results: Most beige markers tested with the exception of TMEM26 can discriminate white from beige adipocytes in culture. Markers FGF21, P2RX5, PAT2, or CAR4 can successfully mark beigeing in whole tissue of younger mice, or in the adipocyte subfraction of older mice. However, markers for the thermoregulatory genes UCP1, CIDEA, and Cox8b displayed the greatest dynamic range and were consistently elevated *in vitro, in vivo*, and in the adipocyte fraction by treatments that induce beige adipogenesis.

Conclusions: While most putative beige markers are clearly expressed in beige adipocytes *in vitro, in vivo* the small dynamic range of most of these markers, the strength of the beigeing stimulus, and the age of the mice may limit their utility, although this limitation may be overcome by specifically evaluating these markers in the adipocyte fraction. Thermoregulatory markers like UCP1, CIDEA, or Cox8b represent the best options to evaluate the beigeing of white adipose tissue *in vivo*.

Keywords: Beige, Brite, Adipocyte marker, Subcutaneous adipose tissue, UCP1, FGF21

Background

Beige or "brite" (brown in white) adipocytes arise in white adipose tissue (WAT) in response to various stimuli including cold exposure and exercise. Unlike white adipocytes, which tend to have a single fat droplet (unilocular morphology) and low mitochondrial density, beige adipocytes have several small fat droplets (multilocular morphology) and a greater mitochondrial density [1]. Beige adipocytes as well as their counterparts in brown adipose tissue express the protein UCP1, which uncouples respiration from energy production resulting in the generation of heat [1]. UCP1 knockout mice reared at thermoneutrality develop obesity [2]. Increased activity of beige or brown adipocytes in transgenic animal models results in resistance to obesity [3]. When the amount of brown adipose tissue is greatly reduced in mice by genetic means, the induction of beige adipocytes in white adipose tissue can restore the thermogenic response to cold and prevent the mice from becoming more susceptible to weight gain in response to a high-fat diet [4]. Mice lacking functional beige adipocytes are more prone to developing obesity, insulin resistance, and hepatic steatosis when fed a high-fat diet [5]. In addition, transplantation of subcutaneous adipose tissue where beiging was induced by exercise into mice fed a high-fat diet restored glucose tolerance and insulin sensitivity [6]. Thus, there is interest in the possibility of exploiting the induction of beige cells to address maintenance of a healthy body weight and obesity-related diseases.

Studies seeking to increase beige adipogenesis (beigeing) or determine how it is affected by environmental treatments such as high-fat diets require markers of beige adipocytes. The expression of several thermoregulatory genes such as Uncoupling Protein-1 (UCP1), Cell Death-Inducing DFFA-Like Effector A (CIDEA) or

* Correspondence: rolando.garcia@ars.usda.gov
USDA-ARS, Grand Forks Human Nutrition Research Center, 2420 2nd Ave. N, Grand Forks, ND 58203, USA

Cytochrome C Oxidase Subunit VIIIb (Cox8b) has been employed to evaluate the induction of beige adipocytes in white adipose tissue (WAT). In addition, transcripts of several markers (e.g., TBX1, TMEM26, CD137, FGF21, P2RX5, PAT2, CAR4, and CITED1) have been identified that appear to be specific for beige adipocytes [7–9]. However, it is not yet clear whether employing these beige markers to gauge the extent of beigeing in WAT represents an improvement over the evaluation of the transcripts of thermoregulatory genes. There are also discrepancies as to the specificity of some of these markers to identify beigeing. Wu and coworkers [7] employing microarray screens of immortalized cells lines derived from murine subcutaneous fat identified TBX1, TMEM26, and CD137 as markers for beige adipocytes. However, Ussar and coworkers [9] did not detect the transcripts for TBX1 or TMEM26 to be changed in response to cold adaptation or treatment with a β3 adrenergic agonist [9], while Rosenwald and coworkers found that of these 3 markers only TBX1 was enriched in beige adipocytes and increased by cold stimulation [10]. A recent study [11] performed a comprehensive examination of several proposed beige adipocyte markers, however the focus of that study was to validate markers for identification of adipose tissues such as brown (interscapular), brite (inguinal), and white (epididymal) and not markers of beige adipocytes.

The aim of the present study was to determine differences in expression of classical thermoregulatory genes and putative beige markers under conditions that induce beigeing. The objective was to identify those markers that in general may be most useful to researchers employing mouse models to evaluate changes in beigeing in WAT in response to experimental treatments, or to researchers seeking to differentiate between white and beige adipocytes in cultured cells.

Methods

Animals

All animal protocols were approved by the Institutional Animal Care and Use Committee of the US Department of Agriculture, Agricultural Research Service, Grand Forks Human Nutrition Research Center. Male C57BL/6 mice were purchased from Harlan (Madison, WI), housed in a pathogen-free room on a 12:12 h light–dark cycle with unlimited access to rodent chow (#5015; LabDiet, St. Louis, MO) and water, and maintained at 22 °C unless otherwise specified. We employed the temperature of 22 °C for housing of the mice because it is within the range of the most common room temperatures employed in experiments. We used C57BL/6 mice because they are a strain of mice prone to obesity that is often used in this type of research. To induce beigeing in WAT, groups of mice ($n = 5–6$) were placed at 5 °C for one week in an environmental chamber. We employed cold exposure because it is the classical paradigm for beige adipocyte induction [1]. For the harvesting of tissues mice were euthanized by either CO2 inhalation or cervical dislocation. Tissue samples were frozen and stored at −80 °C until analysis.

Cell culture

Inguinal adipose tissue from male C57Bl/6 mice was minced and digested in 0.5 % type I collagenase (ThermoFisher Scientific, Waltham, MA) in Hank's balanced salt solution (HBSS) for 1 hr. at 37 °C. The digests were filtered through a 100 μm filter and centrifuged at 200 g for 7 min at 4 °C. After removal of the supernatant, the stromal vascular fraction (SVF) cell pellet was subjected to hypotonic RBC lysis buffer to remove erythrocytes. The cells were then cultured on a T25 in 5 mM glucose DMEM with 10 % FBS and 50 U penicillin and 50 μg of streptomycin/ml and subcultured to a 24 well plate. After cells reached confluence they were induced to differentiate into white adipocytes employing the same culture medium containing 0.5 mM Isobutylmethylxanthine (IBMX), 1 uM dexamethasone, 850 nM insulin, and 17 mM glucose (modified from Wu et al., 2012 [7]). For differentiation into beige adipocytes, 1 uM rosiglitazone and 1 nM T3 were also included. We employed rosiglitazone as an inducer of beiging because it is the most often used method for induction of beige adipocytes *in vitro*. After 4 days in differentiation medium, the white adipocytes were cultured for an additional 4 days in maintenance medium containing only insulin, while beige cells were cultured in the same medium containing 1 uM rosiglitazone and 1 nM T3 for an additional 2 days, and then in medium with only insulin for the last 2 days. About 90-95 % of the cells in the plates differentiated into adipocytes. At the end of the eighth day, cells were treated with 1 uM isoproterenol (Iso) for 6 hrs. We employed adrenergic stimulation in our cultures because the induction of beige adipocytes in white adipose tissue by stimuli like cold exposure is mediated by an increase in adrenergic stimulation, and we wished to examine its effects on gene expression markers in both beige and white adipocytes in culture.

Separation of the stromal vascular fraction from the adipocyte fraction

The collagenase digests of inguinal adipose tissue were filtered through a 200 μm filter and diluted ½ with HBSS containing 10 % FBS to stop collagenase activity. After centrifugation (200 g, 7 min, 4 °C) the supernatant containing the floating adipocytes was decanted and centrifuged again before removing the infranatant to obtain the adipocyte fraction. To the cell pellet constituting the SVF 5 ml of HBSS were added and after centrifugation the supernantant was removed. Both the adipocyte and stromal vascular fractions were lyzed with QIAazol lysis reagent (Qiagen, Valencia, CA).

qPCR

Frozen tissue or cells were homogenized in QIAzol lysis reagent and total RNA was isolated from tissue or cell lysates employing the RNeasy Lipid Tissue Mini Kit (Qiagen, Valencia, CA). RNA was converted to cDNA employing the High Capacity cDNA Reverse Trancription kit from Applied Biosystems (Foster City, CA). The transcripts of the thermoregulatory and beige genes evaluated in this study and their function are listed in Table 1. Additional transcripts for the following genes were evaluated: Solute Carrier Family 7 Member 10 (Slc7a10/ASC1 neutral amino acid transporter, y + system), WAP four-disulfide core domain 21 (Wfdc21/Wdnm1-like), and Serine (or Cysteine) Peptidase Inhibitor, Clade A, Member 3 k (Serpina3k). The beige markers evaluated in this study were selected either because they are among the markers most often used in mice, they have a confirmed role in the process of beigeing (FGF21), or the genes code for cell surface proteins that may prove useful in targeting beige or brown adipocytes for diagnostic or therapeutic purposes (PAT2 and P2RX5). Transcripts were evaluated employing a 5' nuclease qPCR assay using the Faststart Universal Probe Master (Rox) from Roche (Indianapolis, IN) and 18S-rRNA as an endogenous control. Primer sets and hydrolysis probes (Table 2) were obtained from Integrated DNA Technologies (Coralville, IA). Ct values were determined using the ABI Prism 7500 PCR system (Applied Biosystems, Foster City, CA). Relative amplification was determined by the $\Delta\Delta$Ct method.

Western blot

White adipose tissue was homogenized in lysis buffer (50 mM HEPES, PH 7.4, 150 mM NaCl, 1 % Triton X-100, 5 mM EGTA) and homogenates were spun at 20,000 g. Supernatants were extracted with 4 volumes of cold acetone and the precipitated protein was resuspended in 10 % SDS, made up to a final SDS concentration of 2 % with water, and spun at 12,000 g for 2 min to obtain the final supernatant. Protein was determined by the BCA protein assay (Thermo Fisher, Rockford, IL). Proteins were separated in 10 % Bis-Tris NuPAGE gels and transferred to PVDF membranes employing the iBlot2 (Thermo Fisher, Rockford, IL). Membranes were blocked and incubated with primary and secondary antibodies in Odyssey blocking buffer (Li-Cor, Lincoln, NE). Primary antibodies were: anti-FGF21, AF3057, and anti-CD137, AF937 (R&D Systems, Minneapolis, MN), anti-P2RX5, sc-398682 (Santa Cruz Biotechnology, Dallas, TX), anti-beta-actin, sc-47778 (Santa Cruz, Dallas, TX), and anti-UCP1, ab10983, (abcam, Cambridge, MA). Dye-conjugated secondary antibodies were from Li-Cor (Lincoln, NE). The bands were detected by immunofluorescence.

Statistics

Statistical analyses were carried out with the SIGMA Plot 13.0 software. Differences between two groups where tested using two-tailed t-tests. Differences between more than 2 groups were tested using two way ANOVAs followed by multiple comparisons using the Holm-Sidak method. If the normality and/or equal variance assumptions of the tests were not met, the data was transformed prior to analysis.

Table 1 List or thermoregulatory or beige markers employed in this study and their function

Thermoregulatory or Beige marker	Function
UCP1 (Uncoupling protein 1)	Uncouples respiration from energy production
CIDEA (Cell Death-Inducing DFFA-Like Effector A)	Modulates uncoupling action of UCP1
Cox8b (Cytochrome C Oxidase Subunit VIIIb)	Subunit of oxidase involved in respiratory electron transport
FGF21 (Fibroblast Growth Factor 21)	Modulates glucose, lipid, and energy homeostasis: induces beigeing in WAT
Car4 (Carbonic Anhydrase 4)	Acid–base balance (bicarbonate/CO2 equilibrium)
P2RX5 (Purinergic Receptor P2X, Ligand-Gated Ion Channel 5)	Purinergic Signaling
PAT-2 (Proton-Coupled Amino Acid Transporter-2)	Amino acid transport
CITED1 (Cbp/p300-Interacting Transactivator with Glu/Asp-rich Carboxy-Terminal Domain 1)	Transcriptional coactivator
CD137/Tnfrs9 (Tumor Necrosis Factor Receptor Superfamily, Member 9)	Inflammatory reactions
TBX1 (T-Box 1)	Transcription factor (proliferation and differentiation of cells during organogenesis)
TMEM26 (Transmembrane Protein 26)	Unknown

Table 2 List of primer/probe sets

Gene	Forward primer	Reverse primer	Probe
UCP1	GCATTCAGAGGCAAATCAGC	GCCACACCTCCAGTCATTAAG	56-FAM/ACTGAGTCG/Zen/TAGA GGCCAATCCTGA/3IABkFQ
CIDEA	CATACATGCTCCGAGTACTGG	CATCCCACAGCCTATAACAGAG	56-FAM/TAACCAGGG/Zen/CACA GCTACAGAGG/3IABkFQ
Cox8b	AGCCAAAACTCCCACTTCC	TCTCAGGGATGTGCAACTTC	56-FAM/AGATCCCCA/Zen/C AGCCTGCTCC/3IABkFQ
Serpina3k	GCCAAAGTCAATAACCCCAAG	CTTTGCAACAGCCAATCAGAG	56-FAM/AGCCCTGGA/Zen/C AGAATCATGAGAAC/3IABkFQ
Wdnm1-like	GCCAGAGGAACAATGTGTCAG	GTAATCTCCATACATGGCCTCC	56-FAM/TGGTCACAG/Zen/AGCT CCAAACAGACAC/3IABkFQ
ASC1	TCTTCATTTCCATCCCACTGG	ATGACCCACGAAAAGTAGCC	56-FAM/ATGTCGCCT/Zen/ACTT CACTGCCATGT/3IABkFQ
FGF21	CAAATCCTGGGTGTCAAAGC	CATGGGCTTCAGACTGGTAC	56-FAM/CTCCATCTG/Zen/GCTG TTGGCAAAGAAA/3IABkFQ
P2RX5	TGATAGTTAATGGCAAGGCGG	TTGTCTCGGTAAAACTCGCTC	56-FAM/CCAGGTCAC/Zen/A GAAGAAAGCCCCA/3IABkFQ
PAT2	AGCCACCCCTCTCAATCT	TGCCTTTGACCAGATGAACC	56-FAM/CCAGGATCC/Zen/C AGTCCAGCGAATG/3IABkFQ/
CITED1	ATTTATCGGACTTCTGCCCAG	TTGCGATCCTTCACTCCAAG	56-FAM/AGGCCTCGA/Zen/CATA GTTGGCATTTCA/3IABkFQ
CAR4	CAGAGCACAGTATTGATGGGAG	CTTGTTCACCTTGTCTCCTACC	56-FAM/TTGTCCTTC/Zen/GAGT CCTCCTTGCTAGA/3IABkFQ
TBX1	TGGGACGAGTTCAATCAGC	TGTCATCTACGGGCACAAAG	56-FAM/TCCCCACGT/Zen/TCCA AGTGAAGCTTTT/3IABkFQ
CD137	CCTGTGATAACTGTCAGCCTG	TCTTGAACCTGAAATAGCCTGC	56-FAM/TGCCCTCCA/Zen/AGTA CCTTCTCCAG/3IABkFQ
TMEM26	GCACCATCACTAGAGACCAAC	ACAAGAATGCCAGAGACCAG	56-FAM/CGCCGTCCC/Zen/C ACAAACATCAGA/3IABkFQ
PDGFR-α	GTTGCCTTACGACTCCAGATG	TCACAGCCACCTTCATTACAG	56-FAM/TCCCAAAAT/Zen/CCGA CCAAGCACGA/3IABkFQ

Criteria for validation of beige adipocyte markers

We defined the following criteria for a putative marker to be a valid beige adipocyte marker: *In vitro*, the marker must be expressed in beige adipocytes at statistically significant greater levels than white adipocytes. The marker must be statistically significantly increased in subcutaneous white adipose tissue in response to stimuli that give rise to beige adipocytes and have a dynamic range of at least two fold. The marker should be expressed at statistically significantly greater levels in the adipocyte fraction compared to the SVF, and must be statistically significantly increased in the adipocyte fraction in response to stimuli that give rise to beige adipocytes.

Results

Beige adipocyte marker gene expression differences after white and beige adipocyte differentiation

Expression of the thermoregulatory genes UCP1, CIDEA, and Cox8b was elevated 147, 178-, and 4-fold, respectively, in cells treated with rosiglitazone (Fig. 1a-c), and hereafter referred to as beige adipocytes. In comparison, markers associated with white adipocytes, Serpina3k [12], Wdnm1-like [8], and ASC1 [9] were greater in the cells that were not treated with rosiglitazone (Fig. 1d-f), and hereafter referred to as white adipocytes. With the notable exception of TMEM26, putative beige markers were elevated in beige adipocytes (Fig. 2a-h). However, only CAR4, FGF21, CITED1, CD137, and P2RX5 displayed a more than 2-fold elevation with CAR4 exhibiting the greatest elevation (23-fold: Fig. 2e). Hence all markers but TMEM26 fulfil the criteria of being expressed at higher levels in beige vs white adipocytes (Table 3).

Beige adipocyte marker gene expression in white and beige adipocytes after adrenergic stimulation

Adrenergic stimulation increased UCP1 mRNA expression in both white and beige adipocytes with 11-fold greater expression in the beige compared to white adipocytes (Fig. 1a). Adrenergic stimulation reduced levels of white adipocyte markers as well as those of the transcript for Cox8b (Fig. 1c) in both white and beige cells. CIDEA mRNA levels did not change with adrenergic stimulation in both white and beige adipocytes (Fig. 1b). Adrenergic stimulation affected the levels of beige markers in complex ways in both white and beige cells. The levels of the transcript for P2RX5 and TBX1 where decreased in both cells types by stimulation (Fig. 2b and f), while those of PAT2 were decreased only in white adipocytes (Fig. 2c), and those of CAR4 and CD137 were increased only in white adipocytes (Fig. 2e and g). FGF21 was increased both in white and beige cells (Fig. 2a), but the levels were 8-fold greater in beige cells. Despite these changes the capacity to distinguish between beige and white adipocytes was maintained by all the markers except CITED1, which was increased in white adipocytes to such an extent that it lost the capacity to discriminate between both cell types Fig. 2d). Beige marker CAR4 was changed the least by adrenergic stimulation (Fig 2e). While not part of the *a priori* defined criteria for beige adipocyte markers, the responses of the different gene transcripts to adrenergic stimulation are summarized in Table 3.

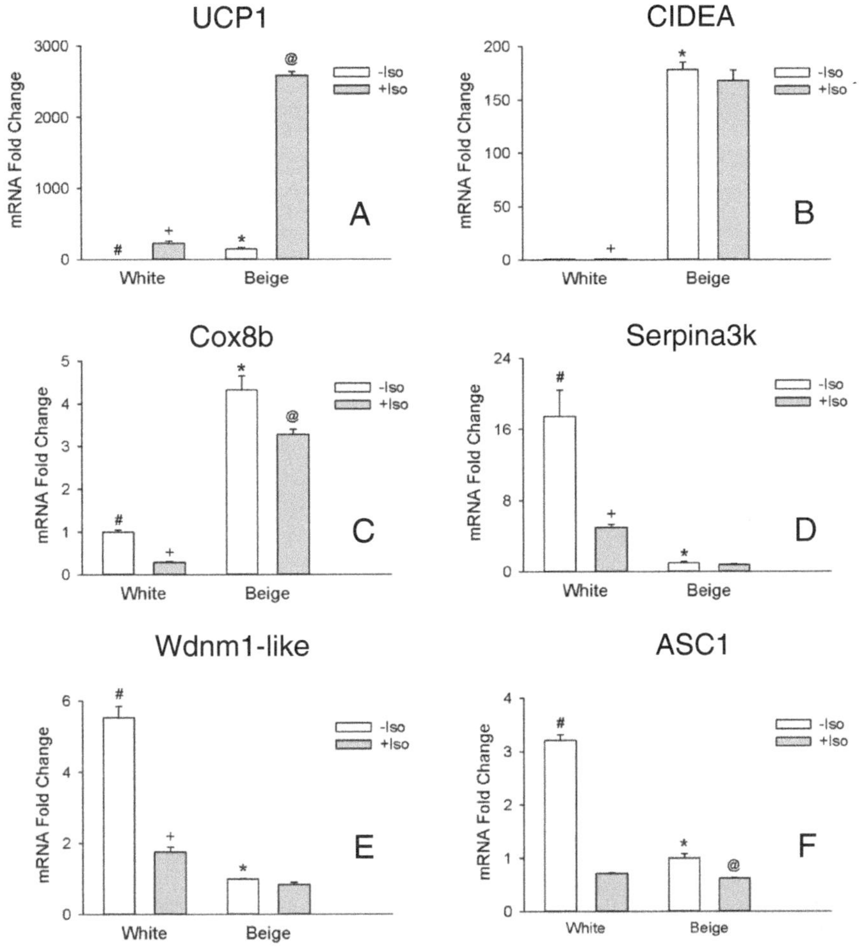

Fig. 1 Thermoregulatory genes and white adipocyte markers *in vitro*. The transcripts for UCP1 **a**, CIDEA **b**, Cox8b **c**, Serpina3k **d**, Wdnm1-like **e**, and ASC1 (**f**) were evaluated in white and beige adipocytes in culture treated with isoproterenol (+ Iso) or without (– Iso) for 6 hrs. before harvesting the cells. Thermoregulatory gene transcripts were normalized to white –Iso, whereas white adipocyte gene transcripts were normalized to beige – Iso. Values are means ± SEM ($n = 3$). (*) different from white – Iso, (#) different from white + Iso, (+) different from beige + Iso, (@) different from beige – Iso, $p \leq 0.05$, two way ANOVA followed by multiple comparisons using the Holm-Sidak method

Age-dependent beige adipocyte marker gene expression in response to cold exposure

We employed mice 2 to 4 months of age to evaluate the possible effect of age on beigeing in WAT. Figures 3 and 4 show the result of 3 such experiments with mice that were 2 months and 10 days (experiment-1), 2 months and 23 days (experiment 2), or 4 months and 10 days (experiment 3) of age by the end of the experiment. In the 3 experiments the transcripts for UCP1, CIDEA, and Cox8b were significantly increased by cold treatment compared to room temperature (Fig. 3a-c). From the younger (Exp-1) to the older (Exp-3) mice there was a trend toward a decrease in the levels of the transcripts both in the mice kept at room temperature as well as those exposed to the cold, suggesting that the number of beige adipocytes decrease with age in mice. As shown in Fig. 4, the transcripts for FGF21, P2RX5, PAT2, and CAR4 were significantly elevated in the first two experiments. Of these, FGF21 displayed the greatest dynamic range, whereas the rest of the transcripts with the exception of P2RX5 and CITED1 in experiment 2 were elevated less than 2-fold, if at all. TBX1, CD137, and TMEM26 were not elevated by cold treatment in either experiment, and TMEM26 was significantly decreased in all 3 experiments. None of the beige markers including FGF21 were significantly increased over baseline in experiment 3 (Fig. 4) which employed older mice.

Therefore only the thermoregulatory gene transcripts meet the criteria that a beige marker should be increased in WAT in response to a beigeing stimulus and display a

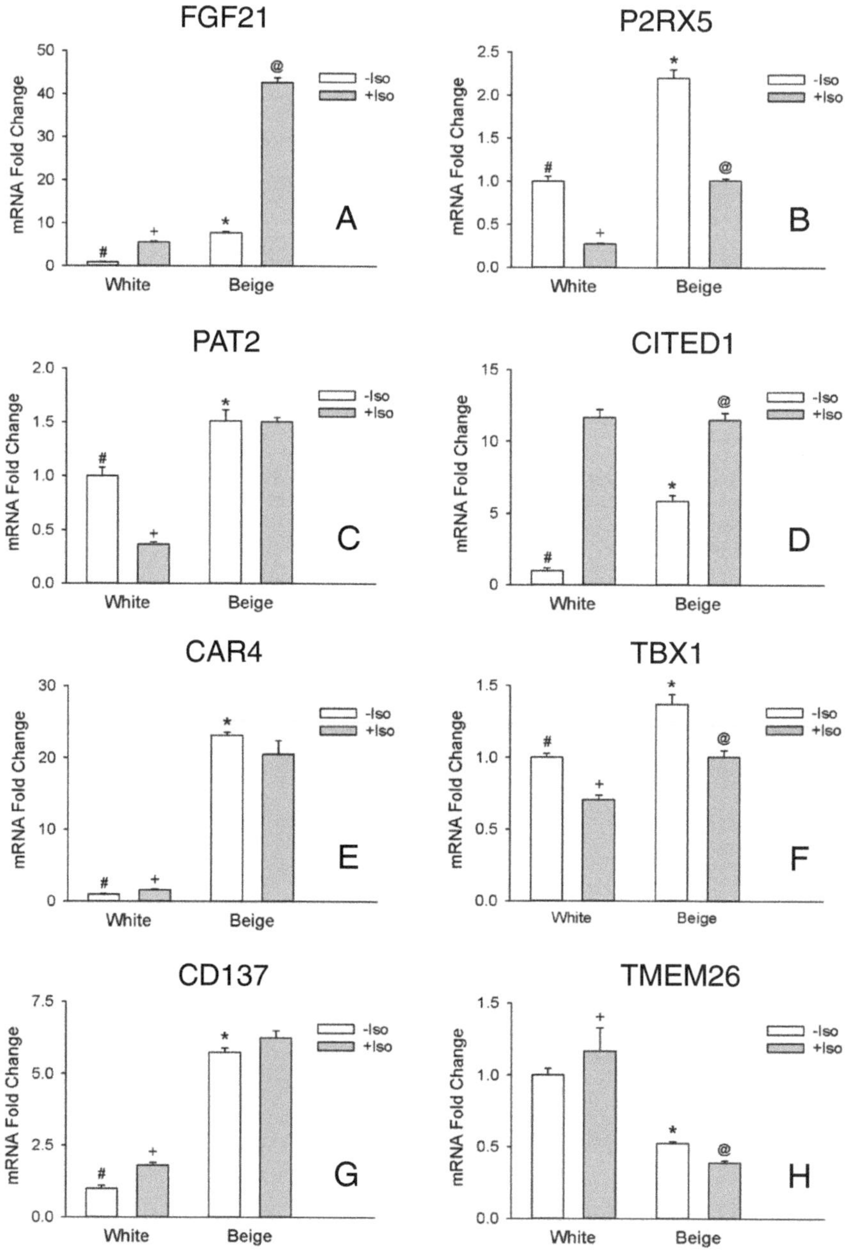

Fig. 2 Markers of beige adipocytes *in vitro*. The transcripts for FGF21 **a**, P2RX5 **b**, PAT2 **c**, CITED1 **d**, CAR4 **e**, TBX1 **f**, CD137 **g**, and TMEM26 (**h**) were evaluated in white and beige adipocytes in culture treated with isoproterenol (+ Iso) or without (– Iso) for 6 hrs. before harvesting the cells. Transcripts were normalized to white – Iso. Values are means ± SEM ($n = 3$). (*) different from white – Iso, (#) different from white + Iso, (+) different from beige + Iso, (@) different from beige – Iso, $p \leq 0.05$, two way ANOVA followed by multiple comparisons using the Holm-Sidak method

sufficiently high dynamic range in the mice of different ages evaluated here, whereas a distinction has to be made between young adult mice and older mice in the case of the proposed beige markers (Table 3).

We attempted to detect by Western blot UCP1, P2RX5, and FGF21 because they were among the markers that were consistently increased in the younger mice in response to cold treatment, and CD137 because

Table 3 Summary of beigeing criteria met by the thermoregulatory genes and putative beige markers when studied under *in vitro* and *in vivo* conditions

Condition	UCP1	CIDEA	Cox8b	FGF21	P2RX5	PAT2	CITED1	CAR4	TBX1	CD137	TMEM26
(A) Beige > white cell culture*	✓	✓	✓	✓	✓	✓	✓	✓	✓	✓	
(B) Beige > white cell culture (adrenergic stimulation)	✓	✓	✓	✓	✓	✓		✓	✓	✓	
(C) Least changed by adrenergic stimulation cell culture		✓						✓			
(D) Elevated in WAT by cold exposure* (young adult mice)	✓	✓	✓	✓	✓	✓		✓			
(E) Large dynamic range in WAT* (young adult mice)	✓	✓	✓	✓							
(F) Elevated in WAT by cold exposure* (older mice)	✓	✓	✓								
(G) Adipocyte fraction > SVF*		✓	✓	✓	✓	✓					
(H) Elevated in adipocyte fraction by cold exposure*	✓	✓	✓	✓	✓	✓	✓	✓	✓		
(I) Beige adipocyte > SVF cells cell culture	✓	✓	✓	✓	✓	✓	✓	✓		✓	

A check mark indicates whether the thermoregulatory genes (columns 2 to 4) or beige transcripts (columns 5 to 12) denoted across the top row met the conditions of a beigeing marker detailed in the first column. The conditions are: A) the marker is significantly elevated in beige over white adipocytes in cell culture, B) the marker is significantly elevated in beige over white adipocytes in cell culture in the presence of adrenergic stimulation, C) the marker was least changed by adrenergic stimulation in beige and white adipocytes in cell culture, D) the marker was significantly elevated by cold exposure in the subcutaneous adipose tissue of young adult mice, E) the marker displayed at least a 2 fold dynamic range in the subcutaneous adipose tissue of young adult mice exposed to cold, F) the marker was significantly elevated by cold exposure in the subcutaneous adipose tissue of older mice, G) the marker was expressed at a significantly higher level in the adipocyte fraction compared to the stromal vascular fraction of subcutaneous adipose tissue of older mice reared at room temperature, H) the marker was significantly elevated by cold exposure in the adipocyte fraction of subcutaneous adipose tissue of older mice exposed to the cold, and I) the marker was expressed at significantly higher levels in SVF cells differentiated into beige adipocytes compared to undifferentiated SVF cells in culture. Conditions marked with an asterisk (*) denote criteria defined *a priori* to be met for a beigeing marker. The remaining conditions, B, C, and I were added based either on results employing adrenergic stimulation in cultured cells or differential expression of the markers in cultured SVF cells and beige adipocytes

of the disparate results we obtained *in vitro* vs *in vivo*. As expected, a large increase in UCP1 was detected in the inguinal adipose tissue of the mice exposed to the cold; however, the levels of the proteins for FGF21, P2RX5, and CD137 were below the limits of detection (see Additional file 1). Ussar et al., 2014, had previously reported that P2RX5 was undetectable in the inguinal adipose tissue of mice [9].

Beige adipocyte marker gene expression in SVF cells and adipocytes

We separated the SVF from the adipocyte fraction of the 4 month and 10 day old mice from Experiment-3 (Figs. 3 and 4) to gauge whether beigeing in white adipose tissue can be better evaluated employing the isolated adipocyte fraction, and to determine the extent of the expression of the markers in both fractions and how it is changed by cold treatment. Transcripts for the markers of white adipocytes ASC1 and Wdnm1-like were 135- and 78-fold greater, respectively, in the adipocyte fraction, whereas the transcript for PDGFR-α, a marker for bipotential adipocyte precursors [13], was 25-fold greater in the SVF (see Additional file 2). This indicates that, at least in terms of the adipocytes and some of their precursors, the two fractions were successfully separated with minimal cross-contamination.

The transcripts for CIDEA and Cox8b, but not UCP1, were expressed at greater abundance in the adipocyte fraction compared to the SVF of mice housed at room temperature (Fig. 5a-c). Of all the beige markers tested only FGF21, P2RX5, and PAT2 (Fig. 6a-c) were expressed at greater levels (5-, 8-, and 28-fold greater, respectively) in the adipocyte fraction compared to the SVF from mice housed at room temperature. Levels of CAR4 did not differ between fractions (Fig. 6e). However TBX1 (Fig. 6f), CITED1 (Fig. 6d), and CD137 and TMEM26 (Fig. 6g-h) were expressed at lower levels (2.5-, 8-, 14-, and 33-fold lower, respectively) in the adipocyte fraction compared to the SVF in mice housed at room temperature. So only 2 thermoregularoty genes (CIDEA and Cox8b), and 3 beige markers (FGF21, P2RX5, and PAT2), meet the criteria of being expressed at a higher level in the adipocyte fraction of mice at room temperature (Table 3).

Beige adipocyte marker gene expression in SVF cells and adipocytes in Response to Cold Exposure

The transcript for UCP1 was upregulated (173-fold) by cold stimulation in the adipocyte fraction, and the transcripts for CIDEA, and Cox8b were also increased by cold exposure, although to a lesser extent (Fig. 5). The beige markers CAR4 (Fig. 6e), P2RX5 (Fig. 6b), CITED1 (Fig. 6d), TBX1 (Fig. 6f), PAT2 (Fig. 6c), and FGF21 (Fig. 6a) were increased (128, 111, 83, 68, 52, and 50 %, respectively) in the adipocyte fraction by cold treatment. Only the transcripts for CD137 and TMEM26 (Fig. 6g-h) did not display a significant increase in the adipocyte fraction of those animals exposed to cold treatment. The net change in the levels of the transcripts in the SVF were small for most markers except for TBX1 where expression was increased to an extent comparable to that in

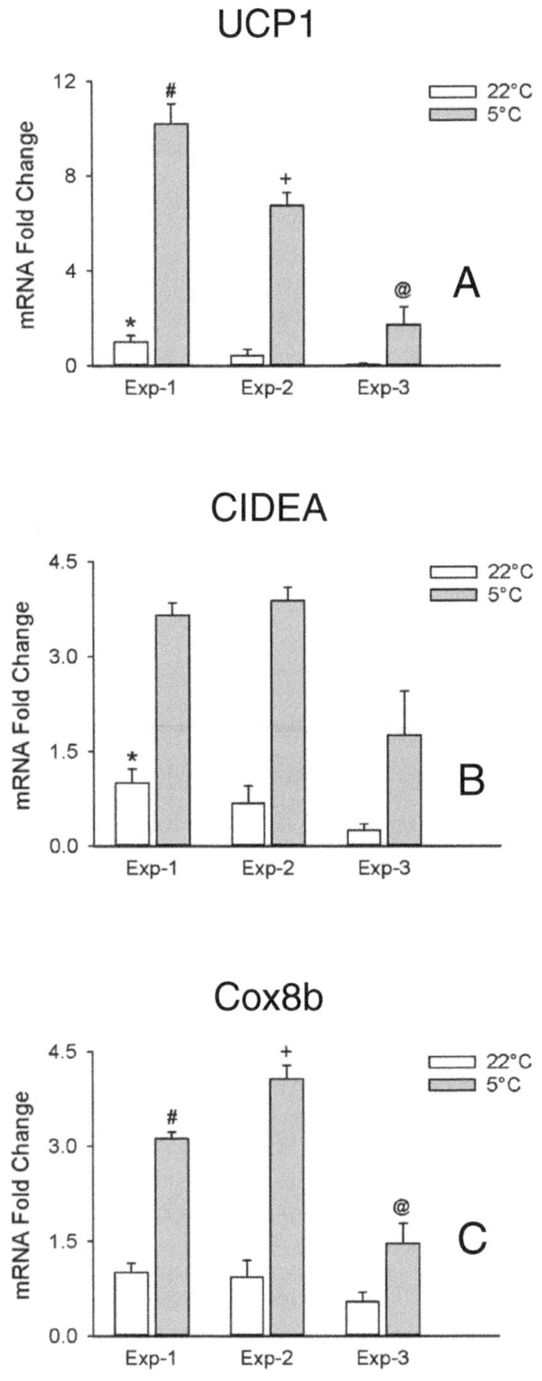

Fig. 3 Transcripts of thermoregulatory genes in inguinal adipose tissue. The transcripts for UCP1 **a**, CIDEA **b**, and Cox8b (**c**) were evaluated in inguinal adipose tissue from mice maintained at room temperature (22 °C) or exposed to cold (5 °C) for one week in 3 separate experiments where the ages of the mice at the end of the experiments were 2 months and 10 days (Exp-1), 2 months and 23 days (Exp-2), and 4 months and 10 days (Exp-3). Transcripts were normalized to 22 °C in Experiment-1. Values are means ± SEM ($n = 4–5$). Comparisons of 22 °C vs 5 °C within each experiment for all transcripts were statistically significantly different ($P \leq 0.05$) and are not marked with a symbol. (*) different from Exp-3, 22 °C, (#) different from Exp-2, 5 °C, (+) different from Exp-3, 5 °C, (@) different from Exp-1, 5 °C, $p \leq 0.05$, two way ANOVA followed by multiple comparisons using the Holm-Sidak method

the adipocyte fraction (Fig. 6f), and TMEM26 where the expression was decreased (Fig. 6h). Thus all gene transcripts but those of CD137 and TMEM26 meet the criteria of increased expression in the adipocyte fraction from subcutaneous WAT in response to a beigeing stimulus (Table 3).

Beige adipocyte marker gene expression in cells from the SVF and beige adipocytes in culture

The results obtained with the differential expression of the beige markers in the SVF and the adipocyte fraction led us to perform an additional experiment to evaluate the expression of beige markers *in vitro* in beige adipocytes and the cells from the SVF. Differentiation of cultured SVF cells into beige adipocytes should result in an increase in the levels of beige adipocyte markers. As expected the abundance of the transcripts for CIDEA, Cox8b, and UCP1 was much higher in beige adipocytes compared to the undifferentiated SVF cells (see Additional file 3). As shown in Fig. 7, the abundance of the transcripts of most beige adipocyte markers, including CD137, was significantly increased in beige adipocytes over that of undifferentiated SVF cells with the exception of TBX1, which did not increase, or TMEM26, which was reduced. While not part of the *a priori* defined criteria for beige adipocyte markers, these results are summarized in Table 3.

Discussion

In this work we evaluated the expression of the transcripts for thermoregulatory genes and putative beige markers in cultured murine SVF cells differentiated into white and beige adipocytes, and in whole subcutaneous (inguinal) white adipose tissue, and its two major fractions (adipocyte fraction and SVF) of mice exposed to cold temperature to induce beigeing. Each of these approaches by itself has shortcomings. Cell culture conditions may generate results that differ from *in vivo* models. The results obtained from whole tissue represent the sum of the contributions of all cell types in the

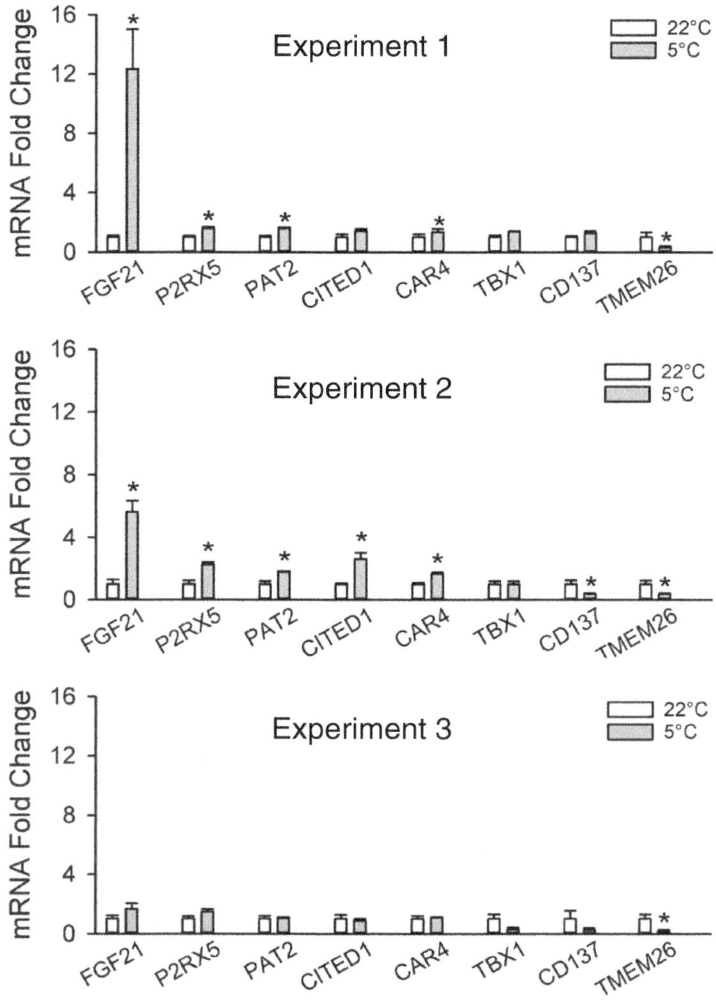

Fig. 4 Markers of beige adipocytes in inguinal adipose tissue. The transcripts for FGF21, P2RX5, PAT2, CITED1, CAR4, TBX1, CD137, and TMEM26 were evaluated in inguinal adipose tissue from mice maintained at room temperature (22 °C) or exposed to cold (5 °C) for one week in 3 separate experiments were the ages of the mice at the end of the experiment were 2 months and 10 days (Exp-1), 2 months and 23 days (Exp-2), and 4 months and 10 days (Exp-3). The levels of the transcripts at 5 °C were normalized to the transcript of the same gene at 22 °C. Values are means ± SEM ($n = 4–5$). (*) different from 22 °C, $p \leq 0.05$, two-tailed t-test

tissue. And the processing and time involved in the separation of the adipocytes and SVF may introduce changes to the relative levels of transcripts present in the cells *in vivo*. However, by characterizing and comparing the changes in gene expression obtained when employing each approach we can determine the best markers to evaluate beigeing.

TMEM26, CD137, and TBX1 were identified as beige adipocyte markers by Wu and coworkers [7], but other labs have had mixed success in validating these markers [9, 10]. Our data indicate that TBX1 may have some utility as a marker to discriminate beige and white adipocytes *in vitro*, or if the assay is performed on the adipocyte fraction from white adipose tissue. On the other hand, TMEM26 did not meet any of the criteria defined a priori or otherwise for a beige marker, and CD137 did not meet the criteria of being increased by a beigeing stimulus *in vivo*, but it seems to be an acceptable marker for beige adipocytes *in vitro*. One possibility to explain the limitations of TMEM26 and CD137 as beige markers is that suggested by Lee and coworkers, 2015. These authors found that the levels of CD137 and TMEM26 in cultured adipocyte precursors are decreased when differentiated into beige adipocytes [14]. The authors suggest that CD137 and TMEM26 may work better to identify beige adipocyte precursors rather than

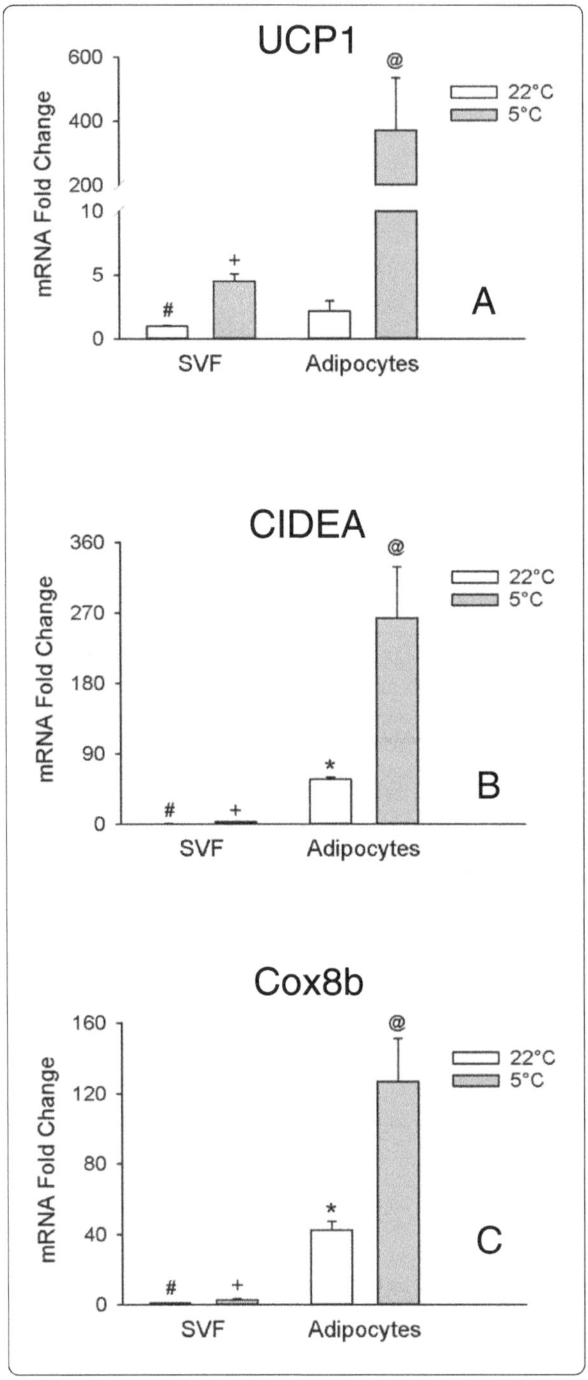

Fig. 5 Transcripts of thermoregulatory genes in the adipocyte and SVF derived from inguinal adipose tissue. The transcripts for UCP1 **a**, CIDEA **b**, and Cox8b (**c**) were evaluated in the adipocyte and SVF of the 4 month and 10 day old mice from Experiment-3 (Figs. 3 and 4) kept at room temperature (22 °C) or exposed to the cold (5 °C) for one week. Transcripts were normalized to 22 °C, SVF. Values are means ± SEM ($n = 3–5$). (*) different from SVF 22 °C, (#) different from SVF 5 °C, (+) different from adipocytes 5 °C, (@) different from adipocytes 22 °C, $p \leq 0.05$, two way ANOVA followed by multiple comparisons using the Holm-Sidak method

differentiated beige adipocytes in white adipose tissue. In agreement with these authors we found that TMEM26 was decreased when cultured cells from the SVF were differentiated into beige adipocytes. Therefore TMEM26 could be expressed at a higher abundance in the precursors of beige adipocytes in the SVF, and its levels decreased by the stimuli that produce beige adipocytes.

However, unlike the results of Lee and coworkers, 2015, we found that the expression of CD137 was increased when cultured cells from the SVF were differentiated into beige adipocytes, which is what would be expected of a beige adipocyte marker. Additional explanations as for why the use of CD137 may be challenging as a beige marker *in vivo* is that the transcript of this gene is expressed at a 10 fold higher abundance in the cells of the SVF and is regulated by other stimuli besides beigeing. CD137 is a member of the tumor necrosis factor (TNF) receptor superfamily of proteins which is expressed in immune cells like activated T cells and macrophages. CD137 participates in proinflamatory processes [15] and its levels are modified by inflammatory stimuli [16]. Thus, the large background signal due to the high expression of CD137 in the SVF, and its fluctuation in response to the inflammatory state of the tissue may make it difficult to evaluate the changes in the levels of the transcript exclusively due to beigeing.

FGF21, CAR4, and CITED1 were identified as beige adipocyte markers by microarray analyses of SVF cells induced to differentiate into brown, beige, or white adipocytes [8], and P2Rx5 and PAT2 were identified as brown/beige adipocyte markers employing a combination of *in silico*, *in vitro*, and *in vivo* methods [9]. We found that these markers can all be used to discriminate beige from white adipocytes *in vitro*. We also found that, with the exception of CITED1, the specificity of these markers is maintained even in the presence of adrenergic stimulation. The fact that short-term adrenergic stimulation modified the levels of most transcripts even in cells fully differentiated into a beige phenotype suggests that fluctuations in the levels of these transcripts can occur in a way that is independent of beige cell numbers. In this sense CIDEA and CAR4 may be useful markers because their expression was least affected by short-term adrenergic stimulation in either beige or

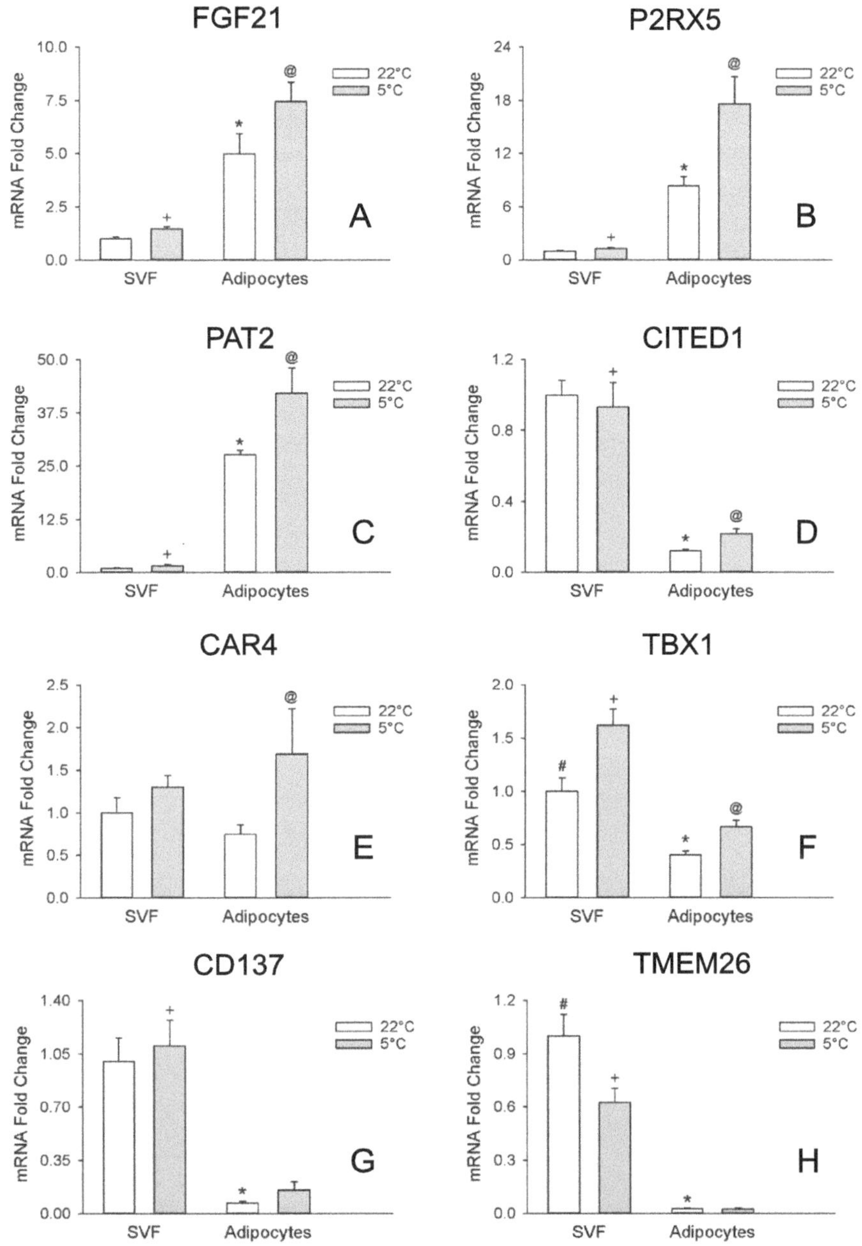

Fig. 6 Markers of beige adipocytes in the adipocyte and SVF derived from inguinal adipose tissue. The transcripts for FGF21 **a**, P2RX5 **b**, PAT2 **c**, CITED1 **d**, CAR4 **e**, TBX1 **f**, CD137 **g**, and TMEM26 (**h**) were evaluated in the adipocyte and SVF of 4 month old mice kept at room temperature (22 °C) or exposed to the cold (5 °C) for one week. Transcripts were normalized to 22 °C, SVF. Values are means ± SEM ($n = 3$–5). (*) different from SVF 22 °C, (#) different from SVF 5 °C, (+) different from adipocytes 5 °C, (@) different from adipocytes 22 °C, $p \leq 0.05$, two way ANOVA followed by multiple comparisons using the Holm-Sidak method

white cells. Even though adrenergic stimulation increased the levels of UCP1 in both beige and white cells, it decreased the levels of the transcript for Cox8b. This may represent a negative feedback mechanism involved in regulating the cell's response to a strong adrenergic stimulus.

Our data also indicated that, at least in the younger mice, FGF21, P2RX5, PAT2, and CAR4 are also markers

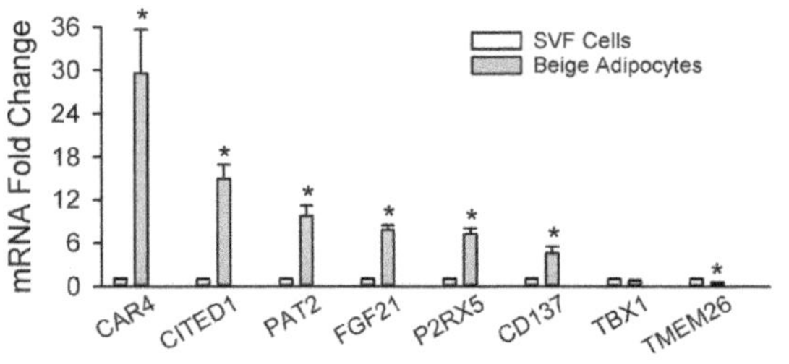

Fig. 7 Beige markers in preadipocytes and SVF cells *in vitro*. The transcripts for CAR4, CITED1, PAT2, FGF21, P2RX5, CD137, TBX1, and TMEM26 were evaluated in SVF cells and beige adipocytes in culture. Transcripts were normalized to SVF cells. Values are means ± SEM ($n = 3$). (*) different from SVF, $p \leq 0.05$, two-tailed t-test

of beige adipocytes, although only FGF21 exhibited a large dynamic range. It is interesting that all the beige markers that were consistently elevated in the first two *in vivo* experiments in response to the cold (FGF21, P2RX5, PAT2, and CAR4) were also the markers that were either expressed at greater (FGF21, P2RX5, and PAT2) or the same (CAR4) level in the adipocyte fraction compared to the SVF of animals kept at room temperature. In contrast the markers that either displayed no consistent increase (CITED1: increased in experiment 2, but not experiment 1) or no increase at all (TBX1, CD137, and TMEM26) in these two experiments were all expressed in the SVF at a greater abundance. A greater expression of a marker in the cells comprising the SVF may create a higher background that can make it harder for increases in expression of a beige marker in the adipocyte fraction to be detected in the intact tissue.

In experiment 3 performed with older animals the data were more variable than in experiments 1 or 2, and although the thermogenic markers UCP1, CIDEA, and Cox8b were significantly elevated by cold treatment, no significant elevations of beige markers were detected. The comparative evaluation of the expression of the transcripts for UCP1, CIDEA, and Cox8b among these experiments suggested that the extent of beigeing in the older mice was lower compared to younger mice, which would explain the decrease in the beige markers. A loss of UCP1 and multilocular adipocytes in subcutaneous adipose tissue with age has been reported in mice [17], so it is also possible that the capacity for beigeing in WAT of older mice in response to a stimulus such as cold exposure is reduced. This indicates that the use of beige markers in older mice may have limited validity. However, when we evaluated the markers in the adipocyte fractions of older mice, we were able to detect significant elevations of most markers in response to cold treatment with the exception of CD137 and TMEM26. So, evaluating the markers in the isolated adipocyte fraction may be one way to overcome this limitation.

Species-dependent difference, age differences, and animal housing temperature may contribute to differences in beige adipocyte marker gene expression across published studies. In a recent study to validate markers of adipose tissue depots by de Jong and coworkers [11], the authors used NMRI mice which are less prone to diet-induced obesity compared to the strain we used, C57BL/6 [18], and they exposed their mice to thermoneutral (30 °C) or cold temperatures (5 °C) for 3 weeks (compared to 22 °C and 5 °C for one week in our study). Despite these differences, the authors also found that in inguinal adipose tissue TBX1, CD137, and TMEM26 were not increased by cold treatment (they were significantly decreased) while FGF21, P2RX5, and PAT2 were increased with FGF21 having the greatest dynamic range. Although our current work has further contributed by highlighting the possible limitations of using beige markers (the age of the animals) as well as their differential expression among the adipocyte and SVFs, the agreement between our data and that of de Jong and coworkers indicate that our results are not specific to one strain of mice and one set of conditions.

While not technically markers of beige adipocytes, the transcripts of thermoregulatory genes like UCP1, CIDEA, and Cox8b can also be employed to evaluate beigeing in mouse WAT. We found that UCP1, CIDEA, and Cox8b fulfilled all of the criteria we defined for beige markers. Because of this and the fact that the stimulus we employed, cold exposure, is a powerful stimulus to induce beigeing, these thermoregulatory genes are likely better markers than the specific beige markers in studies where milder beigeing stimuli and/or older mice are employed. Nevertheless, the use of beige marker FGF21 may provide additional information about the dynamics of the beigeing process. FGF21 is a factor that induces beige cell differentiation in white adipose tissue, and its upregulation in the tissue may stimulate beige adipocyte differentiation through autocrine or paracrine effects [19].

Finally we must consider the applicability of our findings to humans. Our study clearly shows that even in the mouse the effectiveness of some beige markers may vary depending on several variables (*in vitro* vs *in vivo*, adrenergic stimulation, whole tissue vs fractions, age, etc.). Thus the results obtained from the application of beige markers validated in rodents to human samples should be interpreted with caution. There is a need for studies that evaluate these markers in human tissues exposed to beigeing stimuli. For example Kern and coworkers, 2014, found that in human subjects the thermoregulatory markers UCP1 and PGC1-α and the beige markers TMEM26 and TBX1 (but not CD137) were increased during winter in subcutaneous adipose tissue biopsies [20]. It is only through studies like these and the evaluation of in vitro differentiated cells and subcellular fractions in different physiological conditions that beige markers for humans will be fully validated.

Conclusions

Researchers seeking to discriminate between cultured white and beige adipocytes or studying their possible interconversion can use any of the thermoregulatory genes or beige markers described herein with the exception of TMEM26. Researchers including adrenergic stimulation paradigms in their cell culture methodology should consider how even short-term stimulation can change the levels of the markers and note that CIDEA and CAR4 were the genes whose expression was least affected, whereas CITED1 lost its capacity to discriminate between beige and white adipocytes. Researchers seeking to evaluate the degree of beigeing in whole WAT of mouse models in response to experimental manipulations can employ UCP1, CIDEA, or Cox8b. The best beige markers for this purpose are FGF21, P2RX5, PAT2, or CAR4, but the low dynamic range of some of these markers, the age of the mice, and the strength of the beigeing stimulus may represent a limitation, which may be overcome by their evaluation in the adipocyte fraction.

Additional files

Additional file 1: Western blots of UCP1, beta-actin, FGF21, P2RX5, and CD137 in WAT of control mice (22 °C) and mice exposed to cold (5 °C). (PPTX 332 kb)

Additional file 2: Distribution of markers of white adipocytes and preadipocytes between the adipocyte fraction and SVF. The transcripts for ASC1 and Wdnm1-like (A) or PDGFR-alpha (B) were evaluated in the adipocyte fraction and SVF of 4 month and 10 days old mice kept at room temperature (22 °C). Transcripts were normalized to SVF. Values are means ± SEM ($n = 3$–5). (*) different from SVF, $p \leq 0.05$, two-tailed t-test. (PPTX 97 kb)

Additional file 3: Thermoregulatory markers in cells from the SVF and beige adipocytes *in vitro*. The transcripts for CIDEA, Cox8b, and UCP1 were evaluated in SVF cells and beige adipocytes in culture. Transcripts were normalized to SVF cells. Values are means ± SEM ($n = 3$). (*) different from SVF cells, $p \leq 0.05$, two-tailed t-test. (PPTX 71 kb)

Abbreviations

IBMX: isobutylmethylxanthine; Iso: isoproterenol; SVF: stromal vascular fraction; WAT: white adipose tissue.

Competing interests

The authors declare that they have no competing interests.

Authors' contributions

RAG contributed to the design, acquisition of data, analysis and interpretation of results, and drafting of the manuscript. KJC contributed to the design, analysis and interpretation of results, and revision of the manuscript. JNR contributed to the design, analysis and interpretation of results, and revision of the manuscript. All authors read and approved the final manuscript.

Acknowledgements

The authors acknowledge the technical assistance of Phillip Blomberg in the acquisition of the data.

This work was supported by USDA Agricultural Research Service Project #3062-51000-052-00D. The funders had no role in study design, data collection and analysis, decision to publish, or preparation of the manuscript.

References

1. Merlin J, Evans BA, Dehvari N, Sato M, Bengtsson T, Hutchinson DS. Could burning fat start with a brite spark? Pharmacological and nutritional ways to promote thermogenesis. Mol Nutr Food Res. 2015. doi:10.1002/mnfr.201500251.
2. Feldmann HM, Golozoubova V, Cannon B, Nedergaard J. UCP1 ablation induces obesity and abolishes diet-induced thermogenesis in mice exempt from thermal stress by living at thermoneutrality. Cell Metab. 2009;9(2):203–9. doi:10.1016/j.cmet.2008.12.014.
3. Harms M, Seale P. Brown and beige fat: development, function and therapeutic potential. Nat Med. 2013;19(10):1252–63. doi:10.1038/nm.3361.
4. Schulz TJ, Huang P, Huang TL, Xue R, McDougall LE, Townsend KL, et al. Brown-fat paucity due to impaired BMP signalling induces compensatory browning of white fat. Nature. 2013;495(7441):379–83. doi:10.1038/nature11943.
5. Cohen P, Levy JD, Zhang Y, Frontini A, Kolodin DP, Svensson KJ, et al. Ablation of PRDM16 and beige adipose causes metabolic dysfunction and a subcutaneous to visceral fat switch. Cell. 2014;156(1–2):304–16. doi:10.1016/j.cell.2013.12.021.
6. Stanford KI, Middelbeek RJ, Townsend KL, Lee MY, Takahashi H, So K, et al. A novel role for subcutaneous adipose tissue in exercise-induced improvements in glucose homeostasis. Diabetes. 2015;64(6):2002–14. doi:10.2337/db14-0704.
7. Wu J, Bostrom P, Sparks LM, Ye L, Choi JH, Giang AH, et al. Beige adipocytes are a distinct type of thermogenic fat cell in mouse and human. Cell. 2012;150(2):366–76. doi:10.1016/j.cell.2012.05.016.
8. Sharp LZ, Shinoda K, Ohno H, Scheel DW, Tomoda E, Ruiz L, et al. Human BAT possesses molecular signatures that resemble beige/brite cells. PLoS One. 2012;7(11):e49452. doi:10.1371/journal.pone.0049452.
9. Ussar S, Lee KY, Dankel SN, Boucher J, Haering MF, Kleinridders A, et al. ASC-1, PAT2, and P2RX5 are cell surface markers for white, beige, and brown adipocytes. Sci Transl Med. 2014;6(247):247ra103. doi:10.1126/scitranslmed.3008490.
10. Rosenwald M, Perdikari A, Rulicke T, Wolfrum C. Bi-directional interconversion of brite and white adipocytes. Nat Cell Biol. 2013;15(6):659–67. doi:10.1038/ncb2740.
11. de Jong JM, Larsson O, Cannon B, Nedergaard J. A stringent validation of mouse adipose tissue identity markers. Am J Physiol Endocrinol Metab. 2015. doi:10.1152/ajpendo.00023.2015. ajpendo 00023 2015.
12. Kajimura S, Seale P, Tomaru T, Erdjument-Bromage H, Cooper MP, Ruas JL, et al. Regulation of the brown and white fat gene programs through a PRDM16/CtBP transcriptional complex. Genes Dev. 2008;22(10):1397–409. doi:10.1101/gad.1666108.
13. Lee YH, Petkova AP, Mottillo EP, Granneman JG. In vivo identification of bipotential adipocyte progenitors recruited by beta3-adrenoceptor activation and high-fat feeding. Cell Metab. 2012;15(4):480–91. doi:10.1016/j.cmet.2012.03.009.
14. Lee MW, Odegaard JI, Mukundan L, Qiu Y, Molofsky AB, Nussbaum JC, et al. Activated type 2 innate lymphoid cells regulate beige fat biogenesis. Cell. 2015;160(1–2):74–87. doi:10.1016/j.cell.2014.12.011.
15. Kim CS, Kim JG, Lee BJ, Choi MS, Choi HS, Kawada T, et al. Deficiency for costimulatory receptor 4-1BB protects against obesity-induced inflammation and metabolic disorders. Diabetes. 2011;60(12):3159–68. doi:10.2337/db10-1805.
16. Tu TH, Kim CS, Goto T, Kawada T, Kim BS, Yu R. 4-1BB/4-1BBL interaction promotes obesity-induced adipose inflammation by triggering bidirectional inflammatory signaling in adipocytes/macrophages. Mediators Inflamm. 2012;2012:972629. doi:10.1155/2012/972629.
17. Rogers NH, Landa A, Park S, Smith RG. Aging leads to a programmed loss of brown adipocytes in murine subcutaneous white adipose tissue. Aging Cell. 2012;11(6):1074–83. doi:10.1111/acel.12010.
18. Matyskova R, Maletinska L, Maixnerova J, Pirnik Z, Kiss A, Zelezna B. Comparison of the obesity phenotypes related to monosodium glutamate

effect on arcuate nucleus and/or the high fat diet feeding in C57BL/6 and NMRI mice. Physiol Res. 2008;57(5):727–34.
19. Fisher FM, Kleiner S, Douris N, Fox EC, Mepani RJ, Verdeguer F, et al. FGF21 regulates PGC-1alpha and browning of white adipose tissues in adaptive thermogenesis. Genes Dev. 2012;26(3):271–81. doi:10.1101/gad.177857.111.
20. Kern PA, Finlin BS, Zhu B, Rasouli N, McGehee Jr RE, Westgate PM, et al. The effects of temperature and seasons on subcutaneous white adipose tissue in humans: evidence for thermogenic gene induction. J Clin Endocrinol Metab. 2014;99(12):E2772–9. doi:10.1210/jc.2014-2440.

Effects of exogenous ketone supplementation on blood ketone, glucose, triglyceride, and lipoprotein levels in Sprague–Dawley rats

Shannon L. Kesl[1*], Angela M. Poff[1], Nathan P. Ward[1], Tina N. Fiorelli[1], Csilla Ari[1], Ashley J. Van Putten[1], Jacob W. Sherwood[1], Patrick Arnold[2] and Dominic P. D'Agostino[1]

Abstract

Background: Nutritional ketosis induced by the ketogenic diet (KD) has therapeutic applications for many disease states. We hypothesized that oral administration of exogenous ketone supplements could produce sustained nutritional ketosis (>0.5 mM) without carbohydrate restriction.

Methods: We tested the effects of 28-day administration of five ketone supplements on blood glucose, ketones, and lipids in male Sprague–Dawley rats. The supplements included: 1,3-butanediol (BD), a sodium/potassium β-hydroxybutyrate (βHB) mineral salt (BMS), medium chain triglyceride oil (MCT), BMS + MCT 1:1 mixture, and 1,3 butanediol acetoacetate diester (KE). Rats received a daily 5–10 g/kg dose of their respective ketone supplement via intragastric gavage during treatment. Weekly whole blood samples were taken for analysis of glucose and βHB at baseline and, 0.5, 1, 4, 8, and 12 h post-gavage, or until βHB returned to baseline. At 28 days, triglycerides, total cholesterol and high-density lipoprotein (HDL) were measured.

Results: Exogenous ketone supplementation caused a rapid and sustained elevation of βHB, reduction of glucose, and little change to lipid biomarkers compared to control animals.

Conclusions: This study demonstrates the efficacy and tolerability of oral exogenous ketone supplementation in inducing nutritional ketosis independent of dietary restriction.

Keywords: Ketogenic diet, Ketone ester, Ketone supplement, Appetite, β-hydroxybutyrate, Hyperketonemia, Triglycerides

Background

Emerging evidence supports the therapeutic potential of the ketogenic diet (KD) for a variety of disease states, leading investigators to research methods of harnessing the benefits of nutritional ketosis without the dietary restrictions. The KD has been used as an effective non-pharmacological therapy for pediatric intractable seizures since the 1920s [1–3]. In addition to epilepsy, the ketogenic diet has elicited significant therapeutic effects for weight loss and type-2 diabetes (T2D) [4]. Several studies have shown significant weight loss on a high fat, low carbohydrate diet without significant elevations of serum cholesterol [5–12]. Another study demonstrated the safety and benefits of long-term application of the KD in T2D patients. Patients exhibited significant weight loss, reduction of blood glucose, and improvement of lipid markers after eating a well-formulated KD for 56 weeks [13]. Recently, researchers have begun to investigate the use of the KD as a treatment for acne, polycystic ovary syndrome (PCOS), cancer, amyotrophic lateral sclerosis (ALS), traumatic brain injury (TBI) and Alzheimer's disease (AD) with promising preliminary results [14–26].

* Correspondence: skesl@health.usf.edu
[1]Department of Molecular Pharmacology and Physiology, Morsani College of Medicine, University of South Florida, 12901 Bruce B. Downs Blvd. MDC8, Tampa, FL 33612, USA
Full list of author information is available at the end of the article

The classical KD consists of a 4:1 ratio of fat to protein and carbohydrate, with 80–90 % of total calories derived from fat [27]. The macronutrient ratio of the KD induces a metabolic shift towards fatty acid oxidation and hepatic ketogenesis, elevating the ketone bodies acetoacetate (AcAc) and β-hydroxybutyrate (βHB) in the blood. Acetone, generated by decarboxylation of AcAc, has been shown to have anticonvulsant properties [28–32]. Ketone bodies are naturally elevated to serve as alternative metabolic substrates for extra-hepatic tissues during the prolonged reduction of glucose availability, suppression of insulin, and depletion of liver glycogen, such as occurs during starvation, fasting, vigorous exercise, calorie restriction, or the KD. Although the KD has clear therapeutic potential, several factors limit the efficacy and utility of this metabolic therapy for widespread clinical use. Patient compliance to the KD can be low due to the severe dietary restriction - the diet being generally perceived as unpalatable - and intolerance to high-fat ingestion. Maintaining ketosis can be difficult as consumption of even a small quantity of carbohydrates or excess protein can rapidly inhibit ketogenesis [33, 34]. Furthermore, enhanced ketone body production and tissue utilization by the tissues can take several weeks (keto-adaptation), and patients may experience mild hypoglycemic symptoms during this transitional period [35].

Recent studies suggest that many of the benefits of the KD are due to the effects of ketone body metabolism. Interestingly, in studies on T2D patients, improved glycemic control, improved lipid markers, and retraction of insulin and other medications occurred before weight loss became significant. Both βHB and AcAc have been shown to decrease mitochondrial reactive oxygen species (ROS) production [36–39]. Veech et al. have summarized the potential therapeutic uses for ketone bodies [28, 40]. They have demonstrated that exogenous ketones favorably alter mitochondrial bioenergetics to reduce the mitochondrial NAD couple, oxidize the co-enzyme Q, and increase the ΔG' (free enthalpy) of ATP hydrolysis [41]. Ketone bodies have been shown to increase the hydraulic efficiency of the heart by 28 %, simultaneously decreasing oxygen consumption while increasing ATP production [42]. Thus, elevated ketone bodies increase metabolic efficiency and as a consequence, reduce superoxide production and increase reduced glutathione [28]. Sullivan et al. demonstrated that mice fed a KD for 10–12 days showed increased hippocampal uncoupling proteins, indicative of decreased mitochondrial-produced ROS [43]. Bough et al. showed an increase of mitochondrial biogenesis in rats maintained on a KD for 4–6 weeks [44, 45]. Recently, Shimazu et al. reported that βHB is an exogenous and specific inhibitor of class I histone deacetylases (HDACs), which confers protection against oxidative stress [38]. Ketone bodies have also been shown to suppress inflammation by decreasing the inflammatory markers TNF-a, IL-6, IL-8, MCP-1, E-selectin, I-CAM, and PAI-1 [8, 46, 47]. Therefore, it is thought that ketone bodies themselves confer many of the benefits associated with the KD.

Considering both the broad therapeutic potential and limitations of the KD, an oral exogenous ketone supplement capable of inducing sustained therapeutic ketosis without the need for dietary restriction would serve as a practical alternative. Several natural and synthetic ketone supplements capable of inducing nutritional ketosis have been identified. Desrochers et al. elevated ketone bodies in the blood of pigs (>0.5 mM) using exogenous ketone supplements: (R, S)-1,3 butanediol and (R, S)-1,3 butanediol-acetoacetate monoesters and diester [48]. In 2012, Clarke et al. demonstrated the safety and efficacy of chronic oral administration of a ketone monoester of R-βHB in rats and humans [49, 50]. Subjects maintained elevated blood ketones without dietary restriction and experienced little to no adverse side effects, demonstrating the potential to circumvent the restrictive diet typically needed to achieve therapeutic ketosis. We hypothesized that exogenous ketone supplements could produce sustained hyperketonemia (>0.5 mM) without dietary restriction and without negatively influencing metabolic biomarkers, such as blood glucose, total cholesterol, HDL, LDL, and triglycerides. Thus, we measured these biomarkers during a 28-day administration of the following ketone supplements in rats: naturally-derived ketogenic supplements included medium chain triglyceride oil (MCT), sodium/potassium -βHB mineral salt (BMS), and sodium/potassium -βHB mineral salt + medium chain triglyceride oil 1:1 mixture (BMS + MCT) and synthetically produced ketogenic supplements included 1, 3-butanediol (BD), 1, 3-butanediol acetoacetate diester/ ketone ester (KE).

Methods

Synthesis and formulation of ketone supplements

KE was synthesized as previously described [29]. BMS is a novel agent (sodium/potassium- βHB mineral salt) supplied as a 50 % solution containing approximately 375 mg/g of pure βHB and 125 mg/g of sodium/potassium. Both KE and BMS were developed and synthesized in collaboration with Savind Inc. Pharmaceutical grade MCT oil (~65 % caprylic triglyceride; 45 % capric triglyceride) was purchased from Now Foods (Bloomingdale, IL). BMS was formulated in a 1:1 ratio with MCT at the University of South Florida (USF), yielding a final mixture of 25 % water, 25 % pure βHB mineral salt and 50 % MCT. BD was purchased from Sigma-Aldrich (Prod # B84785, Milwaukee, WI).

Daily gavage to induce dietary ketosis

Animal procedures were performed in accordance with the University of South Florida Institutional Animal

Care and Use Committee (IACUC) guidelines (Protocol #0006R). Juvenile male Sprague–Dawley rats (275–325 g, Harlan Laboratories) were randomly assigned to one of six study groups: control (water, $n = 11$), BD ($n = 11$), KE ($n = 11$), MCT ($n = 10$), BMS ($n = 11$), or BMS + MCT ($n = 12$). Caloric density of standard rodent chow and dose of ketone supplements are listed in Table 1. On days 1–14, rats received a 5 g/kg body weight dose of their respective treatments via intragastric gavage. Dosage was increased to 10 g/kg body weight for the second half of the study (days 15–28) for all groups except BD and KE to prevent excessive hyperketonemia (ketoacidosis). Each daily dose of BMS would equal ~1000–1500 mg of βHB, depending on the weight of the animal. Intragastric gavage was performed at the same time daily, and animals had *ad libitum* access to standard rodent chow 2018 (Harlan Teklad) for the duration of the study. The macronutrient ratio the standard rodent chow was 62.2, 23.8 and 14 % of carbohydrates, protein and fat respectively.

Measurement and analysis of blood glucose, ketones, and lipids

Every 7 days, animals were briefly fasted (4 h, water available) prior to intragastric gavage to standardize levels of blood metabolites prior to glucose and βHB measurements at baseline. Baseline (time 0) was immediately prior to gavage. Whole blood samples (10 μL) were taken from the saphenous vein for analysis of glucose and βHB levels with the commercially available glucose and ketone monitoring system Precision Xtra™ (Abbott Laboratories, Abbott Park, IL). Blood glucose and βHB were measured at 0, 0.5, 1, 4, 8, and 12 h after test substance administration, or until βHB returned to baseline levels. Food was returned to animals after blood analysis at time 0 and gavage. At baseline and week 4, whole blood samples (10 μL) were taken from the saphenous vein immediately prior to gavage (time 0) for analysis of total cholesterol, high-density lipoprotein (HDL), and triglycerides with the commercially available CardioChek™ blood lipid analyzer (Polymer Technology Systems, Inc., Indianapolis, IN). Low-density lipoprotein (LDL) cholesterol was calculated from the three measured lipid levels using the Friedewald equation: (LDL Cholesterol = Total Cholesterol - HDL - (Triglycerides/5)) [51, 52]. Animals were weighed once per week to track changes in body weight associated with hyperketonemia.

Organ weight and collection

On day 29, rats were sacrificed via deep isoflurane anesthesia, exsanguination by cardiac puncture, and decapitation 4–8 h after intragastric gavage, which correlated to the time range where the most significantly elevated blood βHB levels were observed. Brain, lungs, liver, kidneys, spleen and heart were harvested, weighed (AWS-1000 1 kg portable digital scale (AWS, Charleston, SC)), and flash-frozen in liquid nitrogen or preserved in 4 % paraformaldehyde for future analysis.

Statistics

All data are presented as the mean ± standard deviation (SD). Data analysis was performed using GraphPad PRISM™ version 6.0a and IBM SPSS Statistics 22.0. Results were considered significant when $p < 0.05$. Triglyceride and lipoprotein profile data were analyzed using One-Way ANOVA. Blood ketone and blood glucose were compared to control at the applicable time points using a Two-Way ANOVA. Correlation between blood βHB and glucose levels in ketone supplemented rats was compared to controls using ANCOVA analysis. Organ and body weights were analyzed using One-Way ANOVA. Basal blood ketone and blood glucose levels were analyzed using Two-Way ANOVA. All mean comparisons were carried out using Tukey's multiple comparisons post-hoc test.

Results

Effect of ketone supplementation on triglycerides and lipoproteins

Baseline measurements showed no significant changes in triglycerides or the lipoproteins (data not shown). Data represent triglyceride and lipoprotein concentrations measured after 4 weeks of daily exogenous ketone supplementation. No significant change in total cholesterol was observed at 4 weeks for any of the ketone treatment groups compared to control. (Fig. 1a). No

Table 1 Caloric density and dose of ketone supplements

Macronutrient Information	Standard Diet	Water	BMS + MCT	BMS	MCT	KE	BD
% Cal from Fat	18.0	0.0	50.0	N/A	100.0	N/A	N/A
% Cal from Protein	24.0	0.0	N/A	N/A	0.0	N/A	N/A
% Cal from Carbohydrates	58.0	0.0	N/A	N/A	0.0	N/A	N/A
Total Caloric Density (Kcal/g)	3.1	0.0	5.1	1.9	8.3	5.6	6.0
Dose 0–14 Days (g/kg)	*ad libitum*	N/A	5.0	5.0	5.0	5.0	5.0
Dose 15–28 Days (g/kg)	*ad libitum*	N/A	10.0	10.0	10.0	5.0	5.0

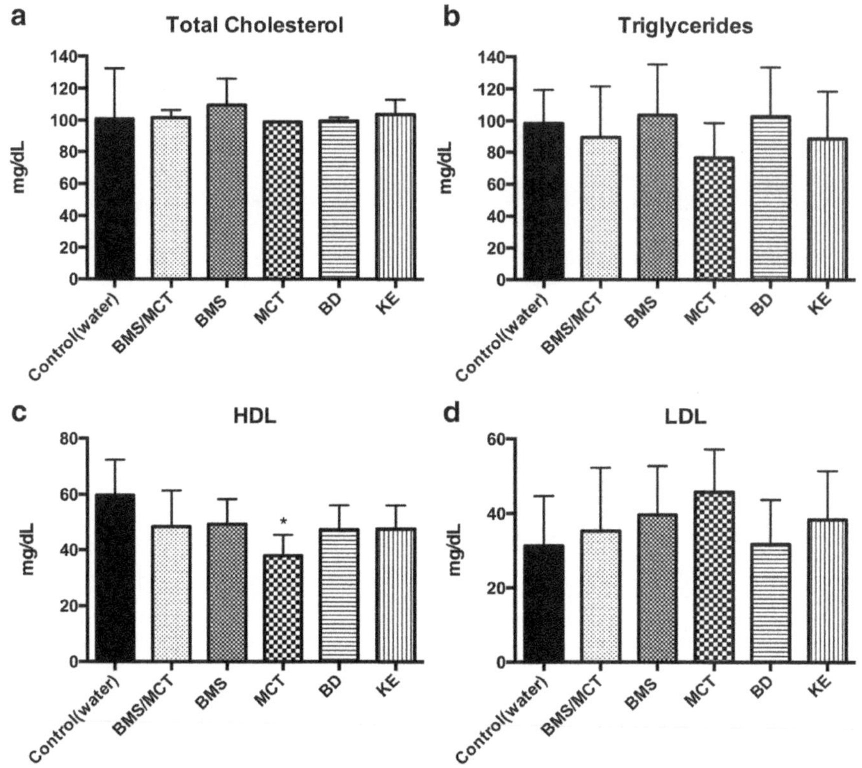

Fig. 1 Effects of ketone supplementation on triglycerides and lipoproteins: Ketone supplementation causes little change in triglycerides and lipoproteins over a 4-week study. Graphs show concentrations at 4-weeks of total cholesterol (**a**), Triglycerides (**b**), LDL (**c**), and HDL (**d**). MCT supplemented rats had signfiicantly reduced concentration of HDL blood levels compared to control ($p < 0.001$) (**b**). One-Way ANOVA with Tukey's post hoc test, results considered significant if $p < 0.05$. Error bars represent mean (SD)

significant difference was detected in triglycerides for any ketone supplement compared to control (Fig. 1b). MCT supplemented animals had a significant reduction in HDL blood levels compared to control (p < 0.001) (Fig. 1c). LDL levels in ketone-supplemented animals did not significantly differ from controls (Fig. 1d).

Ketone supplementation causes rapid and sustained elevation of βHB

Over the 28-day experiment, ketone supplements administered daily significantly elevated blood ketone levels without dietary restriction (Fig. 2a, b). Naturally derived ketogenic supplements including MCT (5 g/kg) elicited a significant rapid elevation in blood βHB within 30–60 min that was sustained for 8 h. BMS + MCT (5 g/kg) elicited a significant elevation in blood βHB at 4 h, which was no longer significant at 8 h. BMS (5 g/kg) did not elicit a significant elevation in blood βHB at any time point. For days 14–28, BMS + MCT (10 g/kg) and MCT (10 g/kg) elevated blood βHB levels within 30 min and remained significantly elevated for up to 12 h. We observed a delay in the peak elevation of blood βHB: BMS + MCT peaked at 8 h instead of at 4 h and MCT at 4 h instead of at 1 h. Blood βHB levels in the BMS group did not show significant elevation at any time point, even after dose escalation (Fig. 2a). Synthetically derived ketogenic supplements including KE and BD supplementation rapidly elevated blood βHB within 30 min and was sustained for 8 h. For the rats receiving ketone supplementation in the form of BD or the KE, dosage was kept at 5 g/kg to prevent adverse effects associated with hyperketonemia. The Precision Xtra™ ketone monitoring system measures βHB only; therefore, total blood ketone levels (βHB + AcAc) would be higher than measured. For each of these groups, the blood βHB profile remained consistent following daily ketone supplementation administration over the 4-week duration. (Fig. 2b).

Ketone supplementation causes a significant decrease of blood glucose

Administration of ketone supplementation significantly reduced blood glucose over the course of the study (Fig. 3a, b). MCT (5 g/kg) decreased blood glucose compared to control within 30 min which was sustained for

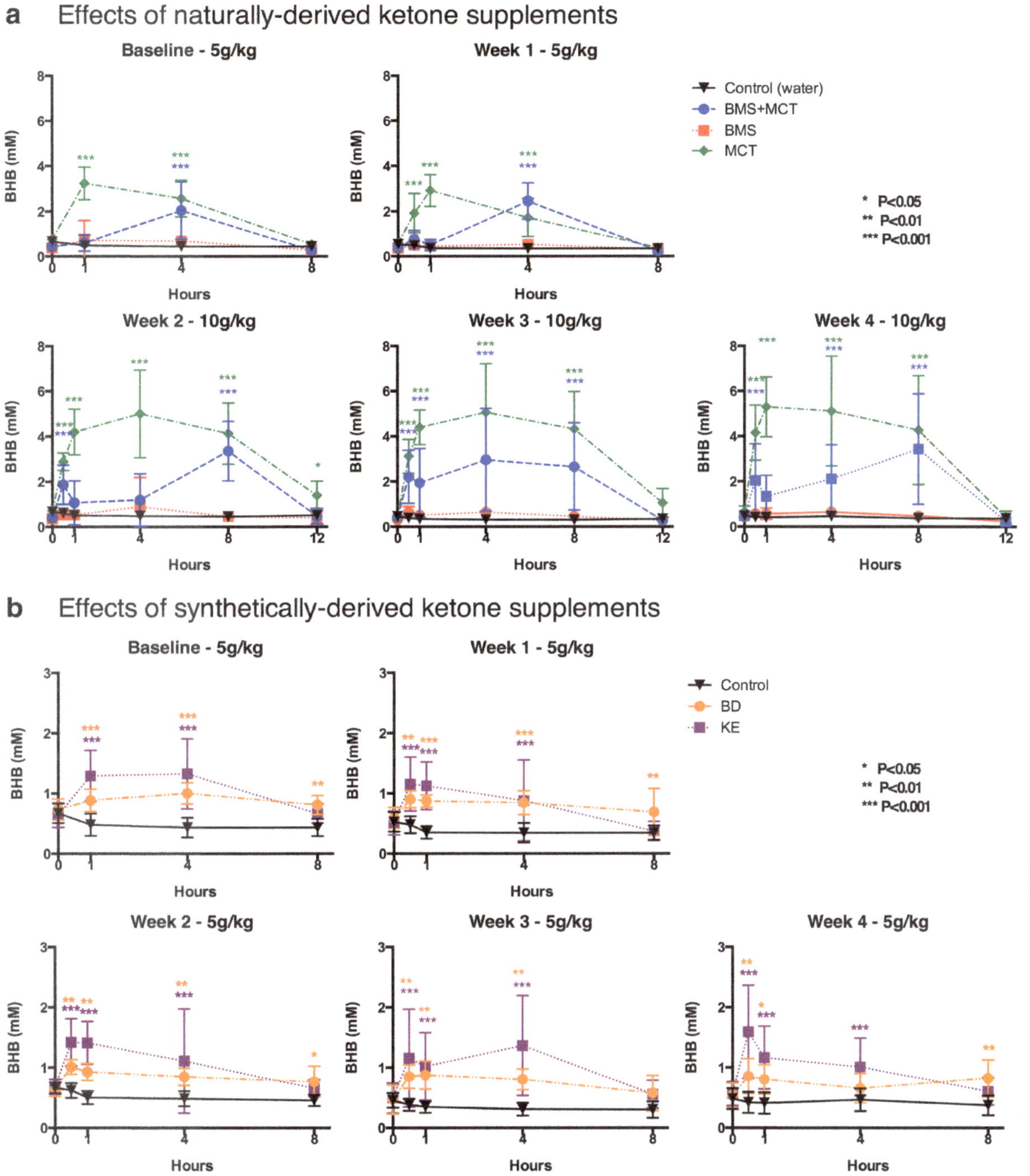

Fig. 2 Effects of ketone supplementation on blood βHB. **a**, **b** Blood βHB levels at times 0, 0.5, 1, 4, 8, and 12 h post intragastric gavage for ketone supplements tested. **a** BMS + MCT and MCT supplementation rapidly elevated and sustained significant βHB elevation compared to controls for the duration of the 4-week dose escalation study. BMS did not significantly elevate βHB at any time point tested compared to controls. **b** BD and KE supplements, maintained at 5 g/kg, significantly elevated βHB levels for the duration of the 4-week study. Two-Way ANOVA with Tukey's post hoc test, results considered significant if $p < 0.05$. Error bars represent mean (SD)

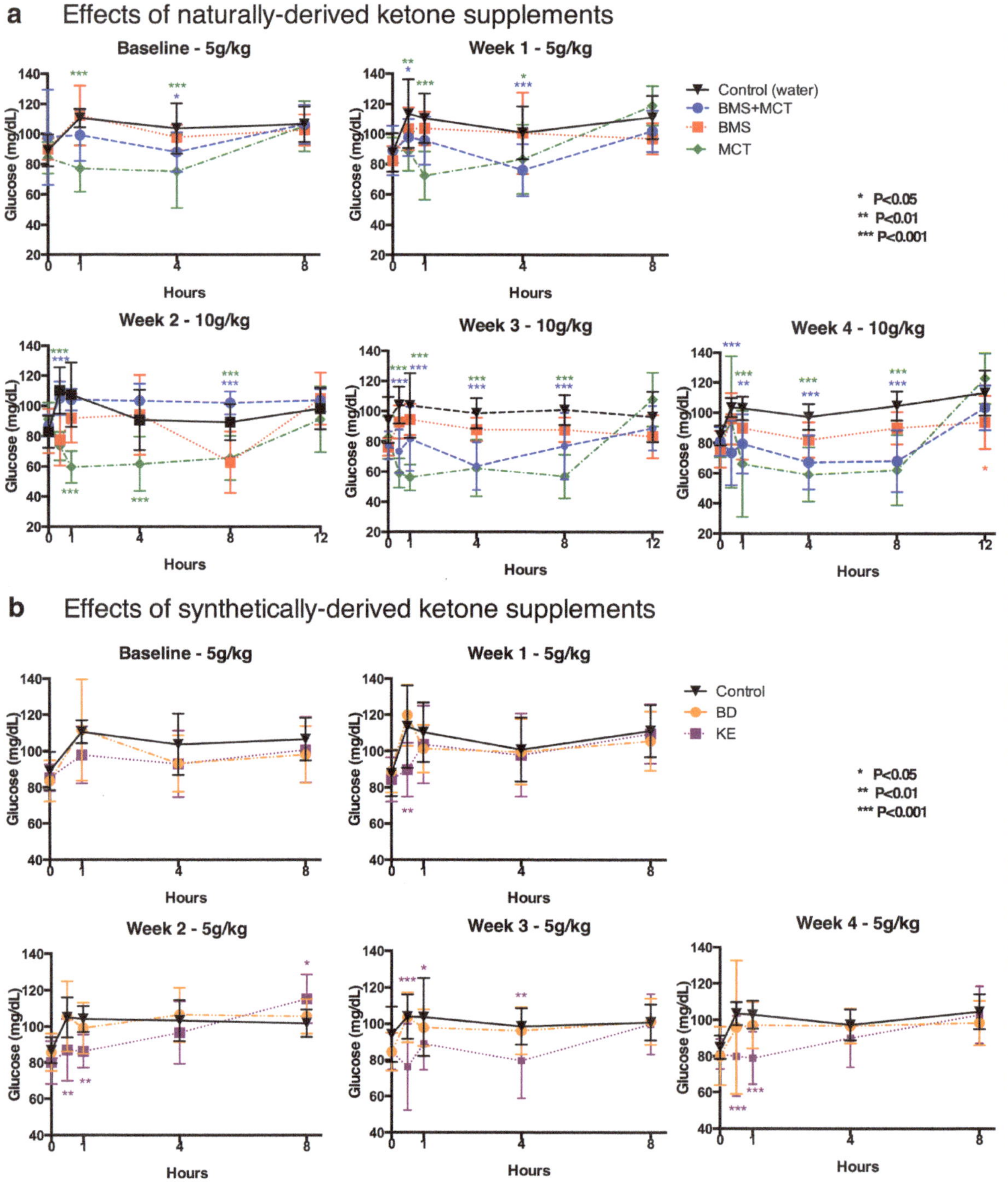

Fig. 3 Effects of ketone supplementation on blood glucose. **a**, **b** Blood glucose levels at times 0, 0.5, 1, 4, 8, and 12 h (for 10 dose) post intragastric gavage for ketone supplements tested. **a** Ketone supplements BMS + MCT and MCT significantly reduced blood glucose levels compared to controls for the duration of the 4-week study. BMS significantly lowered blood glucose only at 8 h/week 1 and 12 h/week 3 (**b**) KE, maintained at 5 g/kg, significantly reduced blood glucose compared to controls from week 1–4. BD did not significantly affect blood glucose levels at any time point during the 4-week study. Two-Way ANOVA with Tukey's post hoc test, results considered significant if $p < 0.05$. Error bars represent mean (SD)

8 h at baseline and at week 1. MCT (10 g/kg) likewise decreased blood glucose within 30 min and lasted through the 12 h time point during weeks 2, 3, and 4. BMS + MCT (5 g/kg) lowered blood glucose compared to control from hours 1–8 only at week 1. BMS + MCT (10 g/kg) lowered blood glucose compared to control within 30 min and remained low through the 12 h time point at weeks 2, 3, and 4. Rats supplemented with BMS had lower blood glucose compared to control at 12 h in week 4 (10) (Fig. 3a). Administration of BD did not significantly change blood glucose levels at any time point during the 4-week study. KE (5 g/kg) significantly lowered blood glucose levels at 30 min for week 1, 2, 3, and 4 and was sustained through 1 h at weeks 2–4 and sustained to 4 h at week 3. (Fig. 3b).

Hyperketonemia suppresses blood glucose levels

At baseline, 4 h after intragastric gavage, the elevation of blood ketones was inversely related to the reduction of blood glucose compared to controls following the administration of MCT (5 g/kg) (p = 0.008) and BMS + MCT (5 g/kg) (p = 0.039) . There was no significant correlation between blood ketone levels and blood glucose levels compared to controls for any other ketone supplemented group at baseline (Fig. 4a). At week 4, 4 h after intragastric gavage, there was a significant correlation between blood ketone levels and

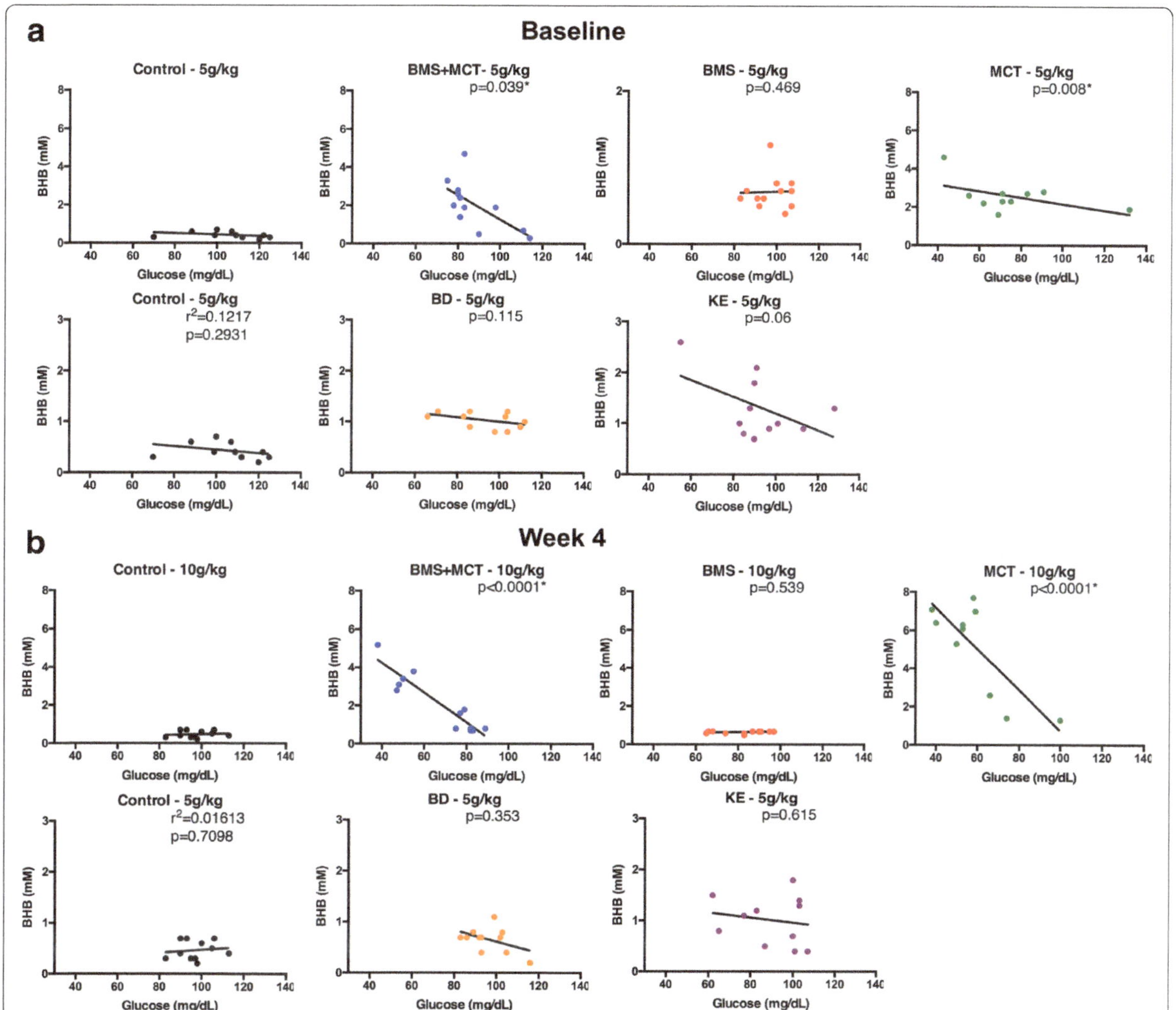

Fig. 4 Relationship between blood ketone and glucose levels: **a** BMS + MCT (5 g/kg) supplemented rats demonstrated a significant inverse relationship between elevated blood ketone levels and decreased blood ketone levels ($r^2 = 0.4314$, p = 0.0203). **b** At week 4, BMS + MCT (10 g/kg) and MCT (10 g/kg) showed a significant correlation between blood ketone levels and blood glucose levels (r2 = 0.8619, $p < 0.0001$; $r^2 = 0.6365$, p = 0.0057). Linear regression analysis, results considered significant if $p < 0.05$

blood glucose levels compared to controls in MCT (10 g/kg) and BMS + MCT (10 g/kg) ($p < 0.0001$, $p < 0.0001$) (Fig. 4b).

Ketone supplementation changes organ weight and decreases body weight

At day 29 of the study, animals were euthanized and brain, lungs, liver, kidneys, spleen and heart were harvested and weighed. Organ weights were normalized to body weight. Ketone supplementation did not significantly change brain, lung, kidney, or heart weights compared to controls (Fig. 5a, b, d, f). MCT supplemented animals had significantly larger livers compared to their body weight ($p < 0.05$) (Fig. 5c). Ketone supplements BMS + MCT, MCT and BD caused a significant reduction in spleen size (BMS + MCT $p < 0.05$, MCT $p < 0.001$, BD $p < 0.05$) (Fig. 5e). Rats administered KE gained significantly less weight over the entire study compared to controls. BMS + MCT, BMS, and BD supplemented rats gained significantly less weight than controls during weeks 2 – 4, and MCT animals gained less

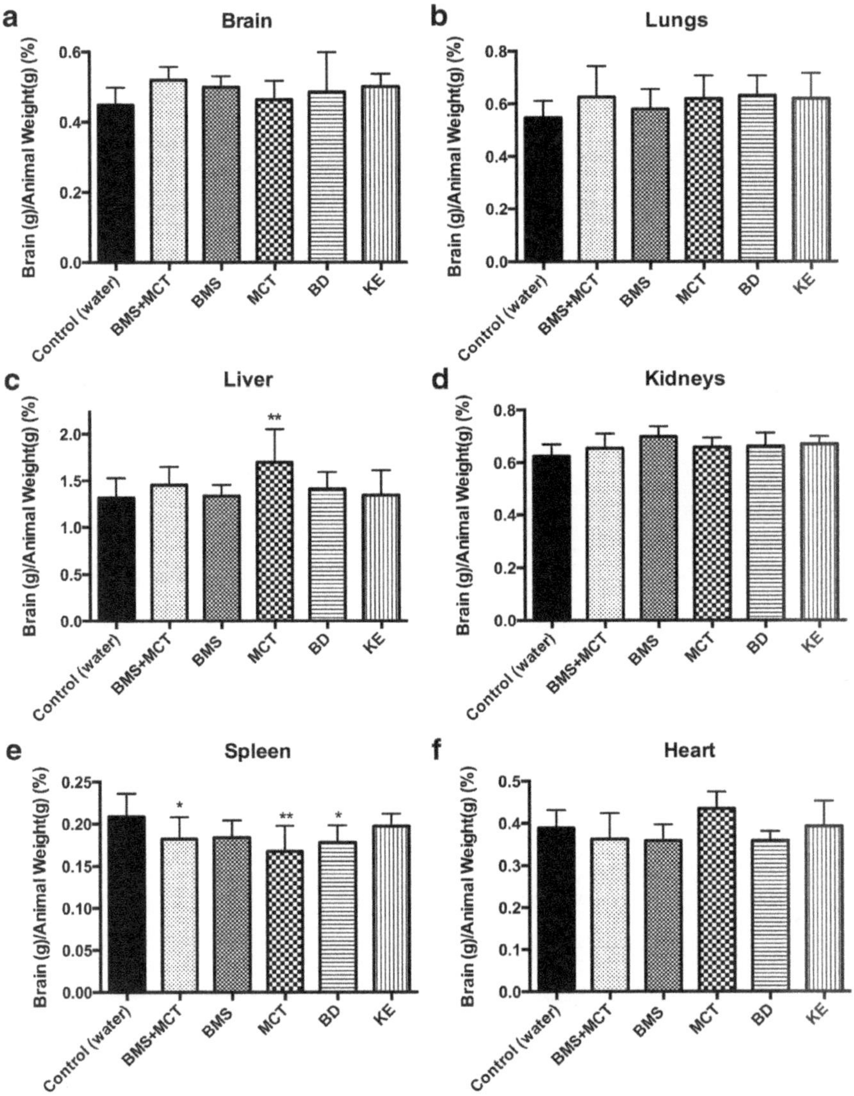

Fig. 5 Effects of ketone supplementation on organ weight: Data is represented as a percentage of organ weight to body weight. **a**, **b**, **d**, **f** Ketone supplements did not significantly affect the weight of the brain, lungs, kidneys or heart. **c** Liver weight was significantly increased as compared to body weight in response to administered MCT ketone supplement compared to control at the end of the study (day 29) ($p < 0.001$). **e** Rats supplemented with BMS + MCT, MCT, and BD had significantly smaller spleen percentage as compared to controls ($p < 0.05$, $p < 0.001$, $p < 0.05$). Two-Way ANOVA with Tukey's post-hoc test; results considered significant if $p < 0.05$. Error bars represent mean (SD)

weight than controls at weeks 3 – 4 (Fig. 6). Increased gastric motility (increased bowel evacuation and changes to fecal consistency) was visually observed in rats supplemented with 10 g/kg MCT, most notably at the 8 and 12-h time points. All animals remained in healthy weight range for their age even though the rate of weight gain changed with ketone supplementation [53–54]. Food intake was not measured in this study. However, there was not a significant change in basal blood glucose or basal blood ketone levels over the 4 week study in any of the rats supplemented with ketones (Fig. 7).

Discussion

Nutritional ketosis induced with the KD has proven effective for the metabolic management of seizures and potentially other disorders [1–26]. Here we present evidence that chronic administration of ketone supplements can induce a state of nutritional ketosis without the need for dietary carbohydrate restriction and with little or no effect on lipid biomarkers. The notion that we can produce the therapeutic effects of the KD with exogenous ketone supplementation is supported by our previous study which demonstrated that acutely administered KE supplementation delays central nervous system (CNS) oxygen toxicity seizures without the need for dietary restriction [29]. We propose that exogenous ketone supplementation could provide an alternative method of attaining the therapeutic benefits of nutritional ketosis, and as a means to further augment the therapeutic potential of the KD.

Ketone supplementation causes little to no change in triglycerides and lipoproteins

One common concern regarding the KD is its purported potential to increase the risk of atherosclerosis by elevating blood cholesterol and triglyceride levels [55, 56]. This topic remains controversial as some, but not all, studies have demonstrated that the KD elevates blood levels of cholesterol and triglycerides [57–62]. Kwitervich and colleagues demonstrated an increase in low-density lipoprotein (LDL) and a decrease in high-density lipoprotein (HDL) in epileptic children fed the classical KD for two years [27]. In this study, total cholesterol increased by ~130 %, and stabilized at the elevated level over the 2-year period. A similar study demonstrated that the lipid profile returned to baseline in children who remained on the KD for six years [63]. Children typically remain on the diet for approximately two years then return to a diet of common fat and carbohydrate ingestion [64]. The implications of these findings are unclear, since the influence of cholesterol on cardiovascular health is controversial and macronutrient sources of the diet vary per study. In contrast to these studies, the majority of recent studies have suggested that the KD can actually lead to significant benefits in biomarkers of metabolic health, including blood lipid profiles [65–72]. In these studies, the

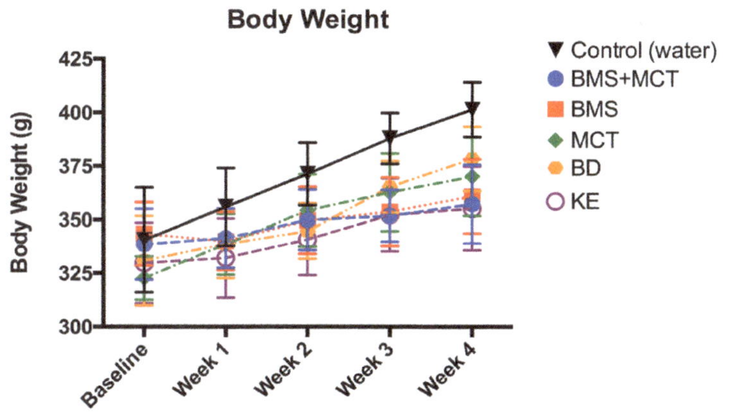

	Baseline	Week 1	Week 2	Week 3	Week 4
BMS+MCT	NS	NS	**	***	***
BMS	NS	NS	**	***	***
MCT	NS	NS	NS	**	***
BD	NS	NS	***	**	**
KE	NS	**	***	***	***

Fig. 6 Effects of ketone supplementation on body weight: Rats administered ketone supplements gained less weight over the 4-week period; however, did not lose weight and maintained healthy range for age. KE supplemented rats gained significantly less weight during the entire 4-week study compared to controls. BMS + MCT, BMS, and BD supplemented rats gained significantly less weight than controls over weeks 2–4.MCT supplemented rats gained significantly less weight than controls over weeks 3–4, Two-Way ANOVA with Tukey's post hoc test, results considered significant if $p < 0.05$. Error bars represent mean (SD)

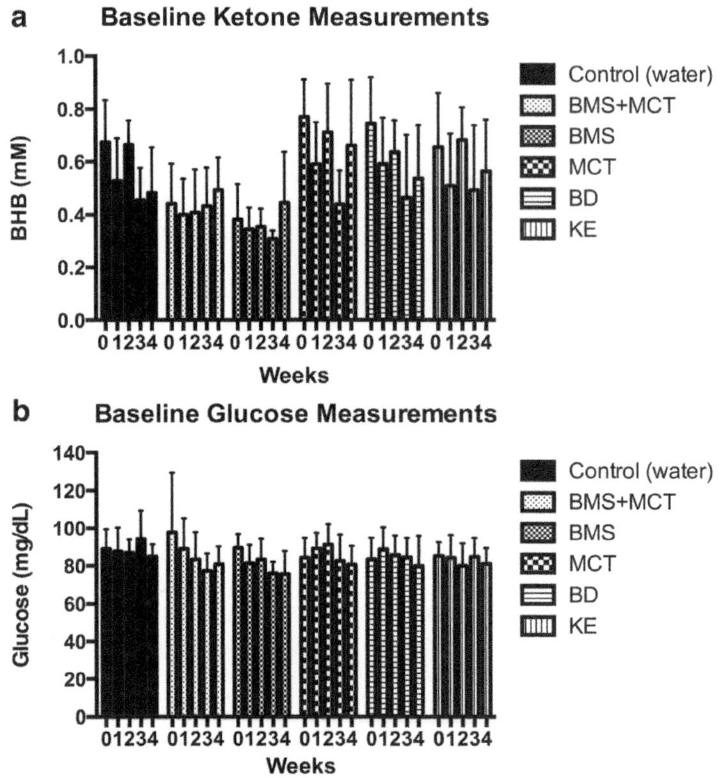

Fig. 7 Effects of ketone supplementation on basal blood ketone and basal blood glucose levels: Rats administered ketone supplements did not have a significant change in basal blood ketone levels (**a**) or basal blood glucose levels (**b**) for the four week study. Two-Way ANOVA with Tukey's post-hoc test, results considered significant if $p < 0.05$. Error bars represent mean (SD)

KD positively altered blood lipids, decreasing total triglycerides and cholesterol while increasing the ratio of HDL to LDL [68–77]. Although, the KD is well-established in children, it has only recently been utilized as a strategy to control seizures in adults. In 2014, Schoeler and colleagues reported on the feasibility of the KD for adults, concluding that 39 % of individuals achieved > 50 % reduction in seizure frequency, similar to the results reported in pediatric studies. Patients experienced similar gastrointestinal adverse advents that have been previously described in pediatric patients, but they did not lead to discontinuation of the diet in any patient [78].

With oral ketone supplementation, we observed a significant elevation in blood βHB without dietary restriction and with little change in lipid biomarkers (Fig. 1). Over the 4 week study, MCT-supplemented rats demonstrated decreased HDL compared to controls. No significant changes were observed in any of the triglycerides or lipoproteins (HDL, LDL) with any of the remaining exogenously applied ketone supplements. It should be noted that the rats used for this study had not yet reached full adult body size [79]. Their normal growth rate and maturation was likely responsible for the changes in triglyceride and lipoprotein levels observed in the control animals over the 4 week study (baseline data not shown, no significant differences) [80, 81]. Future studies are needed to investigate the effect of ketone supplementation on fully mature and aged animals. Overall, our study suggests that oral ketone supplementation has little effect on the triglyceride or lipoprotein profile after 4 weeks. However, it is currently unknown if ketone supplementation would affect lipid biomarkers after a longer duration of consumption. Further studies are needed to determine the effects of ketone supplements on blood triglyceride and lipoproteins after chronic administration and as a means to further enhance the hyperketonemia and improve the lipid profile of the clinically implemented (4:1) KD.

LDL is the lipoprotein particle that is most often associated with atherosclerosis. LDL particles exist in different sizes: large molecules (Pattern A) or small molecules (Pattern B). Recent studies have investigated the importance of LDL-particle type and size rather than total concentration as being the source for cardiovascular risk [56]. Patients whose LDL particles are predominantly small and dense (Pattern B) have a greater risk of cardiovascular disease (CVD). It is thought that small, dense LDL particles are more able to penetrate the endothelium and cause in damage and inflammation [82–85]. Volek et al. reported that the KD increased the pattern and volume of LDL particles, which is considered to reduce cardiovascular risk [73]. Though we did not show a significant effect on LDL levels for ketone supplements, future chronic feeding studies will investigate the effects of ketone supplementation on lipidomic profile and LDL particle type and size.

Therapeutic levels of hyperketonemia suppress blood glucose levels

We demonstrated that therapeutic ketosis could be induced without dietary (calorie or carbohydrate) restriction and that this acute elevation in blood ketones was significantly correlated with a reduction in blood glucose (Figs. 2, 3 and 4). The BMS ketone supplement did not significantly induce blood hyperketonemia or reduced glucose in the rats. The KE supplemented rats trended towards reduced glucose levels; however, the lower dose of this agent did not lower glucose significantly, as reported previously in acute response of mice [59]. MCTs have previously been shown to elicit a slight hypoglycemic effect by enhancing glucose utilization in both diabetic and non-diabetic patients [86–88]. Kashiwaya et al. demonstrated that both blood glucose and blood insulin decreased by approximately 50 % in rats fed a diet where 30 % of calories from starch were replaced with ketone esters for 14 days, suggesting that ketone supplementation increases insulin sensitivity or reduced hepatic glucose output [89]. This ketone-induced hypoglycemic effect has been previously reported in humans with IV infusions of ketone bodies [90, 91]. Recently, Mikkelsen et al. showed that a small increase in βHB concentration decreases glucose production by 14 % in post-absorptive health males [92]. However, this has not been previously reported with any of the oral exogenous ketone supplements we studied. Ketones are an efficient and sufficient energy substrate for the brain, and will therefore prevent side effects of hypoglycemia when blood levels are elevated and the patient is keto-adapted. This was most famously demonstrated by Owen et al. in 1967 wherein keto-adapted patients (starvation induced therapeutic ketosis) were given 20 IU of insulin. The blood glucose of fasted patients dropped to 1–2 mM, but they exhibited no hypoglycemic symptoms due to brain utilization of ketones for energy [93]. Therefore, ketones maintain brain metabolism and are neuroprotective during severe hypoglycemia. The rats in the MCT group had a correlation of blood ketone and glucose levels at week 4, whereas the combination of BMS + MCT produced a significant hypoglycemic correlation both at baseline and at week 4. No hypoglycemic symptoms were observed in the rats during this study. Insulin levels were not measured in this study; however, future ketone supplementation studies should measure the effects of exogenous ketones on insulin sensitivity with a glucose tolerance test. An increase in insulin sensitivity in combination with our observed hypoglycemic effect has potential therapy implications for glycemic control in T2D [40]. Furthermore, it should be noted that the KE metabolizes to both AcAc and βHB in 1:1 ratio [29]. The ketone monitor used in this study only measures βHB as levels of AcAc are more difficult to measure due to spontaneous decarboxylation to acetone; therefore, the total ketone levels (βHB + AcAc) measured were likely higher, specifically for the KE [14]. Interestingly, the 10 g/kg dose produced a delayed blood βHB peak for ketone supplements MCT and BMS + MCT. The higher dose of the ketogenic supplements elevated blood levels more substantially, and thus reached their maximum blood concentration later due to prolonged metabolic clearance. It must be noted that the dosage used in this study does not translate to human patients, since the metabolic physiology of rats is considerably higher. Future studies will be needed to determine optimal dosing for human patients.

Effects of ketone supplementation on organ weight and body weight percentage

Ketone supplementation did not affect the size of the brain, lungs, kidneys or heart of rats. As previously mentioned, the rats were still growing during the experimental time frame; therefore, organ weights were normalized to body weight to determine if organ weight changed independently to growth. There could be several reasons why ketones influenced liver and spleen weight. The ratio of liver to body weight was significantly higher in the MCT supplemented animals (Fig. 5). MCTs are readily absorbed in the intestinal lumen and transported directly to the liver via hepatic portal circulation. When given a large bolus, such as in this study, the amount of MCTs in the liver will likely exceed the β-oxidation rate, causing the MCTs to be deposited in the liver as fat droplets [94]. The accumulated MCT droplets in the liver could explain the higher liver weight to body weight percentage observed with MCT supplemented rats. Future toxicology and histological studies will be needed to determine the cause of the observed hepatomegaly. It should be emphasized that the dose in this study is not optimized in humans. We speculate that an optimized human dose would be lower and may not cause hepatomegaly or potential fat accumulation. Nutritional ketosis achieved with the KD has been shown to decrease inflammatory markers such as TNF-α, IL-6, IL-8, MCP-1, E-selectin, I-CAM, and PAI-1 [8, 46], which may account for the observed decrease in spleen weight. As previously mentioned, Veech and colleagues demonstrated that exogenous supplementation of 5 mM βHB resulted in a 28 % increase in hydraulic work in the working perfused rat heart and a significant decrease in oxygen consumption [28, 41, 42]. Ketone bodies have been shown to increase cerebral blood flow and perfusion [95]. Also, ketone bodies have been shown to increase ATP synthesis and enhance the efficiency of ATP production [14, 28, 40]. It is possible that sustained ketosis results in enhanced cardiac efficiency and O_2 consumption. Even though the size of the heart did not change for any of the ketone supplements, further analysis of tissues harvested from the ketone-supplemented rats will be needed to determine any morphological changes and to understand changes in organ size. It should be noted that the Harlan standard rodent chow 2018 is nutritionally complete and formulated with high-quality ingredients to optimize gestation, lactation, growth, and overall health of the animals. The same cannot be said for the standard American diet (SAD). Therefore, we plan to investigate the effects of ketone supplements administered with the SAD to determine if similar effects will be seen when the micronutrient deficiencies and macronutrient profile mimics what most Americans consume.

MCT oil has recently been used to induce nutritional ketosis although it produces dose-dependent gastrointestinal (GI) side effects in humans that limit the potential for its use to significantly elevate ketones (>0.5 mM). Despite these limitations, Azzam and colleagues published a case report in which a 43-year-old-man had a significant decrease in seizure frequency after supplementing his diet with 4 tablespoons of MCT oil twice daily [96]. An attempt to increase his dosage to 5 tablespoons twice daily was halted by severe GI intolerance. Henderson et al. observed that 20 % of patients reported GI side effects with a 20 g dose of ketogenic agent AC-1202 in a double blind trial in mild to moderate Alzheimer's patients [24]. We visually observed similar gastrointestinal side effects (loose stools) in the rats treated with MCT oil in our study. Rats were closely monitored to avoid dehydration, and gastric motility returned to normal between 12–24 h. Interestingly, the BMS + MCT supplement elevated βHB similarly to MCT oil alone, without causing the adverse gastrointestinal effects seen in MCT-supplemented rats. However, this could be due to the fact in a 10 g/kg dose of BMS + MCT, only 5 g/kg is MCT alone, which is less than the 10 g/kg dose that elicits the GI side effects. This suggests that this novel combination may provide a more useful therapeutic option than MCT oil alone, which is limited in its ability to elevate ketones in humans.

Exogenously delivered ketone supplements significantly altered rat weight gain for the duration of the study (Fig. 6). However, rats did not lose weight and maintained a healthy range for their age. Rats have been shown to effectively balance their caloric intake to prevent weight loss/gain [97–99]. Due to the caloric density of the exogenous ketone supplements (Table 1) it is possible for the rats to eat less of the standard rodent chow and therefore less carbohydrates while maintaining their caloric intake. Food intake was not measured for this study. However, if there was a significant carbohydrate restriction there would be a signifcant change in basal blood ketone and blood glucose levels. As the hallmark to the KD, carbohydrate restriction increases blood ketone levels and reduces blood glucose levels. Neither an increase in basal blood ketone levels nor a decrease in basal blood glucose levels was observed in this study (Fig. 7). Additionally, if there were an overall blood glucose decrease due to a change in food intake, this would not explain the rapid reduction (within 30 min) in blood glucose correlated with an elevation of blood ketone levels after an intragastric bolus of ketone supplement (Figs. 2, 3 and 4).

Conclusions

Several studies have investigated the safety and efficacy of ketone supplements for disease states such as AD and Parkinson's disease, and well as for parenteral nutrition [40, 48–50, 100–103]. Our research demonstrates that several forms of dietary ketone supplementation can effectively elevate blood ketone levels and achieve deleted: therapeutic nutritional ketosis without the need for dietary carbohydrate restriction. We also demonstrated that ketosis achieved with exogenous ketone supplementation can reduce blood glucose, and this is inversely associated with the blood ketone levels. Although preliminary results are encouraging, further studies are needed to determine if oral ketone supplementation can produce the same therapeutic benefits as the classic KD in the broad-spectrum of KD-responsive disease states . Additionally, further experiments need to be conducted to see if the exogenous ketone supplementation affects the same physiological features as the KD (i.e. ROS, inflammation, ATP production). Ketone supplementation could be used as an alternative method for inducing ketosis in patients uninterested in attempting the KD or those who have previously had difficulty implementing the KD because of palatability issues, gall bladder removal, liver abnormalities, or intolerance to fat. Additional experiments should be conducted to see if ketone supplementation could be used in conjunction with the KD to assist and ease the transition to nutrition ketosis and enhance the speed of keto-adaptation. In this study we have demonstrated the ability of several ketone supplements to elevate blood ketone levels, providing multiple options to induce therapeutic ketosis based on patient need. Though additional studies are needed to determine the therapeutic potential of ketone supplementation, many patients that previously were unable to benefit from the KD may now have an alternate method of achieving therapeutic ketosis. Ketone supplementation may also represent a means to further augment ketonemia in those responsive to therapeutic ketosis, especially in those individuals where maintaining low glucose is important.

Abbreviations

AcAc: acetoacetate; ALS: amyotrophic lateral sclerosis; AD: Alzheimer's; βHB: beta-hydroxybutyrate; BMS: sodium/potassium βHB mineral salt; BMS + MCT: BMS + MCT 1:1 mixture; BD: 1,3-butanediol; CNS: central nervous system; HDL: high density lipoprotein; HDACs: histone deacetylases; LDL: low density lipoprotein; KD: ketogenic diet; KE: 1, 3-butanediol acetoacetate diester/ketone ester; MCT: medium chain triglyceride oil; PCOS: polycystic ovary syndrome; ROS: reactive oxygen species; SAD: standard American diet; TBI: traumatic brain injury; T2D: type-2 diabetes.

Competing interests

International Patent # PCT/US2014/031237, University of South Florida, D.P. D'Agostino, S. Kesl, P. Arnold, *"Compositions and Methods for Producing Elevated and Sustained Ketosis"*. P. Arnold (Savind) has received financial support (ONR N000140610105 and N000140910244) from D.P. D'Agostino (USF) to synthesize ketone esters. The remaining authors have no conflicts of interest.

Authors' contributions

Conceived and designed the experiments: SK, AP, NW, TF, DP. Performed the experiments: SK, AP, NW, TF, CA, JS, AVP. Analyzed the data: SK, AP, DP. Contributed reagents/materials/analysis tools: PA. Helped draft the manuscript: SK, AP, NW, CA, DP. All authors read and approved the final manuscript.

Acknowledgements

The authors would like to thank Savind Inc for manufacturing some of the ketone supplements, Jay Dean for the use of his Hyperbaric Research Laboratory, and the ONR and Scivation Inc. for funding the project.

Grants

This study was supported by the Office of Naval Research (ONR) Grant N000140610105 (DPD); and a Morsani College of Medicine Department of Molecular Pharmacology and Physiology departmental grant.

Author details

[1]Department of Molecular Pharmacology and Physiology, Morsani College of Medicine, University of South Florida, 12901 Bruce B. Downs Blvd. MDC8, Tampa, FL 33612, USA. [2]Savind Inc, 205 South Main Street, Seymore, IL 61875, USA.

References

1. Sirven J, Whedon B, Caplan D, Liporace J, Glosser D, O'Dwyer J, et al. The ketogenic diet for intractable epilepsy in adults: preliminary results. Epilepsia. 1999;40(12):1721–6. doi:10.1111/j.1528-1157.1999.tb01589.x.
2. Wilder R. The effect of ketonemia on the course of epilepsy. Mayo Clin Bulletin. 1921;2:307–8.
3. Thiele E. Assessing the efficacy of antiepileptic treatments: the ketogenic diet. Epilepsia. 2003;44 Suppl 7:26–9. doi:10.1046/j.1528-1157.44.s7.4.x.
4. Paoli A, Rubini A, Volek JS, Grimaldi KA. Beyond weight loss: a review of the therapeutic uses of very-low-carbohydrate (ketogenic) diets. Eur J Clin Nutr. 2013;67(8):789–96. doi:10.1038/ejcn.2013.116.
5. Foster GD, Wyatt HR, Hill JO, McGuckin BG, Brill C, Mohemmed BS, et al. A randomized trial of a low-carbohydrate diet for obesity. N Engl J Med. 2003; 348:2082–90.
6. Westman EC, Feinman RD, Mavropoulos JC, Vernon MC, Volek JS, Wortman JA, et al. Low-carbohydrate nutrition and metabolism. Am J Clin Nutr. 2007; 86:276–84.
7. Westman EC, Yancy WS, Edman JS, Tomlin KF, Perkins CE. Effect of 6-month adherence to a very low carbohydrate diet program. Am J Med. 2002; 113(1):30–6.
8. Forsythe C, Phinney S, Fernandez M, Quann E, Wood R, Bibus D, et al. Comparison of low fat and low carbohydrate diets on circulating fatty acid composition and markers of inflammation. Lipids. 2008;43(1):65–77. doi:10.1007/s11745-007-3132-7.
9. Boden G, Sargrad K, Homko C, Mozzoli M, Stein T. Effect of a low-carbohydrate diet on appetite, blood glucose levels, and insulin resistance in obese patients with type 2 diabetes. Ann Intern Med. 2005;142(6):403–11.
10. Gumbiner B, Wendel J, McDermott M. Effects of diet composition and ketosis on glycemia during very-low-energy-diet therapy in obese patients with non-insulin-dependent diabetes mellitus. Am J Clin Nutr. 1996;63(1):110–5.
11. Nielsen J, Joensson E. Low-carbohydrate diet in type 2 diabetes: stable improvement of bodyweight and glycemic control during 44 months follow-up. Nutr Metab. 2008;5:14. doi:10.1186/1743-7075-5-14.
12. Yancy W, Foy M, Chalecki A, Vernon M, Westman E. A low-carbohydrate, ketogenic diet to treat type 2 diabetes. Nutr Metab. 2005;2:34. doi:10.1186/1743-7075-2-34.
13. Dashti HM, Al-Zaid NS, Mathew TC, Al-Mousawi M, Talib H, Asfar SK, et al. Long term effects of ketogenic diet in obese subjects with high cholesterol level. Mol Cell Biochem. 2006;286(1–2):1–9. doi:10.1007/s11010-005-9001-x.
14. Maalouf M, Rho JM, Mattson MP. The neuroprotective properties of calorie restriction, the ketogenic diet, and ketone bodies. Brain Res Rev. 2009;59(2): 293–315. doi:10.1016/j.brainresrev.2008.09.002.
15. Mavropoulos JC, Yancy WS, Hepburn J, Westman EC. The effects of a low-carbohydrate, ketogenic diet on the polycystic ovary syndrome: a pilot study. Nutr Metab. 2004;2:35. doi:10.1186/1743-7075-2-35.
16. Seyfried T, Flores R, Poff A, D'Agostino D. Cancer as a metabolic disease: implications for novel therapeutics. Carcinogenesis. 2014;35:515–27. doi:10.1093/carcin/bgt480.
17. Poff AM, Ari C, Arnold P, Seyfried TN, D'Agostino DP. Ketone supplementation decreases tumor cell viability and prolongs survival of mice with metastatic cancer. Int J Cancer. 2014;135:1711–20. doi:10.1002/ijc.28809.
18. Poff A, Ari C, Seyfried T, D'Agostino D. The ketogenic diet and hyperbaric oxygen therapy prolong survival in mice with systemic metastatic cancer. PLoS ONE. 2013;8(6), e65522. doi:10.1371/journal.pone.0065522.
19. Seyfried T, Shelton L. Cancer as a metabolic disease. Nutr Metab. 2010;7:7. doi:10.1186/1743-7075-7-7.
20. Fine E, Segal-Isaacson C, Feinman R, Herszkopf S, Romano M, Tomuta N, et al. Targeting insulin inhibition as a metabolic therapy in advanced cancer: a pilot safety and feasibility dietary trial in 10 patients. Nutrition. 2012;28(10):1028–35. doi:10.1016/j.nut.2012.05.001.
21. Zhao Z, Lange D, Voustianiouk A, MacGrogan D, Ho L, Suh J, et al. A ketogenic diet as a potential novel therapeutic intervention in amyotrophic lateral sclerosis. BMC Neurosci. 2006;7:29. doi:10.1186/1471-2202-7-29.
22. White H, Venkatesh B. Clinical review: ketones and brain injury. Crit Care. 2011;15(2):219. doi:10.1186/cc10020.
23. Prins M. Cerebral metabolic adaptation and ketone metabolism after brain injury. J Cereb Blood Flow Metab. 2008;28(1):1–16. doi:10.1038/sj.jcbfm.9600543.
24. Henderson S, Vogel J, Barr L, Garvin F, Jones J, Costantini L. Study of the ketogenic agent AC-1202 in mild to moderate Alzheimer's disease: a randomized, double-blind, placebo-controlled, multicenter trial. Nutr Metab. 2009;6:31. doi:10.1186/1743-7075-6-31.
25. Brownlow M, Benner L, D'Agostino D, Gordon M, Morgan D. Ketogenic diet improves motor performance but not cognition in two mouse models of Alzheimer's pathology. PLoS ONE. 2013;8(9), e75713. doi:10.1371/journal.pone.0075713.g008.
26. Kossoff EH, Hartman AL. Ketogenic diets: new advances for metabolism-based therapies. Curr Opin Neurol. 2012;25:173–8. doi:10.1097/WCO.0b013e3283515e4a.
27. Kwiterovich P, Vining E, Pyzik P, Skolasky R, Freeman J. Effect of a high-fat ketogenic diet on plasma levels of lipids, lipoproteins, and apolipoproteins in children. JAMA. 2003;290(7):912–20. doi:10.1001/jama.290.7.912.
28. Veech RL, Chance B, Kashiwaya Y, Lardy HA, Cahill Jr GF. Ketone bodies, potential therapeutic uses. IUBMB Life. 2001;51(4):241–7. doi:10.1080/152165401753311780.
29. D'Agostino D, Pilla R, Held H, Landon C, Puchowicz M, Brunengraber H, et al. Therapeutic ketosis with ketone ester delays central nervous system oxygen toxicity seizures in rats. Am J Physiol Regul Integr Comp Physiol. 2013;304(10):R829–36. doi:10.1152/ajpregu.00506.2012.

30. Gasior M, French A, Joy M, Tang R, Hartman A, Rogawski M. The anticonvulsant activity of acetone, the major ketone body in the ketogenic diet, is not dependent on its metabolites acetol, 1,2-propanediol, methylglyoxal, or pyruvic acid. Epilepsia. 2007;48(4):793–800. doi:10.1111/j.1528-1167.2007.01026.x.
31. Likhodii S, Nylen K, Burnham W. Acetone as an anticonvulsant. Epilepsia. 2008;49 Suppl 8:83–6. doi:10.1111/j.1528-1167.2008.01844.x.
32. Seymour K, Bluml S, Sutherling J, Sutherling W, Ross B. Identification of cerebral acetone by 1H-MRS in patients with epilepsy controlled by ketogenic diet. Magma. 1999;8(1):33–42.
33. Halevy A, Peleg-Weiss L, Cohen R, Shuper A. An update on the ketogenic diet, 2012. Rambam Maimonides Med J. 2012;3(1), e0005. doi:10.5041/RMMJ.10072.
34. Amari A, Grace N, Fisher W. Achieving and maintaining compliance with the ketogenic diet. J Appl Behav Anal. 1995;28(3):341–2. doi:10.1901/jaba.1995.28-341.
35. Zhang Y, Kuang Y, LaManna J, Puchowicz M. Contribution of brain glucose and ketone bodies to oxidative metabolism. Adv Exp Med Biol. 2013;765: 365–70. doi:10.1007/978-1-4614-4989-8_51.
36. Maalouf M, Sullivan P, Davis L, Kim D, Rho J. Ketones inhibit mitochondrial production of reactive oxygen species production following glutamate excitotoxicity by increasing NADH oxidation. Neuroscience. 2007;145(1): 256–64. doi:10.1016/j.neuroscience.2006.11.065.
37. Milder J, Patel M. Modulation of oxidative stress and mitochondrial function by the ketogenic diet. Epilepsy Res. 2012;100(3):295–303. doi:10.1016/j.eplepsyres.2011.09.021.
38. Shimazu T, Hirschey M, Newman J, He W, Shirakawa K, Le Moan N, et al. Suppression of oxidative stress by β-hydroxybutyrate, an endogenous histone deacetylase inhibitor. Science. 2013;339:211–4. doi:10.1126/science.1227166.
39. Kim DY, Davis L, Sullivan P, Maalouf M, Simeone T, van Brederode J, et al. Ketone bodies are protective against oxidative stress in neocortical neurons. J Neurochem. 2007;101(5):1316–26. doi:10.1111/j.1471-4159.2007.04483.x.
40. Veech R. The therapeutic implications of ketone bodies: the effects of ketone bodies in pathological conditions: ketosis, ketogenic diet, redox states, insulin resistance, and mitochondrial metabolism. Prostaglandins Leukot Essent Fat Acids. 2004;70(3):309–19. doi:10.1016/j.plefa.2003.09.007.
41. Sato K, Kashiwaya Y, Keon C, Tsuchiya N, King M, Radda G, et al. Insulin, ketone bodies, and mitochondrial energy transduction. FASEB J. 1995;9(8):651–8.
42. Kashiwaya Y, Sato K, Tsuchiya N, Thomas S, Fell D, Veech R, et al. Control of glucose utilization in working perfused rat heart. J Biol Chem. 1994;269(41): 25502–14.
43. Sullivan P, Rippy N, Dorenbos K, Concepcion R, Agarwal A, Rho J. The ketogenic diet increases mitochondrial uncoupling protein levels and activity. Ann Neurol. 2004;55(4):576–80. doi:10.1002/ana.20062.
44. Bough K, Rho J. Anticonvulsant mechanisms of the ketogenic diet. Epilepsia. 2007;48(1):43–58. doi:10.1111/j.1528-1167.2007.00915.x.
45. Bough K, Wetherington J, Hassel B, Pare J, Gawryluk J, Greene J, et al. Mitochondrial biogenesis in the anticonvulsant mechanism of the ketogenic diet. Ann Neurol. 2006;60(2):223–35. doi:10.1002/ana.20899.
46. Ruskin D, Kawamura M, Masino S. Reduced pain and inflammation in juvenile and adult rats fed a ketogenic diet. PLoS ONE. 2009;4(12), e8349. doi:10.1371/journal.pone.0008349.
47. Paoli A, Moro T, Bosco G, Bianco A, Grimaldi KA, Camporesi E, et al. Effects of n-3 polyunsaturated fatty acids (ω-3) supplementation on some cardiovascular risk factors with a ketogenic Mediterranean diet. Marine drugs. 2015;13(2):996–1009. doi:10.3390/md13020996.
48. Desrochers S, Dubreuil P, Brunet J, Jetté M, David F, Landau BR, et al. Metabolism of (R, S)-1,3-butanediol acetoacetate esters, potential parenteral and enteral nutrients in conscious pigs. Am J Physiol. 1995; 268(4 Pt 1):E660–7.
49. Clarke K, Tchabanenko K, Pawlosky R, Carter E, Knight N, Murray A, et al. Oral 28-day and developmental toxicity studies of (R)-3-hydroxybutyl (R)-3-hydroxybutyrate. Regul Toxicol Pharmacol. 2012;63(2):196–208. doi:10.1016/j.yrtph.2012.04.001.
50. Clarke K, Tchabanenko K, Pawlosky R, Carter E, Todd King M, Musa-Veloso K, et al. Kinetics, safety and tolerability of (R)-3-hydroxybutyl (R)-3-hydroxybutyrate in healthy adult subjects. Regul Toxicol Pharmacol. 2012; 63(3):401–8. doi:10.1016/j.yrtph.2012.04.008.
51. Warnick G, Knopp R, Fitzpatrick V, Branson L. Estimating low-density lipoprotein cholesterol by the Friedewald equation is adequate for classifying patients on the basis of nationally recommended cutpoints. Clin Chem. 1990;36(1):15–9.
52. Friedewald W, Levy R, Fredrickson D. Estimation of the concentration of low-density lipoprotein cholesterol in plasma, without use of the preparative ultracentrifuge. Clin Chem. 1972;18(6):499–502.
53. Harlan Laboratories Inc U. Sprague Dawley Outbred Rat. In: http://www.harlan.com/products_and_services/research_models_and_services/research_models/sprague_dawley_outbred_rat.hl. 2008. http://www.harlan.com/products_and_services/research_models_and_services/research_models/sprague_dawley_outbred_rat.hl. Accessed date January 30, 2014.
54. Inc TB. Sprague Dawley Rat. In: http://www.taconic.com/sd. 2014. http://www.taconic.com/user-assets/documents/spraguedawley_booklet.pdf. Accessed date January 30, 2014.
55. McPherson P, McEneny J. The biochemistry of ketogenesis and its role in weight management, neurological disease and oxidative stress. J Physiol Biochem. 2012;68(1):141–51. doi:10.1007/s13105-011-0112-4.
56 Moore J, Eric C, Westman M. Cholesterol Clarity: What the HDL is Wrong With my Numbers. Las Vegas: Victory Belt Publishing Inc; 2013.
57 Dekaban A. Plasma lipids in epileptic children treated with the high fat diet. Arch Neurol. 1966;15(2):177–84.
58 Chesney D, Brouhard B, Wyllie E, Powaski K. Biochemical abnormalities of the ketogenic diet in children. Clin Pediatr. 1999;38(2):107–9. doi:10.1177/000992289903800207.
59. Schwartz R, Boyes S, Aynsley-Green A. Metabolic effects of three ketogenic diets in the treatment of severe epilepsy. Dev Med Child Neurol. 1989;31(2):152–60.
60. Katyal N, Koehler A, McGhee B, Foley C, Crumrine P. The ketogenic diet in refractory epilepsy: the experience of Children's Hospital of Pittsburgh. Clin Pediatr. 2000;39(3):153–9. doi:10.1177/000992280003900303.
61. Ellenbroek J, van Dijck L, Töns H, Rabelink T, Carlotti F, Ballieux B, et al. Long-term ketogenic diet causes glucose intolerance and reduced beta and alpha cell mass but no weight loss in mice. Am J Physiol Endocrinol Metab. 2014;306(5):E552–8. doi:10.1152/ajpendo.00453.2013.
62. Bergqvist A. Long-term monitoring of the ketogenic diet: Do's and Don'ts. Epilepsy Res. 2012;100(3):261–6. doi:10.1016/j.eplepsyres.2011.05.020.
63. Groesbeck D, Bluml R, Kossoff E. Long-term use of the ketogenic diet in the treatment of epilepsy. Dev Med Child Neurol. 2006;48(12):978–81. doi:10.1017/s0012162206002143.
64. Patel A, Pyzik P, Turner Z, Rubenstein J, Kossoff E. Long-term outcomes of children treated with the ketogenic diet in the past. Epilepsia. 2010;51(7): 1277–82. doi:10.1111/j.1528-1167.2009.02488.x.
65. Brehm BJ, Seeley RJ, Daniels SR, D'Alessio DA. A randomized trial comparing a very low carbohydrate diet and a calorie-restricted low fat diet on body weight and cardiovascular risk factors in healthy women. J Clin Endocrinol Metab. 2003;88(4):1617–23. doi:10.1210/jc.2002-021480.
66. Shai I, Schwarzfuchs D, Henkin Y, Shahar DR, Witkow S, Greenberg I, et al. Weight loss with a low-carbohydrate, Mediterranean, or low-fat diet. N Engl J Med. 2008;359(3):229–41. doi:10.1056/NEJMoa0708681.
67. Volek JS, Phinney SD, Forsythe CE, Quann EE, Wood RJ, Puglisi MJ, et al. Carbohydrate restriction has a more favorable impact on the metabolic syndrome than a low fat diet. Lipids. 2009;44(4):297–309. doi:10.1007/s11745-008-3274-2.
68. Feinman RD, Volek JS. Low carbohydrate diets improve atherogenic dyslipidemia even in the absence of weight loss. Nutr Metab. 2006;3:24. doi:10.1186/1743-7075-3-24.
69. Sharman MJ, Gomez AL, Kraemer WJ, Volek JS. Very low-carbohydrate and low-fat diets affect fasting lipids and postprandial lipemia differently in overweight men. J Nutr. 2004;134(4):880–5.
70. Sharman MJ, Kraemer WJ, Love DM, Avery NG, Gomez AL, Scheett TP, et al. A ketogenic diet favorably affects serum biomarkers for cardiovascular disease in normal-weight men. J Nutr. 2002;132(7):1879–85.
71. Westman EC, Mavropoulos J, Yancy WS, Volek JS. A review of low-carbohydrate ketogenic diets. Curr Atheroscler Rep. 2003;5(6):476–83.
72. Wood RJ, Volek JS, Davis SR, Dell'Ova C, Fernandez ML. Effects of a carbohydrate-restricted diet on emerging plasma markers for cardiovascular disease. Nutr Metab. 2006;3:19. doi:10.1186/1743-7075-3-19.
73. Volek JS, Sharman MJ, Forsythe CE. Modification of lipoproteins by very low-carbohydrate diets. J Nutr. 2005;135(6):1339–42.
74. Volek JS, Westman EC. Very-low-carbohydrate weight-loss diets revisited. Cleve Clin J Med. 2002;69(11):849. 53, 56–8 passim.
75. Volek JS, Sharman MJ, Gomez AL, DiPasquale C, Roti M, Pumerantz A, et al. Comparison of a very low-carbohydrate and low-fat diet on fasting lipids, LDL subclasses, insulin resistance, and postprandial lipemic responses in overweight women. J Am Coll Nutr. 2004;23(2):177–84.

76. Volek JS, Sharman MJ. Cardiovascular and hormonal aspects of very-low-carbohydrate ketogenic diets. Obes Res. 2004;12 Suppl 2:115s–23. doi:10.1038/oby.2004.276.
77. Volek JS, Sharman MJ, Gomez AL, Scheett TP, Kraemer WJ. An isoenergetic very low carbohydrate diet improves serum HDL cholesterol and triacylglycerol concentrations, the total cholesterol to HDL cholesterol ratio and postprandial pipemic responses compared with a low fat diet in normal weight, normolipidemic women. J Nutr. 2003;133(9):2756–61.
78. Schoeler NE, Wood S, Aldridge V, Sander JW, Cross JH, Sisodiya SM. Ketogenic dietary therapies for adults with epilepsy: feasibility and classification of response. Epilepsy & behavior : E&B. 2014;37:77–81. doi:10.1016/j.yebeh.2014.06.007.
79. Sengupta P. The laboratory Rat: relating its Age with Human's. Int J Prev Med. 2013;4(6):624–30.
80. Tsuchiya N, Harada Y, Taki M, Minematsu S, Maemura S, Amagaya S. Age-related changes and sex differences on the serum chemistry values in Sprague–Dawley rats–I. 6–30 weeks of age. Exp Anim. 1995;43(5):671–8.
81. Saito K, Ishikawa M, Murayama M, Urata M, Senoo Y, Toyoshima K, et al. Effects of sex, age, and fasting conditions on plasma lipidomic profiles of fasted Sprague–Dawley rats. PLoS ONE. 2013;9(11):e112266. doi:10.1371/journal.pone.0112266.
82. Ellington A, Kullo I. Atherogenic lipoprotein subprofiling. Adv Clin Chem. 2008;46:295–317.
83. Mudd J, Borlaug B, Johnston P, Kral B, Rouf R, Blumenthal R, et al. Beyond low-density lipoprotein cholesterol: defining the role of low-density lipoprotein heterogeneity in coronary artery disease. J Am Coll Cardiol. 2007;50(18):1735–41. doi:10.1016/j.jacc.2007.07.045.
84. Sacks F, Campos H. Clinical review 163: cardiovascular endocrinology: Low-density lipoprotein size and cardiovascular disease: a reappraisal. J Clin Endocrinol Metab. 2003;88(10):4525–32. doi:10.1210/jc.2003-030636.
85. Wierzbicki A. Quality as well as quantity? Beyond low-density lipoprotein-cholesterol - the role of particle size. Int J Clin Pract. 2007;61(11):1780–2. doi:10.1111/j.1742-1241.2007.01571.x.
86. Tantibhedhyangkul P, Hashim S, Van Itallie T. Effects of ingestion of long-chain triglycerides on glucose tolerance in man. Diabetes. 1967;16(11):796–9. doi:10.2337/diab.16.11.796.
87. Eckel R, Hanson A, Chen A, Berman J, Yost T, Brass E. Dietary substitution of medium-chain triglycerides improves insulin-mediated glucose metabolism in NIDDM subjects. Diabetes. 1992;41(5):641–7. doi:10.2337/diab.41.5.641.
88. Yost T, Erskine J, Gregg T, Podlecki D, Brass E, Eckel R. Dietary substitution of medium chain triglycerides in subjects with non-insulin-dependent diabetes mellitus in an ambulatory setting: impact on glycemic control and insulin-mediated glucose metabolism. J Am Coll Nutr. 1994;13(6):615–22. doi:10.1080/07315724.1994.10718457.
89. Kashiwaya Y, Pawlosky R, Markis W, King MT, Bergman C, Srivastava S, et al. A ketone ester diet increases brain malonyl-CoA and Uncoupling proteins 4 and 5 while decreasing food intake in the normal Wistar Rat. J Biol Chem. 2010;285(34):25950–6. doi:10.1074/jbc.M110.138198.
90. Senior B, Loridan L. Direct regulatory effect of ketones on lipolysis and on glucose concentrations in man. Nature. 1968;219(5149):83–4.
91. Miles JM, Haymond MW, Gerich JE. Suppression of glucose production and stimulation of insulin secretion by physiological concentrations of ketone bodies in man. J Clin Endocrinol Metab. 1980;52(1):34–7. doi:10.1210/jcem-52-1-34.
92. Kristian HM, Thomas S, Niels HS, Thomas G, Gerrit van H. Systemic, cerebral and skeletal muscle ketone body and energy metabolism during acute hyper-D-β-hydroxybutyrataemia in post-absorptive healthy males. J Clin Endocrin Metabol. 2014. doi:10.1210/jc.2014-2608
93. Owen OE, Morgan AP, Kemp HG, Sullivan JM, Herrera MG, Cahill GF. Brain metabolism during fasting. J Clin Invest. 1967;46(10):1589–95. doi:10.1172/JCI105650.
94. Papamandjaris AA, MacDougall DE, Jones PJ. Medium chain fatty acid metabolism and energy expenditure: obesity treatment implications. Life Sci. 1997;62(14):1203–15.
95. Linde R, Hasselbalch S, Topp S, Paulson O, Madsen P. Global cerebral blood flow and metabolism during acute hyperketonemia in the awake and anesthetized rat. J Cereb Blood Flow Metab. 2006;26(2):170–80. doi:10.1038/sj.jcbfm.9600177.
96. Azzam R, Azar N. Marked seizure reduction after MCT supplementation. Case reports in neurological medicine. 2013;2013:809151. doi:10.1155/2013/809151.
97. Corwin RL. Binge-type eating induced by limited access in rats does not require energy restriction on the previous day. Appetite. 2004;42(2):139–42. doi:10.1016/j.appet.2003.08.010.
98. Keenan KP, Ballam GC, Dixit R, Soper KA, Laroque P, Mattson BA, et al. The effects of diet, overfeeding and moderate dietary restriction on Sprague–Dawley rat survival, disease and toxicology. J Nutr. 1997;127(5 Suppl):851S–6.
99. Keenan KP, Smith PF, Hertzog P, Soper K, Ballam GC, Clark RL. The effects of overfeeding and dietary restriction on Sprague–Dawley Rat survival and early pathology biomarkers of aging. Toxicol Pathol. 1994. doi:10.1177/019262339402200308.
100. Kashiwaya Y, Bergman C, Lee J-H, Wan R, King M, Mughal M, et al. A ketone ester diet exhibits anxiolytic and cognition-sparing properties, and lessens amyloid and tau pathologies in a mouse model of Alzheimer's disease. Neurobiol Aging. 2013;34(6):1530–9. doi:10.1016/j.neurobiolaging.2012.11.023.
101. Birkhahn R, McCombs C, Clemens R, Hubbs J. Potential of the monoglyceride and triglyceride of DL-3-hydroxybutyrate for parenteral nutrition: synthesis and preliminary biological testing in the rat. Nutrition. 1997;13(3):213–9. doi:10.1016/s0899-9007(96)00404-2.
102. Puchowicz M, Smith C, Bomont C, Koshy J, David F, Brunengraber H. Dog model of therapeutic ketosis induced by oral administration of R, S-1,3-butanediol diacetoacetate. J Nutr Biochem. 2000;11(5):281–7.
103. Brunengraber H. Potential of ketone body esters for parenteral and oral nutrition. Nutrition. 1997;13(3):233–5.

4

High-fructose and high-fat diet-induced disorders in rats: impact on diabetes risk, hepatic and vascular complications

Iona Lozano[1], Remmelt Van der Werf[1,2], William Bietiger[1], Elodie Seyfritz[1], Claude Peronet[1], Michel Pinget[3], Nathalie Jeandidier[3], Elisa Maillard[1], Eric Marchioni[2], Séverine Sigrist[1*] and Stéphanie Dal[1]

Abstract

Background: As a result of the increased consumption of sugar-rich and fatty-products, and the increase in preference for such products, metabolic disorders are becoming more common at a younger age. Fructose is particularly used in prepared foods and carbonated beverages. We investigated the impact of regular consumption of fructose, in combination or not with fatty food, on the onset of metabolic syndrome and type 2 diabetes (T2D). We evaluated the metabolic, oxidative, and functional effects on the liver and blood vessels, both related to diabetes complications.

Methods: High-fat diet (HFD), high-fructose beverages (HF) or both (HFHF) were compared to rats fed with normal diet (ND) for 8 months to induce T2D and its metabolic, oxidative, and functional complications. Metabolic control was determined by measuring body weight, fasting blood glucose, C-peptide, HOMA2-IR, leptin, and cholesterol; oxidative parameters were studied by lipid peroxidation and total antioxidant capacity in plasma and the use of ROS labelling on tissue. Histological analysis was performed on the liver and endothelial function was performed in main mesenteric artery using organ-baths.

Results: After 2 months, HFHF and HFD increased body weight, leptin, HOMA2-IR associated to steatosis, oxidative stress in plasma and tissues, whereas HF had only a transient increase of leptin and c-peptide. Only HFHF induced fasting hyperglycaemia after 6 months and persistent hyperinsulinaemia and fasting hyperglycaemia with complicated steatosis (inflammation and fibrosis) after 8 months. HFHF and HFD induced endothelial dysfunction at 8 months of diet.

Conclusions: Six months, high fat and high carbohydrate induced T2D with widespread tissues effects. We demonstrated the role of oxidative stress in pathogenesis as well as in complications (hepatic and vascular), reinforcing interest in the use of antioxidants in the prevention and treatment of metabolic diseases, including T2D.

Keywords: High-fat high-fructose diet, Metabolic syndrome, Type 2 diabetes, Oxidative stress, Hepatic complications, Vascular complications, Endothelial dysfunction

* Correspondence: s.sigrist@ceed-diabete.org
[1]UMR DIATHEC, EA 7294, Centre Européen d'Etude du Diabète, Université de Strasbourg, Fédération de Médecine Translationnelle de Strasbourg, Bld René Leriche, 67200 Strasbourg, France
Full list of author information is available at the end of the article

Background

Food and beverages rich in energy, fat, and/or sugar are now commonly consumed in modern societies [1]. In addition to genetic predisposition [2], physical inactivity [1], and perinatal environment [1, 3], such diets are recognized as major causes of the obesogenic environment in humans [1]. The consumption of large amounts of added sugar, a prominent source of low-nutrient calories in processed or prepared foods and caloric beverages (i.e. soft drinks, colas) is a relatively new phenomenon [4]. In the mid-19th century, these sweeteners became widely available and their consumption began to increase dramatically [5]. Fructose is used commercially as a sweetening substitute (fructose corn syrup) for glucose or sucrose, in the preparation of desserts, condiments, and carbonated beverages [6]. It has been recently confirmed [7] that the consumption of high amounts of refined carbohydrates in food and beverage increases the risk of dyslipidaemia [8], obesity [4, 6], insulin resistance [9], and heart disease [10]. A recent epidemiological analysis in humans also found an association between diabetes prevalence and sugar availability [11]. Moreover, chronic consumption of a Western diet, characterized by foods rich in sugar and abundant in total and saturated fat, has been suggested to play a role in the development of type 2 diabetes (T2D) [12].

Diabetes is known to produce substantial changes in intracellular metabolism in most tissues, including liver [13]. Insulin resistance and excessive accumulation of lipids is strongly associated with non-alcoholic fatty liver disease (NAFLD), which represents the hepatic manifestation of a systemic impairment of the insulin network [14].

In addition to being a secondary consequence of metabolic syndrome, NAFLD is also in itself a major risk factor for diabetes [15], and also contributes to cardiovascular morbidity and mortality, with a two-fold increase in the risk of death [16]. One of the alterations that characterize NAFLD is hepatic steatosis, associated with obesity, insulin resistance, diabetes mellitus, and metabolic syndrome. Hepatic steatosis is characterized by the presence of hepatic fat accumulation, which, unlike non-alcoholic steatohepatitis (NASH), is not accompanied by ballooning of hepatocytes [17]. NAFLD includes a spectrum of diseases, ranging from simple fatty liver to NASH, which may progress to end-stage liver disease (cirrhosis) and hepatocellular carcinoma, requiring hepatic transplantation. This pathogenesis is multifactorial and includes lipid metabolism alterations, with an aberrant accumulation of triglycerides, mitochondrial dysfunction, inflammation, and oxidative stress (OS) [18].

OS, defined as an impaired balance between free radical production and antioxidant capacity resulting in accumulation of oxidative products [19], is a well-recognized mechanism that plays important roles in many pathological conditions. Several human diseases have been closely associated with OS [20], including aging [21], metabolic syndrome [20], and diabetes [20]. Several studies, which have proposed mechanisms to explain the increased OS in both forms of diabetes, suggest that diabetes is a bipolar process in which, on one hand, there is an increase in generation of reactive oxygen species (ROS), and, on the other hand, a decrease in the levels of plasma antioxidants levels such as vitamin E, vitamin C, lipoic acid, and glutathione [22]. Recent studies have shown that OS induces changes in redox balance resulting in dysregulation of redox biology [19, 20], and plays an important role in liver disease [18]. Moreover, OS has been closely related to cardiovascular diseases [20] linked with diabetes.

Diabetes-related vascular complications are an important pathological issue which lead to the functional deterioration of several organs, and cause micro- and macro-angiopathy [23]. Large clinical studies of both forms of diabetes have demonstrated that hyperglycaemia plays an important role in the pathogenesis of microvascular complications [23]. Moreover, there is considerable evidence demonstrating impairment of endothelium-dependent vasodilatation in cardiovascular diseases. This impairment of microvascular blood flow occurs early in the pathogenesis of T2D, with evidence at the time of diagnosis [24]. Dysfunction of the endothelium is regarded as an important factor in diabetes [24] and has gained increasing attention in the study of vascular disease.

Animal models have contributed greatly to the study of diabetes. Such models allow researchers to control, in vivo, genetic, and environmental factors that may influence the development of the disease and its secondary complications, therefore gaining useful information on its management and treatment in humans. There are many animal models of obesity and T2D [25], some of which show a genetic predisposition to the disease [26], while others may develop the disease spontaneously [27] or in a diet-induced manner [28]. The most commonly used non-genetic rodent models of diabetes are those induced by streptozotocine or alloxan, in addition to diet [29], or models obtained by partial pancreatectomy [25] which leads to insulin deficiency, hyperglycaemia, and ketosis. Although these models are useful for the study of diabetes, they are not representative of diet-induced human metabolic syndrome and T2D. Diet composition has been considered an important factor in the impairment of insulin activity [28]. Our previous study showed that the administration of a high-fat diet (HFD) to rats for 2 months is a fast and easy way to induce metabolic syndrome, associated with metabolic and oxidative disorders, without modulation of glycaemia [30]. However, recent epidemiological studies of sugar consumption and diabetes prevalence [11] suggest that a diet rich in fat as well as sugar is a greater risk factor for these disorders than a diet that is rich in either fats or sugars.

The aim of our study was to determine the impact of sugar on the development of metabolic syndrome and its evolution into T2D, as well as on the development of related secondary complications. We compared the impact of a diet rich in both sugar and fat with that of a sugar-rich diet without the addition of fat. We measured metabolic parameters such as insulin resistance, glucose tolerance, fasting glycaemia, and compared hepatic (steatosis, inflammation) and vascular (endothelial function) complications.

Methods

Chemicals

2,2′-Azino-bis-(3-ethylbenzthioazoline-6-sulfonic acid) (ABTS) was purchased from VWR (Fontenay sous Bois, France), amyloglucosidase (AMGD) from Roche Diagnostic (Meylan, France), glucose and phosphate-buffered saline (PBS) from Fisher Scientific (Illkirch, France), eosin, Harris hematoxylin, paraffin, ethanol and toluene from Labonord (Templemars, France). The (+)-6-hydroxy-2,5,7,8-tetramethylchroman-2-carboxylic acid (Trolox) and all other products were purchased from Sigma-Aldrich (St Quentin Fallavier, France).

Ethics statement

The study was performed in accordance with the "Guide for the Care and Use of Laboratory Animals" published by the US National Institutes of Health (NIH publication No. 85–23, revised 1996), and the present protocol was approved by the local ethics committee (Comité Régional d'Ethique en Matière d'Expérimentation Animale CREMEAS, approval AL/02/11/05/12). All efforts were made to minimize animal suffering and reduce the number of animals used.

Animals and induction of diabetes

Sixty-five male Wistar rats (8 weeks old; 204 ± 1 g), supplied by Depré (Saint Doulchard, France), were housed in a temperature-controlled room, in a 12-h-light/dark cycle environment with *ad libitum* access to water and food. At the beginning of the study, 5 rats were sacrificed (Ctr-rats, M0). After 2 weeks, the rats (312 ± 2 g) were randomly divided into four groups of 15 rats each. The first group had free access to a standard diet "Normal Diet" (ND) from SAFE (Augy, France), with the following macronutrient composition: 3.1 % fat, 16.1 % protein, 3.9 % fibre, and 5.1 % ash (minerals). The second group "High Fructose" (HF) had the same normal diet, but with an additional 25 % of fructose (Sigma, France) in water. The third group, "High Fat Diet" (HFD), received a purified laboratory hypercaloric rodent diet "WESTERN RD" (SDS, Special Diets Services, Saint Gratien, France) containing 21.4 % fat, 17.5 % protein, 50 % carbohydrate, 3.5 % fibre, and 4.1 % ash. The fourth group, "High Fat High Fructose" (HFHF), had both the enriched diet and fructose in water. Both groups had free access to water. The body weight and calorie intake of each animal was recorded once a week. 5 rats were sacrificed at the beginning of the study (M0), and then 5 rats of all groups were sacrificed at 2 and 8 months (M) after starting administration of each diet.

Sacrifice

Before anaesthesia, body weight was recorded, capillary glucose levels were measured, and tail vein blood samples were taken to estimate metabolic parameters. After anaesthesia with an intraperitoneal injection of 50 mg/kg pentobarbital (Centravet, France), blood was drawn from the abdominal aorta, and plasma and serum were frozen in liquid nitrogen and stored at −80 °C after centrifugation (4 °C, 2 min, 10,000 × *g*) for later biochemical analysis. Liver tissue was cleaned, weighed and embedded in Tissue-Tek® OCT (Optimal Cutting Temperature compound, Leica Microsystem SAS, Nanterre, France) or directly frozen in liquid nitrogen and stored at −80 °C. The main superior mesenteric artery was excised and bathed in Krebs bicarbonate solution (119 mM NaCl, 4.7 mM KCl, 1.18 mM KH_2PO_4, 1.18 mM $MgSO_4$, 1.25 mM $CaCl_2$, 25 mM $NaHCO_3$, and 11 mM D-glucose, pH 7.4, 37 °C) for dissection.

Biochemical plasmatic analysis

Plasmatic metabolic parameters

Glucose tolerance was evaluated by measuring intraperitoneal glucose tolerance (IpGTT) of fasting rats. Capillary glycaemia at baseline and 15, 30, 60, and 120 min after an intraperitoneal (IP)-injection of 2 g/kg glucose (20 % solution) was measured with a glucometer (Accu-Chek Performa®, Roche Diagnostic, France). Blood samples were collected from the tail vein at 0 and 60 min after injection, in order to measure blood glucose (glucose RTU®, Biomérieux, France) and C-peptide levels (Elisa C-peptide kit, Mercodia, Uppsala, Sweden) to evaluate insulin sensitivity. Measuring C-peptide was preferred to measuring insulin for evaluating insulinemia, because it is more stable in blood and is not affected by haemolysis [31]. Results were expressed in g/L for plasma glucose and in pmol/L for plasma C-peptide. Fasting leptin was measured by ELISA (Elisa Leptin kit, Linco Research Inc., St Louis, MO, USA) as An index of fat mass [32]. Plasmatic cholesterol was quantified by a colorimetric method Cholesterol RTU™ (BioMérieux, Lyon, France) using a cholesterol calibrator. Insulin resistance was evaluated using the homeostasis model assessment (HOMA2). HOMA2-IR was calculated for fasting plasma glucose and fasting C-peptide using the

HOMA2 model calculator (http://www.dtu.ox.ac.uk/homa-calculator). All parameters were measured once a month.

Plasmatic inflammatory and oxidative parameters

TNFα was assessed on plasma according to the manufacturer's instructions (Rat TNF-α ELISA Kit, Millipore, Fontenay sous Bois, France). Total antioxidant capacity (TAOC) with the radical cation $ABTS^{\bullet+}$ was performed by a trolox equivalent antioxidant capacity method as previously described [30]. Lipid peroxidation as a consequence of OS was estimated by measuring TBARS using a kit (OxiSelect™ TBARS Assay Kit-MDA Quantitation, Cell Biolabs Inc., San Diego, CA, USA) according to the manufacturer's instructions, and expressed in μmol/L TBARS.

Histological and functional studies

Morphological analysis and immunohistochemistry

The degree of hepatic histological changes was assessed by eosin/hematoxylin coloration, Oil Red O (steatosis), and Masson's Trichrome (fibrosis) staining on 10-μm cryosections fixed with 4 % paraformaldehyde. Steatosis was evaluated according to the standard Kleiner Classification [33] of grading and staging. Degree of steatosis was scored as the percentage of hepatocytes per lipid droplet: 0 (less than 5 %), 1 (between 5 and 33 %), 2 (between 33 and 66 %) and 3 (higher than 66 %), complicated or not by fibrosis.

In situ liver macrophages

As previously described by Dal S et al. [34] frozen-embedded liver sections (10 μm) were fixed and incubated with rabbit anti-Iba-1 (Rat, 1:1000, Wako Chemicals GmbH, Germany). Macrophage density was expressed as the percentage of brown pixels per field in comparison to control values (100 %). Six slides were prepared for each animal, and five fields were analysed per slide at a magnification of × 20.

Hepatic triglycerides and glycogen quantification

Extraction of hepatic triglyceride content was performed on piece of fresh liver (100 mg) mixed with a high-speed homogeniser (Polytron PT MR2100, Kinematica AG, Luzern, Switzerland) in a chloroform and methanol buffer ($CHCl_3$/Methanol/H_2O, v/v: 2/1/0,6), and centrifuged (1000 × *g*, 10 min, ambient temperature). The clot was mixed with a fresh solution of chloroform-Triton (X100, 2 %), evaporated (55 °C), and diluted in milli-Q water. Triglycerides were determined using the Triglycerides Quantification Kit (Abcam, Paris, France) according to the manufacturer's instructions. Samples were measured at 550 nm and concentrations were expressed in nmol/mg of liver.

Hepatic glycogen content extraction was performed on piece of fresh liver (100 mg) according to the method described previously [34] and expressed in mg of glycogen/mg of liver.

Tissue oxidative stress

The oxidative fluorescent dye dihydroethidine (DHE) was used to evaluate *in situ* formation of ROS according to a method described by Dal-Ros et al. [34]. Unfixed liver and mesenteric artery were cut into 10-μm-thick sections, treated with DHE (2.5 μM), and incubated in a light-protected humidified chamber at 37 °C for 30 min. The level of ROS was determined using microscopy and whole fluorescence of tissue was quantified with the microscope assistant (NIS-Elements BR, Nikon, France), and expressed as a percentage of that in age-matched ND rats.

As previously described [35], liver tissue (5 mg) from experimental rats was homogenized using NP-40 buffer (NaCl 150 mmol/L, 1.0 % Triton X-100, Tris 50 mmol/L, pH 8) with a protease/phosphatase inhibitor cocktail (Roche Diagnostics, Meylan, France) using an ULTRA-TURRAX. Supernatants were collected and protein contents measured by the Bradford method [36] SOD and catalase activities were performed (50 mg of proteins) according to the manufacturer's instructions (Superoxide dismutase assay kit and Catalase Assay Kit, Abcam, Paris, France) and expressed respectively in % of inhibition rate and (μmol/L). Lipid peroxidation was estimated by measuring TBARS using a kit (OxiSelect™ TBARS Assay Kit-MDA Quantitation, Cell Biolabs Inc., San Diego, CA, USA) according to the manufacturer's instructions, and expressed in μmol/L TBARS/mg of proteins.

Vascular reactivity studies

Mesenteric artery rings were suspended in organ baths for the determination of changes in isometric tension, as described previously [21]. The NO-mediated component of relaxation was determined in the presence of indomethacin (10 μM) and charybdotoxin (CTX) plus apamin (APA) (100 nM each) to rule out the formation of vasoactive prostanoids and EDHF, respectively. The EDHF-mediated component of relaxation was determined in the presence of indomethacin (10^{-5}M) and N^{ω}-nitro-L-arginine (L-NA, 10^{-4}M) to rule out the formation of vasoactive prostanoids and NO, respectively. Levcromakalim- (an ATP-sensitive K^{+}channel opener; 0.1 nM–10 μM) induced relaxations were examined in endothelium-denuded rings of mesenteric artery to test the vascular smooth muscle cells relaxations without EDHF production by endothelial cells.

Statistical analysis

Values are expressed as means ± SEM, and n indicates the number of rats. Statistical analysis was performed with Student's t-test for unpaired data or ANOVA followed by Tukey's protected least-significant difference test, where appropriate (Statistica®, StatSoft, France). $p < 0.05$ was considered to be statistically significant.

Results

Metabolic follow-up

After 3 weeks of diet, HFHF and HFD induced a significant increase in body weight ($p < 0.05$) maintained until the end of the study, in comparison to HF and ND diet (respectively, 863 ± 72 g; 863 ± 70 g; 680 ± 22 g and 617 ± 9 g) (Fig. 1a). After 2 months, fasting glycaemia

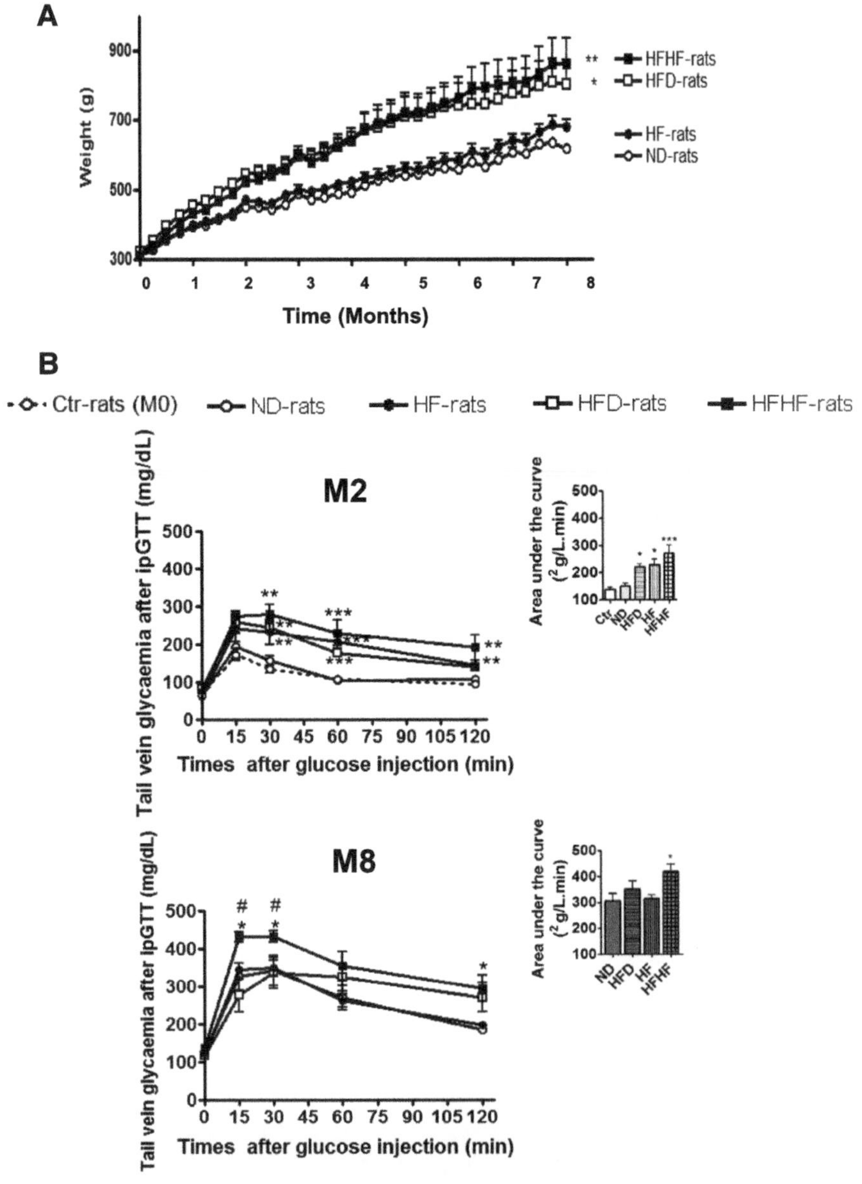

Fig. 1 Weight and glucose tolerance measured during the study. **a** Weight during the study for the normal diet (ND, ○), normal diet + fructose (HF, ●), high fat diet (HFD, □) and HFD + fructose (HFHF, ■) groups. * Global significant results *versus* age-matched ND-rats. **b** Evolution of glycaemia and the area under the curves (AUC) during intraperitoneal glucose tolerance (IpGTT) test on fasting rats (0) and 15, 30, 60, 120 min after glucose injection in all groups and at the beginning (Ctr-rats, M0) and after 2 (M2) and 8 (M8) months of diet. Results are shown as mean ± SEM of 5 different experiments. * Significant results *versus* age-matched ND-rats

(Tables 1, 2 and 3) was higher in HFD and HFHF rats. Moreover, AUC after ipGTT was higher in hypercaloric diet (HF, HFD and HFHF) (respectively: 229 ± 20; 221 ± 12 and 271 ± 30; $p < 0.01$) (Fig. 1b). C-peptide levels in pre- and post-ipGTT were also higher in the 3 groups as compared to those in ND-rats (Tables 1, 2 and 3). After 2 months, HOMA2-IR values were higher than 2.4 in HF, HFD, and HFHF rats, confirming insulin resistance, but only significantly increased in HFD and HFHF rats as compared to ND rats ($p < 0.01$) (Tables 1, 2 and 3). After 4 months, fasting glycaemia was the same in all groups around 104.5 ± 3mg/dL and only HFHF rats shown fasting glycaemia under 126 mg/dL (147 ± 7 mg/dL) after 6 months of diet in comparison to ND, HF and HFD (respectively: 103 ± 2; 114 ± 3 and 105 ± 2 mg/dL) (data not shown).

After 8 months, HFHF maintained all metabolic parameters disorders such as higher fasting leptinaemia, fasting glycaemia, fasting and post-ipGTT C-peptide, as indicated by the AUC ($p < 0.05$) and HOMA2-IR ($p < 0.001$). Glycaemia at 2 h post-ipGTT was increased to greater than 200 mg/dL in HFD rats and associated with a higher level of C-peptide, but without significant increase in fasting glycaemia or HOMA2-IR, as compared to HF or ND rats (Tables 1, 2 and 3). Total cholesterol increased in HFHF rats from 2 months in comparison to ND rats ($p < 0.05$), whereas this effect was not observed for HFD and HF rats (Tables 1, 2 and 3).

Inflammatory and oxidative follow-up

HFHF and HFD induced respectively an increase of five and four times of the plasmatic TNFα after 8 months (Table 4). Moreover, lipid peroxide levels increased also after 8 months in HFHF and HFD rats (Table 4), whereas HF had no effect on these inflammatory and OS parameters. During the study, the total antioxidant capacity was comparable in all groups, in spite of OS (Table 4).

Table 1 Evolution of metabolic parameters during the study

M0		Ctr
Weight (g)		300 ± 6
Fasting Leptin (ng/mL)		3.5 ± 0.4
Fasting glycaemia (mg/dL)		83 ± 3
Peptide-C (pmol/L)	Fasting	860.5 ± 56.8
	Non-fasting	1283.6 ± 115.3
Insulin resistance (HOMA2-IR)		1.22 ± 0.08
Total cholesterol (mM)		2.20 ± 0.49

Effects of diet on body weight and metabolic parameters during the study, at the beginning (M0) of normal diet (ND), normal diet + fructose (HF), high fat diet (HFD) and HFD + fructose (HFHF)

HFHF and hepatic complications

HE analysis of the liver showed marked vacuolar degeneration in HFHF and HFD rats, indicating hepatic fat accumulation (Fig. 2a). Oil-red O-staining confirmed the accumulation of lipid droplets in HFHF and HFD rats. Steatosis increased between 2 and 8 months in HFHF and HFD rats (steatosis score: 1–2 to the maximum 3, according to Kleiner et al. [32]), associated with fibrosis and macrophage infiltration after 8 months only in HFHF rats. In fact, the HFHF diet was found to result in an increase in hepatic macrophages ($p < 0.01$) in comparison to HFD, HF and ND (Fig. 2a and Table 4). Biochemical analysis of the hepatic triglyceride content confirmed lipid accumulation, with a significant increase in triglycerides after 2 months, which was maintained after 8 months (Fig. 2b). The level of hepatic glycogen content was comparable in HFHF and ND rats during the study. HF was found to gradually increase glycogen levels from 2 to 8 months, whereas HFD transiently increased glycogen levels at 2 months (Fig. 2c).

HFHF induced a significant and persistent increase in hepatic ROS levels from 2 months and throughout the study in comparison to ND, without TBARS formation. HFD induced only a transient hepatic ROS formation after 2 months, not associated to TBARS complication. HF induced a transient increase of TBARS ($p < 0.01$) without ROS formation (Fig. 2a and Table 4). In spite of ROS observed in the liver, SOD and catalase activities were comparable in all groups during the study, excepted after 8 months in HF-rats where catalase activity was decreased ($p < 0.01$) (Table 4).

HFHF and vascular function

The cumulative addition of acetylcholine caused concentration-dependent relaxations in isolated mesenteric arteries of Ctr-rats in the presence of indomethacin (10 μM) and N^{ω}-nitro-L-arginine (100 μM) (Fig. 3). This EDHF-mediated component of relaxation is strongly decreased after 8 months in ND and HF rats and abolished in HFHF and HFD rats. The concentration-dependent relaxation induced by levcromakalim (0.1 nM–10 μM), an ATP-sensitive K^+ channel opener, in mesenteric arteries from all groups, was maintained (respectively: relaxant effect at 10 μM, 94.5 ± 7.0 % in mesenteric arteries from Ctr-rats at M0 and at M8: 96.7 ± 0.9 % in ND-rats, 96 ± 2.2 % in HFHF-rats, 98 ± 0.7 % in HFD-rats and 103.5 ± 3.2 % in HF-rats, data not shown). Moreover, in the presence of indomethacin, N^{ω}-nitro-L-arginine, and charybdotoxin plus apamin, acetylcholine-induced relaxations were abolished in all groups (data not shown).

Altogether, these results indicate that the EDHF-mediated component of relaxation is abolished by HFHF and HFD after 8 months, regardless of the age of rats.

Table 2 Evolution of metabolic parameters during the study

M2		ND	HF	HFD	HFHF
Weight (g)		442 ± 610	462 ± 8	**543 ± 14***	**553 ± 14***
Fasting Leptin (ng/mL)		8.19 ± 0.44	**10.84 ± 0.75****	**20.86 ± 0.79*****	**17.05 ± 1.68***a**
Fasting glycaemia (mg/dL)		89 ± 4	102 ± 6	**128 ± 6*****	**112 ± 6****
Peptide-C (pmol/L)	Fasting	1027.8 ± 71.4	**2340.2 ± 73.7*****	**1404.5 ± 73.7*****	**2282.6 ± 187.9*****
	Non-fasting	1974.5 ± 163.8	**5222.9 ± 374.1*****	**3578.2 ± 256*****	**4531.3 ± 432.8*****
Insulin resistance (HOMA2-IR)		2.20 ± 0.15	3.35 ± 0.33	**6.59 ± 0.67*****	**5.36 ± 0.79***
Total cholesterol (mM)		2.92 ± 0.41	4.0 ± 0.80	3.44 ± 0.48	**5.03 ± 0.73***

Effects of diet on body weight and metabolic parameters during the study, after 2 (M2) of normal diet (ND), normal diet + fructose (HF), high fat diet (HFD) and HFD + fructose (HFHF). In bold significant difference with age-matched ND rats and [a]between HFD- and HFHF-rats. *$p<0.05$, **$p<0.01$, ***$p<0.001$

Moreover, HFHF induced a significant and persistent increase in hepatic ROS levels from 2 months and throughout the study, in comparison to ND. HFD induced only a transient hepatic ROS formation after 2 months and HF had no effect on hepatic ROS (Fig. 2a and Table 4).

Discussion

The present study demonstrates that only the combination of sugar and fat, present in beverage and diet (HFHF), allowed the development of T2D associated with long-term metabolic disorders such as maintenance of fasting hyperglycaemia, pre- and post-prandial hyperinsulinaemia, insulin resistance, glucose intolerance, and dyslipidaemia (hypertriglyceridaemia and hypercholesterolaemia). Moreover, HFHF was found to induce T2D-associated complications such as hepatic steatosis complicated by fibrosis, inflammation, and OS in the animals, regardless of their age. In addition, HFHF and HFD induced obesity associated with hyperleptinaemia and endothelial dysfunction. However, HFD alone induced only transient insulin resistance, glucose intolerance, and hypertriglyceridaemia, without any impact on total cholesterol. In contrast, ND rats showed a decrease in insulin sensitivity, associated with glucose intolerance, with increasing age, thus minimizing the effects provided by the HFD. A transient metabolic disorders appears after 2 months of fructose beverage-intake only, characterized by a reduction of insulin sensitivity without abnormal weight gain, which may be due to an expansion of adipose cells [37] suggesting by hyperleptinaemia, even though total calorie intake (food and beverage, data not shown) did not differ between groups. These results are in accordance with the very few studies in humans reporting that the effects of fructose-rich diets, particularly on insulin sensitivity, appear to be dose-dependent [38, 39]. However, the dose of fructose administrated to rodents was higher (50–60 % of the diet) than that administered to humans (10–15 %).

Excessive consumption of fructose may affect the liver [40]. Indeed, this was found to increase the production of glycogen in HF and HFHF rats after 2 and 4 months. The conversion of glucose into glycogen is a key pathway by which the liver removes glucose from the portal vein after a meal, mediated by the bidirectional GLUT2 transporter and through gluconeogenesis [41]. Koo et al. [42] showed that liver glycogen is higher in HF-rats, indicating its conversion by gluconeogenesis. This increase in glycogen may represent a protective mechanism against fat accumulation in the liver [43], and against hyperglycaemia [44], as observed in the HF rats. However, after 8 months of HFHF, hepatic OS resulted in a decrease in the levels of glycogen, as reported by Castro MC et al. [45], throughout a NADPH oxidase pathway. Less significantly, after 2 months of HFD, the hepatic glycogen level was found to have increased through a second mechanism

Table 3 Evolution of metabolic parameters during the study

M8		ND	HF	HFD	HFHF
Weight (g)		617 ± 9	680 ± 22	**863 ± 70*****	**863 ± 72*****
Fasting Leptin (ng/mL)		22.41 ± 1.48	26.13 ± 1.45	**91.17 ± 13.8****	**124.11 ± 5.09**b**
Fasting glycaemia (mg/dL)		124 ± 5	122 ± 4	116 ± 2	**137 ± 2*b**
Peptide-C (pmol/L)	Fasting	1871.8 ± 259	2060.7 ± 180.0	2730 ± 365.1	**3937.3 ± 4953.1***
	Non-fasting	3534.8 ± 185.8	6081.3 ± 987.2	**6615 ± 828.3***	**12411.7 ± 2072.4**a**
Insulin resistance (HOMA2-IR)		4.53 ± 0.62	4.97 ± 0.44	5.7 ± 0.82	**9.78 ± 1.24*****
Total cholesterol (mM)		1.76 ± 0.24	2.44 ± 0.51	3.0 ± 0.59	**4.23 ± 0.47***

Effects of diet on body weight and metabolic parameters during the study, after 8 months (M8) of normal diet (ND), normal diet + fructose (HF), high fat diet (HFD) and HFD + fructose (HFHF). In bold significant difference with * vs. age-matched ND rats and [a, b]between HFD- and HFHF-rats. *$p<0.05$; **$p<0.01$; ***$p<0.001$ and [a]$p<0.05$ and [b]$p<0.001$

Table 4 Evolution of inflammatory and oxidative parameters during the study

M0	Ctr	M0		Ctr
Plasmatic parameters		*Hepatic parameters*		
TNFα (pg/mL)	37.30 ± 13.68	Macrophages (% of area)		1.91 ± 0.4
TAOC (mmol/L trolox equivalent)	10.51 ± 0.29	Oxidative stress (% *vs.* age-matched ND)		100 ± 22.9
Lipids peroxidation (μmol/L TBARS)	20.6 ± 3.2	SOD activity (% inhibition rate)		0.97 ± 0.003
		Catalase activity (μmol/L)		0.272 ± 0.03
		Lipids peroxidation (μmol/L TBARS)		23 ± 0.8
M2	ND	HF	HFD	HFHF
Plasmatic parameters				
TNFα (pg/mL)	23.23 ± 7.82	13.63 ± 3.52	49.03 ± 20.06	13.84 ± 5.46
TAOC (mmol/L trolox equivalent)	7.64 ± 0.15	7.93 ± 0.16	7.58 ± 0.45	8.32 ± 0.25
Lipids peroxidation (μmol/L TBARS)	19.4 ± 2.0	41.9 ± 10.5	26.5 ± 5.3	43.3 ± 13.1
Hepatic parameters				
Macrophages (% of area)	4.34 ± 1.1	2.88 ± 1.2	2.58 ± 0.8	4.10 ± 2.1
Oxidative stress (% *vs.* age-matched ND)	100 ± 11.4	108.1 ± 17.7	**168.2 ± 17.3***	**151 ± 17.9***
SOD activity (% inhibition rate)	1.15 ± 0.13	0.99 ± 0.008	1.17 ± 0.09	1.08 ± 0.07
Catalase activity (μmol/L)	0.243 ± 0.03	0.187 ± 0.02	0.283 ± 0.04	0.257 ± 0.02
Lipids peroxidation (μmol/L TBARS)	20.4 ± 1.1	**23.9 ± 0.1****	19.4 ± 0.7	18 ± 1.4
M8	ND	HF	HFD	HFHF
Plasmatic parameters				
TNFα (pg/mL)	25.63 ± 7.57	48.90 ± 9.74	**97.98 ± 28.42***	**130.7 ± 40.68*****
TAOC (mmol/L trolox equivalent)	11.07 ± 0.08	11.24 ± 0.19	10.96 ± 0.09	11.10 ± 0.27
Lipids peroxidation (μmol/L TBARS)	20.1 ± 2.5	22.5 ± 3.3	**38.8 ± 3.8****	**48.0 ± 6.3***
Hepatic parameters				
Macrophages (% of area)	2.20 ± 1.5	2.37 ± 1.1	5.99 ± 1.9	**11.26 ± 2.4**a**
Oxidative stress (% *vs.* age-matched ND)	100 ± 6.3	110.2 ± 21.5	149.2 ± 15.3	**206 ± 29.1**a**
SOD activity (% inhibition rate)	1.09 ± 0.04	0.94 ± 0.08	1.13 ± 0.14	1.17 ± 0.16
Catalase activity (μmol/L)	0.246 ± 0.03	**0.120 ± 0.03****	0.207 ± 0.03	0.232 ± 0.01
Lipids peroxidation (μmol/L TBARS)	18 ± 1.2	15.7 ± 2.0	18.9 ± 2.1	16.5 ± 1.1

Effects of diet on plasmatic and hepatic inflammation and oxidative parameters during the study, at the beginning (M0) and after 2 (M2) and 8 months (M8) of normal diet (ND), normal diet + fructose (HF), high fat diet (HFD) and HFD + fructose (HFHF). In bold significant difference with age-matched ND rats and [a]between HFD- and HFHF-rats. *$p<0.05$, **$p<0.01$, ***$p<0.001$

involving hyperinsulinaemia [40] and GSK-3 inactivation [46]. Therefore, only this mechanism is involved in glycogen increase in HFD rats, while both mechanisms contribute to increased glycogen levels in rats that were fed fructose.

In our study, only HFHF was found to induce the development and progression of steatosis into NASH. The factors causing progression of NAFLD to fibrosis and cirrhosis have not been defined in humans, in part because of the unavailability of human liver tissue for studies. Nevertheless, a series of mechanisms acting in synergy, or in stages, have been proposed to explain the transition and development of NAFLD to NASH. Factors that appear to be crucial involve increase in the vulnerability of steatotic hepatocytes, OS, alteration in the metabolism of lipids, mitochondrial dysfunction, and insulin resistance. The latter includes not only the metabolic consequences of insulin resistance and hyperinsulinaemia, but also changes in output of adipocytokines in fat tissue, which create a pro-inflammatory and potentially pro-fibrotic state [18, 47]. In fact, HFHF-induced NASH in this model is associated with fibrosis and macrophage infiltration, elevation of hepatic triglyceride level, and OS. Moreover the level of leptin, which also has pro-inflammatory properties and is considered an essential mediator of hepatic fibrosis [48], was significantly higher in HFHF than in HFD rats, despite the same weight gain for each group. This may highlight a body fat abnormality leading to higher hepatic complications [49]. These results are in accordance with the 'two-hits' hypothesis of Day and James [50], in which the accumulation of hepatic triglycerides constitutes the first hit of NASH pathogenesis,

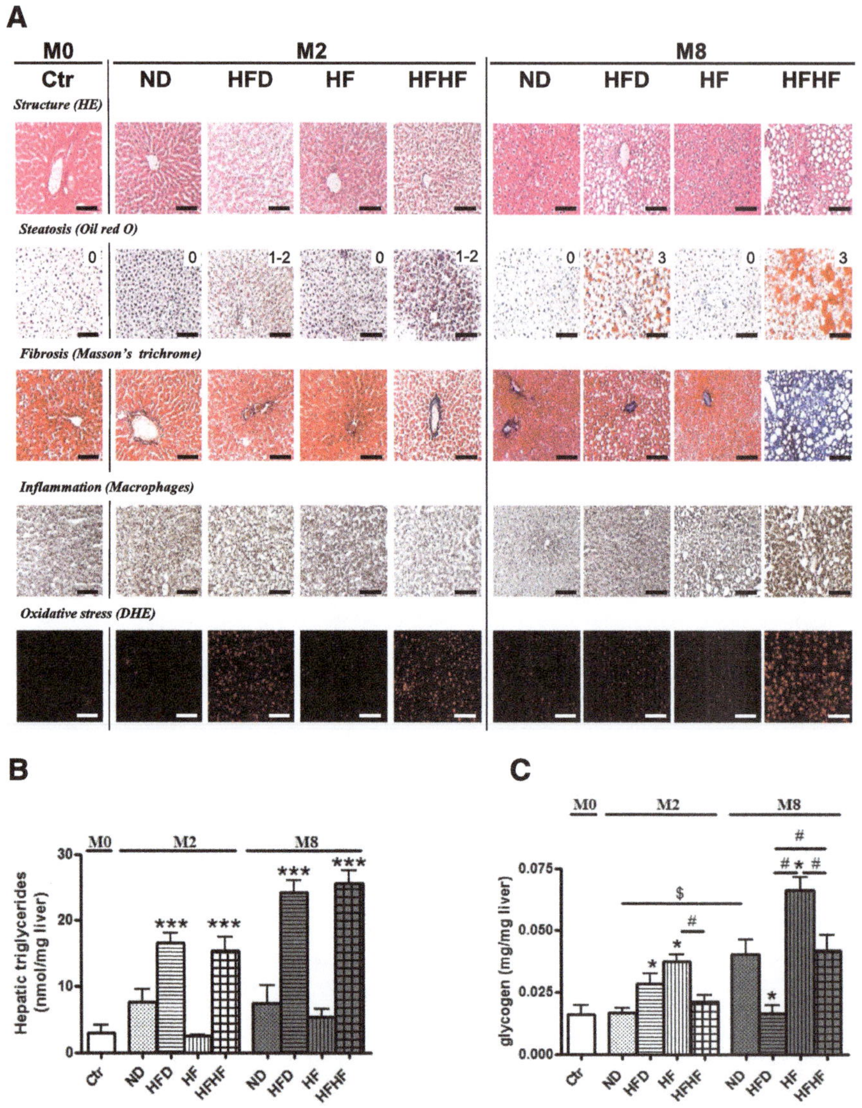

Fig. 2 Evolution of hepatic complications. **a** Severity of hepatic complications was assessed by eosin/hematoxylin coloration and Oil-Red O for steatosis, Masson's Trichrome for fibrosis, macrophages infiltration and oxidative stress by dihydroethidine (DHE) at the beginning (M0), after 2 (M2) and 8 (M8) months of normal diet (ND), normal diet + fructose (HF), high fat diet (HFD) and HFD + fructose (HFHF). The score of steatosis is noted under the picture (0, 1, 2, or 3). Results for 5 different experiments are shown. Bar scale = 100 μm. **b-c** Quantification of hepatic triglycerides (**b**) and glycogen (**c**) in frozen-liver tissue, at the beginning (M0), after 2 (M2) and 8 (M8) months of normal diet (ND), normal diet + fructose (HF), high fat diet (HFD) and HFD + fructose (HFHF). Results are shown as mean ± SEM of 5 different experiments. * Significant results *versus* age-matched ND-rats and # between two groups

and OS followed by inflammation represents the second hit.

Hepatocytes have an elaborate system of enzymatic and non-enzymatic antioxidant defences to remove or neutralize ROS [51]. However, excessive levels of ROS may overwhelm the hepatocellular antioxidant defences, resulting in OS, hepatocyte injury, and cell death. In our model, HFHF and HFD rapidly induced hepatic OS, highlighting that OS as an important inducer of hepatic steatosis, whereas HF alone was neither associated with OS nor with steatosis. Short periods of hyperglycaemia are also able to induce OS [52], as observed after 2 months of HFD (higher but not significant fasting glycaemia), associated with steatosis. However, chronic hyperglycaemia, in addition to fluctuations in glucose level and hyperinsulinaemia (particularly in fasting conditions),

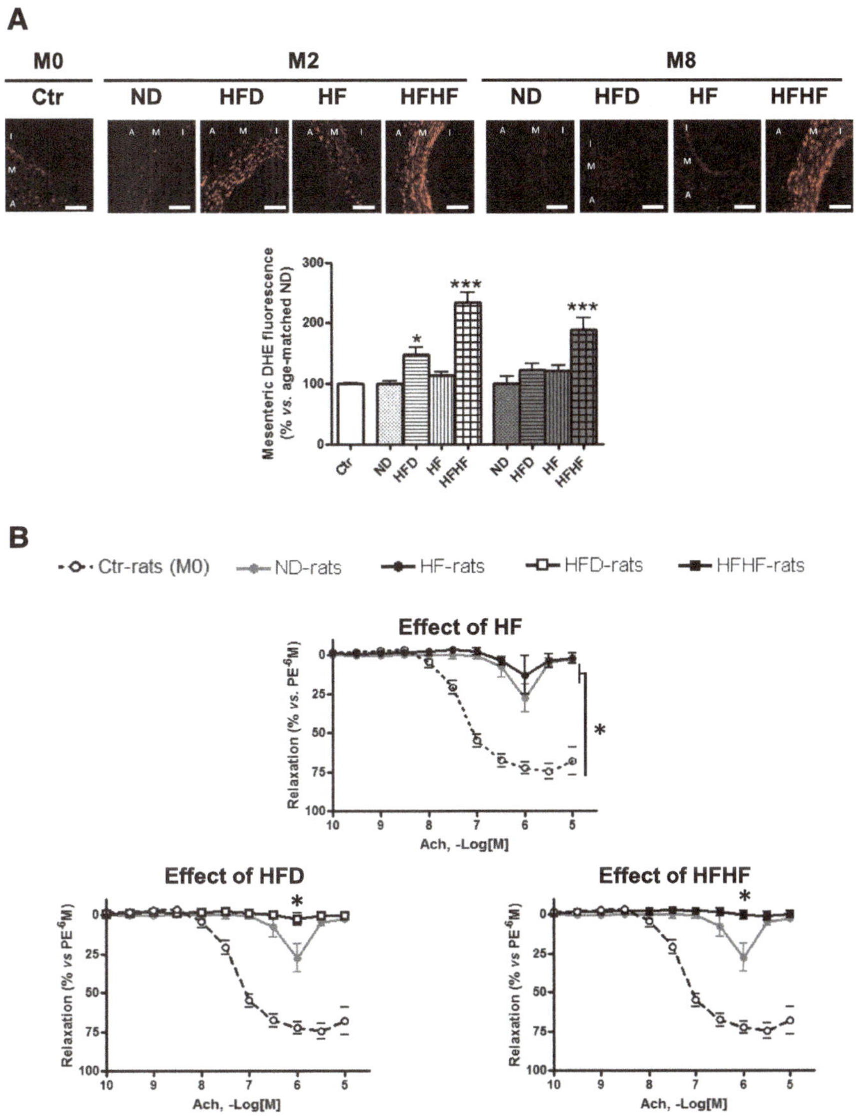

Fig. 3 Evolution of vascular complications: oxidative stress and vascular reactivity of mesenteric artery. **a** *Higher panel.* Visualization of dihydroethidine (DHE) representative immunofluorescent staining of ROS in rats' liver (**a**) and mesenteric artery (**b**) during the study, at the beginning (M0) and after 2 (2M) and 8 (8M) months of normal diet (ND), normal diet + fructose (HF), high fat diet (HFD) and HFD + fructose (HFHF). *Bottom panel.* Corresponding cumulative data. Results are shown as mean ± SEM of 5 different experiments. * Significant results *versus* age-matched ND-rats and # between HFD- and HFHF-rats. Bar scale = 100 μm. **b** Concentration–relaxation curves to acetylcholine (ACh) in mesenteric artery rings with endothelium from control-rats (M0), normal diet-rats (ND, ●) after 8 months of diet and normal diet + fructose (HF, •), high fat diet (HFD, □) and HFD + fructose (HFHF, ■). Experiments were performed in the presence of indomethacin (10^{-5} M) and N$^{\omega}$-nitro-L-arginine (L-NA, 10^{-4} M) to rule out the formation of vasoactive prostanoids and NO, respectively (EDHF-mediated component). Results are shown as means ± SEM of 5 different rats. *$P < 0.05$ represents a significant effect

leptin resistance, and inflammation exacerbate ROS formation and maintain OS [20]. ROS are understood to be important for the stimulating the production of type I collagen by hepatic stellate cells, therefore increasing extracellular matrix deposition during fibrogenesis [53]. These various disorders, which were observed in the HFHF-rats, but not the HF rats, after 8 months, explain the progression of NAFLD into NASH. Our results on liver complications are in accordance with the study of Rector et al. who demonstrated that mitochondrial dysfunction progressively contributes to the development of obesity-associated NAFLD in OLETF rats [54]. It can therefore be concluded that OS plays an important role in both the initial stages of steatosis, as well as its progression, especially in fibrosis and NASH.

Several studies have reported an association between NAFLD and cardiovascular disease-related complications (i.e. atherosclerosis) and hypothesise that common inflammatory and/or OS mediators are involved in inducing hepatic and peripheral vascular alterations [55]. In our study, EDHF-mediated relaxations were found to be blunted in the mesenteric artery of HFHF- and HFD-rats after 8 months of diet, but no significant similar effects were observed in rats fed the HF diet. Moreover, while ageing induced blunted NO-mediated relaxation, neither HF, HFD nor HFHF exacerbate this dysfunction (data not shown). So, NO-mediated relaxations were not affected by diets. These results are in accordance with the reduction of EDHF observed in other models of T2D (Goto-Katizaki rats, Zucker obese rats, and OLETF rats) [56], which do not show any effect on NO. However, studies of NO that report an increase, maintenance, or reduction in relaxation [56] in other types of arteries, species, and animals models may explain this variability. Another factor that influences endothelial function is the age of the animal. Indeed, previous studies have shown that aging is associated with a rapid (20 weeks) and progressive loss of endothelial function in rats [21]. In our study, after 8 months of treatment (at 10 months of age), ND rats developed endothelial dysfunction characterised by reduced NO- and EDHF-mediated relaxations in mesenteric arteries, without any effect on pathways involved in the relaxation of smooth muscle cells (data not shown). The same results were obtained for the aorta, where NO is the most important relaxant factor (data not shown). Therefore, in our study, only the EDHF component of relaxation was found to be blunted by HFHF and HFD after 8 months, in addition to age-induced endothelial dysfunction. Recent studies have reported that two factors are related to glucose-induced OS: the glucose variability and the glucose memory. Therefore, the endothelial dysfunction observed in HFD rats after 8 months may be explained in part by the long-lasting deleterious effects of glucose, which persist beyond the period of hyperglycaemia (observed only at 2 months), whereas HFHF rats have longer-lasting glycaemic fluctuation due to the persistence of glucose intolerance and hyperglycaemia in these rats. In addition, a number of disorders may induce endothelial dysfunction, such as obesity, visceral fat distribution [57], impaired fasting glucose, hyperglycaemia [58], insulin resistance [59], oxidative stress [60], and inflammation [61] all of which were observed in our models, and reported in other studies [62].

Conclusions

Increased fat intake and Western diets have been linked to insulin resistance, impaired postprandial lipid metabolism, and the development or progression of NAFLD. However, data from recent animal experiments and human studies additionally implicate sugar consumption (primarily in the form of soft drinks, worldwide) in the development of diabetes mellitus and related metabolic diseases that raise cardiovascular risk. The latest WHO guidelines advise reducing sugar intake by 10 to 5 % of the daily calorie intake, in order to provide additional benefits. For many years, sugars (mainly fructose) have been added to processed foods, and our taste preferences are progressively shaped by more pronounced sweet flavours. Recent scientific reports identify fructose as the major player in the risk of developing T2D [62]. Therefore, fructose is an essential and indispensable element to consider for the development of an in vivo model of T2D that is most representative of the pathophysiology of the disease in humans. In our study, while the intake of fructose alone was found to accelerate metabolic disturbances associated with increasing age (insulin resistance and glucose intolerance), its association with HFD was found to result in the development of metabolic syndrome in T2D and liver and vascular complications. The administration of a combination of fructose and lipids was found to be ideal for the development of an experimentally induced T2D model. These different in vivo models (HF, HFD, and HFHF) should be useful as tools for testing candidates (natural or synthetic) in drug development for a broad spectrum of metabolic diseases.

Abbreviations

DHE: dihydroethidine; EDHF: endothelium-derived-hyperpolarizing factor; HF: high-fructose beverages; HFD: high-fat diet; HFHF: high-fat-high fructose; IpGTT: intraperitoneal glucose tolerance; NAFLD: non-alcoholic fatty liver disease; NASH: non-alcoholic steatohepatitis; ND: normal diet; NO: nitric oxide; OS: oxidative stress; ROS: reactive oxygen species; T2D: type 2 diabetes; TAOC: total antioxidant capacity.

Competing interests

The authors declare that they have no conflicts of interest.

Authors' contributions

IL performed some experiments, WB and CP assisted technicians with animal sacrifice, ES assisted a technician, and RV, MP, NJ, EM, and EMP approved the final version. SS reviewed the manuscript. All authors read and approved the final manuscript. SD conceived and designed the study, acquired data, interpreted the results, and drafted and revised the manuscript.

Acknowledgements

We are grateful to the CRA (Conseil Regional d'Alsace), the foundation "Vaincre le Diabète", and the company ASDIA (Assistance Service Diabète) for funding this project. The authors would also like to express their gratitude to Pr Valerie Schini-Kerth (UMR 7175 Centre National de la Recherche Scientifique, Université de Strasbourg, Département de Pharmacologie et Physicochimie, Faculté de Pharmacie, Illkirch, France) for lending us the isolated-organ chamber.

Author details
[1]UMR DIATHEC, EA 7294, Centre Européen d'Etude du Diabète, Université de Strasbourg, Fédération de Médecine Translationnelle de Strasbourg, Bld René Leriche, 67200 Strasbourg, France. [2]Equipe de Chimie Analytique des Molécules BioActives, IPHC-LC4, UMR 7178, Faculté de Pharmacie, Ilkirch, France. [3]Structure d'Endocrinologie, Diabète, Nutrition et Addictologie, Pôle NUDE, Hôpitaux Universitaires de Strasbourg, (HUS), 67000 Strasbourg, France.

References

1. Nolan CJ, Damm P, Prentki M. Type 2 diabetes across generations: from pathophysiology to prevention and management. Lancet. 2011;378(9786):169–81.
2. Schwenk RW, Vogel H, Schurmann A. Genetic and epigenetic control of metabolic health. Mol Metab. 2013;2(4):337–47.
3. Dabelea D, Pettitt DJ. Intrauterine diabetic environment confers risks for type 2 diabetes mellitus and obesity in the offspring, in addition to genetic susceptibility. J Pediatr Endocrinol Metab. 2001;14(8):1085–91.
4. Ludwig DS. Dietary glycemic index and obesity. J Nutr. 2000;130(2S Suppl): 280S–3S.
5. Tappy L, Le KA. Metabolic effects of fructose and the worldwide increase in obesity. Physiol Rev. 2010;90(1):23–46.
6. Elliott SS, Keim NL, Stern JS, Teff K, Havel PJ. Fructose, weight gain, and the insulin resistance syndrome. Am J Clin Nutr. 2002;76(5):911–22.
7. Ruxton CH, Gardner EJ, McNulty HM. Is sugar consumption detrimental to health? A review of the evidence 1995–2006. Crit Rev Food Sci Nutr. 2010;50(1):1–19.
8. Welsh JA, Sharma A, Abramson JL, Vaccarino V, Gillespie C, Vos MB. Caloric sweetener consumption and dyslipidemia among US adults. JAMA. 2010;303(15):1490–7.
9. Dekker MJ, Su Q, Baker C, Rutledge AC, Adeli K. Fructose: a highly lipogenic nutrient implicated in insulin resistance, hepatic steatosis, and the metabolic syndrome. Am J Physiol Endocrinol Metab. 2010;299(5):E685–94.
10. Vasdev S, Longerich L, Gill V. Prevention of fructose-induced hypertension by dietary vitamins. Clin Biochem. 2004;37(1):1–9.
11. Basu S, Yoffe P, Hills N, Lustig RH. The relationship of sugar to population-level diabetes prevalence: an econometric analysis of repeated cross-sectional data. PLoS One. 2013;8(2):e57873.
12. van Dam RM, Willett WC, Rimm EB, Stampfer MJ, Hu FB. Dietary fat and meat intake in relation to risk of type 2 diabetes in men. Diabetes Care. 2002;25(3):417–24.
13. RHaP D, editor. Ellenberg and Rifkin's Diabetes Mellitus: Theory and Practice. 4th ed. New York: Elsevier; 1990.
14. Bugianesi E, Moscatiello S, Ciaravella MF, Marchesini G. Insulin resistance in nonalcoholic fatty liver disease. Curr Pharm Des. 2010;16(17):1941–51.
15. Adams LA, Waters OR, Knuiman MW, Elliott RR, Olynyk JK. NAFLD as a risk factor for the development of diabetes and the metabolic syndrome: an eleven-year follow-up study. Am J Gastroenterol. 2009;104(4):861–7.
16. Targher G, Marra F, Marchesini G. Increased risk of cardiovascular disease in non-alcoholic fatty liver disease: causal effect or epiphenomenon? Diabetologia. 2008;51(11):1947–53.
17. Browning JD, Horton JD. Molecular mediators of hepatic steatosis and liver injury. J Clin Invest. 2004;114(2):147–52.
18. Takaki A, Kawai D, Yamamoto K. Multiple hits, including oxidative stress, as pathogenesis and treatment target in non-alcoholic steatohepatitis (NASH). Int J Mol Sci. 2013;14(10):20704–28.
19. Droge W. Free radicals in the physiological control of cell function. Physiol Rev. 2002;82(1):47–95.
20. Valko M, Leibfritz D, Moncol J, Cronin MT, Mazur M, Telser J. Free radicals and antioxidants in normal physiological functions and human disease. Int J Biochem Cell Biol. 2007;39(1):44–84.
21. Dal-Ros S, Zoll J, Lang AL, Auger C, Keller N, Bronner C, et al. Chronic intake of red wine polyphenols by young rats prevents aging-induced endothelial dysfunction and decline in physical performance: role of NADPH oxidase. Biochem Biophys Res Commun. 2011;404(2):743–9.
22. Bloch-Damti A, Bashan N. Proposed mechanisms for the induction of insulin resistance by oxidative stress. Antioxid Redox Signal. 2005;7(11–12):1553–67.
23. Orasanu G, Plutzky J. The pathologic continuum of diabetic vascular disease. J Am Coll Cardiol. 2009;53(5 Suppl):S35–42.
24. Sena CM, Pereira AM, Seica R. Endothelial dysfunction - a major mediator of diabetic vascular disease. Biochim Biophys Acta. 2013;1832(12):2216–31.
25. Islam MS, du Loots T. Experimental rodent models of type 2 diabetes: a review. Methods Find Exp Clin Pharmacol. 2009;31(4):249–61.
26. Kim JH, Nishina PM, Naggert JK. Genetic models for non insulin dependent diabetes mellitus in rodents. J Basic Clin Physiol Pharmacol. 1998;9(2–4):325–45.
27. Liu RH, Mizuta M, Kurose T, Matsukura S. Early events involved in the development of insulin resistance in Zucker fatty rat. Int J Obes Relat Metab Disord. 2002;26(3):318–26.
28. Dourmashkin JT, Chang GQ, Gayles EC, Hill JO, Fried SK, Julien C, et al. Different forms of obesity as a function of diet composition. Int J Obes (Lond). 2005;29(11):1368–78.
29. Lenzen S. The mechanisms of alloxan- and streptozotocin-induced diabetes. Diabetologia. 2008;51(2):216–26.
30. Auberval N, Dal S, Bietiger W, Pinget M, Jeandidier N, Maillard-Pedracini E, et al. Metabolic and oxidative stress markers in Wistar rats after 2 months on a high-fat diet. Diabetol Metab Syndr. 2014;6:130.
31. O'Rahilly S, Burnett MA, Smith RF, Darley JH, Turner RC. Haemolysis affects insulin but not C-peptide immunoassay. Diabetologia. 1987;30(6):394–6.
32. Shapiro A, Mu W, Roncal C, Cheng KY, Johnson RJ, Scarpace PJ. Fructose-induced leptin resistance exacerbates weight gain in response to subsequent high-fat feeding. Am J Physiol Regul Integr Comp Physiol. 2008;295(5):R1370–5.
33. Kleiner DE, Brunt EM, Van Natta M, Behling C, Contos MJ, Cummings OW, et al. Design and validation of a histological scoring system for nonalcoholic fatty liver disease. Hepatology. 2005;41(6):1313–21.
34. Dal S, Jeandidier N, Schaschkow A, Spizzo AH, Seyfritz E, Sookhareea C, et al. Portal or subcutaneous insulin infusion: efficacy and impact on liver inflammation. Fundamental & clinical pharmacology. 2015.
35. Dal S, Jeandidier N, Seyfritz E, Bietiger W, Peronet C, Moreau F, et al. Oxidative stress status and liver tissue defenses in diabetic rats during intensive subcutaneous insulin therapy. Exp Biol Med. 2015.
36. Bradford MM. A rapid and sensitive method for the quantitation of microgram quantities of protein utilizing the principle of protein-dye binding. Anal Biochem. 1976;72:248–54.
37. Du L, Heaney AP. Regulation of adipose differentiation by fructose and GluT5. Mol Endocrinol. 2012;26(10):1773–82.
38. Faeh D, Minehira K, Schwarz JM, Periasamy R, Park S, Tappy L. Effect of fructose overfeeding and fish oil administration on hepatic de novo lipogenesis and insulin sensitivity in healthy men. Diabetes. 2005;54(7):1907–13.
39. Le KA, Faeh D, Stettler R, Ith M, Kreis R, Vermathen P, et al. A 4-wk high-fructose diet alters lipid metabolism without affecting insulin sensitivity or ectopic lipids in healthy humans. Am J Clin Nutr. 2006;84(6):1374–9.
40. Coate KC, Scott M, Farmer B, Moore MC, Smith M, Roop J, et al. Chronic consumption of a high-fat/high-fructose diet renders the liver incapable of net hepatic glucose uptake. Am J Physiol Endocrinol Metab. 2010;299(6):E887–98.
41. Feinman RD, Fine EJ. Fructose in perspective. Nutr Metab. 2013;10(1):45.
42. Koo HY, Wallig MA, Chung BH, Nara TY, Cho BH, Nakamura MT. Dietary fructose induces a wide range of genes with distinct shift in carbohydrate and lipid metabolism in fed and fasted rat liver. Biochim Biophys Acta. 2008;1782(5):341–8.
43. Lopez-Soldado I, Zafra D, Duran J, Adrover A, Calbo J, Guinovart JJ. Liver glycogen reduces food intake and attenuates obesity in a high-fat diet-fed mouse model. Diabetes. 2015;64(3):796–807.
44. Ros S, Garcia-Rocha M, Calbo J, Guinovart JJ. Restoration of hepatic glycogen deposition reduces hyperglycaemia, hyperphagia and gluconeogenic enzymes in a streptozotocin-induced model of diabetes in rats. Diabetologia. 2011;54(10):2639–48.
45. Castro MC, Francini F, Schinella G, Caldiz CI, Zubiria MG, Gagliardino JJ, et al. Apocynin administration prevents the changes induced by a fructose-rich diet on rat liver metabolism and the antioxidant system. Clin Sci. 2012;123(12):681–92.
46. Farese RV, Sajan MP, Standaert ML. Insulin-sensitive protein kinases (atypical protein kinase C and protein kinase B/Akt): actions and defects in obesity and type II diabetes. Exp Biol Med. 2005;230(9):593–605.
47. Sutti S, Jindal A, Locatelli I, Vacchiano M, Gigliotti L, Bozzola C, et al. Adaptive immune responses triggered by oxidative stress contribute to hepatic inflammation in NASH. Hepatology. 2014;59(3):886–97.
48. Tsochatzis E, Papatheodoridis GV, Archimandritis AJ. The evolving role of leptin and adiponectin in chronic liver diseases. Am J Gastroenterol. 2006;101(11):2629–40.

49. Lee UE, Friedman SL. Mechanisms of hepatic fibrogenesis. Best Pract Res Clin Gastroenterol. 2011;25(2):195–206.
50. Day CP, James OF. Steatohepatitis: a tale of two "hits"? Gastroenterology. 1998;114(4):842–5.
51. Masayasu I. Protective mechanism against reactive oxygen species. In: Arias IM, Boyer JL, Fausto, Jakoby WB, Schachter DA, Shafritz DA, editors. The liver: Biology and Pathobiology. New York: Raven Press, Ltd; 1994. p. 443–59.
52. Monnier L, Mas E, Ginet C, Michel F, Villon L, Cristol JP, et al. Activation of oxidative stress by acute glucose fluctuations compared with sustained chronic hyperglycemia in patients with type 2 diabetes. JAMA. 2006;295(14):1681–7.
53. Nieto N, Greenwel P, Friedman SL, Zhang F, Dannenberg AJ, Cederbaum AI. Ethanol and arachidonic acid increase alpha 2(I) collagen expression in rat hepatic stellate cells overexpressing cytochrome P450 2E1. Role of H2O2 and cyclooxygenase-2. J Biol Chem. 2000;275(26):20136–45.
54. Rector RS, Thyfault JP, Uptergrove GM, Morris EM, Naples SP, Borengasser SJ, et al. Mitochondrial dysfunction precedes insulin resistance and hepatic steatosis and contributes to the natural history of non-alcoholic fatty liver disease in an obese rodent model. J Hepatol. 2010;52(5):727–36.
55. Targher G, Chonchol M, Miele L, Zoppini G, Pichiri I, Muggeo M. Nonalcoholic fatty liver disease as a contributor to hypercoagulation and thrombophilia in the metabolic syndrome. Semin Thromb Hemost. 2009;35(3):277–87.
56. Shi Y, Vanhoutte PM. Reactive oxygen-derived free radicals are key to the endothelial dysfunction of diabetes. J Diabetes. 2009;1(3):151–62.
57. Arcaro G, Zamboni M, Rossi L, Turcato E, Covi G, Armellini F, et al. Body fat distribution predicts the degree of endothelial dysfunction in uncomplicated obesity. Int J Obes Relat Metab Disord. 1999;23(9):936–42.
58. Vehkavaara S, Seppala-Lindroos A, Westerbacka J, Groop PH, Yki-Jarvinen H. In vivo endothelial dysfunction characterizes patients with impaired fasting glucose. Diabetes Care. 1999;22(12):2055–60.
59. Steinberg HO, Chaker H, Leaming R, Johnson A, Brechtel G, Baron AD. Obesity/insulin resistance is associated with endothelial dysfunction. Implications for the syndrome of insulin resistance. J Clin Invest. 1996;97(11):2601–10.
60. Griendling KK, FitzGerald GA. Oxidative stress and cardiovascular injury: Part II: animal and human studies. Circulation. 2003;108(17):2034–40.
61. Cleland SJ, Sattar N, Petrie JR, Forouhi NG, Elliott HL, Connell JM. Endothelial dysfunction as a possible link between C-reactive protein levels and cardiovascular disease. Clin Sci. 2000;98(5):531–5.
62. Zhang H, Dellsperger KC, Zhang C. The link between metabolic abnormalities and endothelial dysfunction in type 2 diabetes: an update. Basic Res Cardiol. 2012;107(1):237.

The role of lipid droplet formation in the protection of unsaturated fatty acids against palmitic acid induced lipotoxicity to rat insulin-producing cells

Thomas Plötz, Magnus Hartmann, Sigurd Lenzen and Matthias Elsner*

Abstract

Background: Type 2 diabetes is associated with increased plasma concentrations of non-esterified fatty acids (NEFAs), which trigger pancreatic β-cell dysfunction and apoptosis. Only long-chain saturated NEFAs induced lipotoxicity in rat insulin-producing cells in in vitro experiments, whereas unsaturated NEFAs were not toxic. Some unsaturated NEFAs even protected against lipotoxicity. In former studies it was suggested that long-chain unsaturated NEFAs, which induce the formation of lipid droplets, can cause sequestration of palmitic acid into lipid droplets. In the present structure-activity-relationship study the correlation between lipid droplet formation and the protection against palmitic acid induced lipotoxicity by unsaturated NEFAs in rat insulin-producing cells was examined.

Methods: Rat insulin-producing RINm5F and INS-1E tissue culture cells were incubated in the presence of palmitic acid and unsaturated NEFAs with different chain lengths and different numbers of double bonds. The expression of the lipid droplet associated proteins perilipin 1 and 2 was repressed by the shRNA technique and the expression analyzed by qRT-PCR and Western blotting. Viability was measured by MTT assay and the accumulation of lipid droplets was quantified by fluorescence microscopy after Oil Red O staining.

Results: Long-chain unsaturated NEFAs strongly induce the formation of lipid droplets in rat insulin-producing RINm5F and INS-1E cells. In RINm5F cells incubated with 11-eicosenoic acid (C20:1) 27 % of the cell area was covered by lipid droplets corresponding to a 25-fold increase in comparison with control cells. On the other hand the saturated NEFA palmitic acid only induced minor lipid droplet formation. Viability analyses revealed only a minor toxicity of unsaturated NEFAs, whereas the cells were markedly sensitive to palmitic acid. Long-chain unsaturated NEFAs antagonized palmitic acid induced lipotoxicity during co-incubation, whereby no correlation existed between protection and the ability of lipid droplet formation. Perilipin 1 and 2 expression was decreased after incubation with C20:1 to about 80 % by shRNA. For the protective effect of long-chain unsaturated NEFAs against lipotoxicity of saturated NEFAs repression of perilipin was not of crucial importance.

Conclusions: Long-chain unsaturated fatty acids protected rat insulin-producing cells against lipotoxicity of saturated fatty acids. This protective effect was not dependent on lipid droplet formation. Thus lipid droplet formation is apparently not essential for the protective effect of unsaturated NEFAs against palmitic acid toxicity.

Keywords: Type 2 diabetes, Non-esterified fatty acids, Lipid droplets, Perilipin, Pancreatic β-cell, Peroxisomal β-oxidation

* Correspondence: elsner.matthias@mh-hannover.de
Institute of Clinical Biochemistry, Hannover Medical School, 30623 Hannover, Germany

Background

Type 2 diabetes mellitus (T2DM) is one of the most prevalent metabolic diseases worldwide caused by insulin resistance of the peripheral tissues and impaired insulin secretion of pancreatic β-cells [1]. Physical inactivity and hypercaloric diets, rich in carbohydrates and saturated fats, are thought to be responsible for an increase in body weight and can cause the metabolic syndrome [2–4], which is characterized by obesity, hypertension and dyslipidemia, and often precedes the manifestation of T2DM. Chronically elevated plasma levels of non-esterified fatty acids (NEFAs), which are associated with the metabolic syndrome [5], can suppress insulin secretion and cause β-cell dysfunction and loss by apoptosis. This so-called lipotoxicity is subject to intensive research and scientific debate. Only long-chain saturated NEFAs induce lipotoxicity in rodent insulin-producing cells in in-vitro experiments, whereas unsaturated NEFAs are not toxic [6]. Short- and medium-chain fatty acids are metabolized in the mitochondrial β-oxidation, whereas long-chain fatty acids can be metabolized in the mitochondria but also in the peroxisomes when cells were exposed to high NEFA concentrations [7, 8]. Very long-chain fatty acids are exclusive substrates for the peroxisomal β-oxidation [8–10]. The electron transfer in the first step of the peroxisomal β-oxidation catalyzed by the enzyme acyl-CoA-oxidase results in high concentrations of hydrogen peroxide, which can cause cellular damage [8]. In contrast to other cell types pancreatic β-cells do not express the H_2O_2 inactivating enzyme catalase [11, 12]. This can explain why long-chain saturated fatty acids are harmful to rat insulin-producing β-cells and can cause apoptosis [7].

On the other hand unsaturated NEFAs are not toxic to rat insulin-producing cells and can even protect against lipotoxicity. The molecular mechanism of protection has not yet been fully elucidated, but experimental evidence has been provided that the formation of lipid droplets (LDs) by unsaturated NEFAs may be involved in the protection against lipotoxicity [13]. Specifically it has been suggested that long-chain unsaturated NEFAs can induce the formation of LDs, which may allow the sequestration of the toxic NEFA palmitic acid (PA) into these droplets. NEFAs converted into triglycerides and stored in LDs have been considered to be less toxic than NEFAs, which are readily metabolized [13]. For the formation of LDs perilipins are crucially important [14–17]. These proteins are associated with the LD surface and protect the stored triglycerides against hydrolysis by the hormone-sensitive lipases. Perilipins are thus important regulators of intracellular lipid storage [18, 19]. In the present study we therefore suppressed perilipin 1 and 2 expression in rat insulin-producing cell lines using the shRNA technique and analyzed the effects on LD formation and PA-induced toxicity. In a comprehensive approach we correlated the structural requirements of saturated and unsaturated NEFAs with different chain lengths between C12 and C24 with respect to LD formation and toxicity in rat insulin-producing cells.

Our results show that unsaturated NEFAs were able to antagonize palmitic acid induced lipotoxicity. However, we observed no correlation between protection and the ability of lipid droplet formation in rat insulin-producing cells.

Methods

Tissue culture of insulin-producing cells

The stable insulin-producing RINm5F cell line was established from a radiation-induced rat islet cell tumor by Gazdar et al. [20] and purchased from ATCC (American Type Culture Collection, Manassas, VA, USA; order# ATCC CRL-11605). Cells were cultured in RPMI 1640 medium supplemented with 10 mM glucose, 10 % (v/v) fetal calf serum (Biowest, Nuaillé, France), penicillin and streptomycin in a humidified atmosphere at 37 °C and 5 % CO_2 [12]. The insulin-producing INS-1E cell line was clonally selected from a radiation-induced rat insulinoma and showed a stable phenotype for more than 100 passages [21, 22]. INS-1E cells were kindly provided by Prof. Claes Wollheim (University of Geneva, Switzerland). These cells were cultured in RPMI 1640 medium supplemented with 10 mM glucose, 10 % fetal calf serum (FCS), penicillin and streptomycin, 10 mM Hepes (Serva, Heidelberg, Germany), 2 mM glutamine, 1 mM sodium-pyruvate (Sigma-Aldrich, Munich, Germany), and 50 μM of 2-mercaptoethanol in a humidified atmosphere at 37 °C and 5 % CO_2.

NEFA incubation

For NEFA incubations a 50 mM stock solution was freshly prepared using 90 % ethanol as a solvent. NEFAs are bound to fatty acid free bovine serum albumin (BSA) in RPMI 1640 culture medium supplemented with 1 % fetal calf serum. The ratio between NEFA and BSA is 0.5 mM NEFA to 1 % BSA. For other NEFA concentrations the BSA concentration is adapted according to this ratio. C12:0 (dodecanoic acid/lauric acid), C12:1 (cis-5-dodecenoic acid), C14:0 (tetradecanoic acid/myristic acid), C14:1 (cis-9-tetradecenoic acid/myristoleic acid), C16:0 (hexadecanoic acid/palmitic acid), C16:1 (cis-9-hexadecenoic acid/palmitoleic acid), C18:0 (octadecanoic acid/stearic acid), C18:1 (cis-9-octadecenoic acid/oleic acid), C18:2 (cis-9, 12-octadienoic acid/linoleic acid), α-C18:3 (cis-9, 12, 15-octatrienoic acid/alpha-linolenic acid), γ-C18:3 (cis-6, 9, 12-octatrienoic acid/gamma-linolenic acid), C18:4 (cis-6, 9, 12, 15-octatetraenoic acid/stearidonic acid), C20:0 (eicosanoic acid/arachidic acid), C20:1 (cis-11-eicosenoic acid/gondoic acid), C20:2 (cis-11, 14-eicosadienoic acid), C20:3 (cis-8, 11, 14-eicosatrienoic acid), C20:4 (cis-5, 8, 11, 14-eicosatetraenoic acid/arachidonic acid), C20:5 (cis-5, 8, 11, 14, 17-eicosapentaenoic acid), C22:0 (docosanoic acid/behenic acid), C22:1 (cis-13-docosenoic acid/erucic acid), C22:2 (cis-13, 16-docosadienoic acid), C22:4 (cis-7, 10, 13, 16-docosatetraenoic acid), C22:6 (cis-4, 7, 10, 13, 16, 19-docosahexaenoic acid), C24:0 (tetracosanoic acid/lignoceric acid), C24:1 (cis-15-tetracosenoic acid/nervonic acid) were purchased from Sigma-Aldrich (Munich, Germany) or Larodan (Malmö, Sweden).

Lipid droplet staining with Oil Red O

RINm5F cells were cultured for 24 h and afterwards exposed to 100 μM of different unsaturated NEFAs with different chain lengths and different numbers of double bonds (C18:1 to 18:4, C20:1 to C20:5, C22:1 to C22:6) for another 24 h. Cells were trypsinized and fixed in paraformaldehyde for 15 min at room temperature. Thereafter cells were stained with Oil Red O solution (Sigma-Aldrich, Munich, Germany) and washed twice with PBS (phosphate buffered saline). Lipid droplet formation was analyzed by fluorescence microscopy and the area within the cells was quantified by the use of the Olympus xcellence software (Olympus, Hamburg, Germany) at 546 nm excitation and 580 nm emission. For each incubation condition five to seven coincidentally selected images, each containing 30 to 100 cells, were used to quantify the proportion of the lipid droplet area to the total cell area with the phase analysis module of the xcellence software.

Assessment of cell viability

RINm5F insulin-producing cells were seeded at 2.5×10^4 cells/well in 100 μl culture medium onto 96-well plates and allowed to attach for 24 h before they were incubated at 37 °C with combinations of different unsaturated NEFAs and PA (palmitic acid/hexadecanoic acid/C16:0) for further 24 h. Cell viability and the ability to protect against PA-induced toxicity was determined by a microplate-based MTT assay (3-(4,5-dimethylthiazol-2-yl)-2,5-diphenyl tetrazolium bromide, Serva, Heidelberg, Germany) [23].

Lentivirus preparation and transduction of insulin-producing cells

Lentiviral vector particles were produced as described [24]. In brief, $5x10^6$ 293FT cells were transfected with the packaging plasmid pPAX2 (37.5 μg), the envelope plasmid pcDNA-MDG (7.5 μg), and the transfer plasmids pLV-U6-sh-rPlin1, pLV-U6-sh-rPlin2 or pLV-U6-sh-NTC (22.5 μg) by calcium phosphate precipitation. The transfer plasmids were produced by Sirion Biotech (Munich, Germany) and validated for suppression efficiencies > 85 %. The virus particles were harvested from the culture medium 48 h after transfection and purified by ultrafiltration columns at 3000 g for 25 min (Amicon Ultra Ultracel-100 K, Millipore, Schwalbach, Germany). Virus titers (typically $5x10^7$ infectious particles) were quantified by a TaqMan qPCR assay as described elsewhere [24]. RINm5F-Tet3G and INS-1E-Tet3G cells were transduced with either the sh-rPlin1, sh-rPlin2 or sh-NTC virus with a multiplicity of infection (MOI) followed by a selection with puromycin (2.5 μg/ml).

Gene expression analyses

RNA from RINm5F and INS-1E cells was isolated with the RNeasy Kit (Qiagen, Hilden, Germany) according to the manufacturer's instructions. The quality of the total RNA was verified by comparing the intensities of the 28S and 18S rRNA bands in agarose gel electrophoresis. Two microgram total RNA was reverse transcribed into cDNA using the RevertAid H Minus M-MuLV Reverse Transcriptase (Thermo Fisher Scientific, Schwerte, Germany) and random hexamer primers (Life Technologies, Karlsruhe, Germany). The *Plin1* or *Plin2* expression in 10 ng cDNA was quantified by a SYBR Green based assay (GoTaq Green Master Mix; Promega, Mannheim, Germany) and performed on an Opticon fluorescence detection system (Biorad, Munich, Germany) with the following protocol: Samples were initially denaturated at 95 °C for 2 min followed by up to 40 PCR cycles. Each PCR cycle comprised a denaturation at 94 °C for 30 s, an annealing at 60 °C for 30 s, and an extension at 72 °C for 30 s. The specificity of the amplification was verified by melting point analysis. For each sample amplification was performed in triplicate. The *Plin1* and *Plin2* expression data were normalized against the geometric mean of the three reference genes *actin beta* (*Actb*), peptidylprolyl isomerase A (*PPIA*), and *TATA box binding protein* (*TBP*) with the software qBasePlus (Biogazelle, Zwijnaarde, Belgium). Primers for qPCR analyses were synthesized by Life Technologies (Karlsruhe, Germany): Plin1-fw (5′ GATTCTGCTTTGCA GCGTGAA 3′), Plin1-rv (5′ CAGGACTCTCTGGAGCA CATTC 3′), Plin2-fw (5′ TCGTCTCTCAGCTCTCCTGT 3′), Plin2-rv (5′ TAGGTGGAGCTCACCAAGGG 3′), Actb-fw (5′ GCGTCCACCCGCGAGTACAA 3′), Actb-fw (5′ TTGCACATGCCGGAGCCGTT 3′), PPIA-fw (5′ TT GCAGACGCCGCTGTCTCTT 3′), PPIA-rv (5′ TGGAA CTTTGTCTGCAAACAGCTCG 3′) TBP-fw (5′ CAGCT CGGCGCACCGTACAT 3′), TBP-rv (5′ TCTGGGTTAT CGTCACGCACCA 3′).

Western blot analyses

Whole cell extracts were prepared in radioimmune precipitation assay buffer according to the manufacturer's recommendation (Sigma) supplemented with complete protease inhibitor mixture (Roche Diagnostics, Mannheim, Germany). Protein content was determined by the BCA assay (Thermo Fisher Scientific, Rockford, IL, USA). 30 μg of total protein were separated by a 10 % SDS-PAGE and electroblotted to nitrocellulose membranes (GE Healthcare, Buckinghamshire, UK). Nonspecific binding sites of the membranes were blocked with 5 % nonfat dry milk for 1 h at room temperature. The membranes were incubated with specific primary antibodies overnight at 4 °C. The following antibodies from Santa Cruz Biotechnology (Santa Cruz, CA, USA) were used: anti-Perilipin 1 (H-300, diluted 1:2000), anti-Perilipin 2 (H-80, diluted 1:200), and anti-β-actin (sc-1615, diluted 1:250). The excess of primary antibody was removed by three washing steps with washing buffer (PBS, 0.1 % Tween 20, 0.1 % BSA). Subsequently, the membranes were incubated with peroxidase-labeled secondary anti-rabbit antibodies at a dilution of 1:20,000 at room temperature for 1 h. Protein bands were visualized by chemiluminescence using the ECL detection system (GE Healthcare). As a loading control the expression of β-actin was analyzed after stripping the blots with Reblot Pus solution (Merck-Millipore, Darmstadt, Germany) according to the manufacturer's manual. Protein band intensity was quantified and normalized to β-actin though densitometry with the Gel-Pro Analyzer program (version 6.0, Media Cybernetics, Silver Spring, MD, USA).

Statistical analysis

Data are expressed as means ± SEM. Statistical analyses were performed using ANOVA plus Dunnett's or Bonferroni's test for multiple comparisons, unless stated otherwise (GraphPad Prism5, San Diego, CA, USA).

Results

Induction of lipid droplet formation by NEFAs in insulin-producing cells

Long-chain monounsaturated NEFAs (C18:1, C20:1, C22:1) strongly induced the formation of LDs in rat insulin-producing RINm5F cells. More than 25 % of the cell area of RINm5F cells incubated with the long-chain NEFA gondoic acid (C20:1, 100 μM) was covered by LDs, which corresponds to a 16-fold increase in comparison to untreated cells. On the other hand incubation with medium-chain and long-chain monounsaturated NEFAs (C12:1, C14:1, C16:1) and with a very long-chain NEFA (C24:1) showed no significant increase in LD formation in comparison to control cells (Fig. 1). In contrast to unsaturated NEFAs none of the analyzed saturated NEFAs (C12:0 to C24:0) caused significant increases in LD content in RINm5F cells.

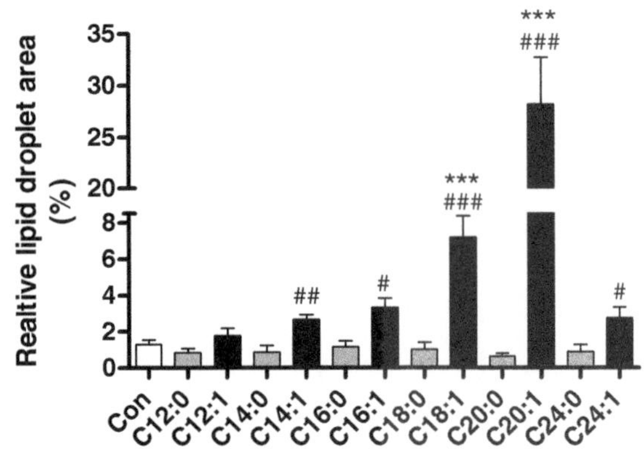

Fig. 1 Lipid droplet formation in rat insulin-producing RINm5F cells after incubation with saturated and monounsaturated NEFAs of increasing chain length. RINm5F cells were incubated with different medium- and long-chain saturated and monounsaturated NEFAs (100 μM) for 24 h. Thereafter cells were fixed and stained with Oil Red O. Lipid droplet formation was analyzed by fluorescence microscopy and quantified using the software xcellence rt. Data are means ± SEM of $n = 3$. ***$p < 0.001$ compared to control cells (Dunnett's Multiple Comparison Test). #$p < 0.05$, ##$p < 0.01$, ###$p < 0.005$ compared to saturated NEFA with the same chain length (Student's t-test)

Effect of saturation level of unsaturated NEFAs on lipid droplet formation in insulin-producing cells

In the group of unsaturated NEFAs with the chain length of C18 with different numbers of double bonds (C18:x) only C18:1 and C18:2 revealed a significant up to 15 % increase in the cell area covered with LDs (Fig. 2a). However, the unsaturated NEFAs C18:3 and C18:4 showed no increase in LD formation compared to the control condition. With 27 % LDs of the cell area C20:1 induced maximal lipid droplet formation. With an increasing number of double bonds the LD area declined to < 4 % after incubation with C20:4 or C20:5 (Fig. 2b), which was not significantly higher than in the control condition. The unsaturated C22:x NEFA group revealed the same tendency with the greatest LD formation after incubation with the monounsaturated C22:1 and a steady decrease with increasing numbers of double bonds up to C22:6 (Fig. 2c).

Antagonistic effect of saturated fatty acids against lipid droplet formation

Long-chain unsaturated NEFAs induced LD formation, whereas long-chain saturated NEFAs were not able to form LDs. A co-incubation experiment of both saturated and unsaturated NEFAs revealed a decline of LD formation typically induced by long-chain unsaturated NEFAs. Palmitic acid (C16:0), which is the physiologically and nutritionally most important saturated fatty acid, antagonized the LD formation by C18:1 and to a lesser extent

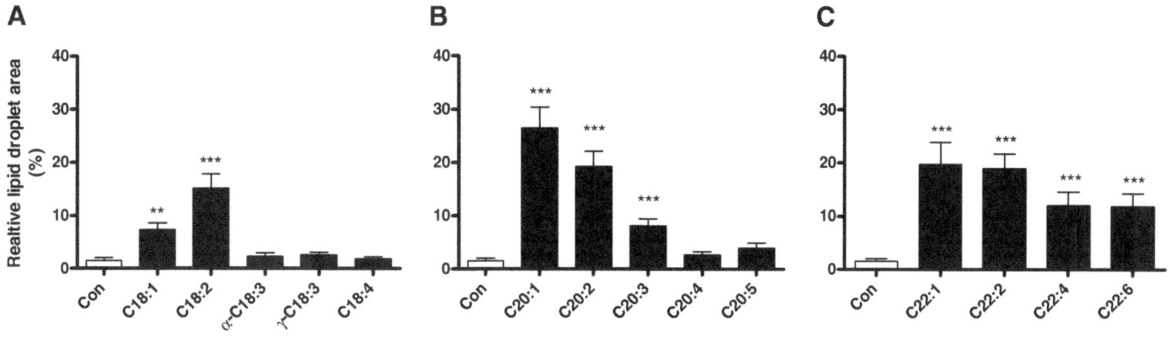

Fig. 2 Lipid droplet formation in rat insulin-producing RINm5F cells after incubation with unsaturated NEFAs with a different degree of unsaturation. RINm5F cells were incubated with C18:x (**a**), C20:x (**b**) and C22:x (**c**) NEFAs (100 μM) with different numbers of double bonds for 24 h. Thereafter cells were fixed and stained with Oil Red O. Lipid droplet formation was analyzed by fluorescence microscopy and quantified using the software xcellence rt. Data are given as means ± SEM from 5 to 8 individual experiments. $^{**}p < 0.01$, $^{***}p < 0.001$ compared with control cells (Dunnett's Multiple Comparison Test)

by C20:1 (Fig. 3a-b). The antagonistic effect increased with the increase of the proportion of C16:0 in the mixtures with C18:1 and C20:1.

Toxicity of long-chain NEFAs in insulin-producing cells

Long-chain saturated NEFAs at a 100 μM concentration were highly toxic to insulin-producing RINm5F cells. On the other hand the corresponding unsaturated NEFAs with the same chain lengths showed only a minimal or no significant toxicity at a concentration of 100 μM compared to the toxic effect of palmitic acid with a viability of 31 % (Additional file 1: Figure S1). Generally no correlation between the toxicity and the number of double bonds could be identified.

Protective capacity of long-chain unsaturated NEFAs against the toxicity of palmitic acid in insulin-producing cells in dependence on chain length and saturation level

The protective capacity of long-chain unsaturated NEFAs was analyzed in co-incubation experiments of 200 μM PA with increasing concentrations of unsaturated NEFAs to determine the unsaturated NEFA concentration necessary to achieve a 50 % viability reduction (Table 1). The best protection against PA-induced toxicity in RINm5F insulin-producing cells was provided by C20:5 with a half-maximally effective protective concentration of 5.4 μM. Generally NEFAs of the C20:x group revealed the highest protective potency. In the NEFA groups of C20:x and C22:x the monounsaturated NEFAs were less protective than the polyunsaturated NEFAs. A concentration of

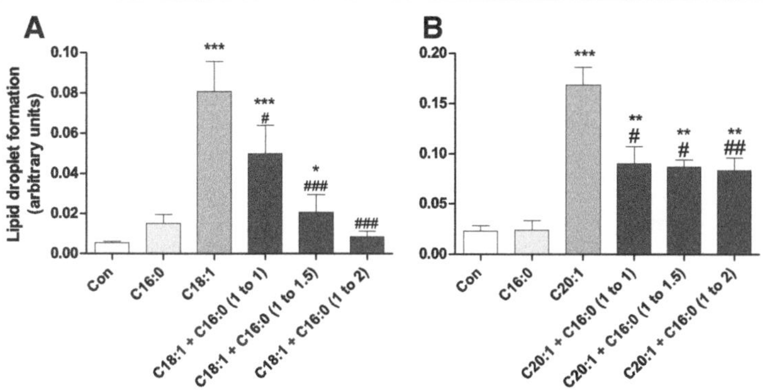

Fig. 3 Lipid droplet formation in co-incubation experiments with unsaturated NEFAs in combination with increasing PA concentrations. RINm5F cells were incubated with 100 μM of the unsaturated NEFAs C18:1 (**a**) or C20:1 (**b**) in combination with increasing concentrations of the saturated NEFA C16:0 for 24 h. Thereafter cells were fixed, stained with Oil Red O and analyzed by fluorescence microscopy. Lipid droplet formation per cell was quantified by the software xcellence rt. $^{*}p < 0.05$, $^{**}p < 0.01$, $^{***}p < 0.001$ compared to control cells (Dunnett's Multiple Comparison Test). $^{\#}p < 0.05$, $^{\#\#}p < 0.01$, $^{\#\#\#}p < 0.005$ compared to unsaturated NEFA only (Student's *t*-test)

Table 1 Protective effect of unsaturated NEFAs against PA-induced toxicity and relative lipid droplet area linked with the correlation coefficient for each group

NEFA	Half-maximal protective concentration (μM)	Lipid droplet area after incubation with 100 μM NEFA (% of cell area)	Correlation coefficient for each group	*P* value for each group
C18:1	32.8 ± 2.2 (6)	7.3 ± 1.3 (5)	C18-FFA: +0.52	C18-FFA: 0.37
C18:2	11.4 ± 1.2 (5)	15.1 ± 2.8 (5)		
α-C18:3	24.0 ± 1.8 (4)	2.4 ± 0.6 (5)		
γ-C18:3	27.2 ± 1.6 (4)	2.6 ± 0.5 (5)		
C18:4	> 100.0 (5)	1.9 ± 0.3 (5)		
C20:1	17.2 ± 1.6 (6)	26.5 ± 4.9 (5)	C20-FFA: −0.63	C20-FFA: 0.25
C20:2	6.0 ± 0.6 (4)	19.2 ± 2.9 (5)		
C20:3	10.4 ± 1.2 (4)	8.1 ± 1.3 (5)		
C20:4	8.6 ± 0.6 (4)	2.7 ± 0.6 (5)		
C20:5	5.4 ± 0.6 (4)	3.9 ± 1.0 (5)		
C22:1	88.6 ± 22.8 (6)	19.7 ± 4.1 (5)	C22-FFA: −0.89	C22-FFA: 0.11
C22:2	42.0 ± 6.8 (4)	18.9 ± 2.7 (5)		
C22:4	8.6 ± 1.4 (5)	12.1 ± 2.5 (5)		
C22:6	10.8 ± 3.2 (5)	11.8 ± 2.4 (5)		
Total value			0.04	0.89

The protective concentration of the unsaturated NEFAs was determined in co-incubation experiments for 24 h with 200 μM PA resulting in a 50 % cell viability measured by MTT assay. The protective effects were calculated by nonlinear regression analyses. Lipid droplet and MTT data are means ± SEM with the number of independent experiments in parenthesis. Correlation coefficients and *P* values were determined by Pearson correlation

17.2 μM for C20:1 and of 88.6 μM for C22:1 respectively was required to antagonize PA toxicity by 50 %. With a rise in the number of double bonds in these two groups the protective potential increased. The group of C18:x unsaturated NEFAs revealed the weakest protection of all tested groups. There were no significant differences in the protective potency against PA-induced toxicity between the omega-9 fatty acid oleic acid (C18:1), the omega-6 fatty acid γ-linolenic acid (γ-C18:3) and the omega-3 fatty acid α-linolenic acid (α-C18:3). The lowest protective potency exhibited the omega-3 fatty acid C18:4.

Lack of correlation between protective potency against PA-induced toxicity and lipid droplet formation in insulin-producing cells

The most efficient unsaturated NEFA with respect to the ability to form lipid droplets was C20:1, which mediated only a moderate protection against PA-induced toxicity. The highest protective potency against PA-induced toxicity revealed C20:5, but it showed no significant increase in lipid droplet formation compared to control conditions without NEFAs. To examine, whether there was a correlation between the protective potency and lipid droplet formation in the different unsaturated NEFA groups (C18:x, C20:x, C22:x) the corresponding correlation coefficients and the p values were calculated. In none of the groups the correlation coefficient was significant (Table 1). A calculation of an overall coefficient between lipid droplet formation and the protective potency of the different NEFA groups revealed a correlation coefficient of 0.04.

Gene expression analyses of perilipin 1 or 2 in insulin-producing cells after suppression of perilipin 1 or 2

To verify the efficiency of the shRNA mediated knockdown of perilipin 1 or 2 (shRNA-Plin1 or shRNA-Plin2) gene expression in insulin-producing RINm5F and INS-1E cells was analyzed after incubation with PA, OA (oleic acid/cis-9-octadecenoic acid/C18:1), a combination of PA and OA, or GA (gondoic acid/cis-11-eicosenoic acid/C20:1). Control INS-1E and RINm5F cells as well as non-target shRNA control cells showed a significant 3- to 4-fold increase in perilipin 1 gene expression after incubation with OA, PA + OA, or GA in comparison to control conditions without NEFAs. In shRNA-Plin1 cells no significant increase was detectable (Fig. 4a-c). Similar results were obtained in shRNA-Plin2 cells. Only in control cells and non-target shRNA control cells a significant increase in perilipin 2 expression was detectable, whereas the gene expression in shRNA-Plin2 was not significantly increased after incubation with OA, PA + OA, or GA in comparison to control conditions (Fig. 4b-d).

In addition to the gene expression quantification the mRNA level, perilipin 1 and 2 protein expression in insulin-producing RINm5F and INS-1E cells was analyzed by immunoblotting (Fig. 5). In Western blot analyses two bands in the range between approx. 60 kDa

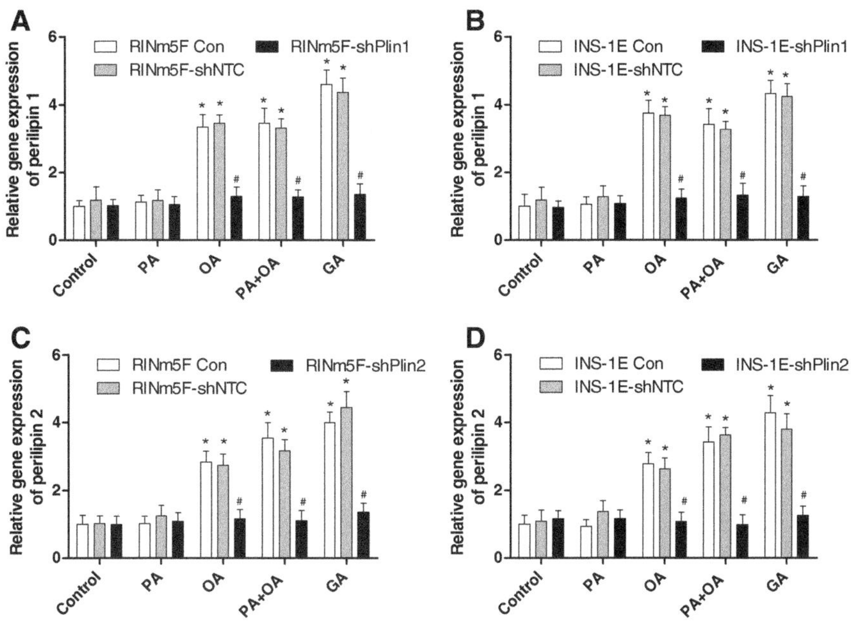

Fig. 4 Gene expression analysis of perilipin 1 or 2 suppressed RINm5F and INS-1E cells. Perilipin 1 and 2 expression in RINm5F (**a**, **c**) and INS-1E (**b**, **d**) cells was stably suppressed by the shRNA technique after lentiviral transduction. Cells were incubated with 100 μM palmitic acid (PA), 100 μM oleic acid (OA), a combination of both, or 100 μM gondoic acid (GA) or without NEFAs (Con) for 24 h. Thereafter RNA was isolated and reverse transcribed into cDNA. Gene expression of perilipin 1 and perilipin 2 was measured by qRT-PCR and normalized to the reference genes *PPIA*, *α-tubulin* and *β-actin* using qBase + software (Biogazelle). Data are means ± SEM of $n = 4$. $^{*}p < 0.01$ compared to control cells without NEFAs (ANOVA/Tukey Multiple Comparison Test). $^{\#}p < 0.01$ compared with control cells (ANOVA/Tukey Multiple Comparison Test)

and 65 kDa were detectable for perilipin 1. This finding confirms earlier immunoblotting analyses of INS-1E cells [13]. For perilipin 2 the immunoblotting revealed a specific band at a molecular weight of 48 kDa. Through shRNA mediated suppression of perilipin 1 or perilipin 2 a 60 to 70 % reduction both on the mRNA and protein level was achieved after incubation with OA, PA + OA, or GA, when compared to non-targeted control cells (Fig. 5). PA alone did not induce expression of perilipin 1 or 2. This low expression level was also not affected by shRNA mediated perilipin suppression.

Quantification of lipid droplet formation in insulin-producing cells after exposure to oleic acid

In order to verify the effect of perilipins on LD formation shRNA-Plin1 or shRNA-Plin2 RINm5F and shRNA-Plin1 or shRNA-Plin2 INS-1E cells were incubated with the physiologically most important NEFAs, the saturated palmitic acid, (PA, C16:0) and the monounsaturated oleic acid (OA, C18:1) as well as a combination of both. Maximal LD formation was induced in RINm5F and INS-1E control cells or shRNA non-target controls (shNTC) after OA incubation in comparison to cells incubated without this NEFA (Fig. 6a and b). In shRNA-Plin1 or shRNA-Plin2 cells C18:1 exposure resulted in a non-significant increase in LD formation in comparison to cells not incubated with OA. Furthermore shRNA-Plin1 or shRNA-Plin2 cells generated significantly fewer LDs in response to OA when compared to non-suppressed perilipin cells. The reduction in LD formation was in INS-1E-shPlin cells approx. 80 % (Fig. 6a) and in RINm5F-shPlin cells approx. 50 % (Fig. 6b). Incubation of RINm5F and INS-1E cells with knockdown of perilipin 1 or 2 in the presence of PA (200 μM) plus OA (100 or 200 μM) also caused a significant reduction of lipid droplet formation in the range of 50–70 % in comparison with the respective shNTC control cells (Fig. 6c and d). PA (200 μm) alone did not cause lipid droplet formation (data not shown).

Palmitic acid-induced lipotoxicity in perilipin suppressed insulin-producing cells

Perilipin suppressed RINm5F and INS-1E cells were used to analyze differences in the sensitivity against PA-induced toxicity. Neither perilipin 1 suppression nor perilipin 2 suppression showed a significantly higher sensitivity when compared to non-target shRNA control cells after incubation with the toxic saturated NEFA PA (C16:0) (Fig. 7a and b). Furthermore the cell lines were co-incubated with

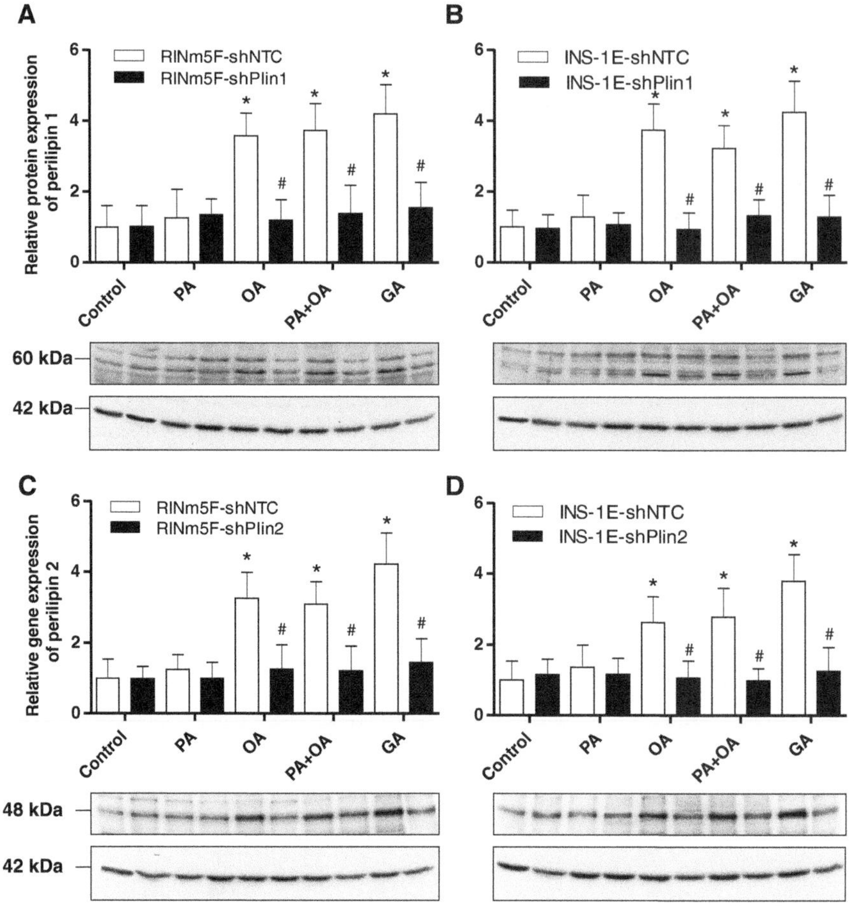

Fig. 5 Western blot analyses of perilipin 1 or 2 suppressed RINm5F and INS-1E cells. Perilipin 1 and 2 expression in RINm5F (**a**, **c**) and INS-1E (**b**, **d**) cells was stably suppressed by the shRNA technique after lentiviral transduction. Cells were incubated with 100 μM palmitic acid (PA), 100 μM oleic acid (OA), a combination of both, or 100 μM gondoic acid (GA) or without NEFAs (Con) for 24 h. Thereafter, 30 μg protein of total whole cell extracts were separated by a SDS-PAGE and electroblotted on nitrocellulose membranes. Specific protein detection was carried out with a primary anti-perilipin 1 or anti-perilipin 2 antibody and a horseradish peroxidase labelled anti-rabbit IGG secondary antibody. After visualization of the protein bands by chemiluminescence the perilipin 1 and 2 bands were quantified and normalized to β-actin bands. Shown are means of ± SEM of $n = 3$ independent immunoblots and one representative blot for each cell line. $^{*}p < 0.01$ compared to control cells without NEFAs (ANOVA/Tukey Multiple Comparison Test). $^{\#}p < 0.01$ compared with control cells (ANOVA/Tukey Multiple Comparison Test)

200 μM PA and increasing concentrations of OA (up to 200 μM) demonstrating the protective effect of the monounsaturated NEFA OA on PA-induced toxicity. In these experiments there were also no significant differences in toxicity detectable between perilipin 1 or 2 suppressed cell lines detectable (Fig. 7c and d). Incubation with OA (up to 500 μM) alone did not induce significant toxicity in the cell lines (data not shown).

Discussion

Obesity and the metabolic syndrome are associated with increased plasma concentrations of non-esterified fatty acids (NEFAs) concentrations in the circulation, which can cause T2DM by inducing insulin resistance in peripheral tissues as well as damage to pancreatic β-cells [1, 2]. In several in vitro studies on lipotoxicity in rodent β-cells long-chain saturated NEFAs were found to be responsible for the induction of apoptosis by ER-stress [25–27] or the formation of toxic reactive oxygen species (ROS) [7, 28–30]. In contrast, long-chain unsaturated NEFAs are less toxic or non-toxic to rat β-cells and can even provide protection against the toxicity induced by long-chain saturated NEFAs. We recently reported that the PA-induced formation of cytotoxic H_2O_2 in the peroxisomal β-oxidation is inhibited by long-chain unsaturated NEFAs [27]. Pancreatic β-cells

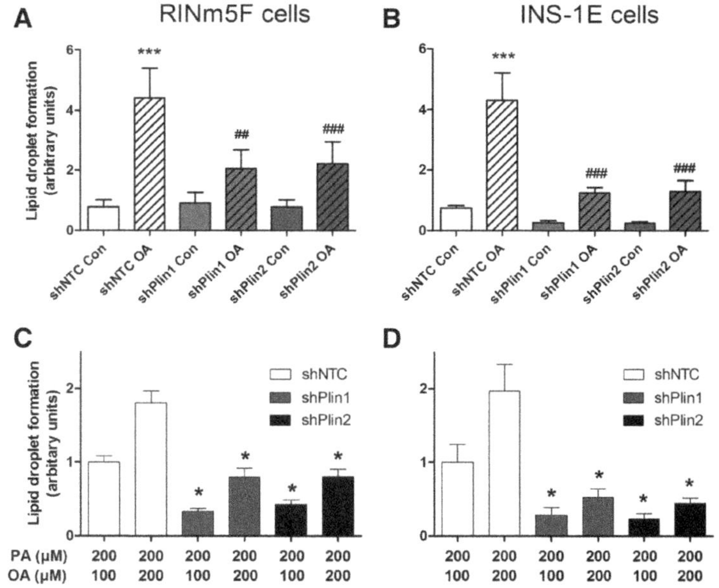

Fig. 6 Effect of perilipin 1 or 2 suppression in insulin-producing RINm5F and INS-1E cells on lipid droplet formation after OA and PA incubation. For the suppression of perilipin 1 and 2 RINm5F (**a**, **c**) and INS-1E (**b**, **d**) cells were transduced lentivirally with the respective shRNA constructs or as a control with a non-target shRNA (shNTC). Cells were incubated with the indicated NEFAs for 24 h and after fixation stained with Oil Red O. Lipid droplet formation was analyzed by fluorescence microscopy and quantified using the software xcellence rt. **a**, **b** Cells were incubated with 100 μM oleic acid (C18:1, OA) or under control conditions (Con). Data are presented as means ± SEM of 4 to 5 independent experiments. ##$p <$ 0.01; ###$p < 0.001$ compared with shNTC cells after incubation with OA (ANOVA/Tukey Multiple Comparison Test). ***$p < 0.001$ compared with non-OA-incubated controls (ANOVA/Tukey Multiple Comparison Test). **c**, **d** Cells were incubated with 200 μM palmitic acid (PA) in combination with 100 or 200 μM OA. Data are presented as means ± SEM of 4 independent experiments. *$p < 0.05$; compared with shNTC cells with the respective PA and OA concentrations (ANOVA/Tukey Multiple Comparison Test)

do not express the H_2O_2 detoxifying enzyme catalase which contributes to the exceptional sensitivity towards ROS mediated toxicity of this cell type [11, 31].

Another concept offered to explain the protection of long-chain unsaturated NEFAs against lipotoxicity is the formation of cytosolic lipid droplets (LDs). NEFAs in the cytosol can be sequestrated to LDs after esterification in triglycerides and could therefore not express their cytotoxic action [13, 32, 33]. PA is known to be incorporated into LDs to a significantly lesser extent and evokes a greater lipotoxic effect than OA [32–34]. Furthermore, when cells are incubated with PA and OA simultaneously, OA induces LD formation and facilitates the incorporation of PA into the LDs, and thereby is thought to decrease the lipotoxic action of PA [33]. It was therefore the aim of the present study to verify if this hypothesis is applicable not only to OA but also to other unsaturated NEFAs with different chain lengths and saturation levels in rat insulin-producing cells.

In a comprehensive experimental approach we analyzed for the first time a group of 16 different saturated as well as mono- and polyunsaturated NEFAs with chain lengths ranging from C12 to C24 by fluorescence microscopy for their ability to form LDs in insulin-producing cells. Only long-chain mono- and polyunsaturated NEFAs were found to cause LD formation whereas the saturated NEFAs were ineffective. Such a difference had been reported in previous studies only between the unsaturated NEFA OA and the unsaturated NEFA PA [13, 32, 33, 35]. Our detailed comparison of different mono- and polyunsaturated NEFAs with chain lengths of C18, C20 and C22 revealed no correlation (correlation coefficient $r = 0.04$) between extent of NEFAs saturation and LD formation.

These results are in disagreement with the previously proposed hypothesis that LD formation is responsible for the protective effect of unsaturated NEFAs against toxicity of long-chain saturated NEFAs [13, 32, 33, 35]. To obtain further evidence for a lack of association between LD formation and a possible protective effect of unsaturated NEFAs against the toxicity of the saturated NEFA PA we determined in RINm5F insulin-producing cells in co-incubation experiments with 200 μM PA the half maximal protective concentration for each of the 14 unsaturated NEFAs with different chain lengths and saturation levels and correlated these data with the LD formation. Interestingly, there was no correlation detectable

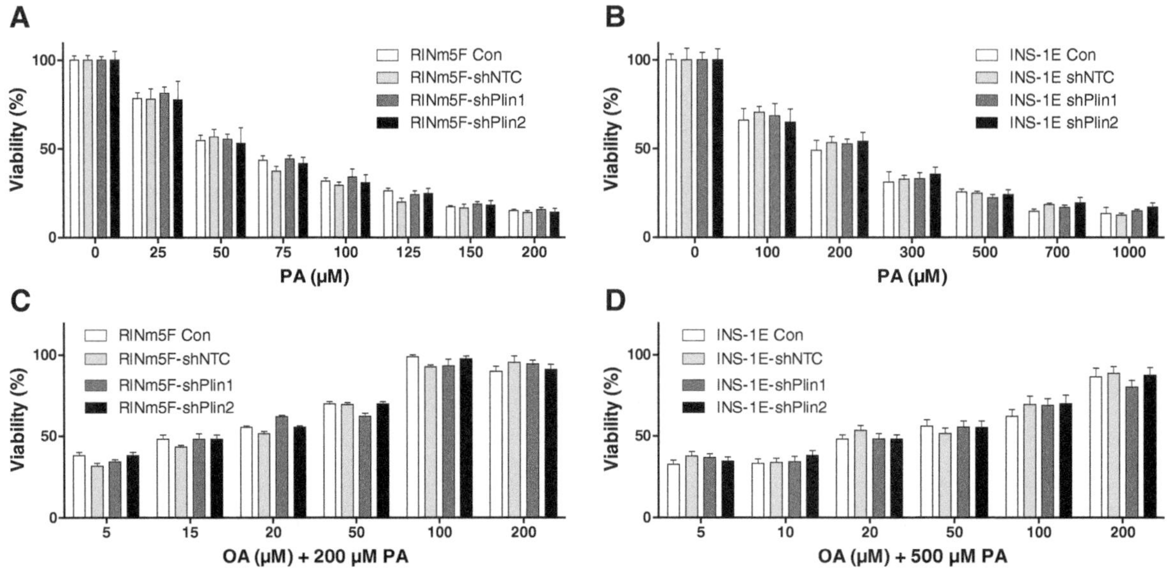

Fig. 7 PA-induced lipotoxicity and OA protection against PA-induced lipotoxicity in perilipin 1 or 2 suppressed insulin-producing RINm5F and INS-1E cells. Perilipin 1 or 2 suppressed RINm5F cells were incubated with increasing concentrations of the saturated NEFA C16:0 (PA) (**a**) or co-incubated with 200 µM PA and increasing concentrations of the monounsaturated NEFA C18:1 (OA) (**c**). Perilipin 1 or 2 suppressed INS-1E cells were incubated with increasing concentrations of the saturated NEFA C16:0 (PA) (**b**) or co-incubated with 500 µM PA and increasing concentrations of the monounsaturated NEFA C18:1 (OA) (**d**). The cell viability was measured by MTT assay after 24 h. Data are means ± SEM of $n = 4$ to 6. Significance was tested against control cells (ANOVA/Tukey Multiple Comparison Test)

between toxicity and LD formation. This conclusion is in contradiction to the hypothesis of a crucial role of LDs for the protection against PA toxicity [13, 31, 32], which was based only on analyses of the effects of PA, OA and linoleic acid [13, 35]. Thus a valid conclusion must be based upon the analyses of more than these three NEFAs.

Additional evidence that LD formation is not a crucial protective mechanism against lipotoxicity was provided by the perilipin 1 and 2 repression experiments in insulin-producing cells. Perilipin repression was used as an additional experimental tool to study the effect of LD formation on lipotoxicity. Perilipins are proteins which are involved in the biogenesis of LDs and located in the phospholipid mono layer of the LDs [16, 17]. Like other investigators [13] we were able to detect perilipin 1 and 2 gene expression in rat insulin-producing RINm5F and INS-1E cells on the mRNA as well as on the protein level. Incubation with OA, PA + OA, or GA led to an approx. 3 to 4-fold increase in perilipin 1 and 2 mRNA and protein expression. This induced perilipin 1 and 2 expression was diminished by the shRNA technique by 60 % to 80 %. This gene suppression caused also a 50-80 % reduction in LD formation in insulin-producing cells indicating that perilipins are involved in LD formation. If LD formation would be of crucial importance for lipotoxicity of long-chain saturated NEFAs it should be expected, that the protection of OA against PA-induced toxicity was reduced in perilipin 1 and 2 repressed cells which was not the case in our experiments. On the other hand we obtained also no experimental evidence for a short-term detrimental effect on cell viability of LD storing unsaturated fatty acids. This does not exclude that long-term intracellular storage of fatty acids in the form of triglycerides may have unfavorable effects on the cellular function; in particular in diseases affecting other organs such as non-alcoholic fatty liver [36] and cardiovascular diseases [37], which go along with pathological intracellular fat accumulation.

Conclusions

The results document convincingly that LD formation plays no essential role in the protective effect of unsaturated NEFAs against the toxicity of palmitic acid in rat insulin-producing cells.

Additional file

Additional file 1: Figure S1. Viability of long-chain unsaturated NEFAs in comparison to the long-chain saturated NEFA PA (C16:0). RINm5F cells were incubated with 100 µM of the long-chain saturated NEFA or 100 µM of the unsaturated NEFAs as depicted for 24 h. Thereafter viability was measured by MTT assay. Data are means ± SEM of $n = 5$ to 8. $^{*}p < 0.05$, $^{**}p < 0.01$, $^{***}p < 0.001$ compared to cells incabated under control condition without NEFAs (Dunnett's Multiple Comparison Test). (DOCX 34 kb)

Abbreviations

GA: gondoic acid; LDs: lipid droplets; MOI: multiplicity of infection; NEFA: non-esterified fatty acid; NTC: non-target control; OA: oleic acid; PA: palmitic acid; ROS: reactive oxygen species; T2DM: type 2 diabetes mellitus.

Competing interests

The authors declare that they have no competing interests

Authors' contributions

TP performed lipid droplet analyses and cell viability assays, participated in data analyses and interpretation. MH carried out the shRNA and qPCR experiments and analyzed the data. TP and ME prepared the manuscript. ME was responsible for the experimental design and the interpretation of the data. SL was responsible for the design of the research and reviewed the manuscript. All authors read and approved the final manuscript.

Acknowledgements

We are grateful to Maren Böger and Martin Wirth for their skillful technical assistance. This work was supported by the European Union (Collaborative Project BetaBAT in the Framework Programme 7, grant agreement 277713), the German Diabetes Association (Hans-Christian-Hagedorn project grant), and the German Research Foundation (DFG) within the Research Training Group (GRK) 1947, project A4.

References

1. Stumvoll M, Goldstein BJ, van Haeften TW. Type 2 diabetes: principles of pathogenesis and therapy. Lancet. 2005;365:1333–46.
2. Vinciguerra F, Baratta R, Farina MG, Tita P, Padova G, Vigneri R, et al. Very severely obese patients have a high prevalence of type 2 diabetes mellitus and cardiovascular disease. Acta Diabetol. 2013;50:443–9.
3. Hamilton MT, Hamilton DG, Zderic TW. Role of low energy expenditure and sitting in obesity, metabolic syndrome, type 2 diabetes, and cardiovascular disease. Diabetes. 2007;56:2655–67.
4. Lottenberg AM, Afonso Mda S, Lavrador MS, Machado RM, Nakandakare ER. The role of dietary fatty acids in the pathology of metabolic syndrome. J Nutr Biochem. 2012;23:1027–40.
5. Sabin MA, De Hora M, Holly JM, Hunt LP, Ford AL, Williams SR, et al. Fasting nonesterified fatty acid profiles in childhood and their relationship with adiposity, insulin sensitivity, and lipid levels. Pediatrics. 2007;120:1426–33.
6. Dhayal S, Welters HJ, Morgan NG. Structural requirements for the cytoprotective actions of mono-unsaturated fatty acids in the pancreatic beta-cell line, BRIN-BD11. Br J Pharmacol. 2008;153:1718–27.
7. Elsner M, Gehrmann W, Lenzen S. Peroxisome-generated hydrogen peroxide as important mediator of lipotoxicity in insulin-producing cells. Diabetes. 2011;60:200–8.
8. Kunau WH, Dommes V, Schulz H. Beta-oxidation of fatty acids in mitochondria, peroxisomes, and bacteria: a century of continued progress. Prog Lipid Res. 1995;34:267–342.
9. Van Veldhoven PP. Biochemistry and genetics of inherited disorders of peroxisomal fatty acid metabolism. J Lipid Res. 2010;51:2863–95.
10. Fransen M, Nordgren M, Wang B, Apanasets O. Role of peroxisomes in ROS/RNS-metabolism: implications for human disease. Biochim Biophys Acta. 1822;2012:1363–73.
11. Lenzen S, Drinkgern J, Tiedge M. Low antioxidant enzyme gene expression in pancreatic islets compared with various other mouse tissues. Free Radic Biol Med. 1996;20:463–6.
12. Tiedge M, Lortz S, Drinkgern J, Lenzen S. Relation between antioxidant enzyme gene expression and antioxidative defense status of insulin-producing cells. Diabetes. 1997;46:1733–42.
13. Borg J, Klint C, Wierup N, Strom K, Larsson S, Sundler F, et al. Perilipin is present in islets of Langerhans and protects against lipotoxicity when overexpressed in the beta-cell line INS-1. Endocrinology. 2009;150:3049–57.
14. Grahn TH, Zhang Y, Lee MJ, Sommer AG, Mostoslavsky G, Fried SK, et al. FSP27 and PLIN1 interaction promotes the formation of large lipid droplets in human adipocytes. Biochem Biophys Res Commun. 2013;432:296–301.
15. McIntosh AL, Senthivinayagam S, Moon KC, Gupta S, Lwande JS, Murphy CC, et al. Direct interaction of Plin2 with lipids on the surface of lipid droplets: a live cell FRET analysis. Am J Physiol Cell Physiol. 2012;303:C728–42.
16. Brasaemle DL. Thematic review series: adipocyte biology. The perilipin family of structural lipid droplet proteins: stabilization of lipid droplets and control of lipolysis. J Lipid Res. 2007;48:2547–59.
17. Hsieh K, Lee YK, Londos C, Raaka BM, Dalen KT, Kimmel AR. Perilipin family members preferentially sequester to either triacylglycerol-specific or cholesteryl-ester-specific intracellular lipid storage droplets. J Cell Sci. 2012; 125:4067–76.
18. Brasaemle DL, Rubin B, Harten IA, Gruia-Gray J, Kimmel AR, Londos C. Perilipin A increases triacylglycerol storage by decreasing the rate of triacylglycerol hydrolysis. J Biol Chem. 2000;275:38486–93.
19. Martinez-Botas J, Anderson JB, Tessier D, Lapillonne A, Chang BH, Quast MJ, et al. Absence of perilipin results in leanness and reverses obesity in Lepr(db/db) mice. Nat Genet. 2000;26:474–9.
20. Gazdar AF, Chick WL, Oie HK, Sims HL, King DL, Weir GC, et al. Continuous, clonal, insulin- and somatostatin-secreting cell lines established from a transplantable rat islet cell tumor. Proc Natl Acad Sci U S A. 1980;77:3519–23.
21. Asfari M, Janjic D, Meda P, Li G, Halban PA, Wollheim CB. Establishment of 2-mercaptoethanol-dependent differentiated insulin-secreting cell lines. Endocrinology. 1992;130:167–78.
22. Merglen A, Theander S, Rubi B, Chaffard G, Wollheim CB, Maechler P. Glucose sensitivity and metabolism-secretion coupling studied during two-year continuous culture in INS-1E insulinoma cells. Endocrinology. 2004;145:667–78.
23. Mosmann T. Rapid colorimetric assay for cellular growth and survival: application to proliferation and cytotoxicity assays. J Immunol Methods. 1983;65:55–63.
24. Elsner M, Terbish T, Jörns A, Naujok O, Wedekind D, Hedrich HJ, et al. Reversal of diabetes through gene therapy of diabetic rats by hepatic insulin expression via lentiviral transduction. Mol Ther. 2012;20:918–26.
25. Cunha DA, Hekerman P, Ladriere L, Bazarra-Castro A, Ortis F, Wakeham MC, et al. Initiation and execution of lipotoxic ER stress in pancreatic beta-cells. J Cell Sci. 2008;121:2308–18.
26. Karaskov E, Scott C, Zhang L, Teodoro T, Ravazzola M, Volchuk A. Chronic palmitate but not oleate exposure induces endoplasmic reticulum stress, which may contribute to INS-1 pancreatic beta-cell apoptosis. Endocrinology. 2006;147:3398–407.
27. Gehrmann W, Würdemann W, Plötz T, Jörns A, Lenzen S, Elsner M. Antagonism between saturated and unsaturated fatty acids in ROS mediated lipotoxicity in rat insulin-producing cells. Cell Physiol Biochem. 2015;36:852–65.
28. Gehrmann W, Elsner M, Lenzen S. Role of metabolically generated reactive oxygen species for lipotoxicity in pancreatic beta-cells. Diabetes Obes Metab. 2010;12 Suppl 2:149–58.
29. Schönfeld P, Wojtczak L. Fatty acids as modulators of the cellular production of reactive oxygen species. Free Radic Biol Med. 2008;45:231–41.
30. Newsholme P, Haber EP, Hirabara SM, Rebelato EL, Procopio J, Morgan D, et al. Diabetes associated cell stress and dysfunction: role of mitochondrial and non-mitochondrial ROS production and activity. J Physiol. 2007;583:9–24.
31. Lenzen S. Oxidative stress: the vulnerable beta-cell. Biochem Soc Trans. 2008;36:343–7.
32. Cnop M, Hannaert JC, Hoorens A, Eizirik DL, Pipeleers DG. Inverse relationship between cytotoxicity of free fatty acids in pancreatic islet cells and cellular triglyceride accumulation. Diabetes. 2001;50:1771–7.
33. Listenberger LL, Han X, Lewis SE, Cases S, Farese Jr RV, Ory DS, et al. Triglyceride accumulation protects against fatty acid-induced lipotoxicity. PNAS. 2003;100:3077–82.
34. Listenberger LL, Ory DS, Schaffer JE. Palmitate-induced apoptosis can occur through a ceramide-independent pathway. The Journal of biological chemistry. 2001;276:14890–5.
35. Moffitt JH, Fielding BA, Evershed R, Berstan R, Currie JM, Clark A. Adverse physicochemical properties of tripalmitin in beta cells lead to morphological changes and lipotoxicity in vitro. Diabetologia. 2005;48:1819–29.
36. Parekh S, Anania FA. Abnormal lipid and glucose metabolism in obesity: implications for nonalcoholic fatty liver disease. Gastroenterology. 2007;132: 2191–207.
37. Kienesberger PC, Pulinilkunnil T, Nagendran J, Dyck JR. Myocardial triacylglycerol metabolism. J Mol Cell Cardiol. 2013;55:101–10.

Replacing carbohydrate with protein and fat in prediabetes or type-2 diabetes: greater effect on metabolites in PBMC than plasma

Minjoo Kim[1], Gayoung Song[2,3], Miso Kang[2,3], Hye Jin Yoo[2,3], Tae-Sook Jeong[4], Sang-Hyun Lee[5] and Jong Ho Lee[1,2,3*]

Abstract

Background: Active metabolism of peripheral blood mononuclear cells (PBMC) could suggest their suitability for metabolomics studies. This study examined whether reductions in PBMCs and plasma lipoprotein-associated phospholipase A_2 (Lp-PLA_2) activities induced by dietary intervention affected the overall metabolic profiles of PBMC and plasma.

Methods: Eighty nonobese subjects aged 40–70 years (18.5 ≤ BMI < 30 kg/m^2) with prediabetes or newly-diagnosed type-2 diabetes were assigned to consume either the usual refined-rice diet (control group, n = 40) or to replace refined rice with whole grains and legumes as carbohydrates (whole-grain group, n = 40) for three meals per day during the 12-week intervention. Fasting PBMC and plasma metabolomes were profiled using UPLC-LTQ-Orbitrap mass spectrometry.

Results: After 12 weeks, changes in fasting glucose, HbA_{1c}, HOMA-IR, MDA, ox-LDL, LDL particle size, plasma Lp-PLA_2 activity, and PBMC enzyme activity in the whole-grain group were significantly different from those in the control group before and after adjusting for baseline levels. The PBMC levels of L-leucine, oleamide, lysoPC (16:0), and lysoPC (18:0) in the whole-grain group showed greater reductions compared with those of the control group. Changes in plasma metabolites were not significantly different between the two groups. Changes in PBMC Lp-PLA_2 activity positively correlated with changes in L-leucine, oleamide, lysoPC (16:0), lysoPC (18:0), glucose, and ox-LDL, and negatively correlated with changes in LDL particle size.

Conclusions: This study showed that dietary intervention in prediabetic or type-2 diabetic patients had a greater effect on PBMC Lp-PLA_2 activity and metabolites compared with those of plasma metabolites.

Trial registration: NCT02191644

Keywords: Metabolites, Peripheral blood mononuclear cells, Prediabetes, Whole-grains and legumes

* Correspondence: jhleeb@yonsei.ac.kr
[1]Research Center for Silver Science, Institute of Symbiotic Life-TECH, Yonsei University, Seoul 03722, Republic of Korea
[2]National Leading Research Laboratory of Clinical Nutrigenetics/Nutrigenomics, Department of Food and Nutrition, College of Human Ecology, Yonsei University, Seoul 03722, Republic of Korea
Full list of author information is available at the end of the article

Background

Diabetes is an epidemic metabolic disorder; about 2.7 million Korean people (8.03 %) aged 30 years or older had type-2 diabetes (T2D) and 25.0 % of adults had prediabetes in 2013 according to Korean Diabetes Fact Sheet 2015. Diabetes-related mortality was steadily decreased since 2003 and ranked as the fifth leading cause of natural death [1]. Prediabetes can be indicated by either impaired fasting glucose (IFG) by the American Diabetes Association criteria [2] or impaired glucose tolerance (IGT) by World Health Organization criteria [3].

Lipoprotein-associated phospholipase A_2 (Lp-PLA_2) independently predicts T2D incidence and may be involved in its etiology [4]. In recent study, an inverse association was observed between protein intake and circulating Lp-PLA_2 activity, suggesting that nutritional factors may influence Lp-PLA_2 activity [5]. An intervention study that replaced refined rice with whole grains and legumes reduced blood glucose, insulin, Lp-PLA_2 activity, and cardiovascular risk factors in patients with prediabetes or T2D [6]. The effects of this intervention diet on plasma and peripheral blood mononuclear cell (PBMC) metabolites have not been determined.

PBMCs include monocytes and lymphocytes which are blood cells having a round nucleus. These blood cells are a critical component in the immune system to fight infection and adapt to intruders. Monocytes have a key role in onset and development of inflammatory reactions by generating bioactive molecules such as Lp-PLA_2 in response to inflammatory stimuli [7]. Lymphocytes are consist of three major types; T cells, B cells, and natural killer cells. T cells and B cells are the major cellular components of the adaptive immune response, whereas natural killer cells are a part of the innate immune system. The production and release of Lp-PLA_2 by lymphocytes may become increased under inflammatory conditions [8]. Dietary intervention induces PBMC gene expression changes, including downregulating genes involved in inflammatory processes [9]. Therefore, changes in PBMC metabolites and Lp-PLA_2 activity after dietary intervention could reflect dynamic responses, which are not detectable in plasma metabolomics analyses. The aim of this 12-week intervention study was to examine whether reductions in PBMC and plasma Lp-PLA_2 activities induced by dietary intervention (replacement of refined rice with whole grains and legumes, and higher intake of vegetables) affected the overall metabolic profiles of PBMC and plasma in nonobese patients that exhibited IFG, IGT, or newly-diagnosed T2D.

Methods

Subjects and study design

Nonobese subjects aged 40–70 years ($18.5 \leq$ BMI < 30 kg/m^2) were recruited from the Health Service Center (HSC) at the Ilsan Hospital, Goyang, Korea, during January–June 2013. Based on the HSC data, subjects who had IFG ($100 \leq$ fasting glucose <126 mg/dL) or newly-diagnosed T2D (fasting glucose ≥ 126 mg/dL) were referred to the Department of Family Medicine or Internal Medicine. Exclusion criteria included: current and/or past history of cardiovascular disease; liver or kidney dysfunction; thyroid or pituitary disease. Subjects who were taking medications or supplements also were excluded. A total of 82 subjects were enrolled. The macronutrient composition of each subject's usual diet corresponded to a typical diet with cooked refined rice. The purpose of the study was carefully explained to all participants, and written consent was obtained prior to their participation. The Institutional Review Board of the NHIC-sponsored Ilsan Hospital and Yonsei University provided ethical approval of the study protocol, which was performed according to the Helsinki Declaration.

The present study was performed in two phases, including a 2-week run-in phase consisting of the usual diet with refined rice, and a 12-week intervention phase. During the run-in period, two subjects who did not maintain their energy intake dropped out. The remaining 80 subjects were randomly subdivided into the two study groups, and were assigned to consume either the usual refined-rice diet (control group, $n = 40$) or to replace refined rice with whole grains and legumes as carbohydrates (whole-grain group, $n = 40$) for three meals per day during the 12-week intervention.

Assessment of dietary intake and physical activity level

All subjects were given written and verbal instructions by a registered dietitian on completion of a 3-day (2 week days and 1 weekend day) dietary record every 2 weeks throughout the study. On the dietary record sheet, subjects were instructed to weigh and record the food amount before and after ingestion. All participants were advised to continue their usual refined-rice diet during a 2-week run-in period. Baseline measurements were performed at the start of the run-in phase. After a run-in period, subjects in the control group maintained the usual refined-rice diet, whereas subjects in the whole-grain group replaced refined rice with a mix of 1/3 legumes, 1/3 barley, and 1/3 wild rice three times per day, and increased vegetable intake to at least 6 units (30–70 g/unit) per day for sufficient dietary fiber intake. The dietitian monitored subject compliance and body-weight changes during the whole study by performing biweekly visits or telephone interviews and all participants were encouraged to maintain their usual lifestyles. Dietary energy values and nutrient contents from 3-day food records were calculated using the CAN-pro 3.0 (Korean Nutrition Society, Seoul, Korea). Total energy expenditures (kcal/day) were calculated from activity patterns including basal metabolic rate, physical activity for 24 h [10], and specific food dynamic action. Basal metabolic rate for each subject was calculated with the Harris–Benedict equation [11].

Anthropometry and blood pressure analysis

Body weight and height of unclothed subjects without shoes were measured in the morning for calculating body mass index (BMI, kg/m^2). Waist circumference was measured on standing subjects at the umbilical level after normal expiration. Blood pressure (BP) of seated subjects after a 20-min rest was measured in the left arm with an automatic BP monitor (FT-200S, Jawon Medical, Gyeongsan, Korea). After a 12-h fasting period, venous blood specimens were collected in EDTA-treated and plain tubes and centrifuged to yield plasma or serum, respectively, which were stored at −70 °C until analysis.

Clinical measurements

Fasting total cholesterol and triglyceride levels were analyzed using a Hitachi 7600 Autoanalyzer (Hitachi Ltd., Tokyo, Japan). ApoB-containing lipoproteins were precipitated with dextran-magnesium sulfate, and high density lipoprotein (HDL)-cholesterol concentrations in patient serum samples were measured enzymatically. For subjects with serum triglyceride levels <400 mg/dL, low density lipoprotein (LDL)-cholesterol concentrations were estimated indirectly using the Friedewald formula. For subjects with serum triglyceride levels ≥400 mg/dL, LDL-cholesterol concentrations were measured directly. Free fatty acids (FFA) were analyzed using the acyl-CoA synthetase – acyl-CoA oxidase enzymatic assay method and a Hitachi 7600 Autoanalyzer.

All subjects underwent an oral glucose-tolerance test at 0 and 12 weeks by ingesting a 75 g glucose solution after a 12-h overnight fast. Venous specimens were collected before glucose loading, at loading, and 30, 60, and 120-min after loading to determine serum glucose levels and responses. Fasting glucose levels were analyzed by the hexokinase method using a Hitachi 7600 Autoanalyzer. Insulin levels were measured using an immunoradiometric assay kit from DIAsource ImmunoAssays S.A. (Louvain, Belgium). Hemoglobin A_{1c} (HbA_{1c}) was measured by immonoturbidimetric analysis. Insulin resistance (IR) was calculated by the homeostasis-model assessment (HOMA) [12].

Whole blood was mixed with the same volume of RPMI 1640 (Gibco, Life Technologies, Gland Island, NY) and gently laid on a histopaque-1077 (Sigma-Aldrich, St. Louis, MO). The sample was then centrifuged at 1800 rpm for 20-min at 10 °C. After the separation, a thin layer of PBMCs was isolated and washed twice with RPMI 1640. The pellet was resuspended in RPMI 1640 with streptomycin. Isolated PBMCs were cultured in RPMI 1640 supplemented with 10 % fetal bovine serum (FBS), seeded in 12-well plates ($1x10^6$ cells/mL; SPL, Gyeonggi-do, Korea), and incubated at 37 °C with 5 % CO_2 for 22.5 h. After a 22.5 h incubation, 10 % FBS was added and incubated for 24.5 h. At third day, PBMC supernatants were collected and stored at −80 °C until Lp-PLA_2 activity levels were assayed. Lp-PLA_2 activity in plasma and PBMC supernatants was measured by using a modification of a previously described high-throughput radiometric activity assay [13].

Serum high-sensitivity C-reactive protein (hs-CRP) was measured with an ADVIA 2400 Clinical Chemistry System (Siemens Ltd., Tarrytown, NY) using a commercially available, hs-CRP-Latex(II) *X*2 kit (Denka-Seiken Co., Ltd., Tokyo, Japan). Plasma malondialdehyde (MDA) was measured from thiobarbituric acid – reactive substances (TBARS) using the TBARS Assay Kit (ZeptoMetrix Co., Buffalo, NY). LDL particles were isolated by sequential flotation ultracentrifugation, and particle size distribution (1.019–1.063 g/mL) was examined using a pore-gradient lipoprotein system (CBS Scientific Company, San Diego, CA) on commercially available, non-denaturing gels containing a linear 2–16 % acrylamide gradient (CBS Scientific Company). Latex-bead (30 nm) conjugated thyroglobulin (17 nm), ferritin (12.2 nm), and catalase (10.4 nm) standards were used to estimate the relative band migration rates. Gels were scanned using a GS-800 Calibrated Imaging Densitometer (Bio-Rad Laboratories, Hercules, CA). Plasma oxidized (ox)-LDL was measured using an enzyme immunoassay (Mercodia AB, Uppsala, Sweden), and the resulting color reaction was determined at 450 nm on a Wallac Victor^2 multilabel counter (Perkin-Elmer Life Sciences, Boston, MA).

Global (nontargeted) metabolic profiling of PBMC and plasma

PBMC and plasma extract sample preparation

Before analysis, 800 μL of 80 % acetonitrile was added to 100 μL of PBMC and plasma, mixed by vortexing, and centrifuged at 10,000 rpm for 5-min at 4 °C. The supernatant was dried with N_2 (l), dissolved in 10 % methanol, mixed by vortexing, and centrifuged at 10,000 rpm for 5-min at 4 °C. The supernatant was transferred into a vial.

Ultra performance liquid chromatography

PBMC and Plasma extract samples (4 μL) were injected into an Acquity UPLC-BEH-C18 column (2.1 × 50 mm, 1.7 μm; Waters, Milford, MA) that was coupled in-line with a UPLC-LTQ-Orbitrap XL (Thermo Fisher Scientific, Waltham, MA). The injected samples were equilibrated with water containing 0.1 % formic acid. Samples were eluted with an acetonitrile gradient containing 0.1 % formic acid at a flow rate of 0.35 mL/min for 20-min. Metabolites were separated by UPLC, analyzed, and assigned by LTQ-

Orbitrap-XL. The mass spectrometer (MS) was operated in ESI-positive mode. The spray voltage was 5 kV. The flow-rate nitrogen sheath gas and the auxiliary gas were 50 and 5 (arbitrary units). The capillary voltage (V), tube-lens voltage (V), and capillary temperature (°C) were kept constant at 35 V, 80 V, and 370 °C. Orbitrap data were collected in the range of *m/z* 50–1,000. MS/MS spectra of metabolites were obtained by a collision-energy ramp from 55–65 eV, and conducted with Xcalibur 2.1 and MS Frontier software (Thermo Fisher Scientific).

Data processing and identification of metabolites

All MS data including retention times, *m/z*, and ion intensities were extracted by SIEVE software (Thermo Fisher Scientific) incorporated into the instrument, and the resulting MS data were assembled into a matrix. SIEVE parameters were set as follows: *m/z* range 50–1,000; *m/z* width 0.02; retention time width 2.5; and *m/z* tolerance 0.005. Metabolites were searched using the following databases: ChemSpider (www.chemspider.com), Human Metabolome (www.hmdb.ca), Lipid MAPS (www.lipidmaps.org), KEGG (www.genome.jp/kegg), and MassBank (www.massbank.jp). Selected metabolites were confirmed by retention times and mass spectra of standard samples.

Statistical analyses

Statistical analyses were performed using SPSS v. 21.0 (IBM SPSS Statistics 21, Chicago, IL). Skewed variables were logarithmically transformed for statistical analyses. A two-tailed P-value of <0.05 was considered statistically significant. Differences in biochemical variables between two groups at baseline and follow-up were tested using Student's independent t-test. General linear model tests were applied to compare parameter changes between the two groups by adjusting for baseline values. Paired t-tests were used to evaluate differences between baseline and follow-up levels in each group. Pearson's and partial correlation coefficients were used to examine the relationships between variables over time. False discovery rate – corrected q-values were computed using the R package 'fdrtool'. Heat map was created to visualize and evaluate correlations among metabolites and conventional risk factors in study populations.

Multivariate statistical analysis was performed using SIMCA-P+ software version 12.0 (Umetrics, Umeå, Sweden). Partial least-squares discriminant analysis (PLS-DA) was used as the classification method for modeling the discrimination between groups by visualizing the score scatter plot or S-plot using the first and second PLS components. The goodness-of-fit was quantified by R^2Y, whereas the predictive ability was quantified by Q^2Y. Generally, R^2Y describes how well the data in the training set were mathematically reproduced and varied between 0 and 1 (a value of 1 indicated a model with a perfect fit). Models with $Q^2Y \geq 0.5$ were considered to have good predictive capabilities.

Results

Clinical characteristics, lipid profiles, and nutrient intake

There were no significant differences between two groups in baseline characteristics including age, gender, smoking, and drinking (data not shown). At baseline, there were no significant differences between two groups in BMI, waist:hip ratio (WHR), systolic BP, diastolic BP, serum triglyceride, total cholesterol, LDL-cholesterol, HDL-cholesterol, FFA, and hs-CRP. BMI, WHR, BP, serum lipid profiles, hs-CRP, total energy expenditure, and total energy intake were similar before and after the study in both groups (data not shown).

Replacement with whole grains and legumes caused significant increase in percent energy intake of protein and fat, and significant decrease in percent energy intake of carbohydrate. The percent energy intake of protein, fat, and carbohydrate significantly differed between the two groups before adjusting for baseline values. The whole-grain group had significant increases in fiber intake and polyunsaturated-to-saturated fatty acids ratio compared with baseline values. After 12-week, the whole-grain group had lower percent energy of carbohydrate, higher percent calorie of protein and fat, and fiber intake than control group (Table 1).

Fasting glucose, insulin, and malondialdehyde

At the end of the study, glucose, HbA_{1c}, and MDA concentrations significantly increased in the control group, whereas glucose, glucose AUC (area under the curve), HbA_{1c}, HOMA-IR, insulin, and MDA significantly decreased in the whole-grain group (Table 1). Changes in glucose, glucose AUC, HbA_{1c}, HOMA-IR, and MDA in the whole-grain group were significantly different from those in the control group before and after adjusting for baseline levels. Post-treatment glucose, HOMA-IR, and MDA in the whole-grain group were significantly lower than those in the control group (Table 1).

Plasma ox-LDL, LDL particle size, Lp-PLA_2 activity in plasma and unstimulated PBMC

At the end of the study, the whole-grain group had lower ox-LDL and Lp-PLA_2 activity in PBMC and larger LDL particle size, whereas the control group had higher Lp-PLA_2 activity in PBMC (Table 1). These changes in ox-LDL, LDL particle size, plasma Lp-PLA_2 activity, and PBMC Lp-PLA_2 activity in the whole-grain group were significantly different from those in the control group before and after adjusting for baseline levels. The post-treatment whole-grain group had lower ox-LDL and

Table 1 Biochemical characteristics and estimates of daily nutrient intake before and after 12-week dietary intervention

	Control group ($n = 40$)		Whole-grain group ($n = 40$)		P^a	P^b	P^c	P^d
	Baseline	Follow-up	Baseline	Follow-up				
Glucose (mg/dL)$^{\int}$	119.8 ± 5.40	126.6 ± 6.02***	119.4 ± 5.31	110.0 ± 4.58***	0.958	0.005		
Change	6.78 ± 1.51		9.45 ± 1.43				<0.001	<0.001
Glucose AUC (mg/dL × h)$^{\int}$	376.8 ± 17.7	390.4 ± 22.9	376.6 ± 18.9	352.0 ± 17.5*	0.923	0.225		
Change	13.6 ± 9.52		24.7 ± 8.75				0.004	0.004
HbA_{1c} (%)$^{\int}$	6.46 ± 0.19	6.60 ± 0.19*	6.41 ± 0.18	6.18 ± 0.15*	0.821	0.061		
Change	0.14 ± 0.06		0.23 ± 0.12				0.007	0.003
HOMA-IR$^{\int}$	2.24 ± 0.15	2.34 ± 0.17	2.18 ± 0.12	1.79 ± 0.12***	0.791	0.006		
Change	0.10 ± 0.11		0.39 ± 0.10				0.002	0.001
Insulin (IU/mL)$^{\int}$	7.58 ± 0.35	7.47 ± 0.43	7.58 ± 0.43	6.72 ± 0.46**	0.798	0.132		
Malondialdehyde (nmol/mL)$^{\int}$	9.24 ± 0.53	10.2 ± 0.61***	9.41 ± 0.39	8.70 ± 0.37**	0.530	0.041		
Change	0.98 ± 0.24		0.71 ± 0.24				0.001	<0.001
Oxidized LDL (U/L)$^{\int}$	49.1 ± 2.14	50.7 ± 2.26	48.2 ± 2.01	43.8 ± 2.00***	0.846	0.036		
Change	1.65 ± 0.90		4.41 ± 0.82				0.001	<0.001
LDL particle size (nm)$^{\int}$	24.1 ± 0.12	24.1 ± 0.13	24.4 ± 0.15	24.6 ± 0.17***	0.214	0.015		
Change	0.05 ± 0.06		0.24 ± 0.05				0.001	0.001
Plasma $Lp\text{-}PLA_2$ activity (nmol/mL/min)$^{\int}$	30.1 ± 1.64	30.3 ± 1.61	28.0 ± 1.20	25.7 ± 1.11	0.874	0.701		
Change	0.24 ± 0.41		2.38 ± 0.55				0.001	<0.001
Unstimulated PBMCLp-PLA_2 activity (nmol/mL/min)$^{\int}$	2.00 ± 0.12	2.28 ± 0.13**	2.16 ± 0.12	1.90 ± 0.12**	0.365	0.046		
Change	0.28 ± 0.08		0.26 ± 0.10				0.001	<0.001
Estimate of daily nutrient intake								
Energy intake (kcal/d)	2,143 ± 40	2,170 ± 38	2,166 ± 36	2,185 ± 38	0.665	0.786		
Carbohydrate (%)	61.9 ± 0.16	61.9 ± 0.17	61.9 ± 0.17	54.6 ± 0.11	0.833	<0.001		
Protein (%)	16.3 ± 0.10	16.3 ± 0.08	16.3 ± 0.10	20.5 ± 0.13	0.851	<0.001		
Fat (%)	22.1 ± 0.16	22.2 ± 0.15	22.1 ± 0.16	24.9 ± 0.15	0.731	<0.001		
Crude fiber (g)$^{\int}$	25.2 ± 1.20	22.8 ± 1.19	24.5 ± 1.21	28.4 ± 1.18	0.713	0.001		
PUFA/SFA	2.10 ± 0.18	2.10 ± 0.16	2.29 ± 0.16	2.98 ± 0.17	0.418	<0.001		

Mean ± SEM.$^{\int}$tested by logarithmic transformation, P^a, values derived from independent *t*-test in baseline. P^b, values derived from independent *t*-test in follow-up. P^c, values derived from independent *t*-test in changed value. P^d, values derived from independent *t*-test in changed value after adjusting for baseline. $^*P < 0.05$, $^{**}P < 0.01$, $^{***}P < 0.001$ derived from paired *t*-test. PBMC, peripheral blood mononuclear cell; AUC, area under the curve; PUFA/SFA, polyunsaturated-to-saturated fatty acids ratio

PBMC $Lp\text{-}PLA_2$ activity, and larger LDL particle size than control group (Table 1).

Metabolic profiling of PBMC and plasma using UPLC-LTQ-orbitrap MS

Nontargeted metabolic pattern analysis

MS data of PBMC and plasma metabolites obtained at baseline and follow-up were analyzed with PLS-DA score scatter plot for the following two combinations: 1) control and whole-grain groups at baseline, control group at follow-up, and whole-grain group at follow-up (Fig. 1a, PBMC; Fig. 1c, plasma); and 2) control and whole-grain groups at follow-up (Fig. 1b, PBMC; Fig. 1d, plasma). The PBMC metabolite PLS-DA score scatter plot showed distinct clustering and clear separation for the following subjects: control and whole-grain groups at baseline, control group at follow-up, and whole-grain group at follow-up [$R^2X(\text{cum}) = 0.124$, $R^2Y(\text{cum}) = 0.34$, $Q^2Y(\text{cum}) = 0.218$] (Fig. 1a). These distinct clusters indicate that PBMC profiling detects metabolic changes induced by dietary intervention. The PBMC metabolite PLS-DA score scatter plot showed distinct clustering for control and whole-grain groups at follow-up [$R^2X(\text{cum}) = 0.125$, $R^2Y(\text{cum}) = 0.809$, $Q^2Y(\text{cum}) = 0.525$] (Fig. 1b).

The plasma metabolite PLS-DA score scatter plot were not as clearly clustered as those for PBMC metabolites [$R^2X(\text{cum}) = 0.124$, $R^2Y(\text{cum}) = 0.376$, $Q^2Y(\text{cum}) = 0.127$] (Fig. 1c). For control and whole-grain groups at follow-up, the plasma metabolite PLS-DA score scatter plot were not as clearly clustered as those for PBMC metabolites [$R^2X(\text{cum}) = 0.201$, $R^2Y(\text{cum}) = 0.704$, $Q^2Y(\text{cum}) = 0.414$] (Fig. 1d). To identify metabolites that differentially

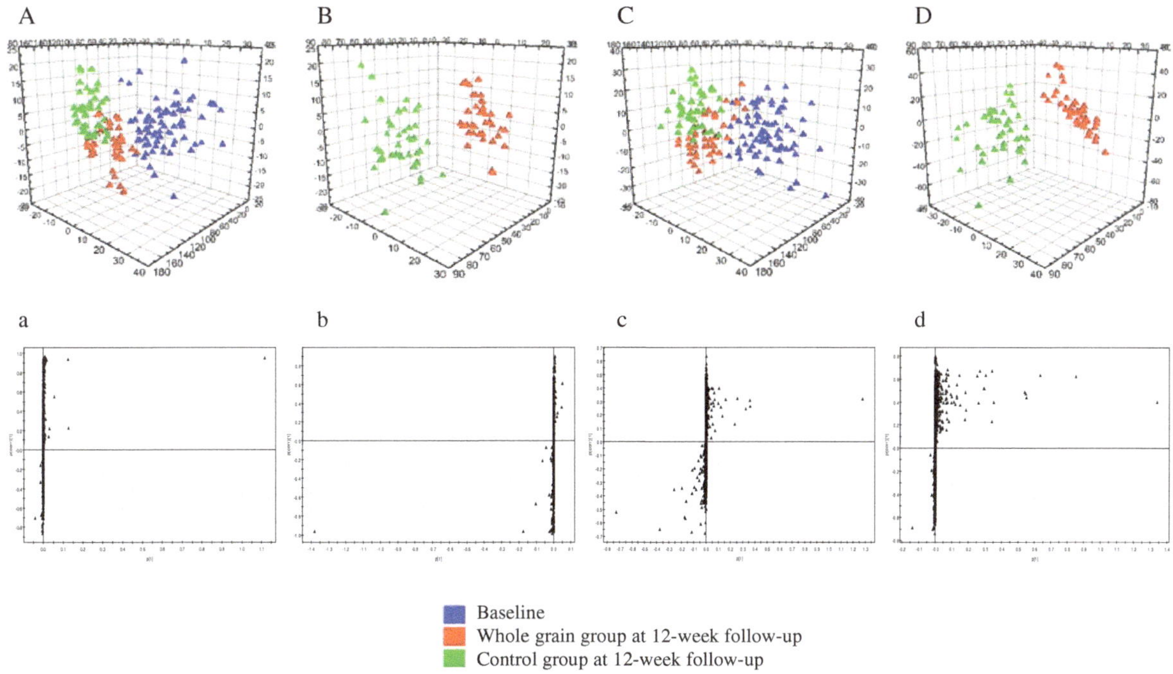

Fig. 1 Identification of PBMC and plasma metabolites that were significantly altered at 12-week follow-up. **a** Partial least squares discriminant analysis score scatter plot (PLS-DA score scatter plot) of PBMC metabolites at baseline ($n = 80$), whole-grain group at follow-up ($n = 40$), and control group at follow-up ($n = 40$). **b** PLS-DA score scatter plot of PBMC metabolites for whole-grain group at follow-up ($n = 40$) and control group at follow-up ($n = 40$). **c** PLS-DA PLS-DA score scatter plot of plasma metabolites at baseline ($n = 80$), whole-grain group at follow-up ($n = 40$), and control group at follow-up ($n = 40$). **d** PLS-DA score scatter plot of plasma metabolites for whole-grain group at follow-up ($n = 40$) and control group at follow-up ($n = 40$)

determined data at baseline and follow-up, *S*-plots of p(1) and p(corr) (1) were generated using centroid scaling. The *S*-plots revealed that metabolites with higher or lower p(corr) values more clearly discriminated between the two groups.

Identification of PBMC metabolites

Of 1,923 PBMC metabolites, those that correlated with separation between the groups were identified by the variable important in the projection (VIP) parameter; VIP values >1.0 were highly relevant for group differences. 51 metabolites had VIP >1.0; 10 of these were previously identified and 41 were unknown. Those 10 PBMC metabolites at baseline and follow-up are shown in Table 2. There were no significant differences in baseline metabolites between two groups. After follow-up, the control group showed significant changes in six PBMC metabolite levels, whereas the whole-grain group showed significant changes in seven PBMC metabolite levels (Table 2).

We compared PBMC metabolite changes between two groups. The whole-grain group had greater reductions in L-leucine ($q = 0.031$), oleamide ($q = 0.032$), lysoPC (16:0) ($q = 0.003$), and lysoPC (18:0) ($q = 0.003$) (Table 2). At follow-up, the whole-grain group had higher peak intensities of L-pyroglutamic acid and ribothymidine, and lower peak intensities of palmitic amide, oleamide, and lysoPCs, compared with those of the control group (Table 2).

Identification of plasma metabolites

Of 4,121 plasma metabolites, those that correlated with separation between the groups were selected by VIP >1.0. 122 plasma metabolites were selected; 20 were previously identified and 102 were unknown (Table 3). There were no significant differences in baseline between two groups. After follow-up, C17 sphinganine significantly increased in the control group, also, there were no significant differences in metabolites between two groups, and no significant differences in metabolite changes with respect to baseline (Table 3).

Correlations among fasting glucose, plasma and PBMC Lp-PLA$_2$ activities, biochemical parameters, and major PBMC metabolites

The correlation matrix of changes in glucose, Lp-PLA$_2$ activities in plasma and PBMC, biochemical parameters, and major PBMC metabolites was computed (Fig. 2).

Table 2 Identification of PBMC metabolites at baseline and 12-week follow-up

Metabolite	Formula $[M+H]^+$	Exact mass (M + H)	Normalized peak intensity				Variable important in the projection		
			Control group ($n = 40$)		Whole-grain group ($n = 40$)		Baseline vs. follow-up		12-weeks
			Baseline	Follow-up	Baseline	Follow-up	Control	Whole-grain	Control vs. whole-grain
Cyclopentanone dimethylhydrazone	$C_7H_{14}N_2$	127.1235	82,551 ± 21,507	101,931 ± 26,693*	43,192 ± 11,728	51,504 ± 14,505*	0.0722	0.1523	1.0119
L-Pyroglutamic acid	$C_5H_7NO_3$	130.0504	2,410,045 ± 108,001	2,075,511 ± 48,362*	2,455,521 ± 70,667	2,484,381 ± 103,907††	0.1241	3.9771	2.6550
L-Leucine	$C_6H_{13}NO_2$	132.1025	7,884,178 ± 309,297	7,922,462 ± 251,819	8,253,845 ± 170,803	7,531,331 ± 171,144**	1.8209	3.1661	5.0363
Change			38,283 ± 198,486		722,514 ± 145,341‡				
L-Phenylalanine	$C_9H_{11}NO_2$	166.0868	2,880,509 ± 113,266	2,755,872 ± 75,646	2,825,355 ± 101,371	2,761,323 ± 56,360	0.5962	0.6567	1.1474
Dihydrobiopterin	$C_9H_{13}N5O_3$	239.1018	432,360 ± 23,845	335,279 ± 14,924***	427,487 ± 16,797	383,280 ± 15,727*	0.4537	1.2616	0.4680
Palmitic amide	$C_{16}H_{33}NO$	256.2640	354,492 ± 50,930	330,909 ± 44,809	490,272 ± 84,177	172,851 ± 26,551**,†	2.7281	0.1468	2.0394
Ribothymidine	$C_{10}H_{14}N_2O_6$	258.0930	302,320 ± 22,108	239,902 ± 12,851**	322,971 ± 16,498	311,114 ± 19,898†	0.0730	0.5966	1.3107
Oleamide	$C_{18}H_{35}NO$	282.2797	2,676,408 ± 412,881	3,257,688 ± 511,380	3,697,245 ± 621,193	1,491,246 ± 235,475*,†	18.4793	8.3202	22.5845
Change			581,279 ± 634,410		2,205,998 ± 651,404‡				
LysoPC(16:0)	$C_{24}H_{50}NO_7P$	496.3403	414,438 ± 44,544	645,199 ± 57,544*	549,155 ± 59,016	383,399 ± 35,718*,††	2.7864	2.8925	3.5066
Change			230,762 ± 72,860		165,756 ± 63,955‡‡				
LysoPC(18:0)	$C_{26}H_{54}NO_7P$	524.3716	285,044 ± 26,648	423,718 ± 34,129**	364,186 ± 33,732	262,585 ± 23,409*,††	1.5197	1.7796	2.0579
Change			138,674 ± 40,222		101,601 ± 42,602‡‡				

Mean ± SEM. $^{*}q < 0.05$, $^{**}q < 0.01$, $^{***}q < 0.001$ derived from paired *t*-test. $^{†}q < 0.05$, $^{††}q < 0.01$, $^{†††}q < 0.001$ derived from independent *t*-test in follow-up. $^{‡}q < 0.05$, $^{‡‡}q < 0.01$, $^{‡‡‡}q < 0.001$ derived from changed values between control and whole-grain groups

Table 3 Identification of plasma metabolites at baseline and 12-week follow-up

Metabolite	Formula [M + H]⁺	Exact mass (M + H)	Normalized peak intensity				Variable important in the projection		
			Control group ($n = 40$)		Whole-grain group ($n = 40$)		Baseline vs. follow-up		12-weeks
			Baseline	Follow-up	Baseline	Follow-up	Control	Whole-grain	Control vs. whole grain
L-Valine	$C_5H_{11}NO_2$	118.0868	1,338,114 ± 39,666	1,323,676 ± 36,213	1,328,470 ± 41,793	1,376,655 ± 34,768	0.7807	0.1901	1.0144
L-Leucine	$C_6H_{13}NO_2$	132.1025	3,130,607 ± 99,839	3,098,031 ± 98,593	3,130,777 ± 107,368	3,166,315 ± 85,278	0.4904	0.5781	0.7853
L-Phenylalanine	$C_9H_{11}NO_2$	166.0868	1,984,169 ± 49,821	1,914,567 ± 45,393	1,997,467 ± 84,582	1,975,319 ± 41,491	0.6137	1.1072	0.7382
Oleamide	$C_{18}H_{35}NO$	282.2797	11,074,949 ± 815,519	11,182,173 ± 1,054,856	11,348,184 ± 805,164	12,102,398 ± 709,965	8.4316	19.2720	6.6270
C17 Sphinganine	$C_{17}H_{37}NO_2$	288.2903	323,013 ± 20,549	441,137 ± 24,748*	333,258 ± 29,775	355,950 ± 25,250	0.9135	1.3462	0.1114
(4E,8E,10E-d18:3) Sphingosine	$C_{18}H_{33}NO_2$	296.2590	420,731 ± 59,507	832,979 ± 152,996	608,061 ± 81,037	754,737 ± 66,758	1.5120	8.8050	2.2736
Anandamide (18:4, n-3)	$C_{20}H_{33}NO_2$	320.2590	170,194 ± 28,584	237,343 ± 31,518	209,059 ± 26,262	213,643 ± 16,101	0.1156	1.4954	0.5840
LysoPC (14:0)	$C_{22}H_{46}NO_7P$	468.3090	480,474 ± 33,898	503,684 ± 38,015	625,962 ± 45,904	537,767 ± 45,983	1.5352	0.7142	0.2242
LysoPC (16:1)	$C_{24}H_{48}NO_7P$	494.3247	1,133,250 ± 77,052	1,033,013 ± 69,288	1,261,066 ± 78,064	1,127,811 ± 88,549	2.3243	1.4177	1.0354
LysoPC (16:0)	$C_{24}H_{50}NO_7P$	496.3403	15,953,932 ± 573,566	15,910,457 ± 684,453	16,830,932 ± 686,817	15,967,767 ± 537,944	15.3974	7.7607	4.7470
LysoPC (17:0)	$C_{25}H_{52}NO_7P$	510.3560	689,578 ± 58,089	710,335 ± 73,384	758,848 ± 49,685	733,637 ± 53,343	0.5841	1.3389	0.1217
LysoPC (18:3)	$C_{26}H_{48}NO_7P$	518.3247	620,814 ± 20,714	591,900 ± 19,836	658,460 ± 22,577	675,799 ± 31,645	0.1217	0.3985	1.1643
LysoPC (18:2)	$C_{26}H_{50}NO_7P$	520.3403	6,388,637 ± 262,115	6,025,486 ± 300,959	6,617,717 ± 260,021	6,878,238 ± 274,508	2.2535	4.8170	15.1889
LysoPC (18:1)	$C_{26}H_{52}NO_7P$	522.3560	5,375,808 ± 229,038	5,364,828 ± 250,194	5,593,899 ± 214,117	5,425,134 ± 241,245	4.2976	3.7059	4.2779
LysoPC (18:0)	$C_{26}H_{54}NO_7P$	524.3716	5,661,866 ± 195,118	5,610,496 ± 261,241	5,976,007 ± 255,107	5,830,224 ± 224,489	2.5863	3.3556	5.4463
LysoPC (20:5)	$C_{28}H_{48}NO_7P$	542.3247	771,884 ± 61,530	784,374 ± 53,112	997,008 ± 89,800	876,925 ± 59,723	2.1218	0.4055	1.2595
LysoPC (20:4)	$C_{28}H_{50}NO_7P$	544.3403	2,512,566 ± 118,266	2,294,343 ± 118,562	2,188,892 ± 126,719	1,958,744 ± 83,560	2.9839	3.3959	6.5629
LysoPC (22:6)	$C_{30}H_{50}NO_7P$	568.3403	1,268,789 ± 89,205	1,160,444 ± 72,253	1,322,936 ± 96,792	1,153,481 ± 79,319	1.8183	1.6819	0.2714
SM (d18:0/16:1)	$C_{39}H_{79}N_2O_6P$	703.5754	918,463 ± 110,095	628,987 ± 81,863	1,046,537 ± 118,533	1,088,608 ± 142,939	0.9346	4.2113	7.9088
Lactosylceramide (d18:1/12:0)	$C_{42}H_{79}NO_{13}$	806.5630	5,977,825 ± 630,100	8,134,712 ± 703,408	6,832,476 ± 741,718	5,908,934 ± 712,523	4.8718	8.3007	5.9197
[1]PCs			44,523,937 ± 2,514,233	44,154,177 ± 1,968,873	43,454,754 ± 2,366,214	50,137,749 ± 2,118,552			

Mean ± SEM. *$q < 0.05$, **$q < 0.01$, ***$q < 0.001$ derived from paired t-test. †$q < 0.05$, ††$q < 0.01$, †††$q < 0.001$ derived from independent t-test in follow-up. ‡$q < 0.05$, ‡‡$q < 0.01$, ‡‡‡$q < 0.001$ derived from changed values between control and whole-grain groups. [1]PCs were detected by Orbitrap MS; therefore, all detected PC amounts were combined. SM, sphingomyelin

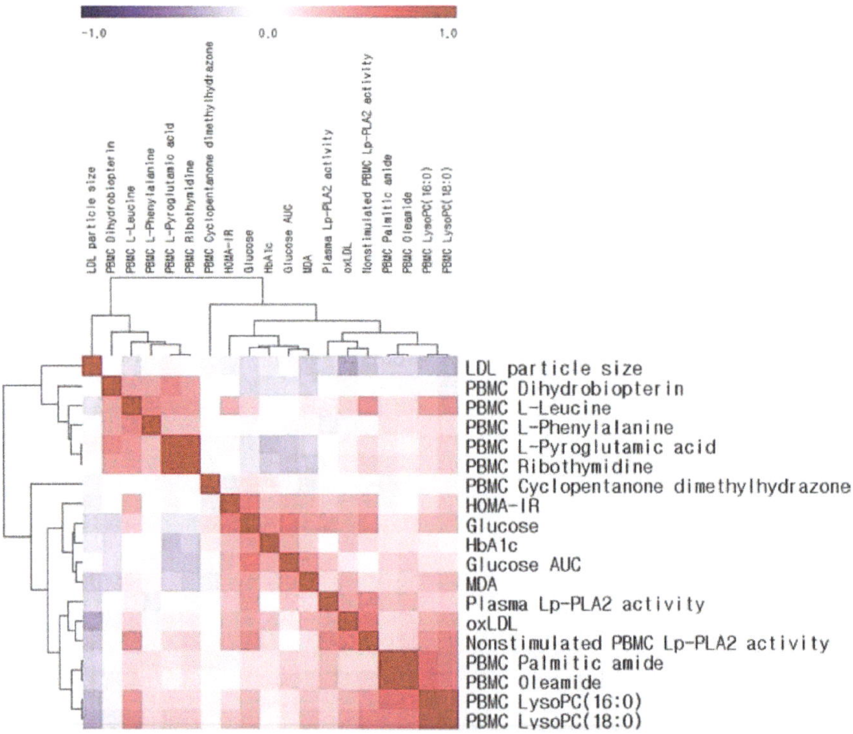

Fig. 2 Correlation matrix for changes in biochemical characteristics and PBMC metabolites in total subjects. Supervised hierarchical clustering identifies the most important 10 metabolites and 9 biochemical characteristics. Correlations were obtained by deriving Spearman correlation coefficients. *Red*, positive correlation. *Purple*, negative correlation

Analysis of metabolic changes including all subjects identified the following correlations: glucose correlated positively with insulin, HOMA-IR, plasma Lp-PLA$_2$ activity ($r = 0.454$, $P < 0.001$), MDA, ox-LDL, Lp-PLA$_2$ in PBMC ($r = 0.511$, $P < 0.001$), glucose AUC, C-peptide, HbA$_{1c}$, and PBMC lysoPCs after adjusting for age, gender, BMI, smoking, and drinking. After adjusting for confounding variables, plasma Lp-PLA$_2$ activity correlated positively with glucose, HOMA-IR, ox-LDL, Lp-PLA$_2$ activity in PBMC ($r = 0.516$, $P < 0.001$), glucose AUC, PBMC palmitic amide, and PBMC oleamide. After adjusting for confounding variables, PBMC Lp-PLA$_2$ activity correlated positively with glucose, HOMA-IR, plasma Lp-PLA$_2$ activity, ox-LDL, PBMC L-leucine, PBMC oleamide, PBMC lysoPCs, and correlated negatively with LDL particle size (Fig. 2).

Discussion

We identified four PBMC metabolites that had statistically significant differences after dietary intervention, including L-leucine, oleamide, lysoPC (16:0), and lysoPC (18:0); however, there were no significant differences in plasma metabolites after dietary intervention. These aspects of results were also shown in both subjects with prediabetes and T2D, respectively. PBMCs may be a useful tool for nutrigenomics and understanding the pathophysiology of chronic disease due to their active metabolism [14, 15]. These results identify PBMC metabolites as powerful metabolomics tools to detect diet-induced metabolic changes.

Improving glycemic control in the whole-grain group decreases ox-LDL, and reduces PBMC Lp-PLA$_2$ activity and PBMC lysoPCs. A strong correlation between PBMC Lp-PLA$_2$ activity and ox-LDL, but not LDL-cholesterol, is consistent with a previous report of a direct effect of ox-LDL on Lp-PLA$_2$ expression in THP-1 monocytes [16]. Ox-LDL may upregulate PBMC Lp-PLA$_2$ expression in smokers [17]. Ox-phospholipids in LDL particles are hydrolyzed by Lp-PLA$_2$ at the *sn*-2 position to produce bioactive ox-FFAs and lysoPCs. Only 1 – 5 % of the total non-ox-LDL PC content is lysoPC; however, up to 40 – 50 % of LDL PC is converted to lysoPC during LDL oxidation [18]. This study identified strongly positive correlations among ox-LDL, PBMC Lp-PLA$_2$ activity, PBMC lysoPCs, which may indicate that ox-LDL and PBMC Lp-PLA$_2$ activity are major determinants of PBMC lysoPC levels.

A negative correlation between PBMC Lp-PLA$_2$ activities, PBMC lysoPCs with LDL particle size is consistent with a previous report of Lp-PLA$_2$ binding preference for small dense LDL [19]. This study and other work [6] reported positive correlations among glucose, PBMC Lp-PLA_2 activity, and plasma Lp-PLA_2 activity. A strongly positive correlation between PBMC and plasma Lp-PLA_2 activities also is observed in healthy subjects [17, 20]. In a porcine diabetes model, PBMC Lp-PLA_2 expression is up-regulated in the presence of glycation end products [21]. Increases in circulating Lp-PLA_2 activity and increased ox-LDL levels in hypercholesterolemic pigs are primarily due to plaque macrophages [22]. These results indicate that the primary sources of plasma Lp-PLA_2 are plaque macrophages [22] and PBMC [17]. This could explain our observations of lower plasma Lp-PLA_2 activity changes compared with that of PBMC Lp-PLA_2 activity, and no significant differences in plasma metabolite changes between two groups.

Reduced Lp-PLA_2 activity in plasma and PBMC in the whole-grain group could be a marker of metabolic changes induced by increased consumption of protein relative to carbohydrate. Diet composition is an important factor in inflammatory processes of blood cells [23]. A study of macronutrient composition determined that increasing dietary protein from 19 % energy intake to 30 % yielded immediate and persistent downregulation of immunological genes in PBMCs [9]. Replacing 5 % of energy from carbohydrates with energy from protein and measured a 2.2 nmol/min/mL reduction in Lp-PLA_2 activity that was independent of other changes in lipid profiles [5]. Our study replaced 7 % of energy from carbohydrate with approximately 4 % energy from protein and 3 % energy from fat.

Whole grains, legumes, and vegetables contain many antioxidants, vitamins, minerals, and phytochemicals [24, 25]. Antioxidants slow the oxidation rate of reduced substrates [24, 26]. Soybean phytochemicals reduce lipid peroxidation *in vivo* and attenuate LDL oxidation [27]. Our observed changes in glucose and HOMA-IR strongly correlated with changes in MDA and ox-LDL in patients with prediabetes or T2D, consistent with a previous report [28]. We observed positive correlation between changes in HOMA-IR and PBMC L-leucine, but not plasma L-leucine. This may be due to a negligible effect of PBMC L-leucine on plasma L-leucine, or the 12-week dietary intervention may not be long enough to change plasma L-leucine. The whole-grain group also had greater reduction in PBMC oleamide, but not in plasma, compared with control group. We identified PBMC oleamide (VIP = 22.5845) as the most important metabolite for evaluating differences between two groups at the end of the study. Recently, Ha et al. [29] identified plasma oleamide as the most important metabolite for distinguishing nondiabetic from diabetic males. Therefore, positive correlations between changes in PBMC oleamide, Lp-PLA_2, PBMC palmitic amide, and PBMC lysoPCs observed in our study could be partly due to dietary-induced effects on blood cell inflammatory processes [23].

This study detected many metabolic markers using UPLC-LTQ-Orbitrap MS, but most are currently unidentified. Endogenous biomolecule databases for use with LC-MS – based metabolomics research are still under construction [30]. Despite this limitation, UPLC-LTQ-Orbitrap MS metabolomics and multivariate data analysis identified greater reductions in PBMC L-leucine, PBMC oleamide, PBMC lysoPCs in the whole-grain group than control group; however, there were no significant differences in plasma metabolites between two groups.

Conclusion

This study demonstrates that replacing refined rice with whole grains and legumes induced greater differences in PBMC Lp-PLA_2 activity and metabolites than in plasma metabolites in nonobese patients with prediabetes or newly-diagnosed T2D. Therefore, consumption of minimally refined grains, legumes, and vegetables should be recommended to control glucose metabolism and reduce cardiovascular risk factors in patients with IFG, IGT, or newly-diagnosed T2D.

Abbreviations

Lp-PLA_2: Lipoprotein-associated phospholipase A_2; T2D: Type-2 diabetes; PBMC: Peripheral blood mononuclear cell; IFG: Impaired fasting glucose; IGT: Impaired glucose tolerance; BMI: Body mass index; BP: Blood pressure; HDL: High density lipoprotein; LDL: Low density lipoprotein; FFA: Free fatty acid; HbA_{1c}: Hemoglobin A_{1c}; IR: Insulin resistance; HOMA: Homeostasis-model assessment; FBS: Fetal bovine serum; hs-CRP: High-sensitivity C-reactive protein; MDA: Malondialdehyde; TBARS: Thiobarbituric acid-reactive substances; Ox: Oxidized; MS: Mass spectrometer; PLS-DA: Partial least-squares discriminant analysis; WHR: Waist-hip ratio; AUC: Area under the curve; VIP: Variable important in the projection.

Competing interests

The authors declare that they have no competing interests.

Authors' contributions

All the authors were involved in the development of the study protocol and the experimental design. GS, MK and JHY collected samples and carried out experiments. MK performed data analysis. T-SJ, S-HL and JHL reviewed data and participated in general discussion. JHL provided the research funding and wrote the manuscript. All the authors read, commented on, and contributed to the submitted manuscript. All authors read and approved the final manuscript.

Acknowledgments

This research was supported by the Bio-Synergy Research Projects (NRF-2012M3A9C4048762) of the National Research Foundation (NRF) funded by the Ministry of Science, ICT & Future Planning, Republic of Korea.

Author details

[1]Research Center for Silver Science, Institute of Symbiotic Life-TECH, Yonsei University, Seoul 03722, Republic of Korea. [2]National Leading Research Laboratory of Clinical Nutrigenetics/Nutrigenomics, Department of Food and Nutrition, College of Human Ecology, Yonsei University, Seoul 03722, Republic of Korea. [3]Department of Food and Nutrition, Brain Korea 21 PLUS Project, College of Human Ecology, Yonsei University, 50 Yonsei-ro, Seodaemun-gu, Seoul 03722, Republic of Korea. [4]National Research Laboratory of Lipid Metabolism and Atherosclerosis, Korea Research Institute of Bioscience and Biotechnology, Daejeon 34141, Republic of Korea. [5]Department of Family Practice, National Health Insurance Corporation Ilsan Hospital, Goyang 10444, Republic of Korea.

References

1. Statistics Korea: Causes of death statistics in 2013. Available from: http://kostat.go.kr (updated 23 Sep 2014).
2. The Expert Committee on the Diagnosis and Classification of Diabetes Mellitus. Report of the expert committee on the diagnosis and classification of diabetes mellitus. Diabetes Care. 1997;20:1183–97.
3. Alberti KG, Zimmet PZ. Definition, diagnosis and classification of diabetes mellitus and its complications. Part 1: diagnosis and classification of diabetes mellitus provisional report of a WHO consultation. Diabet Med. 1998;15:539–53.
4. Nelson TL, Biggs ML, Kizer JR, Cushman M, Hokanson JE, Furberg CD, et al. Lipoprotein-associated phospholipase A2 (Lp-PLA2) and future risk of type 2 diabetes: results from the cardiovascular health study. J Clin Endocrinol Metab. 2012;97:1695–701.
5. Hatoum IJ, Nelson JJ, Cook NR, Hu FB, Rimm EB. Dietary, lifestyle, and clinical predictors of lipoprotein-associated phospholipase A2 activity in individuals without coronary artery disease. Am J Clin Nutr. 2010;91:786–93.
6. Kim M, Jeung SR, Jeong TS, Lee SH, Lee JH. Replacing with whole grains and legumes reduces Lp-PLA2 activities in plasma and PBMCs in patients with prediabetes or T2D. J Lipid Res. 2014;55:1762–71.
7. Dentan C, Lesnik P, Chapman MJ, Ninio E. Phagocytic activation induces formation of platelet-activating factor in human monocyte-derived macrophages and in macrophage-derived foam cells. Relevance to the inflammatory reaction in atherogenesis. Eur J Biochem. 1996;236:48–55.
8. Yang EH, McConnell JP, Lennon RJ, Barsness GW, Pumper G, Hartman SJ, et al. Lipoprotein-associated phospholipase A2 is an independent marker for coronary endothelial dysfunction in humans. Arterioscler Thromb Vasc Biol. 2006;26:106–11.
9. Brattbakk HR, Arbo I, Aagaard S, Lindseth I, de Soysa AK, Langaas M, et al. Balanced caloric macronutrient composition downregulates immunological gene expression in human blood cells-adipose tissue diverges. OMICS. 2013;17:41–52.
10. Christian JL, Greger JL. Energy sources and uses. In: Christian JL, Greger JL, editors. Nutrition for living. Redwood City: Benjamin/Cummings Publishing Co.; 1994. p. 242–66.
11. Butte NF, Caballero B. Energy needs: assessment and requirements. In: Shils ME, Shike M, Ross AC, Caballero B, Cousins RJ, editors. Modern nutrition in health and disease. Philadelphia: Lippincott Williams & Wilkins; 2006. p. 136–48.
12. Matthews DR, Hosker JP, Rudenski AS, Naylor BA, Treacher DF, Turner RC. Homeostasis model assessment: insulin resistance and beta-cell function from fasting plasma glucose and insulin concentrations in man. Diabetologia. 1985;28:412–9.
13. Wilensky RL, Shi Y, Mohler 3rd ER, Hamamdzic D, Burgert ME, Li J, et al. Inhibition of lipoprotein-associated phospholipase A2 reduces complex coronary atherosclerotic plaque development. Nat Med. 2008;14:1059–66.
14. Crujeiras AB, Parra D, Milagro FI, Goyenechea E, Larrarte E, Margareto J, et al. Differential expression of oxidative stress and inflammation related genes in peripheral blood mononuclear cells in response to a low-calorie diet: a nutrigenomics study. OMICS. 2008;12:251–61.
15. Kussmann M, Raymond F, Affolter M. OMICS-driven biomarker discovery in nutrition and health. J Biotechnol. 2006;124:758–87.
16. Wang WY, Li J, Yang D, Xu W, Zha RP, Wang YP. OxLDL stimulated lipoprotein-associated phopholipase A2 expression in THP-1 monocytes via PI3K and p38 MAPK pathways. Cardiovasc Res. 2010;85:845–52.
17. Fratta Pasini A, Stranieri C, Pasini A, Vallerio P, Mozzini C, Solani E, et al. Lysophosphatidylcholine and carotid intima-media thickness in young smokers: a role for oxidized LDL-induced expression of PBMC lipoprotein-associated phospholiase A2? PLoS One. 2013;8, e83092.
18. Matsumono T, Konayashi T, Kamata K. Role of lysophosphatidyl-choline (LPC) in atherosclerosis. Curr Med Chem. 2007;14:3209–20.
19. McNeill AM, Rosamond WD, Girman CJ, Golden SH, Schmidt MI, East HE, et al. The metabolic syndrome and 11-year risk of incident cardiovascular disease in the atherosclerosis risk in communities study. Diabetes Care. 2005;28:385–90.
20. Paik JK, Kim JY, Kim OY, Lee Y, Jeong TS, Sweeney G, et al. Circulating and PBMC Lp-PLA2 associate differently with oxidative stress and subclinical inflammation in nonobese women (menopausal status). PLoS One. 2012;7, e29675.
21. Shi Y, Zhang P, Zhang L, Osman H, Mohler 3rd ER, Macphee C, et al. Role of lipoprotein-associated phospholipase A2 in leukocyte activation and inflammatory responses. Atherosclerosis. 2007;191:54–62.
22. De Keyzer D, Karabina SA, Wei W, Geeraert B, Stengel D, Marsillach J, et al. Increased PAFAH and oxidized lipids are associated with inflammation and atherosclerosis in hypercholesterolemic pigs. Arterioscler Thrombo Vasc Biol. 2009;29:2041–6.
23. Munoz A, Costa M. Nutritionally mediated oxidative stress and inflammation. Oxid Med Cell Longev. 2013;2013:610950.
24. Belobrajdic DP, Bird AR. The potential role of phytochemicals in wholegrain cereals for the prevention of type-2 diabetes. Nutr J. 2013;12:62–74.
25. Liu S, Manson JE, Lee IM, Cole SR, Hennekens CH, Willett WC, et al. Fruit and vegetable intake and risk of cardiovascular disease: the Women's Health Study. Am J Clin Nutr. 2000;72:922–8.
26. Jacobs Jr DR, Andersen LF, Blomhoff R. Whole-grain consumption is associated with a reduced risk of noncardiovascular, noncancer death attributed to inflammatory disease in the Iowa Women's Health Study. Am J Clin Nutr. 2007;85:1606–14.
27. Crujeiras AB, Parra D, Abete I, Martínez JA. A hypocaloric diet enriched in legumes specifically mitigates lipid peroxidation in obese subjects. Free Radic Res. 2007;41:498–506.
28. Chung HK, Chae JS, Hyun YJ, Paik JK, Kim JY, Jang Y, et al. Influence of adiponectin gene polymorphisms on adiponectin level and insulin resistance index in response to dietary intervention in overweight-obese patients with impaired fasting glucose or newly diagnosed type 2 diabetes. Diabetes Care. 2009;32:552–8.
29. Ha CY, Kim JY, Paik JK, Kim OY, Paik YH, Lee EJ, et al. The association of specific metabolites of lipid metabolism with markers of oxidative stress, inflammation and arterial stiffness in men with newly diagnosed type 2 diabetes. Clin Endocrinol. 2012;76:674–82.
30. Skoog T, Dichtl W, Boquist S, Skoglund-Andersson C, Karpe F, Tang R, et al. Plasma tumour necrosis factor-α and early carotid atherosclerosis in healthy middle-aged men. Eur Heart J. 2002;23:376–83.

The effect of cholesteryl ester transfer protein on pancreatic beta cell dysfunction in mice

Wen Guo†, Yingyun Gong†, Zhenzhen Fu†, Jinxiang Fu, Yan Sun, Xianxia Ju, Yina Chang, Wen Wang, Xiaohui Zhu, Beibei Gao, Xiaoyun Liu, Tao Yang and Hongwen Zhou*

Abstract

Background: Cholesterol accumulation causes pancreatic beta cell lipotoxicity and dysfunction. Cholesteryl ester transfer protein (CETP) plays an important role in blood lipid homeostasis. However, its role in tissue lipid metabolism remains unclear. We hypothesized that plasma CETP impact cholesterol homeostasis in the beta cells, thus damaging their functions.

Methods: The adipose tissue-specific CETP expression transgenic (aP2-CETPTg) mice, characterized by high CETP levels in the circulation, were used in this study. Pancreatic islet cholesterol and beta cell function were assessed in mice. We further measured mRNA levels of the genes involved in beta cell proliferation and differentiation, inflammation and cholesterol metabolism. TUNEL assay was applied to investigate beta cell apoptosis in islets.

Results: The aP2-CETPTg mice exhibited glucose intolerance, lower plasma insulin concentrations but increased insulin sensitivity compared with wild type mice. In addition, glucose-stimulated insulin secretion from isolated pancreatic islets significantly decreased, and free cholesterol significantly increased. Moreover, the number and size of islets from aP2-CETPTg mice were significantly decreased. Genes involved in beta cell proliferation, such as Pdx1 and BETA2, were down-regulated; genes involved in inflammation and ER stress, such as IL-1β, CHOP, and Xbp1 were up-regulated, in line with an increase of beta cell apoptosis.

Conclusions: Plasma CETP causes free cholesterol accumulation in islets which could contribute to beta cell dysfunction. Thus, CETP inhibition could be a novel protective strategy for dyslipidemia related to diabetes and obese.

Keywords: Cholesterol ester transfer protein, Free cholesterol, Beta cell function, Glucose metabolism

Background

The increased morbidity, mortality of type 2 diabetes mellitus (T2DM) makes it a crucial public health condition. Islet beta cell dysfunction and insulin resistance are major characteristics of pathophysiology of T2DM. Although insulin resistance occurs earlier during disease onset, beta cell dysfunction predates long before the occurrence of clinical hyperglycemia [1]. Many potential mechanisms for islet beta cell dysfunction have been proposed [2], however it still remains unclear. Lipotoxicity is regarded as one of the possible mechanisms which contribute to beta cell dysfunction. It has been suggested that increased free fatty acids accumulation in beta cells could reduce insulin secretion from beta cell, and induce beta cell apoptosis [3]. Recent studies have indicated that the accumulation of free cholesterol in beta cells may also contribute to lipotoxicity [4] and beta cell dysfunction [5].

Cholesteryl ester transfer protein (CETP) is a hydrophobic plasma glycoprotein that mediates the cholesteryl ester (CE) transfer from high density

* Correspondence: drhongwenzhou@njmu.edu.cn
†Equal contributors
Department of Endocrinology, the First Affiliated Hospital of Nanjing Medical University, 300 Guangzhou Road, Nanjing 210029, China

lipoprotein (HDL) to very low density lipoprotein (VLDL) or low density lipoprotein (LDL) in exchange for triglycerides, leading to lower HDL concentrations and more small dense-LDL particles [6]. In human, CETP is highly expressed in adipose tissue and liver, where it can be secreted into the blood and then participates in cholesterol metabolism [7]. We speculated that circulating CETP may mediate cholesterol homeostasis in islet beta cells. Some studies indicate that CETP may have additional effects on glucose metabolism other than lipid metabolism. A sub-study of the Investigation of Lipid Level Management to Understand Its Impact in Atherosclerotic Events (ILLUMINATE) trial reported that treatment with CETP inhibitor (torcetrapib) improved glycemic control in atorvastatin-treated patients with T2DM [8]. Siebel et al. [9] found that CETP inhibitor increased postprandial insulin and promoted ex vivo beta cell glucose-stimulated insulin secretion, potentially via enhanced beta cell cholesterol efflux. Most clinical studies have shown that CETP mass was increased in patients with T2DM and obesity [10]. CETP activity was positively correlated with fasting blood glucose and HbA1c while negatively correlated with HDL-C in T2DM [11]. Few studies also reported diabetes may suppress hepatic CETP in obese [12, 13]. Our previous study showed that glucose uptake and intracellular cholesterol were increased when 3T3-L1 adipocyte was transfected with CETP [14]. All these studies indicated that CETP might play a role in glucose metabolism.

We previously generated adipose tissue-specific CETP expression transgenic (aP2-CETPTg) mice and demonstrated that this model have the following characteristics: 1) high circulating CETP secreted by adipose tissue; 2) elevated LDL and declined HDL levels compared with WT mice; 3) very low CETP expression in other tissues (including skeletal muscle, liver, lung, kidney, heart, and brain) [15]. Natural flanking region (NFR)-CETPTg mice is another CETP transgenic mouse model with human like CETP concentration in the circulation and tissue distributions (liver, spleen, small intestine, kidney, and adipose tissue) [16]. Recently, Raposo et al. reported physiological levels of CETP (~2 μg/ml) did not affect glucose homeostasis and insulin secretion [17]. Interestingly, we previously found that over-expressed CETP might modulate glucose metabolism and insulin action in addition to its effects on lipoprotein metabolism in 3T3-L1 adipocytes [14]. In order to investigate whether circulating CETP (other than local CETP expression) and elevated CETP activity play roles in regulation of glucose metabolism and beta cell lipid accumulation, we used aP2-CETPTg mouse to explore the effects of CETP on mouse pancreatic beta cell lipid composition and beta cell function.

Methods

Animals

The NFR-CETPTg and aP2-CETPTg mice have C57BL/6J background [15]. Transgenic mice and non-transgenic littermates were fed standard rodent chow diet, housed in cages in a pathogen-free facility, and maintained on a 12 h light/12 h dark cycle. All experiments were performed on 10~16 week-old male mice. All animal experiments were conducted in accord with accepted standards of humane animal care, as outlined in the Ethical Guidelines, and were approved by the Research Animal Care Committee of Nanjing Medical University (IACUC-14030136).

CETP activity measurement

Mouse plasma CETP activity was measured by a fluorescence method as previously described [15]. Briefly, NBD-CE works as the donor, and ultracentrifugation separated human VLDL/LDL works as the acceptor. Reactions were performed in a 100 μl reaction mixture containing 3 μl plasma sample. Finally, fluorescence were measured by fluorescence microplate (SynergyMx, BioTek, United States) under 460 nm excitation wave and 530 nm emission wave. Plasma CETP activity was presented as detected fluorescence value (arbitrary units)/3 μl plasma).

Glucose and insulin tolerance test

Intraperitoneal glucose tolerance test (IPGTT) was performed on 16 h-fasted mice injected with D-glucose at 1 g/kg body weight. Blood glucose levels were measured at 0, 15, 30, 60 and 120 min after glucose injection. Plasma insulin during IPGTT was measured by Mouse Insulin ELISA kit (Millipore-linco, Billerica, MA, USA). Intraperitoneal insulin tolerance test (IPITT) was performed on 5 h-fasted mice injected with recombinant human insulin (Humulin, Eli Lilly and company, China) at 0.75 mU/kg body weight. Blood glucose levels were measured at 0, 15, 30, 60 and 120 min after insulin injection.

Isolation of pancreatic islets

Primary mouse islets were isolated by collagenase V (Sigma-Aldrich Chemie, Steinheim, Germany) digestion and filtration as previously described [18]. Islets used for glucose-stimulated insulin secretion measurement were cultured in RPMI-1640 (Gibco, California, USA) supplemented with 10 % FCS (Gibco, California, USA), 100 U/ml penicillin and 100 μg/ml streptomycin. Islets used for cholesterol measurement and real-time PCR were washed with PBS and frozen down immediately after isolation. Isolated islets number counting was conducted by two persons in a double-blinded fashion, referring to the method used by Ishikawa [19].

Glucose-stimulated insulin secretion assay

After overnight culture, islets were washed and used for glucose-stimulated insulin secretion (GSIS). Islets (eight similar-sized islets per well and eight wells per group) were firstly pre-incubated in Krebs-Ringer bicarbonate HEPES buffer supplemented with 0.2 % BSA for 1 h at 37 °C and 5 % CO_2, then incubated with KRB/HEPES buffer supplemented with 0.2 % BSA containing 3.3 or 16.7 mmol/l glucose for 1 h [18]. After then, islets were incubated with acid-ethanol (1.5 % HCl in 70 % Ethanol) overnight for insulin content measurement. The supernatants were collected after each treatment. Insulin levels were measured by the radioimmunoassay kit (BNIBT, Beijing, China). Insulin secretion ability is calculated by the relative secreted insulin to insulin content.

Plasma lipid measurement

Overnight fasting plasma were collected for plasma lipid measurement. The total cholesterol (TC), free cholesterol (FC) were assayed by enzymatic methods (Applygen Technologies Inc. Beijing, China), according to the instructions provided by the manufacturers. CE concentration is calculated by TC minus FC.

Islet lipid determination

Twenty similar-sized islets were washed five times with PBS and then cellular lipids were extracted by hexane: isopropyl alcohol (2:1 *v/v*) as described [20], using β-sitosterol (5 μg/ml) as an internal standard. Samples were split into two equal fractions to measure FC and TC separately. For TC measurement, CE was firstly transformed into free cholesterol. Finally, CE content is calculated by TC minus FC. To hydrolyze cellular cholesteryl esters prior to gas chromatography, 50 % KOH (200 μl) and methanol (3 ml) were added to dried aliquots and heated to 80 °C for 1 h in argon-capped tubes. After cooling, 3 ml H_2O and 5 ml HPLC grade hexane were added. Samples were centrifuged at 1000 rpm for 5 min and supernatant containing cholesterol was removed and dried under nitrogen. Cholesterol mass was measured by injection of 1 μl aliquots into a 5890 Series II gas chromatograph with a Detector (FID DETECTOR) using a 15 m × 0.53 mm × 1.5 μm cross-linked HP-5 Trace Analysis (5 % Ph Me Siloxane) column. Gas chromatography was performed at an isothermal 260 °C, injection port temperature of 300 °C, and detector temperature of 300 °C with nitrogen carrier flow rate of 30 ml/min. Calibration was achieved by injection of a standard solution of cholesterol (100 μg/ml).

RNA extraction, reverse transcription and gene expression

Total RNA from isolated islets were extracted using the RNAiso Plus (Takara, Dalian, China) and reverse-transcribed into cDNA using the Prime Script RT reagent kit (Takara, Dalian, China). Data for triplex real-time PCR assay were collected with an AB 7500 Real time PCR system (Applied Biosystems, Inc. United States). Reactions were performed with SYBR Green PCR Master Mix (Takara, Dalian, China) under following thermal cycling conditions: 2 min at 50 °C, 10 min at 95 °C, followed by 40 cycles of 95 °C for 15 s and 60 °C for 1 min. Conventional PCR reactions were performed in a 20 μl reaction mixture containing 0.5 μmol/L primers and 12.5 mg/L cDNA. Relative gene expression data were analyzed in the 2-ΔΔCT method, and the results were expressed as the expression fold over the control group. In exception, since there is no CETP mRNA expression in WT mice, the relative CETP mRNA of adipose tissue from aP2-CETPTg mice and NFR-CETPTg mice and of islets from NFR-CETPTg mice were expressed as 2^-ΔCT. The following primer sequences were used:

CETP310-A, 5′-TAGTGTTTACAGCCCTCATGAACAGCAAAG- 3′;

CETP310-B, 5′-CTCCATCTCCGTACTCCTAACCCAACTTCC- 3′.

Ki-67 forward, 5′-ATCATTGACCGCTCCTTTAGGT- 3′;

Ki-67 reverse, 5′-GCTCGCCTTGATGGTTCCT- 3′.

Pdx1 forward, 5′-GATGAAATCCACCAAAGCTCA- 3′;

Pdx1 reverse, 5′-AGAATTCCTTCTCCAGCTCCA- 3′.

BETA2 forward, 5′-ACTCCAAGACCCAGAAACTGTC- 3′;

BETA2 reverse, 5′-ACTGGTAGGAGTAGGGATGCAC- 3′.

IL-1β forward, 5′- TGCAGAGTTCCCCAACTGGTA-CATC- 3′;

IL-1β reverse, 5′- GTGCTGCCTAATGTCCCCTT-GAATC- 3.

TNF-α forward, 5′- CCCTCACACTCAGATCATCTTCT- 3′;

TNF-α reverse, 5′- GCTACGACGTGGGCTACAG- 3′.

IL-6 forward, 5′- CCAAGAGGTGAGTGCTTCCC- 3′;

IL-6 reverse, 5′- CTGTTGTTCAGACTCTCTCCCT- 3′.

IL-10 forward, 5′- GCTCTTACTGACTGGCATGAG- 3′;

IL-10 reverse, 5′- CGCAGCTCTAGGAGCATGTG- 3′.

CHOP forward, 5′-CATACACCACCACACCTGAAAG- 3′;

CHOP reverse, 5′-CCGTTTCCTAGTTCTTCCTTGC- 3′.

Atf6 forward, 5′- GACTCACCCATCCGAGTTGTG- 3′;

Atf6 reverse, 5′- CTCCCAGTCTTCATCTGGTCC- 3′.
Xbp1 forward, 5′- AGCAGCAAGTGGTGGATTTG- 3′;
Xbp1 reverse, 5′- GAGTTTTCTCCCGTAAAAGCTGA-3′.
Ldlr forward, 5′-CTGTTCCCA CCTCTGTTT AC- 3′;
Ldlr reverse, 5′- AGTGAG ATACGGCGA ATA GA- 3′.
HMGCS forward, 5′-TGG GAC CAA CCT TCT ACC TC- 3′;
HMGCS reverse, 5′-CAT CAA GGA CAG CTC ACC AG- 3′.
Srebp2 forward, 5′-TAACCCCTTGACTTCCTTGCT-3′;
Srebp2 reverse, 5′-TGCTCTTAGCCTCATCCTCCA-3′.

Histology and immunohistochemistry

Pancreata were isolated, fixed with 10 % buffered formalin, embedded in paraffin, sectioned and stained with hematoxylin and eosin for histological analysis. Pancreatic sections were scanned by Zeiss microscope at ×200 magnifications and islet size was analyzed with AxioVision software. For analysis of pancreatic islet apoptosis, double staining of in situ cell death detection fluorescence and insulin fluorescent immunohistochemistry were performed. The following primary antibodies were used: Rabbit anti-insulin polyclonal antibody, 1:50 (Proteintech Group, Inc. Chicago, USA); Secondary antibodies DyLight594 rabbit anti-goat IgG[H+L], 1:300 (MultiSciences Biotech, Hangzhou, China). The beta cell apoptosis was assessed by transferase-mediated dUTP nick-end labeling (TUNEL) assay (keyGEN, Nanjing, China) according to the manufacturer's protocol. For the determination of the overall rate of apoptosis, each section stained for insulin, TUNEL, and DAPI were imaged at 400 magnification (40 × objective), and the total number of TUNEL-positive cells per field were quantified. To determine the frequency of beta cell apoptosis, the number of cells positive for TUNEL was quantified in each islet and expressed as percentage of the total number of beta cells (n = ~4000). Beta cells were counted in 16 week old of age male mice per genotype (n = 4–5).

Statistical analysis and calculation

Data are expressed as means ± SD. Differences between groups were calculated by Student's t test. Data were analyzed using GraphPad Prism Software version 5.0, with significance defined as $p < 0.05$ (two-tailed). HOMA-IR is calculated by fasting plasma glucose (mmol/L) × fasting insulin (mIU/L)/22.5; HOMA-β is calculated by 20 × fasting insulin (mIU/L)/(fasting plasma glucose (mmol/L) – 3.5) (%).

Results

Characteristics of CETP transgenic mice

Wild-type (WT), NFR-CETPTg and aP2-CETPTg mice did not show differences in body weight in the age of 8 to 20 week (Fig. 1). The CETP mRNA in the adipose tissue was significantly higher in aP2-CETPTg mice than in NFR-CETPTg mice, but not expressed in WT littermates as expected (Fig. 2a). In consistent with the real-time PCR results, no CETP activity was detected in WT mice whereas high plasma CETP levels in aP2-CETPTg mice (OD value = 12,600 ± 784/μl), which is up to 2.3 folds of that in human plasma (OD value = 5570 ± 171/μl). Moreover, there is no detectable CETP mRNA expression in the isolated islets from WT and aP2-CETPTg mice, while a certain CETP expression in the islets from NFR-CETPTg mice (Fig. 2b).

aP2-CETPTg mice exhibit impaired glucose tolerance and insulin secretion

To study the effects of CETP on systemic glucose metabolism and insulin secretion in NFR-CETPTg and aP2-CETPTg mice, we conducted IPGTT, IPITT in vivo. A glucose challenge (1 g/kg) revealed an impaired glucose tolerance in aP2-CETPTg mice ($p < 0.05$), compared with WT mice, while a glucose intolerance tendency in NFR-CETPTg mice (Fig. 3a). Interestingly, we also found that NFR-CETPTg and aP2-CETPTg mice had an increased sensitivity to insulin compared with WT mice (Fig. 3b). The homeostasis model assessment of insulin resistance (HOMA-IR) of NFR-CETPTg and aP2-CETPTg mice were lower compared with WT mice (4.24 ± 1.19, 2.47 ± 0.54, 6.14 ± 3.14, respectively, $p < 0.05$), which also suggested that insulin sensitivity of aP2-CETPTg mice were higher. Besides, both NFR-CETPTg and aP2-CETPTg mice had significantly decreased plasma fasting insulin than WT mice ($p < 0.001$) (Fig. 3c). We further

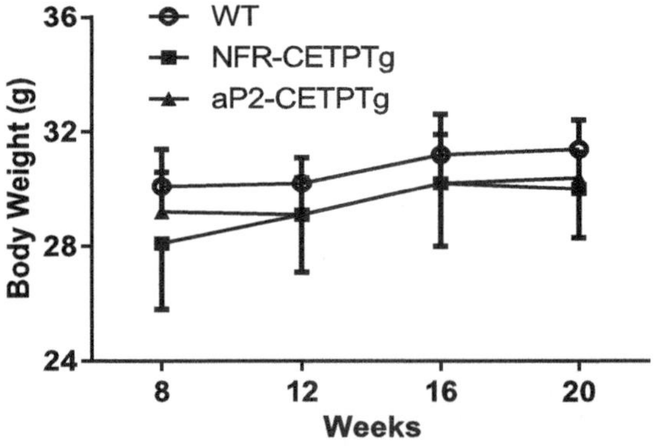

Fig. 1 Body weight of NFR-CETPTg, aP2-CETPTg and WT mice. Body weight records at 8, 12, 16 and 20 week-old mice. No significant difference between NFR-CETPTg, aP2-CETPTg and WT mice (n = 6 per group). Values are expressed as mean ± SD

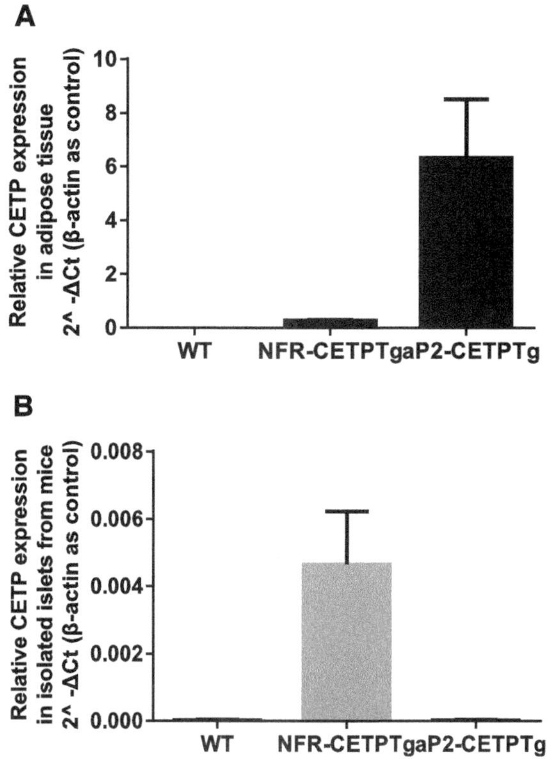

Fig. 2 CETP mRNA expression in adipose tissue and islets. Real-time PCR CETP mRNA analysis in mouse adipose tissue (**a**) and isolated islets (**b**). In aP2-CETPTg mice, CETP is predominantly expressed in adipose tissue but not detectable in islets, while a regular CETP expression in NFR-CETPTg mice. No CETP gene expression is noted in their controls. $n = 6$ per group. Values are expressed as mean ± SD

measured insulin levels after glucose overload, and we found that aP2-CETPTg mice had less insulin secretion than WT mice, especially at 0 and 60 min ($p < 0.05$) (Fig. 3d). Homeostasis model assessment of beta cell function index (HOMA-β) of NFR-CETPTg and aP2-CETPTg mice were lower compared with WT mice (48.7 ± 26.2, 56.9 ± 24.0, 96.6 ± 31.6, repectively, $p < 0.05$), which indicated beta cell dysfunction in aP2-CETPTg mice. Furthermore, we found that islets from aP2-CETPTg mice had a significant reduction in glucose-stimulated insulin secretion in vitro compared with that from WT mice ($p < 0.05$) (Fig. 3e). Collectively, both NFR-CETPTg and aP2-CETPTg mice have impaired glucose tolerance and insulin secretion, but increased insulin sensitivity. Moreover, we also found that there was a CETP dose-dependent effect on glucose tolerance.

aP2-CETPTg mice have fewer and smaller islets

Islets from aP2-CETPTg mice exhibited less islet number (138 ± 14 vs.166 ± 10, $p < 0.05$) (Fig. 4d) and smaller size (6850 ± 6940 vs. 9780 ± 10,100 μm^2, $p < 0.05$) compared with WT mice, which was clearly reflected by frequency distribution and mean area quantification on the pancreatic H-E staining sections (10 sections from two separate levels per mouse, 9–10 mice per group) (Fig. 4a–c).

aP2-CETPTg mice have higher apoptosis rate in beta cell

We next sought to determine whether decreased insulin secretion and smaller sized islets in aP2-CETPTg mice result from increased apoptosis of beta cells? Immunofluorescence stating of pancreas sections were conducted to quantify apoptosis rate of beta cells in aP2-CETP and WT mice. Results showed that the frequency of TUNEL-positive beta cell significantly increased in aP2-CETPTg mice (Fig. 5), indicating that circulating CETP could induce beta cell apoptosis. To further explain the reduction of islet mass, we next measured general proliferation marker Ki-67 and beta cell specific transcription factors, pancreatic and duodenal homeobox 1 (Pdx1) and BETA2. Ki-67 mRNA level was increased but the latter two both were suppressed in aP2-CETPTg mice (Fig. 6).

Circulating CETP promotes free cholesterol accumulation in the islets

To investigate the effect of CETP on islet lipid content, we utilized gas chromatograph to determine the lipid profile in the islets and found that FC (15.6 ± 3.60 vs. 10.3 ± 1.62 mmol/mg protein, $p < 0.05$), FC/CE ratio (2.44 ± 0.640 vs. 1.20 ± 0.430, $p < 0.05$) but not total cholesterol (22.0 ± 3.83 vs. 19.9 ± 2.13 mmol/mg protein, $p = 0.216$) were significantly increased in the transgenic mice islets compared with controls (Fig. 7a). In addition, plasma TC and CE were significantly decreased in aP2-CETPTg mice than WT mice (Fig. 7b), no difference was observed in FC (Fig. 7b) but FC/CE ratio induced (Fig. 7c). ACAT1 converts FC to CE, playing an important role in cellular cholesterol homeostasis, but ACAT1 mRNA in islets did not differ between the two groups (Fig. 7b). We further found that mRNA levels of cholesterol synthesis and uptake related genes, 3-hydroxy-3-methylglutaryl-CoA synthase (HMGCS), sterol regulatory element-binding protein-2 (SREBP-2), and LDL receptor (LDLR) were all significantly reduced (71, 41, 71 %, respectively) (Fig. 8).

The effect of circulating CETP on the expression of genes participated in islet inflammation and ER stress

Islet inflammation is emerging as an important factor that participates in the development of T2DM [21]. Thus, we sought to examine mRNA levels of IL-1β, TNF-α and IL-6, these representative pro-inflammatory cytokines that play key roles in modulating islet cytokine

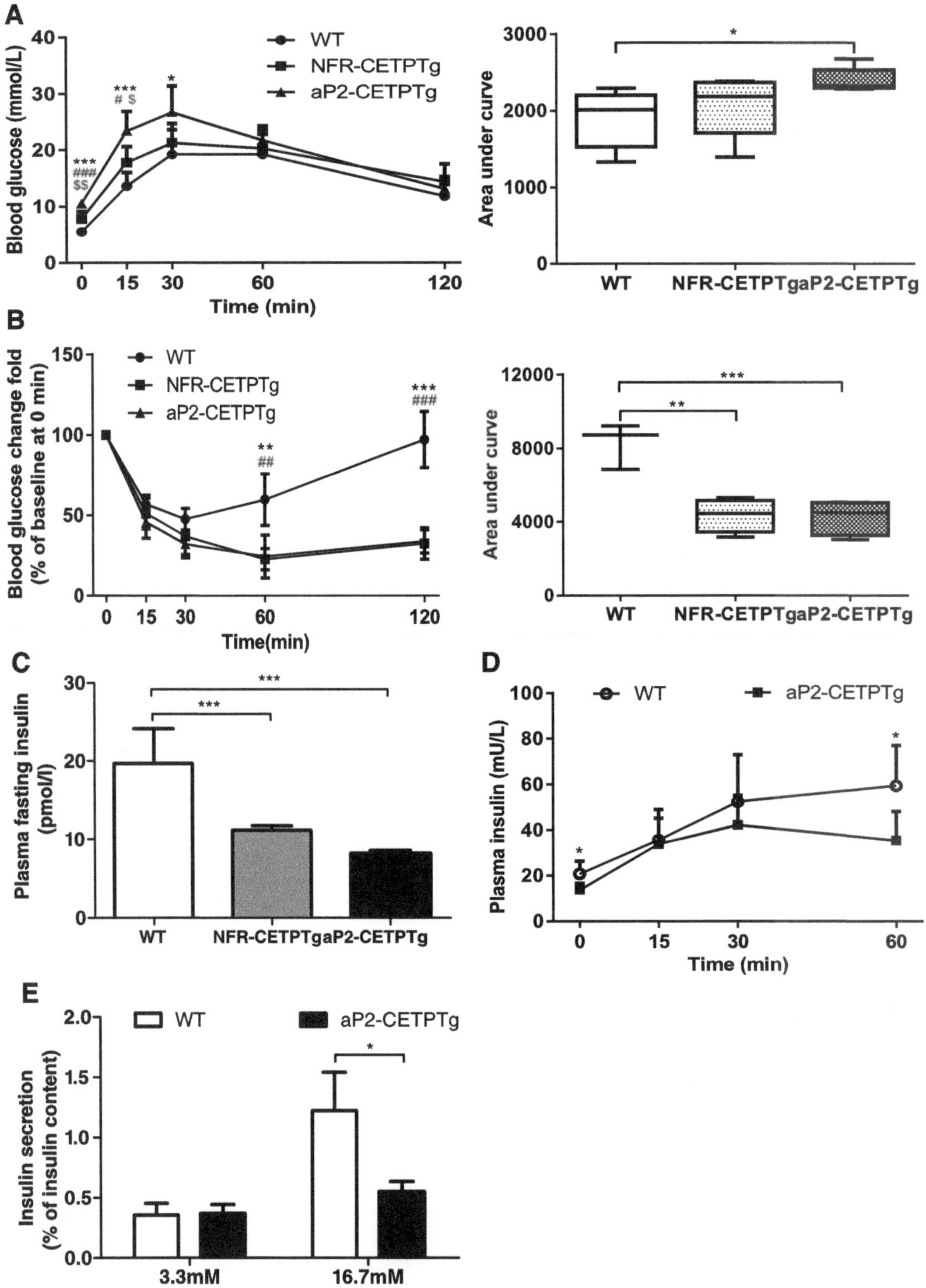

Fig. 3 (See legend on next page.)

(See figure on previous page.)
Fig. 3 Impaired glucose tolerance and decreased insulin secretion in aP2-CETPTg mice in vivo and in vitro. **a** IPGTT was performed in 10–12 week-old mice by intraperitoneal injecting D-glucose (1 g/kg body weight). Blood glucose levels were measured at 0, 15, 30, 60 and 120 min during IPGTT. $n = 6$ per group. Area under curve is calculated and showed (*right*). The aP2-CETPTg mice have impaired glucose tolerance than WT mice. **b** IPITT was performed in 10–12 week-old mice by intraperitoneal injecting insulin (0.75 IU/kg body weight). Blood glucose were recorded at 0, 15, 30, 60 and 120 min during IPITT. $n = 6$ per group. Area under curve is calculated and showed (*right*). The insulin sensitivity is increased in the NFR-CETPTg and aP2-CETPTg mice. **c** Plasma fasting insulin levels in NFR-CETPTg, aP2-CETPTg and WT mice. CETP transgenic mice exhibited decreased fasting insulin secretion than WT mice. $n = 5$ per group. **d** Plasma insulin levels were measured at 0, 15, 30 and 60 min during IPGTT in WT and aP2-CETPTg mice. After glucose challenge, aP2-CETPTg mice secreted less insulin than WT mice. $n = 6$ per group. **e** Insulin secretion ability was measured from isolated islets by glucose-stimulated insulin secretion. Eight islets per well, eight wells per group. Insulin release in response to 16.7 mmol/l glucose was significantly impaired in aP2-CETPTg mice compared with WT mice. Values are expressed as mean ± SD. $^{*}p < 0.05$ compared with control group, $^{**}p < 0.01$ compared with control group. *IPGTT* intraperitoneal glucose tolerance test, *IPITT* intraperitoneal insulin tolerance test

release and impairs islet function [21]. The results indicated that IL-1β mRNA was significantly increased in islets of aP2-CETPTg mice, but without differences in TNF-α, IL-6 or IL-10 mRNA expression (Fig. 9a).

Free cholesterol accumulation in macrophages leads to CHOP-induced ER stress [22]. To investigate whether unfolded protein response is enhanced in the islets from aP2-CETPTg mice, we measured the mRNA expression of CHOP, X-box binding protein 1 (Xbp1) and activating transcription factor 6 (Atf6). Our data showed that the mRNA levels of CHOP and Xbp1 were also increased in aP2-CETPTg mouse islets (Fig. 9b), suggesting that circulating CETP could be cytotoxic to beta cells. Atf6 did not differ between the islets from aP2-CETPTg and WT mice (Fig. 9b).

Discussion

In this study, we demonstrated for the first time that circulating CETP, 1) exacerbate glucose intolerance, lower plasma insulin concentrations but increase insulin sensitivity; 2) increase free cholesterol accumulation in the islets; 3) reduce the expression of the genes which participate in beta cell proliferation and differentiation, resulting in fewer and smaller islet number and size; 4) induced the expression of the genes which are involved in inflammation, ER stress, and apoptosis; and 5) finally and most importantly, circulating CETP decreased insulin secretion from islet beta cells.

It is well known that insulin resistance and insulin deficiency are main factors of glucose intolerance. In our aP2-CETPTg mice, insulin sensitivity is increased, compared with WT mice. This could be due to two reasons, 1) adipocyte size becomes smaller [23], and 2) skeletal muscle takes up more glucose. Although aP2-CETPTg mice had increased insulin sensitivity, they displayed glucose intolerance and this could be due to beta cell dysfunction.

Circulating CETP influences insulin sensitivity and insulin secretion in a dose-dependent fashion. Recently, Raposo et al. [17] reported that CETP expression does not affect glucose homeostasis and insulin secretion. However, our GTT results clearly indicated that there is a CETP dose-dependent effect on mice glucose tolerance impairment and fasting insulin secretion dysfunction. Therefore, the inconsistent results between Raposo et al's and ours' could be mainly due to the different CETP levels in the blood. Raposo et al. utilized a heterozygous CETP transgenic (NFR-CETP-Tg) mice model which is identical to our NFR-CETP-Tg mice, presenting human like plasma levels of CETP (~2 ug/ml). However, our aP2-CETPTg mice have significantly higher levels of CETP in circulation. Therefore, elevated CETP mass and activity in T2DM patients may bring additional damage to insulin secretion.

What is the mechanism for beta cell dysfunction in aP2-CETPTg mice? We hypothesized that free cholesterol accumulation in aP2-CETPTg mice islet induce beta cell dysfunction. It is known that high cholesterol levels in islets interfere with glucose metabolism by inhibiting glucokinase activity, the critical glucose-sensing component of the beta cell, and reducing the effectiveness of the insulin secretory apparatus [4, 24]. ATP-binding cassette transporter A1 (ABCA1) is a cellular cholesterol transporter which participates in cholesterol efflux, mice lacking beta cell ABCA1 exhibited impaired glucose tolerance and decreased insulin secretion due to abnormalities of cholesterol homeostasis in isolated islets [25]. SREBP-2 is another member of the membrane-bound transcription factor SREBP family, and plays a crucial role in the regulation of cholesterol metabolism [19]. Expression of nuclear human SREBP-2 in beta cells resulted in severe diabetes due to defects in glucose- and potassium-stimulated insulin secretion. Cholesterol is a well-known component of both secretory granules and plasma membranes, and cholesterol-rich microdomains in the plasma membrane are thought to be essential for normal cell function, including exocytosis [26, 27]. The cholesterol-rich lipid rafts in beta cell membranes contain calcium channels and the proteins that constitute the secretory apparatus which consists of soluble N-ethylmaleimide-sensitive factor (NST) attachment protein receptor (SNARE), soluble NST attachment

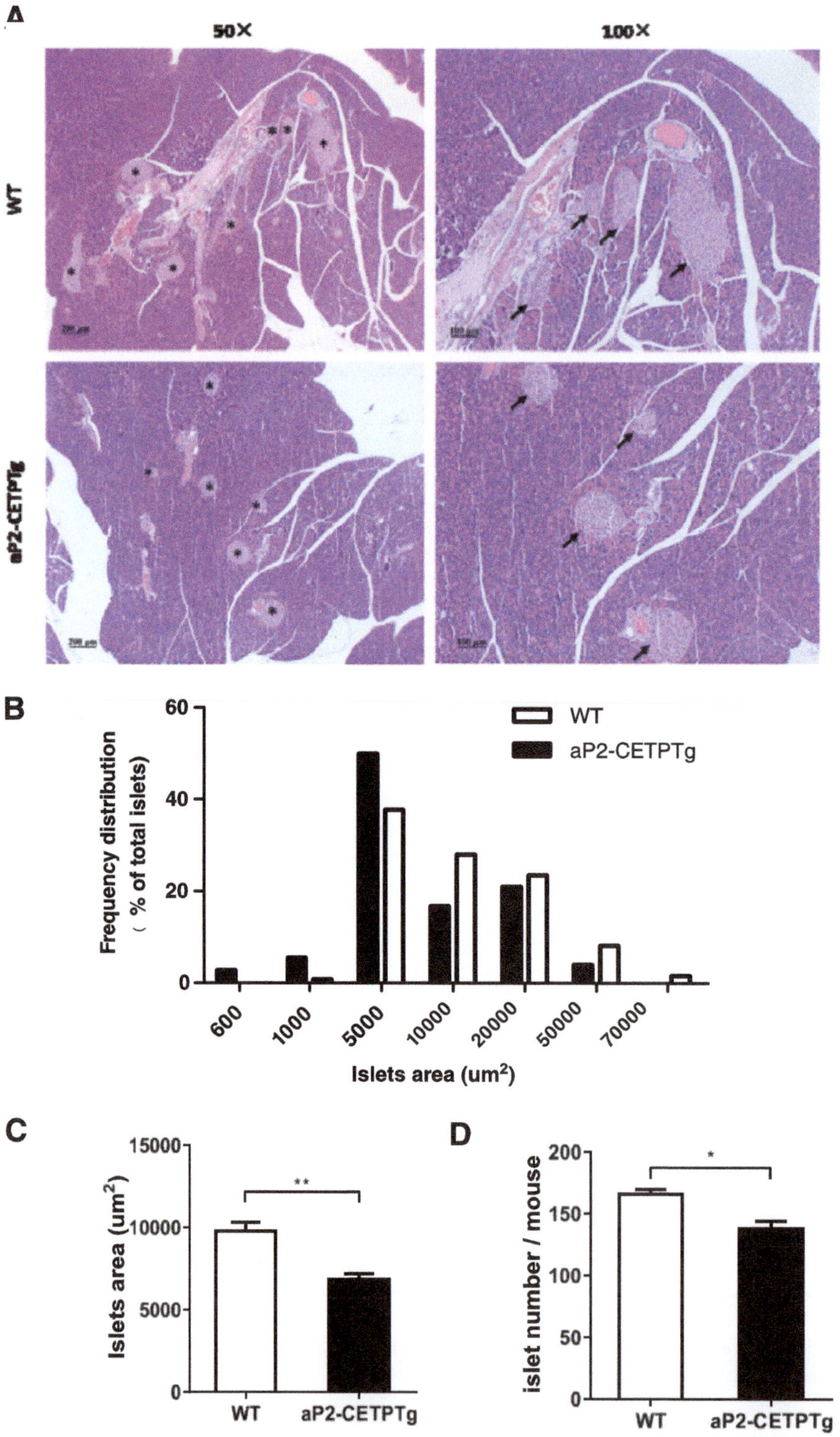

Fig. 4 (See legend on next page.)

(See figure on previous page.)
Fig. 4 Morphology, number and area distribution of islets from aP2-CETPTg mice. **a** Representative pancreas sections of aP2-CETPTg mice and WT mice were stained with hematoxylin and eosin for histological analysis. Original magnification, ×50 (*left panels*); ×100 (*right panels*). Islets are marked with *asterisk* and *arrow*. **b** The area distribution of islets on H-E staining pancreas sections. (aP2-CETPTg, $n = 9$; WT, $n = 10$; 10 sections at two separate levels per mouse pancreas). Islets from aP2-CETPTg mice were smaller in size than that from WT mice. **c** Area quantification of islets on pancreas sections displayed significant decreased area in aP2-CETPTg mice. **d** Pancreatic islets were isolated from aP2-CETPTg mice and WT mice ($n = 6$ per group) and double-blinded counted by two persons. Islets isolated from aP2-CETPTg mice were fewer than that from WT mice. Values are expressed as mean ± SD. $^{**}p < 0.01$, compared with control group

protein-25 (SNAP-25), and synaptobrevin. All of these proteins participate in insulin secretion. The accumulation of cholesterol in beta cell interferes with the effectiveness of the insulin secretory apparatus then decrease insulin secretion. Conversely, lowering beta cell cholesterol levels with methyl-β-cyclodextrin [4, 28], which depletes membrane cholesterol, increases insulin secretion. Our results indicated that FC/CE of islets was increased in the islets from aP2-CETPTg mice when compared with WT mice. Moreover, the free cholesterol accumulation is not directly result from ACAT mRNA level changes. Enrichment of FC changes beta cell membrane lipid composition and this could lead to less efficiency in insulin secretion through exocytosis.

Our study showed that the size of islets from aP2-CETPTg mice were significantly reduced, which could be another reason for the decrease of insulin secretion. These morphologic variations of islets in aP2-CETPTg mice might be a consequence of cholesterol accumulation in the beta cells. Studies in macrophages demonstrated that free cholesterol induces apoptosis by causing stiffening of the ER membrane, with subsequent induction of the unfolded protein response [29]. Our data also showed that beta cell apoptosis was increased, in line with higher expression of ER stress markers, including CHOP and Xbp1. Cholesterol accumulation can decrease expression of the beta cell specific proliferation and differentiation genes, Pdx1 and BETA2, which may be another reason for the decrease of beta cell number and size. Interestingly, Ki-67 mRNA expression was upregulated in aP2-CETPTg mice, which may be a feedback regulation of increased beta cell apoptosis. Islet inflammation has been reported in T2DM, and individuals with elevated serum levels of certain pro-inflammatory cytokines show increased risks for developing T2DM [30]. IL-1β is well established as a pro-inflammatory cytokine involved with the demise of the beta cell [31]. Our results showed that IL-1β mRNA was significantly increased in islets of aP2-CETPTg mice.

The question arises as to how CETP might promote free cholesterol accumulation in pancreatic beta cells. CETP has been reported to exchange lipids between cell membranes and between cell membranes and lipoproteins. For example, CETP can mediate efflux of cholesteryl ester from biological membranes to lipoproteins [32, 33]. CETP can also facilitate HDL-cholesterol selective uptake by adipocytes [34]. It is conceivable that CETP could also facilitate cholesteryl ester efflux out of the plasma membrane of cell, thus causing free cholesterol accumulation in the cells. It has been suggested that CETP could enhance the exchange of lipids during the formation of a ternary collision complex consisting of donor and acceptor lipoproteins, bridged by CETP [35]. By analogy, CETP might bind the HDL to the plasma membrane of cell, and increase the collisions between the membrane and the lipoprotein, allowing lipids to be exchanged in the process. We speculate that circulating CETP could transfer cholesteryl ester but not free cholesterol out of the beta cell to lipoproteins in the

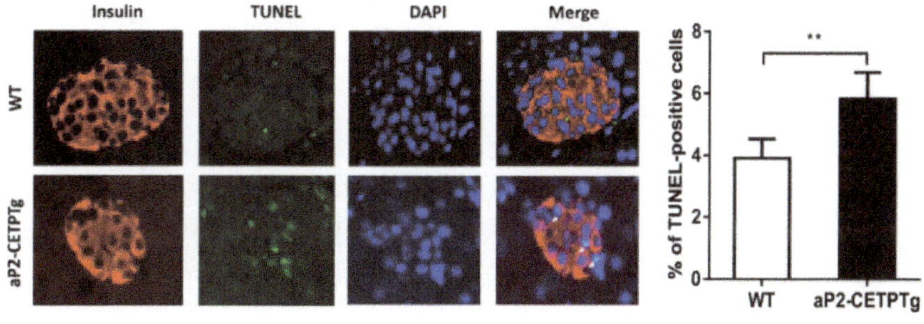

Fig. 5 Increased beta cell apoptosis in aP2-CETPTg mice compared with WT mice by TUNEL. Representative TUNEL-positive beta cells were marked with *white arrows* (*Left*). The number of cells positive for TUNEL was quantified in every single islet and expressed as percentage of the total number of beta cells ($n = \sim 4000$) (*Right*). Beta cells were counted in immunofluorescence staining pancreas section form 16 week-old male mice ($n = 5$ per group). Values are expressed as mean ± SD. $^{**}p < 0.01$, compared with control group

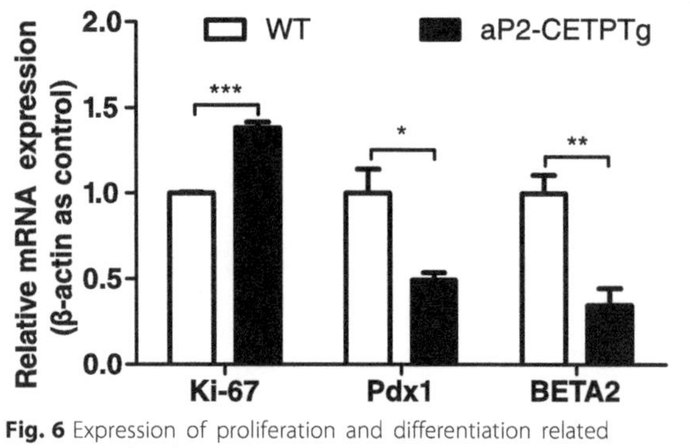

Fig. 6 Expression of proliferation and differentiation related genes in isolated islets from aP2-CETPTg mice. Ki-67 mRNA level was significantly upregulated in islets from aP2-CETPTg mice. The mRNA expression of Pdx1 and BETA2 were decreased compared with WT mice. Values are expressed as mean ± SD. *$p < 0.05$, **$p < 0.01$, and *** $p < 0.001$ compared with control group. $n = 5$ per group. *Pdx1* pancreatic and duodenal homeobox 1

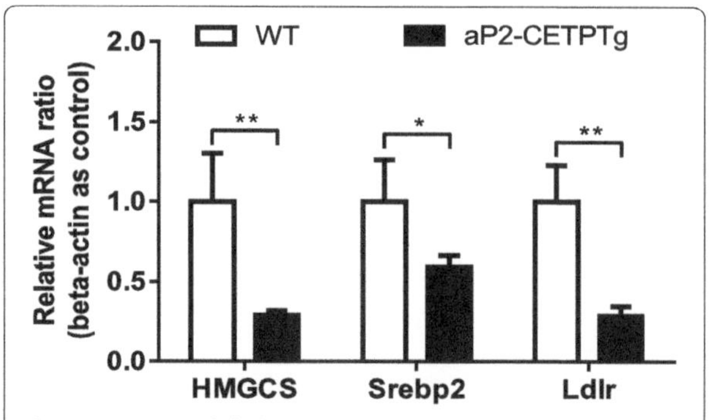

Fig. 8 Expression of cholesterol synthesis and uptake related genes in isolated islets from aP2-CETPTg mice. Relative mRNA levels of HMGCS, Srebp2 and Ldlr in isolated islets. $n = 5$ per group. Values are expressed as mean ± SD. *$p < 0.05$ and **$p < 0.01$, compared with control group. *HMGCS* 3-hydroxy-3-methylglutaryl-CoA synthase, *Srebp2* sterol regulatory element-binding protein 2, *Ldlr* LDL receptor

circulation, resulting in elevation of FC/CE ratio in the islets, and the precise mechanism needs further study.

Conclusions

In summary, our data show that circulating CETP have an impact on beta cell cholesterol homeostasis by accumulation of free cholesterol, thus reducing beta cell insulin secretion. These data provide further evidence to the concept that regulation of beta cell cholesterol homeostasis is essential for normal islet function. CETP inhibition could be a potential promising approach to improve beta cell function in T2DM by decreasing islet cholesterol accumulation and inflammation.

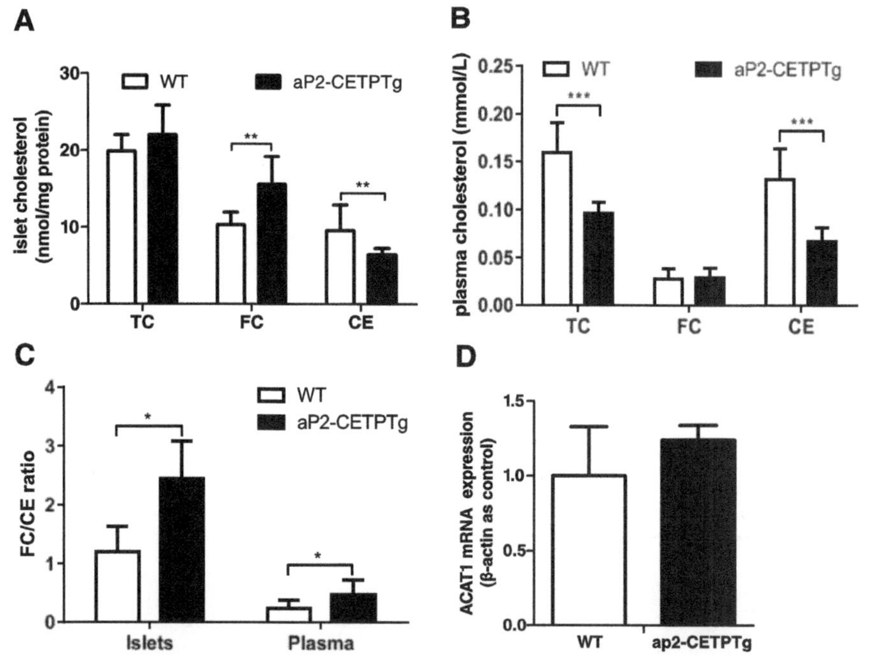

Fig. 7 Lipid profile in plasma and islets from ap2-CETPTg mice. **a** Total cholesterol, free cholesterol, and cholesteryl ester of islets isolated from aP2-CETPTg mice and WT mice (20 islets per mice, 5 mice per group) were extracted and measured as described in the Methods. **b** Plasma cholesterol profile in aP2-CETPTg and WT mice ($n = 10$ per group). **c** The FC/CE ratio in plasma and islets. **d** ACAT1 mRNA expression does not differ in the two groups. Values are expressed as mean ± SD. *$p < 0.05$ and **$p < 0.01$, ***$p < 0.001$, compared with control group

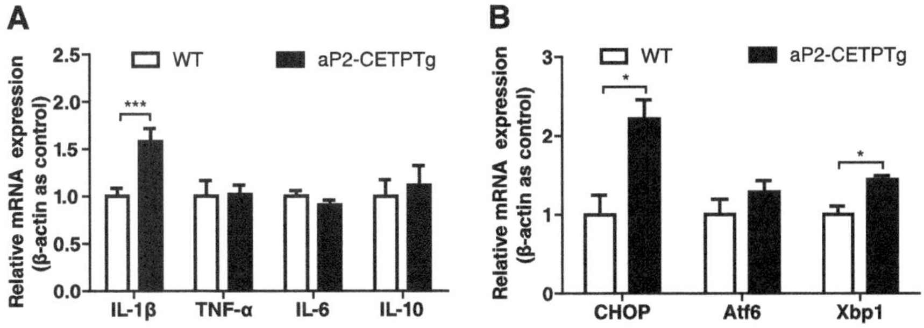

Fig. 9 Expression of inflammation and ER stress related genes in isolated islets from aP2-CETPTg mice. **a** As for the mRNA level of pro-inflammatory markers, IL-1β was higher in aP2-CETPTg mice than their control, but TNF-α and IL-6 mRNA expression did not differ between the two groups. For the anti-inflammatory marker, IL-10 mRNA level had an increasing tendency in aP2-CETPTg mice. **b** Relative mRNA levels of CHOP and Xbp1 in isolated islets were increased in aP2-CETPTg mice. $n = 4$–6 per group. Values are expressed as mean ± SD. *$p < 0.05$, and *** $p < 0.001$ compared with control group. *Xbp1* X-box binding protein 1, *Atf6* activating transcription factor 6

Ethics approval

All animal experiments were conducted in accord with accepted standards of humane animal care, as outlined in the Ethical Guidelines, and were approved by the Research Animal Care Committee of Nanjing Medical University (IACUC-14030136).

Consent for publication

Not applicable.

Abbreviations

ABCA1: ATP-binding cassette transporter A1; Atf6: activating transcription factor 6; aP2-CETPTg: adipose tissue-specific CETP expression transgenic; CE: cholesteryl esters; CETP: cholesteryl ester transfer protein; FC: free cholesterol; GSIS: glucose-stimulated insulin secretion; HDL: high density lipoprotein; HMGCS: 3-hydroxy-3-methylglutaryl-CoA synthase; IPGTT: intraperitoneal glucose tolerance test; LDL: low density lipoprotein; LDLR: LDL receptor; Pdx1: pancreatic and duodenal homeobox 1; SNAP: soluble N-ethylmaleimide-sensitive factor attachment protein; SNARE: soluble N-ethylmaleimide-sensitive factor attachment protein receptor; SREBP-2: sterol regulatory element-binding protein-2; T2DM: type 2 diabetes mellitus; TUNEL: transferase-mediated dUTP nick-end labeling; VLDL: very low density lipoprotein; WT: wild type; Xbp1: X-box binding protein 1.

Competing interests

The authors declare that they have no competing interests.

Authors' contributions

WG, ZF, XJ and HZ participated in the study design. WG, YG, ZF, JF, YS, XJ, YC, WW, XZ, BG and HZ were involved in the conduct of the study. WG, YG, XL, TY and HZ mainly contributed to the writing of the manuscript. All authors participated in the analysis and interpretation of the data and approved the final version.

Acknowledgements

None.

Fundings

National Natural Sciences Foundation of China (81170747).
Health Promotion Foundation of Jiangsu Province, China (H201106).
This two grants support this study in the design of the study and collection, analysis, and interpretation of data and in writing the manuscript.

References

1. Cerf ME. Beta cell dysfunction and insulin resistance. Front Endocrinol (Lausanne). 2013;4:37.
2. Prentki M, Nolan CJ. Islet beta cell failure in type 2 diabetes. J Clin Invest. 2006;116:1802–12.
3. Poitout V, Robertson RP. Glucolipotoxicity: fuel excess and beta-cell dysfunction. Endocr Rev. 2008;29:351–66.
4. Hao M, Head WS, Gunawardana SC, Hasty AH, Piston DW. Direct effect of cholesterol on insulin secretion: a novel mechanism for pancreatic beta-cell dysfunction. Diabetes. 2007;56:2328–38.
5. Fryirs M, Barter PJ, Rye KA. Cholesterol metabolism and pancreatic beta-cell function. Curr Opin Lipidol. 2009;20:159–64.
6. Yamashita S, Hirano K, Sakai N, Matsuzawa Y. Molecular biology and pathophysiological aspects of plasma cholesteryl ester transfer protein. Biochim Biophys Acta. 2000;1529:257–75.
7. Jiang XC, Moulin P, Quinet E, Goldberg IJ, Yacoub LK, Agellon LB, Compton D, Schnitzer-Polokoff R, Tall AR. Mammalian adipose tissue and muscle are major sources of lipid transfer protein mRNA. J Biol Chem. 1991;266:4631–9.
8. Barter PJ, Rye KA, Tardif JC, Waters DD, Boekholdt SM, Breazna A, Kastelein JJ. Effect of torcetrapib on glucose, insulin, and hemoglobin A1c in subjects in the Investigation of Lipid Level Management to Understand its Impact in Atherosclerotic Events (ILLUMINATE) trial. Circulation. 2011;124:555–62.
9. Siebel AL, Natoli AK, Yap FY, Carey AL, Reddy-Luthmoodoo M, Sviridov D, Weber CI, Meneses-Lorente G, Maugeais C, Forbes JM, Kingwell BA. Effects of high-density lipoprotein elevation with cholesteryl ester transfer protein inhibition on insulin secretion. Circ Res. 2013;113:167–75.
10. de Vries R, Perton FG, Dallinga-Thie GM, van Roon AM, Wolffenbuttel BH, van Tol A, Dullaart RP. Plasma cholesteryl ester transfer is a determinant of intima-media thickness in type 2 diabetic and nondiabetic subjects: role of CETP and triglycerides. Diabetes. 2005;54:3554–9.
11. Smaoui M, Hammami S, Attia N, Chaaba R, Abid N, Kilani N, Kchaou H, Mahjoub S, Abid M, Hammami M. Modulation of plasma cholesteryl ester transfer protein activity by unsaturated fatty acids in Tunisian type 2 diabetic women. Nutr Metab Cardiovasc Dis. 2006;16:44–53.
12. Dallinga-Thie GM, Dullaart RP, van Tol A. Concerted actions of cholesteryl ester transfer protein and phospholipid transfer protein in type 2 diabetes: effects of apolipoproteins. Curr Opin Lipidol. 2007;18:251–7.
13. MacLean PS, Vadlamudi S, MacDonald KG, Pories WJ, Barakat HA. Suppression of hepatic cholesteryl ester transfer protein expression in obese humans with the development of type 2 diabetes mellitus. J Clin Endocrinol Metab. 2005;90:2250–8.
14. Ju X, Cui Q, Zhang M, Wang W, Jiang J, Chang Y, Wang K, Yang T, Zhou H. Human cholesteryl ester transfer protein enhances insulin-mediated glucose uptake in adipocytes. Life Sci. 2011;89:479–84.

15. Zhou H, Li Z, Hojjati MR, Jang D, Beyer TP, Cao G, Tall AR, Jiang XC. Adipose tissue-specific CETP expression in mice: impact on plasma lipoprotein metabolism. J Lipid Res. 2006;47:2011–9.
16. Jiang XC, Agellon LB, Walsh A, Breslow JL, Tall A. Dietary cholesterol increases transcription of the human cholesteryl ester transfer protein gene in transgenic mice. Dependence on natural flanking sequences. J Clin Invest. 1992;90:1290–5.
17. Raposo HF, Vanzela EC, Berti JA, Oliveira HC. Cholesteryl Ester Transfer Protein (CETP) expression does not affect glucose homeostasis and insulin secretion: studies in human CETP transgenic mice. Lipids Health Dis. 2016;15:9.
18. Zhu SS, Ren Y, Zhang M, Cao JQ, Yang Q, Li XY, Bai H, Jiang L, Jiang Q, He ZG, Chen Q. Wld(S) protects against peripheral neuropathy and retinopathy in an experimental model of diabetes in mice. Diabetologia. 2011;54:2440–50.
19. Ishikawa M, Iwasaki Y, Yatoh S, Kato T, Kumadaki S, Inoue N, Yamamoto T, Matsuzaka T, Nakagawa Y, Yahagi N, et al. Cholesterol accumulation and diabetes in pancreatic beta-cell-specific SREBP-2 transgenic mice: a new model for lipotoxicity. J Lipid Res. 2008;49:2524–34.
20. Rumsey SC, Galeano NF, Lipschitz B, Deckelbaum RJ. Oleate and other long chain fatty acids stimulate low density lipoprotein receptor activity by enhancing acyl coenzyme A:cholesterol acyltransferase activity and altering intracellular regulatory cholesterol pools in cultured cells. J Biol Chem. 1995; 270:10008–16.
21. Kashiwagi A, Takahashi H, Ishikawa H, Yoshida S, Kazuta K, Utsuno A, Ueyama E. A randomized, double-blind, placebo-controlled study on long-term efficacy and safety of ipragliflozin treatment in patients with type 2 diabetes mellitus and renal impairment: results of the long-term ASP1941 safety evaluation in patients with type 2 diabetes with renal impairment (LANTERN) study. Diabetes Obes Metab. 2015;17:152–60.
22. Feng B, Yao PM, Li Y, Devlin CM, Zhang D, Harding HP, Sweeney M, Rong JX, Kuriakose G, Fisher EA, et al. The endoplasmic reticulum is the site of cholesterol-induced cytotoxicity in macrophages. Nat Cell Biol. 2003;5:781–92.
23. Zhou H, Li Z, Silver DL, Jiang XC. Cholesteryl ester transfer protein (CETP) expression enhances HDL cholesteryl ester liver delivery, which is independent of scavenger receptor BI, LDL receptor related protein and possibly LDL receptor. Biochim Biophys Acta. 2006;1761:1482–8.
24. Vikman J, Jimenez-Feltstrom J, Nyman P, Thelin J, Eliasson L. Insulin secretion is highly sensitive to desorption of plasma membrane cholesterol. FASEB J. 2009;23:58–67.
25. Brunham LR, Kruit JK, Pape TD, Timmins JM, Reuwer AQ, Vasanji Z, Marsh BJ, Rodrigues B, Johnson JD, Parks JS, et al. Beta-cell ABCA1 influences insulin secretion, glucose homeostasis and response to thiazolidinedione treatment. Nat Med. 2007;13:340–7.
26. Salaun C, James DJ, Chamberlain LH. Lipid rafts and the regulation of exocytosis. Traffic. 2004;5:255–64.
27. Wang Y, Thiele C, Huttner WB. Cholesterol is required for the formation of regulated and constitutive secretory vesicles from the trans-Golgi network. Traffic. 2000;1:952–62.
28. Xia F, Gao X, Kwan E, Lam PP, Chan L, Sy K, Sheu L, Wheeler MB, Gaisano HY, Tsushima RG. Disruption of pancreatic beta-cell lipid rafts modifies Kv2.1 channel gating and insulin exocytosis. J Biol Chem. 2004;279:24685–91.
29. Yao PM, Tabas I. Free cholesterol loading of macrophages is associated with widespread mitochondrial dysfunction and activation of the mitochondrial apoptosis pathway. J Biol Chem. 2001;276:42468–76.
30. Spranger J, Kroke A, Mohlig M, Hoffmann K, Bergmann MM, Ristow M, Boeing H, Pfeiffer AF. Inflammatory cytokines and the risk to develop type 2 diabetes: results of the prospective population-based European Prospective Investigation into Cancer and Nutrition (EPIC)-Potsdam Study. Diabetes. 2003;52:812–7.
31. Dinarello CA, Donath MY, Mandrup-Poulsen T. Role of IL-1beta in type 2 diabetes. Curr Opin Endocrinol Diabetes Obes. 2010;17:314–21.
32. Stein O, Halperin G, Stein Y. Cholesteryl ester efflux from extracellular and cellular elements of the arterial wall. Model systems in culture with cholesteryl linoleyl ether. Arteriosclerosis. 1986;6:70–8.
33. Stein Y, Stein O, Olivecrona T, Halperin G. Putative role of cholesteryl ester transfer protein in removal of cholesteryl ester from vascular interstitium, studied in a model system in cell culture. Biochim Biophys Acta. 1985;834:336–45.
34. Vassiliou G, McPherson R. Role of cholesteryl ester transfer protein in selective uptake of high density lipoprotein cholesteryl esters by adipocytes. J Lipid Res. 2004;45:1683–93.
35. Tall A. Plasma lipid transfer proteins. Annu Rev Biochem. 1995;64:235–57.

8

Short chain acyl-CoA dehydrogenase deficiency and short-term high-fat diet perturb mitochondrial energy metabolism and transcriptional control of lipid-handling in liver

Sujoy Ghosh[1,2], Claudia Kruger[1], Shawna Wicks[1], Jacob Simon[1], K. Ganesh Kumar[1,3], William D. Johnson[1], Randall L. Mynatt[1], Robert C. Noland[1] and Brenda K. Richards[1*]

Abstract

Background: The liver is an important site of fat oxidation, which participates in the metabolic regulation of food intake. We showed previously that mice with genetically inactivated *Acads*, encoding short-chain acyl-CoA dehydrogenase (SCAD), shift food consumption away from fat and toward carbohydrate when tested in a macronutrient choice paradigm. This phenotypic eating behavior suggests a link between fat oxidation and nutrient choice which may involve an energy sensing mechanism. To identify hepatic processes that could trigger energy-related signals, we have now performed transcriptional, metabolite and physiological analyses in *Acads-/-* mice following short-term (2 days) exposure to either high- or low-fat diet.

Methods and Results: Metabolite analysis revealed 25 acylcarnitine species that were altered by diet and/or genotype. Compared to wild-type mice, phosphorylated AMP-activated protein kinase was 40 % higher in *Acads-/-* mice after short-term high-fat diet, indicating a low ATP/AMP ratio. Metabolite analyses in isolated liver mitochondria from *Acads-/-* mice during ADP-linked respiration on butyrate demonstrated a reduced oxygen consumption rate (OCR) compared to wild-type, an effect that was not observed with succinate or palmitoylcarnitine substrates. Liver transcriptomic responses in *Acads-/-* mice fed high- vs. lowfat diet revealed increased RXR/PPARA signaling, up-regulation of lipid handling pathways (including beta and omega oxidation), and increased mRNA expression of Nfe2l2 target genes.

Conclusions: Together, these results point to an oxidative shortage in this genetic model and support the hypothesis of a lower hepatic energy state associated with SCAD deficiency and high-fat diet.

Keywords: Short chain acyl-CoA dehydrogenase deficiency, Fatty acid beta-oxidation, Mitochondrial

Background

Acads encodes short-chain acyl-CoA dehydrogenase (SCAD), a member of the family of four enzymes that catalyzes the first of four sequential steps in the mitochondrial fatty acid oxidation spiral which produces acetyl-CoA for the tricarboxylic acid cycle. The optimum substrate for SCAD is butyryl-CoA, a fatty acid with four carbon units. Fatty acids are an important source of energy, particularly for tissues with high metabolic demands such as the liver, which plays a major role in the regulation of energy homeostasis in mammals.

Previously we reported that mice with a global, genetic inactivation of the gene encoding short-chain acyl-CoA dehydrogenase (*Acads−/−*) shift consumption away from fat and toward carbohydrate when offered a choice between macronutrient-rich diets [1]. As the mice avoid eating fat, they apparently compensate by eating more carbohydrate, thus preventing a reduction in caloric intake. Our observation provides evidence for a link

* Correspondence: richarbk@pbrc.edu
[1]Pennington Biomedical Research Center, Louisiana State University System, 6400 Perkins Road, Baton Rouge, LA 70808-4124, USA
Full list of author information is available at the end of the article

between fatty acid oxidation and fat selection. Furthermore, the potential for altered fatty acid oxidation to affect the selection of fat-rich diets could be dependent on hepatic energy status, as changes in ATP/ADP ratio are quite likely sensed by the brain [2–5] to ultimately influence feeding behavior. Thus it is reasonable to postulate the liver as a site where signals related to fatty acid-derived energy may originate. Based on this proposition, the current study addressed the metabolic consequences of short-chain acyl-coenzyme A (CoA) dehydrogenase (SCAD) deficiency and dietary fat content on liver metabolism, including effects on tissue acylcarnitines, mitochondrial oxidative metabolism, hepatic pAMPK level, and genome-wide transcription. These studies were performed in the liver of *Acads−/−* and *Acads+/+* mice fed high- or low-fat diet for 2 days.

Methods

Animals and diets

The BALB/cByJ (*Acads−/−*) and BALB/cByKZ (*Acads+/+*) mice were obtained from breeding colonies maintained at the Pennington Biomedical Research Center (PBRC). Mice were singly housed in filter-top cages and kept in a specific-pathogen free facility, under 12 h light/12 h dark cycle and at an ambient temperature of 22–23 °C. All animals were fed standard rodent chow (no. 5001, LabDiets, Richmond, IN) until initiation of experimental diets. All animal experiments were approved by the Institutional Animal Care and Use Committee of the PBRC. The BALB/cByJ mouse strain carries a spontaneous 278-bp deletion at the 3' end of the structural gene for *Acads* [6, 7], resulting in missplicing of RNA and a truncated, unstable SCAD enzyme with no residual activity [8]. This mutation occurred in the BALB/cByJ subline around 1982 [9] after it was separated from the BALB/cBy subline. Although the BALB/cByJ or *Acads−/−* mice have no detectable butyryl-CoA dehydrogenase activity [8], they appear to be normal [8, 10]. Their primary clinical phenotype is an impaired adaptation to prolonged fasting, due to the rapid depletion of hepatic glycogen stores [8]. The BALB/cBy line is considered the best *Acads+/+* control for the *Acads−/−* BALB/cByJ [11]. Our BALB/cByKZ.*Acads+/+* substrain was separated from the research colonies at The Jackson Laboratory in 1996.

Several days prior to each experiment, bedding was removed and replaced with stainless steel wire floor inserts, to permit measurement of spilled food. Polyvinylchloride nesting tubes were provided to reduce time spent on wire flooring. The experimental diets were equivalent for both micronutrients and for protein (16.4 % of energy). The balance of calories was contributed by 58 % fat and 25.5 % carbohydrate in D12331 and by 10.5 % fat and 73.1 % carbohydrate in D12329 (Research Diets, Inc., New Brunswick, NJ). The diets obtain most of their fat content from medium chain fatty acids. Tissues were harvested on day 2 after initiation of the high-fat (D12331) or low-fat (D12329) diet. Thus, there was no diet choice in the current study design. We selected the day 2 time point for tissue harvest to coincide with the time at which animals begin to avoid eating fat in a diet selection paradigm [1].

Measurement of acylcarnitines

Twelve week old male BALB/cByJ (*Acads−/−*) and BALB/cByKZ (*Acads+/+*) mice were fed the experimental high- (HF) and low-fat (LF) diets for two days and then killed by CO_2 inhalation followed by cervical dislocation. The liver was rapidly excised, frozen in liquid nitrogen, then powdered under liquid nitrogen and stored at −80 °C. Measurement of liver acylcarnitine content was performed by the Metabolomics Core of the University of Michigan. Liver samples were extracted and proteins precipitated by addition of solvent containing labeled internal standards (Cambridge Isotopes, labeled carnitine standards set B, cat#NSK-B1). Weighed samples were sonicated briefly (10 % duty cycle, 2 min, on ice) in the extraction solvent (Methanol-Chloroform-Water (8:1:1). Acylcarnitine species were measured by MRM transitions using an Agilent 1260 HPLC and 6430 Triple Quadrupole LC/MS system (Agilent Technologies, Santa Clara, CA). All data were acquired and analyzed using Agilent Masshunter Quantitative software, version 6.0. Standard curves were generated and acylcarnitines were measured using isotope dilution internal standards. Data were normalized to wet tissue weight and analyzed using 2-way analysis of variance in SAS v9.4 (SAS Institute Inc., Cary, NC, USA).

Protein analysis by western blotting

Male, *Acads−/−* and *Acads+/+* mice were fed the HF and LF experimental diets for 0, 1, or 2 days. On the day of tissue harvest, mice were euthanized with CO_2 between 10:00 and 11:00 am; the liver was quickly removed, frozen in liquid nitrogen and stored at −80 °C. Total protein was isolated using Lysis buffer (25 mM HEPES pH 7.8, 1 % Nonidet P-40, 50 mM KCl, 125 μM DTT, 1 mM PMSF, 5 mM NaPPi, 1 mM EDTA, 50 mM NaF including protease inhibitor cocktail). The samples were centrifuged and protein concentrations of the supernatants were determined using the BCA Protein Assay (Pierce Biotechnology, Rockford, IL). Electrophoretic separations were carried out on Mini-Protean II electrophoresis cells (Bio-Rad Laboratories, Inc., Hercules, CA). Supernatants (45 μg) were resolved by 10 % SDS-PAGE and subjected to immunoblotting. The protein was detected with antibodies against AMPKp(Thr^{172}), AMPK (Abcam Inc., Cambridge, MA) and beta Actin (HRP) (Abcam) using Chemiluminescence Reagent Plus (Perkin-Elmer Life Sciences). Signal intensity was quantified by densitometry analysis using ImageJ Software [12].

Preparation of mouse liver mitochondria

Male *Acads-/-* and *Acads+/+* mice were fed the high fat (HF) diet for two days, as described above. On the morning of the experiment, mice were euthanized using CO_2 inhalation and liver tissue was collected in ice cold isolation buffer and subsequently homogenized according to the detailed method of Frezza et al. [13]. Mitochondrial protein content was measured using the BCA Protein Assay (Pierce Biotechnology, Rockford, IL). The preparation was kept on ice at all times and used within 6 h of isolation for mitochondrial bioenergetic measurements.

Measurement of mitochondrial respiration

The oxygen consumption rate (OCR) of mitochondria during respiration was measured in the assay solution (MAS-1, 1X): 70 mM sucrose, 220 mM mannitol, 10 mM KH_2PO_4, 5 mM $MgCl_2$, 2 mM HEPES, 1 mM EGTA and 0.2 % BSA, using a Seahorse XF24 Extracellular Flux Analyzer (Seahorse Bioscience, North Billerica MA, USA) [14]. Ten (10) μg of freshly prepared mitochondria were added to each well in an initial volume of 50ul, and the plate was centrifuged at 1800 g, 4 °C for 10 min to insure that mitochondria adhered to the bottom of the well. Substrate mix was added and the plate was brought to equilibrium at 37 °C for 10 min before loading it into the XF24-3 and initiating the experiment. State 4 respiration was determined in the presence of either succinate/rotenone (5.5 mM/2.2uM), butyrate/malate (900uM/2 mM), or palmitoylcarnitine/malate (80uM/2 mM) as substrates. The substrates butyrate/malate and palmitoylcarnitine/malate were used to involve short- and long-chain acyl-CoA dehydrogenases, respectively. First, two baseline measurements of oxygen consumption rate (OCR) were obtained. Next, ADP (4 mM) was injected to determine state 3 respiration, followed by sequential injections of oligomycin (2uM), FCCP (4uM) and antimycin A (4uM). Collectively, this injection series allowed for determination of ATP-linked OCR (ADP), proton leak (oligomycin), maximal respiration (FCCP) and non-mitochondrial or residual oxygen consumption (antimycin A). Samples from individual animals were run in 2–3 replicates using typical mix and measurement cycle times [14]. Respiratory control ratios (RCR) were calculated as the state 3 respiratory rate divided by the state 4 respiratory rate, obtained from the ADP-linked/oligomycin OCR readings [15]. Data are displayed as absolute, point-to-point oxygen consumption rates (pmol/min/well) and were analyzed using the XF software and Microsoft Excel. OCR data represent the mean of 2–3 replicate wells ± SE. Differences in OCR between genotype groups were tested using a two-tailed Student's *t*-test, with P values less than 0.05 considered to be statistically significant.

Measurement of mitochondrial DNA (mtDNA) content

Mitochondrial DNA was quantified by determining the ratios of encoded mitochondrial cytochrome c oxidase (*mt-Co2*) and cytochrome b (*mt-Cybt*) to nuclear intron of hemoglobin beta (*Hbb*) and glucagon (*Gcg*), respectively, by qRT–PCR of isolated DNA. Total DNA was extracted from liver using the DNeasy Qiagen Kit (Qiagen, Germantown, MD) and amplified using published primer sequences [16] and quantitative PCR (7900HT Sequence Detection System; Life Technologies, Carlsbad, CA). All primers were synthesized by Sigma-Aldrich (St. Louis, MO, USA).

Microarray studies

Mice used for tissue harvest in the microarrays showed no statistically significant differences in baseline body weight or total energy intake between the genotype (*Acads-/-*, *Acads+/+*) or diet (HF, LF) groups (Additional file 1: Table S1). Animals were euthanatized with CO_2 between 10:00 and 11:00 am on the morning of dissection. The liver was quickly removed, frozen in liquid nitrogen and stored at −80 °C. Total RNA from 12 animals (3 biological replicates in each of four diet-genotype comparisons) was isolated from liver using TRI Reagent (Molecular Research Center, Inc., Cincinnati, OH, USA), and assessed for quality in an Agilent Bioanalyzer 2100 (Agilent Technologies, Santa Clara, CA, USA). One μg of total RNA was used to transcribe DIG-labeled cRNA using AB Chemiluminescent RT-IVT Kit v2.0. Hybridization of 10 μg fragmented DIG-labeled cRNA to AB Mouse Genome Survey microarray (version 2.0), processing, chemiluminescence detection, imaging, auto-gridding, and image analysis were performed according to AB protocols, using the 1700 Chemiluminescent Microarray Analyzer Software v. 1.0.3. The AB Expression system software V2.0 was used to extract assay signal and signal-to-noise ratios from the images as previously described [17].

Microarray data analysis

Signal intensities across microarrays were log transformed (base 2) and quantile normalized using the BRB-Array Tools software [18]. Statistical significance of the differentially expressed (DE) genes was ascertained via a regularized *t*-test based on the Bayesian statistical framework [19]. The magnitude of gene over-expression or under-expression was quantified by the difference in the $\log_2$ average signals between the treatment and control groups. Using analysis of variance, gene expression profiles in liver were analyzed for main effects involving diet and genotype, as well as diet by genotype interactions [18]. The MIAME guidelines compliant microarray data have been deposited in the National Center for Biotechnology Information (NCBI) Gene Expression Omnibus (GEO) repository, under accession number GSE35180.

Ingenuity pathway analysis

Over-representation analysis (ORA) of canonical pathways was carried out by subjecting a pre-filtered list of differentially expressed genes with $P < 0.01$ and absolute fold-change ≥1.5-fold to Ingenuity Pathway Analysis (IPA). The Ingenuity Knowledge Base was used as the source for the reference genes. Fisher's exact test p-values were used to estimate the significance of over-representation and corrections for multiple testing were made using the Benjamini-Hochberg procedure for false discovery rate [20]. Significantly enriched pathways were compared across treatments by 2-way clustering and then color coded according to the negative logarithm of their Fisher's exact *P*-value.

IPA was further utilized to identify 'upstream regulators' whose activation/inhibition could explain the observed gene expression results. An overrepresentation analysis (Fisher's exact test) was first performed to determine whether a regulator was enriched for differential expression of its target genes (the list of regulators and their target genes were obtained from the Ingenuity Knowledge Base). The overall activation/inhibition status of the regulator was inferred from the degree of consistency (up- or down-regulation) in the expression patterns of its target genes, expressed as a z-score. Regulators with $z \geq 2$ or $z \leq -2$ were considered to be activated or inhibited, respectively. A new score (C), combining the magnitude of the z-score with significance of overlap (*P*-value), was created according to the relationship: $C = z\text{-}score * -logP$. The C score was used to summarize the predicted effects from the upstream regulators.

Quantitative real-time PCR

Complementary DNA (cDNA) was obtained by reverse transcription (SuperScript III First-Strand Synthesis System for RT-PCR, Invitrogen, Carlsbad, CA, USA) of 4 μg of RNA from each liver sample. cDNA was subjected to QIAquick PCR purification columns (Qiagen, Valencia, CA, USA). For qRT-PCR, samples from 6–12 individuals were tested for the *Acads−/−* and *Acads+/+* strains, respectively, using the microarray samples (3 per strain and condition) and additional samples collected under the same conditions.

Primers for amplification were designed using gene sequences obtained from the National Center for Biotechnology Information (NCBI) and Primer Express Software v3.0 (Life Technologies). Primers were synthesized by IDT (Integrated DNA Technologies, Coralville, IA, USA). The locations and sequences of primers are listed in Additional file 2: Table S2.

Gene expression levels were measured using the ABI PRISM 7900HT Sequence Detection System. Individual samples were run in triplicate. As an endogenous reference for normalization, we used the measurement of Cyclophilin (*Ppia*) cDNA in the same sample; *Ppia* levels were unaffected by diet and genotype on the arrays. Analysis was performed using SDS Software v2.3 for the 7900HT (Life Technologies). Relative quantification was calculated using the comparative C_T method (AB: User Bulletin #2: Relative quantification of gene expression. P/N 4303859 [21]. A two-tailed Student's *t*-test was performed on ΔC_T values to evaluate strain differences in gene expression. *P* values of ≤ 0.05 were considered statistically significant.

Results/Discussion

We investigated the effects of SCAD deficiency and high-fat diet in the liver. Our approach included analyses of mitochondrial oxidative function and nutrient-sensing signaling mechanisms, metabolic profiling of acylcarnitine levels and genome-wide transcriptional profiling. In each case, tissue was harvested from *Acads−/−* or *Acads+/+* mice only 2 days after initiating a single, high- or low-fat diet, to coincide with the time point at which the *Acads* mutants begin to eat less fat in a macronutrient diet selection paradigm [1]. Our overall aim was to uncover hepatic processes affected by fuel oxidation and ATP generation [3] that potentially could be linked to feeding behavior [17].

Acads genotype and HF diet increase acylcarnitine levels in the liver

Acylcarnitines are intermediary metabolites derived from mitochondrial acyl-CoA metabolism. To examine the biochemical effects of SCAD deficiency and dietary fat on lipid substrate metabolism in the liver, we measured acylcarnitines of *Acads−/−* and *Acads+/+* mice fed either HF or LF fat diet for 2 days. The analysis of variance (ANOVA) revealed significant main effects of diet on twenty (20) acylcarnitines, and of genotype on twenty-five (25) acylcarnitines (Additional file 3: Table S3). For example, on HF diet, the liver content of C4 (butyryl) and C5 (isovaleryl) was 30-fold ($P < 0.0001$) and 2-fold ($P < 0.0001$) higher, respectively, in *Acads−/−* compared with *Acads+/+* mice (Fig. 1), demonstrating the metabolic block. On LF diet however, the liver C4 content ($P < 0.01$) was only 4-fold higher in mutant animals. Six acylcarnitine species showed a significant diet-by-genotype interaction (see Additional file 3: Table S3). The accumulation of excess medium-chain and long-chain lipid byproducts, e.g., 3-fold higher levels of C12:0 and C14:0 acylcarnitines in HF-fed *Acads−/−* compared to HF-fed *Acads+/+* could have resulted, in part, from the enrichment of medium chain fatty acids from coconut oil in the HF diet. In liver, 20–25 acylcarnitine species were affected by genotype or diet, compared to only 5 species in plasma, as shown previously [17], suggesting a dysregulation of hepatic mitochondrial beta oxidation.

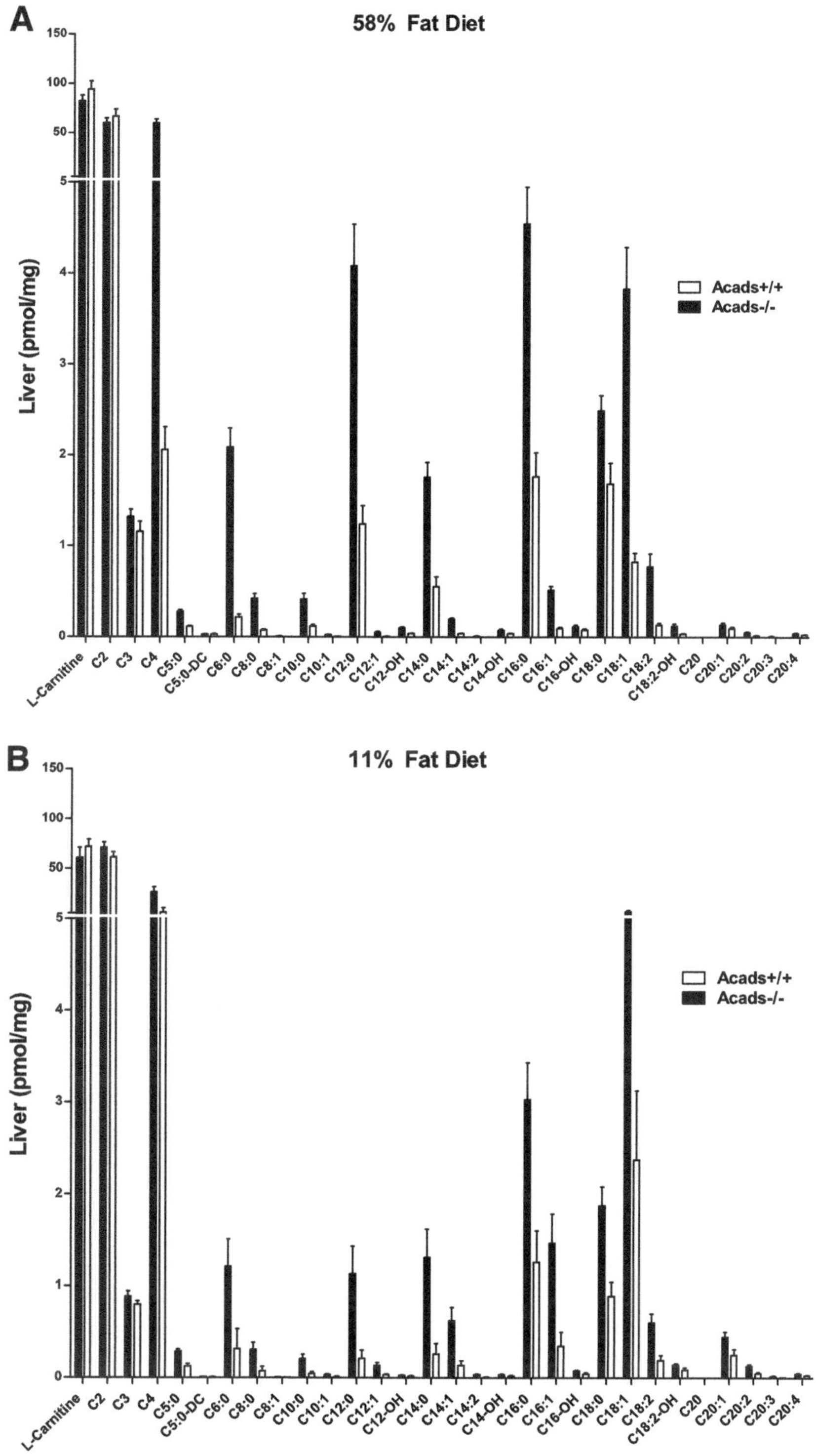

Fig. 1 Effects of genotype and dietary fat level on liver acylcarnitine levels. Legend: Acylcarnitines were measured by tandem mass-spectrometry in liver tissue from Acads−/− and Acads+/+ fed high- (**a**) or low-fat (**b**) diet for 2 days. Values are means (pmol/mg protein) ± SEM. *n* = 6 animals per group. See Additional file 3: Table S3 for a summary of ANOVA results

Acads genotype and HF diet increase pAMPK in the liver

Phosphorylation of AMP-kinase (pAMPK) is a key signal in the response to changes in energy balance including consumption of HF diet [22]. Cellular conditions that inhibit ATP production will result in a change in the AMP:ATP ratio and thus activate the AMPK signaling pathway. We therefore examined the effects of SCAD deficiency on hepatic pAMPK in *Acads−/−* mice fed HF diet for 2 d. Immunoblot analysis of liver tissue showed enhanced pAMP-kinase, compared to wild type controls, as evidenced by the ~40 % increase in (Thr-172) phosphorylation of the AMPK protein (Fig. 2). The adenosine monophosphate (AMP)-activated protein kinase (AMPK) phosphorylates numerous intracellular proteins and alters the transcription of genes involved in the regulation of energy metabolism including the transcriptional co-activation of PPAR-alpha. The net effect of AMPK activation is to turn off biosynthetic pathways such as lipogenesis and to activate catabolic pathways that produce ATP (e.g., fatty acid oxidation) [23]. This finding is consistent with a cellular "switch" from energy storage to energy release/use, suggesting that ATP availability is reduced under the conditions of impaired short chain fatty acid oxidation and high-fat diet, and agrees with our previous observation of AMPK activation in the hypothalamus of high-fat fed *Acads−/−* animals [17]. Finally, in light of previous reports that SCAD-deficient (also known as *Acads−/−*) mice are prone to fasting induced hypoglycemia [8], the animals in this experiment were tested a few hours

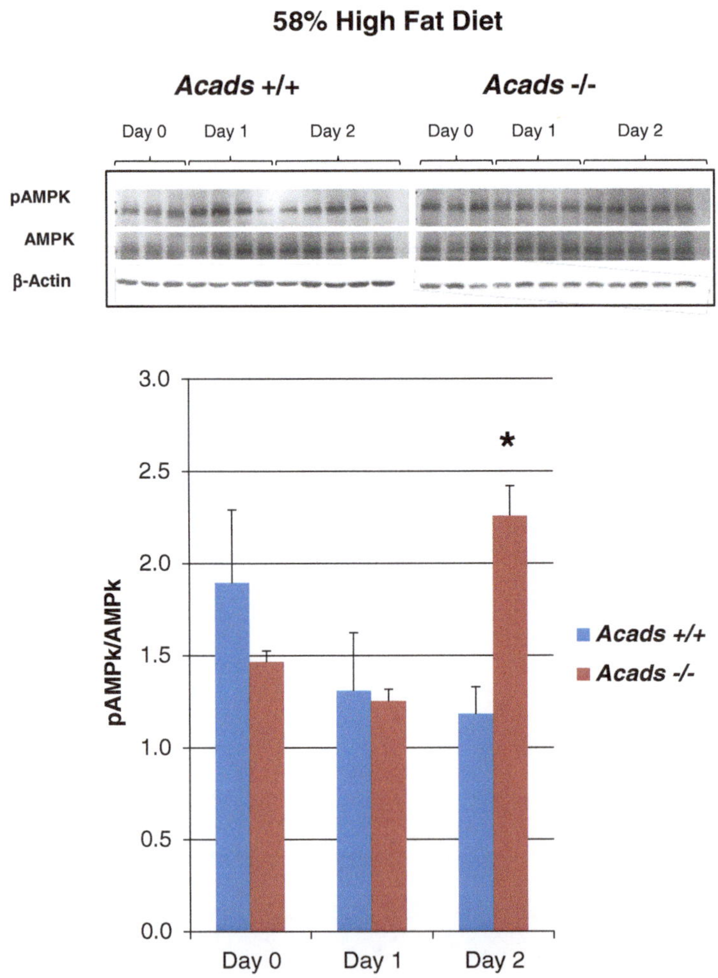

Fig. 2 Effect of *Acads* genotype on pAMPK in the liver of mice fed high-fat diet. Legend: On chow (day 0) and after one day of high-fat diet, there was no effect of genotype on pAMPK level in liver. However, on day 2 of high-fat diet, pAMPK level was increased by ~40 % in *Acads−/−* compared to *Acads+/+* mice. Food was removed at 0700, animals were euthanized and tissues were harvested at 0900. Immunoblots for total AMPK, pAMPK and beta actin are shown. $n = 3–5$ per genotype and day. $^*P < 0.005$, genotype comparison

after their most recent meal, when plasma glucose concentrations were similar between genotypes (data not shown). The absence of hypoglycemia in this study suggests that the observed AMPK activation in liver results from the metabolic effects of impaired short-chain fatty acid catabolism.

Acads inactivation inhibits oxygen consumption rate of isolated liver mitochondria in a substrate-specific manner

We found that pAMPK was significantly elevated in the liver of HF-fed, *Acads*–/– mice, suggesting a depletion of ATP. Mitochondria are the main sites of cellular ATP production from substrate oxidative phosphorylation [24] and play a critical role in fatty acid oxidation. Thus, we investigated the effects of SCAD deficiency on mitochondrial respiration in isolated hepatic mitochondria from *Acads*–/– mice fed HF diet. Because the SCAD protein is the first enzyme involved in the short-chain fatty acid beta oxidation spiral, we tested mitochondria for their ability to oxidize exogenously added fatty acids.

Acads–/– mitochondria function normally

To test the hypothesis of differences in mitochondrial efficiency between *Acads*–/– and *Acads*+/+ mice, we measured real-time oxygen consumption rates (OCR) in isolated liver mitochondria using an extra-organelle flux assay. OCR was measured in the presence (state 3) or the absence (state 4) of ADP, along with the ratio of these two rates—the respiratory control ratio (RCR) [25]. We first tested the function of complex II (a.k.a. succinate dehydrogenase), which is an enzyme complex bound to the inner mitochondrial membrane that participates in both the citric acid cycle and the electron transport chain. The results showed that in the presence of succinate + rotenone (complex II), basal respiration, leak respiration, uncoupled respiration and non-mitochondrial respiration were similar between mitochondria from *Acads*–/– and wild-type mice (Fig. 3a). Additionally, the RCR values indicate that the mitochondria used in these experiments were intact and functional; there were no differences between genotype groups (Fig. 3d), demonstrating that SCAD deficiency does not result in systemic mitochondrial dysfunction.

Acads–/– mitochondria have impaired ability to oxidize butyrate

Mitochondria isolated from the liver of *Acads*–/– mice were also tested for their ability to respire on a short chain lipid using butyrate combined with the anaplerotic substrate malate. We found that both ADP-stimulated and uncoupled respiration were significantly reduced in *Acads*–/– mitochondria compared with *Acads*+/+ (Fig. 3b). However, neither basal nor leak (oligomycin inhibited) respiration were significantly different between genotypes. These changes resulted in a slight, although not statistically significant, decrease in the RCR obtained from *Acads*–/– mitochondria (Fig. 3d), suggesting the possibility of a substrate-specific impairment in *Acads*–/– mitochondrial function when using butyrate/malate. Importantly, the *Acads*–/– mitochondria retained their capacity to respond to both ADP and an uncoupling agent, although at lower rates than wild-type mitochondria. This result is consistent with the different but overlapping substrate-chain-length specificities of acyl-CoA dehydrogenases, e.g., that medium chain acyl-CoA dehydrogenase (MCAD) may be active toward some esters of short-chain fatty acids such as C6, but not toward those of long-chain fatty acids [26]. To examine more fully the implications of SCAD deficiency on energy production, we then measured mitochondrial respiration using long-chain fatty acids as the substrate.

Maximal, but not ADP-linked, long chain fatty acid respiration was reduced by SCAD deficiency

We measured OCR in liver mitochondria from *Acads*–/– mice using palmitoylcarnitine/malate as substrates and found no difference in basal, resting or ADP-stimulated respiration (Fig. 3c), or in RCR (Fig. 3d), compared to controls. The absence of a significant difference in palmitoylcarnitine OCR under these conditions is somewhat surprising but may indicate that partial oxidation of long-chain fatty acids is sufficient to meet the energy demands of the cell under most conditions. When mitochondria from wild type liver were fed fatty acids as substrate, respiratory control by the phosphorylation of ADP acted to limit activity of the electron transport chain. Then, when the chemical uncoupler FCCP was applied and electron transfer was no longer controlled by the proton gradient, we observed an increase in oxygen consumption that was 39 % greater than ADP-stimulated respiration, providing evidence for enhanced mitochondrial spare capacity under conditions of heightened energy demand. However in isolated mitochondria from *Acads*–/– liver, maximal uncoupled respiration merely reached levels similar to those observed in ADP-stimulated respiration, indicating a nearly complete decrement in spare respiratory capacity when using a traditional long chain fatty acid substrate. Therefore, it appears that under normal circumstances the long and medium chain acyl-CoA dehydrogenases can supply sufficient reducing equivalents to the electron transport chain [27]. This residual activity may help explain the reports of weaker clinical symptoms for SCAD deficiency than for VLCAD deficiency [28, 29]. Nevertheless, in the absence of functional SCAD enzyme, a decrement in the beta-oxidation of C4-C6 fatty acids may exceed the mitochondrial capacity for energy production under conditions of greater energy demand, such as that induced by FCCP,

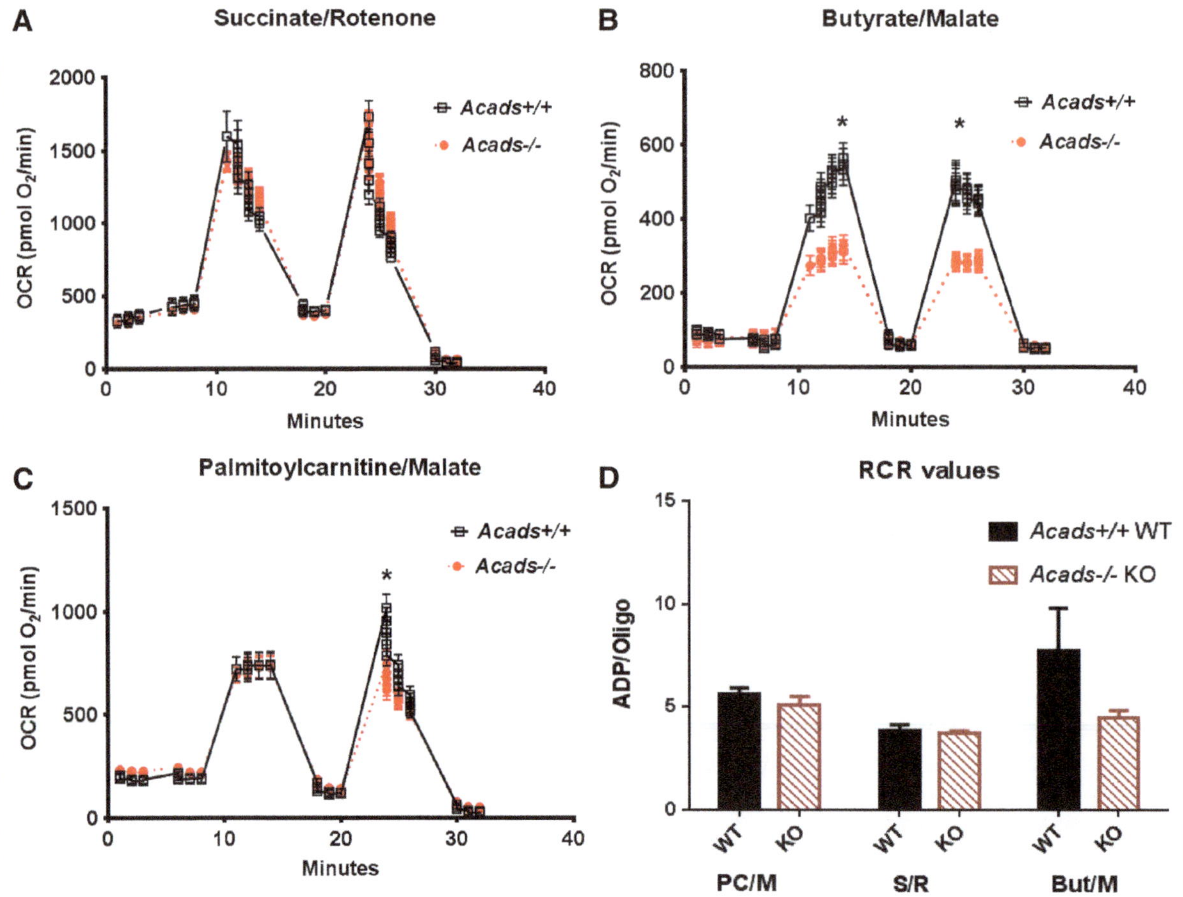

Fig. 3 Mitochondrial oxygen consumption rate. Legend: Mitochondrial oxygen consumption rate in isolated liver mitochondria in the presence of various substrates. Experiments were run on a SeaHorse XF24 extracellular flux analyzer to obtain bioenergetics profiles from *Acads−/−* and +/+ mice. OCR, oxygen consumption rate. Data are displayed as absolute, point-to-point oxygen consumption rates (pmol/min/well). **a** OCR in the presence of succinate/rotenone. **b** OCR with butyrate/malate. **c** OCR with palmitoylcarnitine/malate. **d** respiratory control ratio (RCR); calculated as the state 3 respiratory rate divided by the state 4 respiratory rate, obtained from the ADP-linked/oligomycin OCR readings. Samples were run in triplicate. Data represent means ± SE for $n = 3$-9 animals. $^*P < 0.05$, *Acads−/−* vs. *Acads+/+*

supporting our finding that mitochondrial oxidative phosphorylation is impaired in isolated hepatic mitochondria from *Acads−/−* animals.

Mitochondrial copy number

The induction of AMPK by energy restriction is known to activate the transcription coactivator peroxisome proliferator-activated receptor gamma, coactivator 1 alpha (PPARGC1A, also known as PGC1-a) and to enhance mitochondrial biogenesis [23]. Additionally, prolonged high-fat diet intake has been shown to induce changes in mtDNA content [30]. Here we measured the hepatic mtDNA content of *Acads−/−* and *Acads+/+* mice using qRT-PCR and found no significant differences in mtDNA content (Additional file 4: Figure S1), in mice that were fed HF diet for 2 days. Thus we can exclude the possibility that differential mitochondrial proliferation is responsible for the observed genotype difference in mitochondrial OCR.

Acads genotype and high-fat diet alter gene expression in the liver

Energy balance is maintained by changes in feeding behavior and metabolism which can be regulated by gene expression. To identify the transcriptional responses to *Acads* inactivation and dietary fat, we used microarrays to profile the expression of 32,381 transcripts in the liver of *Acads−/−* and *Acads+/+* mice fed either high- or low-fat diet. We found more pronounced differences in transcript abundance (absolute fold-change ≥ 1.5 and nominal *P*-value of <0.01) between the two diet comparisons than between the two genotype comparisons (Table 1).

Table 1 Summary of differentially expressed genes

Experimental comparison	Total	Increased	Decreased
HF: *Acads−/−* vs. *Acads+/+*	182	108	74
LF: *Acads−/−* vs. *Acads+/+*	72	31	41
Acads+/+: HF vs. LF	284	97	187
Acads−/−: HF vs. LF	287	145	142

The Applied Biosystems Mouse Genome Survey Microarray v2.0 was used to identify in liver the differential expression of genes by genotype or diet. A total of 12 arrays were used. Lists of differentially expressed genes for each comparison are based on a fold change of ≥1.5 and a *P* value of <0.05

Acads genotype alters hepatic gene expression

Microarray analysis of gene expression in the liver, under the HF diet condition, revealed changes in 182 genes due to genotype, of which 108 genes showed increased levels in *Acads−/−* mice (Table 1). LF diet resulted in a considerably weaker transcriptional response, as only 72 genes were differentially expressed, with 31 increased in *Acads−/−* mice. Of these, 20 were common to both the HF and LF diets, with an equal number of up- and down-regulated transcripts (Fig. 4a and b). The extent of this overlap was statistically significant, based on the hypergeometric test ($p < 2.92e\text{-}13$). For example, we uncovered the genotype-regulated induction of *Glo1*, encoding glyoxalase 1, with both the HF and LF diets, by a factor of 2.0 and 2.5, respectively. The glyoxalase system acts to degrade endogenous reactive dicarbonyls such as glyoxal formed by lipid peroxidation and/or methylglyoxal derived from glycolysis [31]. Glyoxal and methylglyoxal are toxic byproducts of metabolism, which if not neutralized, can produce deleterious modifications of protein and DNA through glycation [32]. Activation of the hepatic glyoxalase pathway in *Acads* mutants, compared to wild type controls, suggests an enzymatic

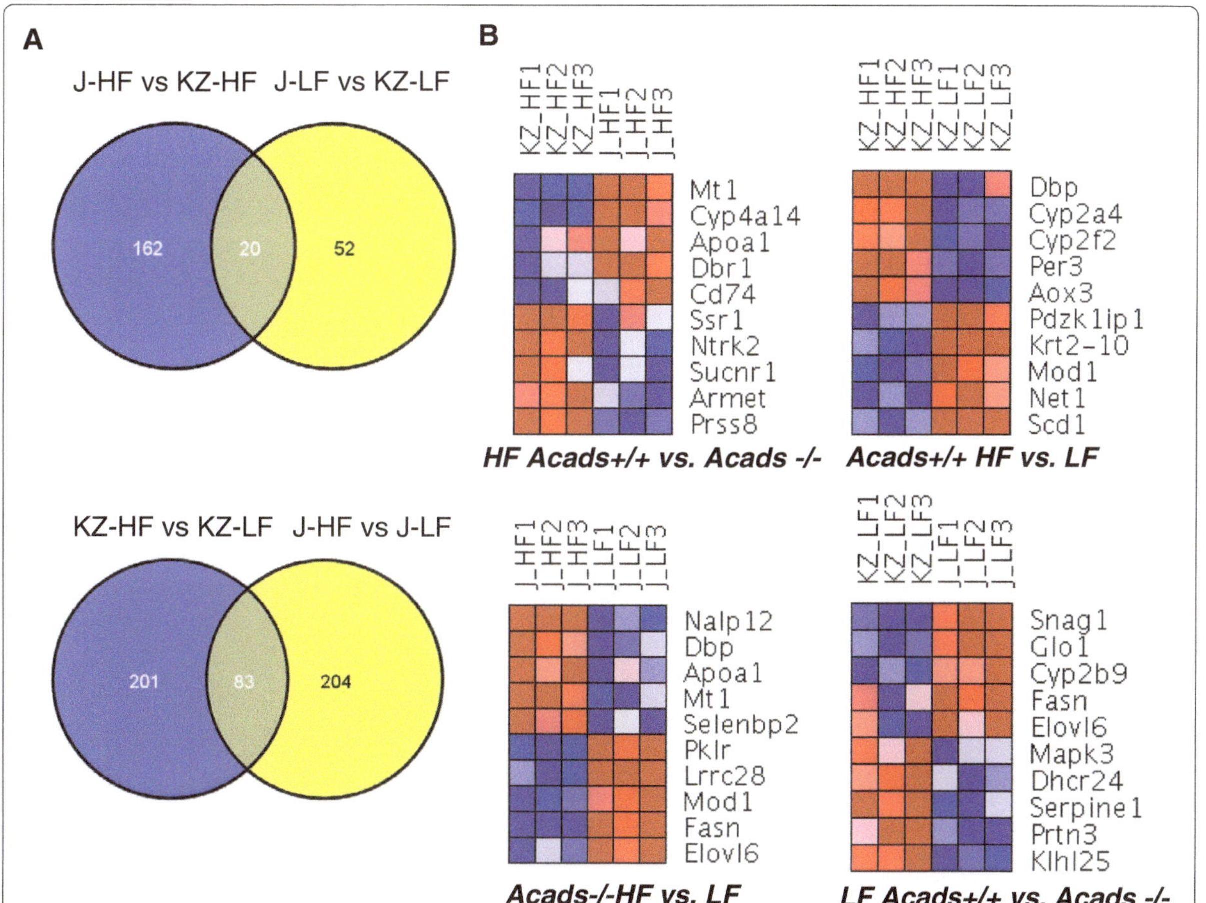

Fig. 4 Venn diagrams of differentially expressed genes affected by diet and genotype along with two-way Ward clustering of top 5 increased and top 5 decreased genes. Legend: **a** Overlap among significantly differentially expressed (DE) genes from each treatment (genotype, diet). Genes with an absolute fold change ≥ 1.5-fold and a nominal p-value <0.01 were considered to be significantly DE. **b** Two-way Ward clustering of top significantly DE genes. Treatments are organized by columns and genes by rows (expression levels in the heatmap are color-coded with blue representing lower and red representing higher levels of mRNA abundance). J, BALB/cByJ or *Acads−/−*; KZ, BALB/ByKZ, or *Acads+/+*

response to the accumulation of intermediates brought about by SCAD deficiency. The observed *Glo1* induction in this model is consistent with the inferred activation of *Nfe2l2/Nrf2* (see "Predicted Upstream Regulators" below), an oxidative stress response gene and transcriptional regulator of *Glo1* [32]. A more detailed list of the top 25 up- and down-regulated genes for each of the above treatments is provided in Additional file 5: Table S4.

High-fat diet alters hepatic gene expression

Two hundred and eighty-seven (287) diet-responsive genes were differentially expressed in *Acads−/−* mice, with 142 of them decreased in the HF fed group. By contrast in wild type controls, two hundred and eighty-four genes (284) were differentially expressed, with 187 genes down-regulated in the HF fed group. Eighty-three (83) genes were altered by high-fat diet in both *Acads−/−* and *Acads+/+* mice (Fig. 4a) and of these, 50 were down-regulated. The overlap in these 83 genes was highly significant by the hypergeometric test ($P < 9.87e-12$).

Diet-modified genes involved in fatty acid (FA) synthesis and elongation were strongly decreased by HF (vs. LF) diet in both mouse strains, usually with greater fold changes noted in *Acads−/−* animals. For example, *Me1* (malic enzyme; also known as *Mod1*) was decreased by 5.8-fold in *Acads−/−* and by 3.5-fold in *Acads+/+* mice. *Me1* induction by carbohydrate consumption in the LF diet groups, independent of genotype, may be responsible for this outcome (Fig. 4b), producing enzymatic action that links the glycolytic and citric acid cycles. As another example, *Elovl6* (elongation of very long chain fatty acids) was reduced by 25-fold in *Acads−/−* but only by 3.3-fold in wild type controls, suggesting a consequence of impaired SCFA oxidation in the mutants.

Genotype x diet interaction effects

A total of 137 genes demonstrated significant diet x genotype interactions at the $P < 0.01$ level (Additional file 6: Table S5). For nearly all of these transcripts, the

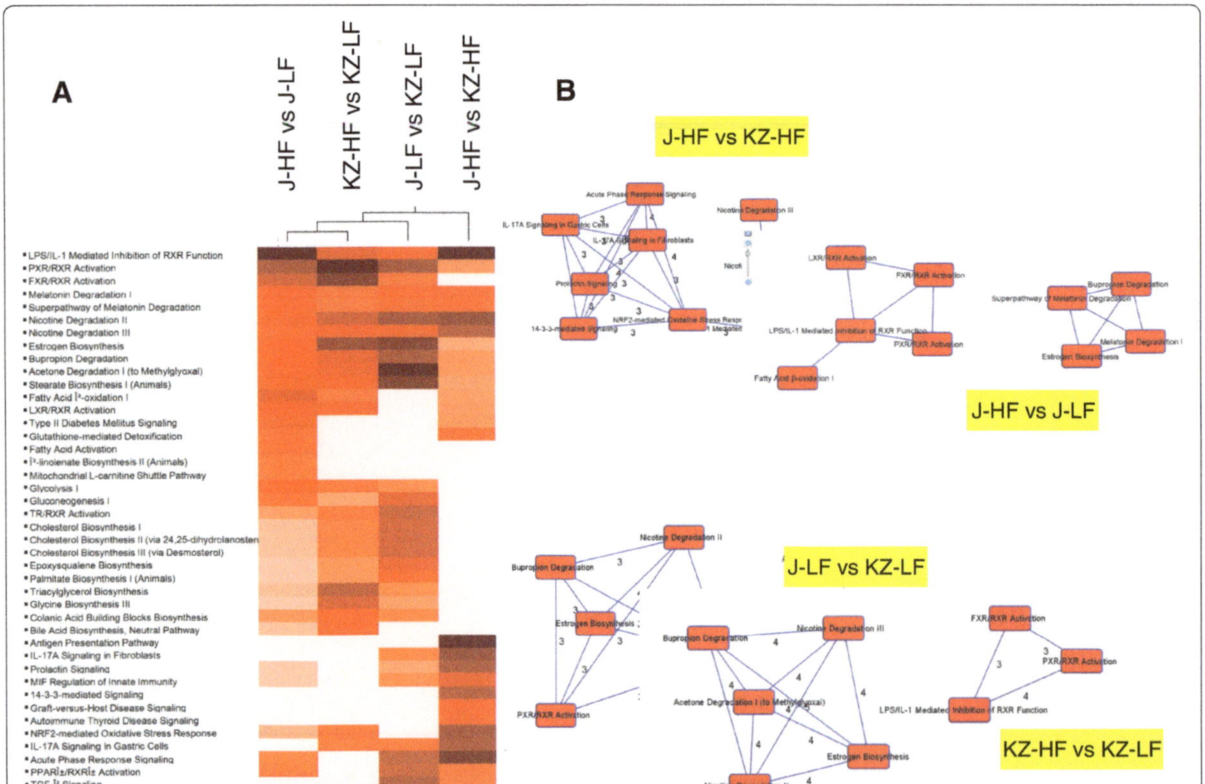

Fig. 5 Enrichment of canonical pathways for diet- and genotype-specific comparisons. Legend: Analysis was conducted using the Ingenuity Pathway Analysis tool, based on the Ingenuity Knowledge Base. **a** 2-way clustering based on pathway significance levels (Fisher's exact test). Heatmap is color-coded from white to red according to an ascending scale of negative $\log_{10}$P-value. Pathways with a negative $\log_{10}P \geq 3$ in at least one comparison are shown. **b** Sharing of common genes among top-ranking pathways in each comparison. Pathways sharing at least 3 genes for any pathway-pair are shown. The number of genes shared between any two pathways are also indicated. J, BALB/cByJ or *Acads−/−*; KZ, BALB/cByKZ or *Acads+/+*

interaction model explained substantially more of the variation in expression than did a model based only on main effects. Twenty-nine (29) of these transcripts encode for mitochondrial proteins, e.g., *Acsl3* (activates LCFAs for both synthesis and beta oxidation), *Cyp27a1* (drug metabolism, cholesterol synthesis), *Gpx1* (glutathione peroxidase), *Ndufc2* (complex I mitochondrial enzyme), *Uqcrfs1* (complex III), as well as three cytochrome c oxidase (*Cox*) components of complex IV: *Cox5b*, *Cox7c* and *Cox11*. Notably, genes in three complexes of the electron transport chain were affected by a genotype x diet interaction, and of these, *Ndufc2*, *Uqcrfs1*, and *Cox11* were more responsive to genotype. The possibility that these specific results may reflect a secondary defect in oxidative phosphorylation, and thus ATP production, in the *Acads−/−* mice [33], remains speculative.

Biological pathways are altered by *Acads* and dietary fat level

Canonical pathway analysis using IPA highlighted key alterations associated with short term high-fat diet and/or genotype (Fig. 5a), e.g., a significant inhibition of fatty acid and triacylglycerol synthesis in both *Acads+/+* and *Acads−/−* liver. This process was reflected by the decreased expression of *Scd1, Fasn, Srebf1,* and *Mod1* (fatty acid synthesis), as well as *Gpam* and *Elovl6* (fatty acid storage and elongation). IPA analysis also found strong enrichment of "Fatty Acid Beta Oxidation" in HF-fed *Acads−/−* mice, e.g., genes involved in long-chain FA degradation (*Acsl3, Acsl5, Slc17a2, Slc17a5*) and in peroxisomal beta oxidation (see below).

In *Acads−/−* mice fed HF diet for 2 days, all three top enriched pathways involved *Rxra* (retinoid X receptor alpha), which forms heterodimers with other nuclear receptors such as PPARs [34], and is required for *Ppara* transcriptional activity on fatty acid oxidation genes [34, 35]. A potential mechanism for the induction of RXRA/PPARA pathways is butyryl CoA buildup in the cell [36], which is expected to occur with SCAD deficiency. Additionally, the transcriptional regulation of other genes is consistent with activation of alternate lipid handling pathways in the liver, including both beta- (mitochondria, peroxisomes) and omega-oxidation (microsomes). Long-chain fatty acids (C14-C20) are catabolized by either mitochondrial or peroxisomal beta-oxidation pathways, whereas very long-chain fatty acids (C22) are chain-shortened through peroxisomal beta-oxidation before being completely oxidized in the mitochondria [37]. The increased expression of *Acaa1a, Ehhadh* and *Decr2,* genes encoding key enzymes of peroxisomal beta-oxidation [38], provides evidence that peroxisomal oxidation was enhanced in *Acads−/−* mice, but not in wild type. Further support for alternate lipid handling was indicated by the 3-fold induction of *Acot1* (acyl-CoA thioesterase 1) which predominantly hydrolyzes long-chain (C12-C16) acyl-CoA molecules. Evidence for an adaptive metabolic response was also observed in the 5 to 6-fold induction in *Cyp4a14* and *Cyp4a10* in *Acads −/−* liver by HF diet. The CYP4A subfamily of

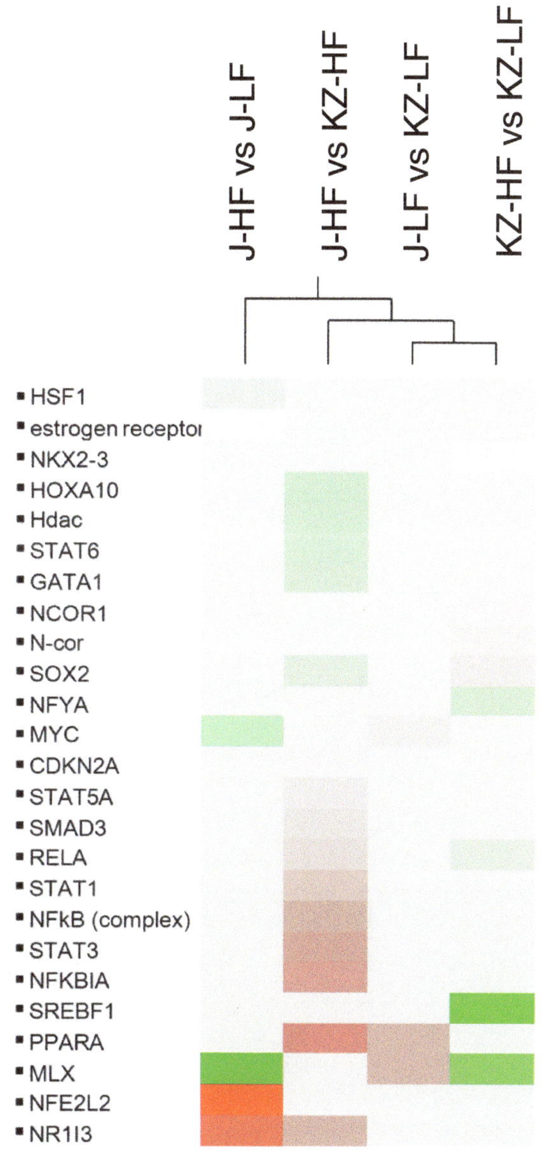

Fig. 6 Clustering of candidate upstream activators. Legend: Average-linkage clustering of candidate upstream regulators identified as significantly activated or inhibited in at least one of the four treatments ($|z| \geq 2$). Clustering was performed based on the *C* score and visualized by a heat-map. Predicted activations and inhibitions are shown in red and green, respectively, and shaded by the magnitude of the *C* score. J, BALB/cByJ or *Acads−/−*; KZ, BALB/cByKZ or *Acads+/+*

cytochrome P450 enzymes, located in the endoplasmic reticulum, function in microsomal omega oxidation, i.e., they metabolize medium and long chain length fatty acids at their omega-carbon atom to produce dicarboxylates as an alternative route to mitochondrial beta oxidation [39]. Normally, omega oxidation accounts for less than 10 % of total fatty acid oxidation in the liver [40], but when beta oxidation is defective, microsomal omega-oxidation may provide a means for eliminating toxic levels of free fatty acids [41]. For example, this pathway includes mitochondrial aldehyde dehydrogenase (*Aldh2*), encoding an antioxidant defense protein, which was induced by 5-fold in *Acads−/−* animals.

A comprehensive list of all the significantly enriched IPA pathways in each experimental comparison is provided in Additional file 7: Table S6.

Predicted upstream regulators of gene expression

To better understand the possible molecular basis for the observed transcriptomic changes, we investigated the predicted activation or inhibition of upstream transcription factors (TF) with at least 5 target genes in the list of differentially expressed genes (absolute fold change ≥ 1.5 and nominal p-value of <0.01) for a given diet or genotype comparison. In the diet comparison involving *Acads−/−* mice, we noted the significant,

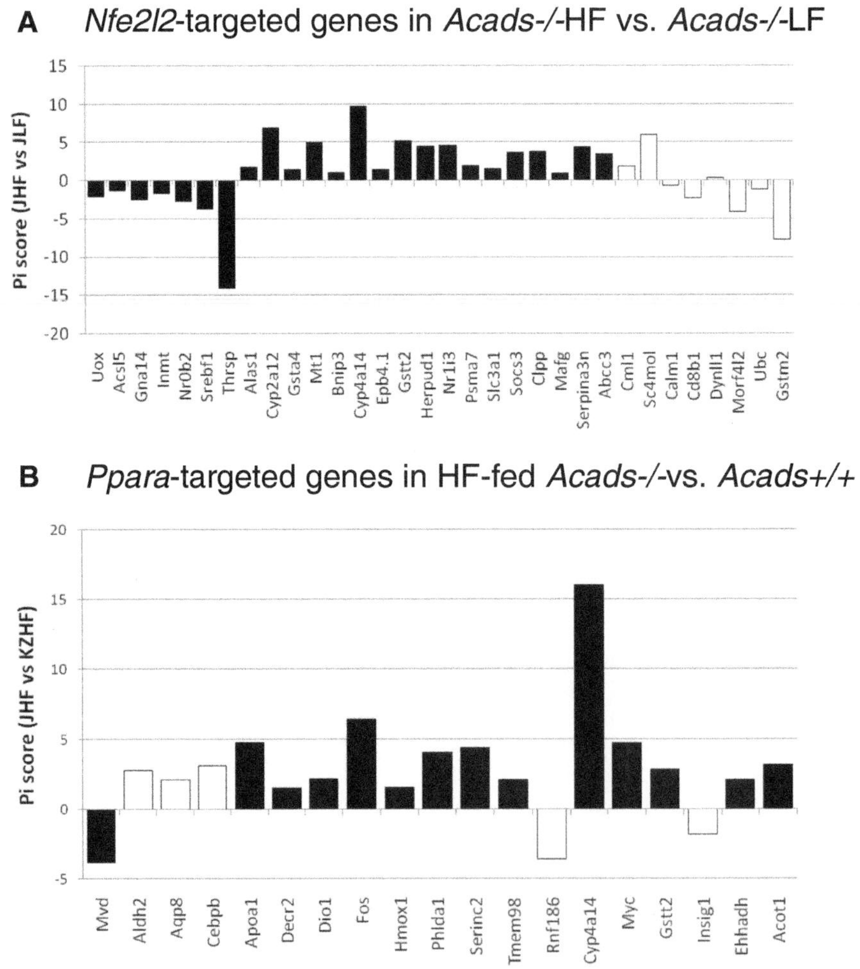

Fig. 7 Predicted upstream regulators of gene expression in microarray. Legend: Upstream regulator analysis on gene expression in microarray was restricted to transcription factors with at least 5 target genes in the list of differentially expressed genes (absolute fold change ≥ 1.5 and nominal *P*-value ≤ 0.01) for a given diet or genotype comparison. **a** *Nfe2l2*-targeted genes in *Acads−/−* mutant mice fed high-fat (HF) vs. low-fat (LF) diet. **b** *Ppara*-targeted genes in HF-fed *Acads−/−* vs. *Acads+/+* mice. Pi = neglogP*logratio. Genes whose direction of expression was consistent with activation of *Nfe2l2* (**a**) or *Ppara* (**b**) are colored in black and those with inconsistent direction of expression are shown in white. J, BALB/cByJ or *Acads−/−*; KZ, BALB/cByKZ or *Acads+/+*

predicted activation of *Nfe2l2* (nuclear factor, erythroid derived 2, like 2) as well as the significant inhibition of *Mlx* (MAX-like protein X), a transcriptional activator of glycolytic target genes (Fig. 6). The predicted activation or inhibition status for the full list of upstream regulators (beyond TFs) is shown in Additional file 8: Table S7. The similarities and dissimilarities in upstream regulator activation or inhibition across the 4 treatment groups are shown via hierarchical clustering in Additional file 9: Figure S2.

Using differentially expressed genes obtained from the diet comparison (HF vs. LF) in *Acads−/−* animals, upstream regulator analysis revealed 24 significantly differentially expressed genes whose direction of expression was consistent with activation of the transcription factor *Nfe2l2* (Fig. 7a). *Nfe2l2* (synonymous with *Nrf2*) binds to antioxidant response elements (ARE) in the upstream promoter region and initiates the transcription of a variety of cyto-protective target genes involved in the response to oxidative stress caused by xenobiotic exposure and other factors [42]. Several of these genes (e.g., *Gsta4*, *Cyp4a14*) are also known to regulate various aspects of lipid metabolism, e.g., the alpha class of glutathione S-transferases, e.g., *Gsta4*, functions to detoxify products of lipid peroxidation, as illustrated by significant enrichment of the "Glutathione-mediated Detoxification" pathway, when both SCAD deficiency and HF diet are involved (Fig. 5a). As well, dysregulation of the cytochrome P450 (*Cyp*) 4a subfamily of genes by HF diet may be related to the demands for transformation of excess fatty acids which are substrates for *Cyp4* isoforms. Overall, the inferred activation of *Nfe2l2*/ARE and the explicit induction of the *Cyp4a* subfamily in *Acads−/−* liver, appear to be directed at processing the incomplete products of mitochondrial beta oxidation [43]. Confirmation of this result will require a direct test of NFE2L2 activity or studies using *Nfe2l2−/−* mice.

Upstream regulator analysis also was performed on differentially expressed transcripts obtained by comparing

Table 2 Gene expression analyses by qRT-PCR for diet and genotype comparisons

Gene Symbol	Diet comparisons				Gene Symbol	Genotype comparisons			
	Microarray		qRT-PCR			Microarray		qRT-PCR	
	FC	*p*-value	FC	*p*-value		FC	*p*-value	FC	*p*-value
Acads−/− HF vs. LF					HF *Acads−/−* vs. *Acads+/+*				
Acacb	ND	ND	−2.86	0.001	Acacb	4.02	0.230	1.14	0.652
G6pc	−3.20	0.000	−2.94	0.000	G6pc	ND	ND	−1.07	0.606
Nr0b2 (SHP-1)	−1.87	0.000	1.40	0.063	Nr0b2	ND	ND	1.33	0.253
Nr1h3 (LXR)	ND	ND	1.15	0.234	Nr1h3	ND	ND	−1.08	0.512
Nr1h4 (FXR)	ND	ND	−1.10	0.619	Nr1h4	ND	ND	1.22	0.308
Nr1i2 (PXR)	ND	ND	−1.31	0.081	Nr1i2	ND	ND	−1.38	0.024
Nr1i3 (CAR)	2.40	0.000	4.23	0.001	Nr1i3	ND	ND	1.43	0.161
Pklr	−5.28	0.000	−3.93	0.000	Pklr	ND	ND	1.18	0.372
Rxra	2.28	0.000	1.56	0.004	Rxra	ND	ND	1.00	0.981
Srebf1	−2.03	0.000	−1.61	0.095	Srebf1	ND	ND	−1.04	0.829
Sult1a1(Phase II DME)	2.55	0.000	3.28	0.000	Sult1a1	ND	ND	1.40	0.666
Acads+/+ HF vs. LF					LF *Acads−/−* vs. *Acads+/+*				
Acacb	−5.13	0.000	−2.99	0.003	Acacb	ND	ND	1.09	0.704
G6pc	ND	ND	−1.67	0.001	G6pc	ND	ND	1.64	0.000
Nr0b2 (SHP-1)	ND	ND	−1.12	0.719	Nr0b2	ND	ND	−1.18	.551
Nr1h3 (LXR)	ND	ND	1.07	0.757	Nr1h3	ND	ND	−1.17	0.457
Nr1h4 (FXR)	ND	ND	1.16	0.568	Nr1h4	ND	ND	1.56	0.125
Nr1i2 (PXR)	ND	ND	1.32	0.197	Nr1i2	ND	ND	1.25	0.311
Nr1i3 (CAR)	1.87	0.000	2.60	0.002	Nr1i3	ND	ND	−1.14	0.688
Pklr	−3.56	0.000	−3.65	0.000	Pklr	ND	ND	1.27	0.188
Rxra	ND	ND	1.31	0.034	Rxra	ND	ND	−1.19	0.147
Srebf1	−1.71	0.009	−1.56	0.070	Srebf1	ND	ND	−1.01	0.974
Sult1a1(Phase II DME)	ND	ND	1.67	0.009	Sult1a1	ND	ND	−1.41	0.046

Representative genes were selected to validate the microarray results in liver. Overall, we observed concordant changes in the array and the qPCR. With the diet comparisons alone, 12 PCR assays reached statistical significance in a two-tailed Student's *t*-test performed on ΔCt values
ND, not detected

genotypes (*Acads*−/− vs. *Acads*+/+) in HF-fed animals. Fourteen (14) gene targets were identified whose direction of expression suggested PPARA activation, including *Cyp4a14* whose mRNA was elevated by nearly 9-fold (Fig. 7b). The predicted target genes represent the diverse functions of *Ppara*, including lipoprotein metabolism (*Apoa1*), microsomal omega oxidation (*Cyp4a10*, *Cyp4a14*), peroxisomal beta oxidation (*Ehhadh*), hydrolysis of fatty acyl-CoAs by thioesterases (*Acot1*), and biotransformation (*Gstt2*). Overall, these effects are consistent with the regulatory role of PPAR-alpha in energy metabolism, including all three hepatic fatty acid oxidation systems, i.e., mitochondrial and peroxisomal beta oxidation, as well as microsomal omega oxidation in the endoplasmic reticulum [38].

Both chronic high-fat feeding and fasting activate PPARA signaling in mouse liver, as part of the physiological response to an increased need for fatty acid oxidation [44]. In our short-term feeding experiment, the inferred PPARA activation may have been triggered by accumulated acylcarnitines, both in the circulation [17] and in liver tissue [45]. This result follows the pattern of PPARA induction reported previously for both the *Lcad*−/− and *Vlcad*−/− mouse strains with chow feeding [46]. It is also possible that PPARA signaling and fatty acid oxidation pathways were activated by a low energy state, as indicated by the enhanced hepatic pAMPK (Fig. 2) and reduced mitochondrial OCR in HF-fed *Acads*−/− mice (Fig. 3b).

Quantitative RT-PCR validation of gene expression in liver

To investigate the potential evidence for RXR-alpha activation and determine the effects of high-fat diet and

Table 3 Gene expression analyses by qRT-PCR for diet comparison in *Acads*−/− mice

		Microarray		qRT-PCR	
Gene Symbol	Gene Name	Fold change	p-value	Fold change	p-value
Aacs	acetoacetyl-CoA synthetase	−3.34	0.000	−3.34	0.001
Abcc3	ATP-binding cassette, sub-family C (CFTR/MRP), member 3	1.98	0.004	2.07	0.003
Acaa1a	acetyl-Coenzyme A acyltransferase 1A	1.82	0.003	1.59	0.041
Acot1	acyl-CoA thioesterase 1	3.11	0.039	4.15	0.011
Apol9b	apolipoprotein L 9b	3.00	0.022	2.34	0.000
Decr2	2-4-dienoyl-Coenzyme A reductase 2, peroxisomal	2.04	0.003	2.04	0.011
Dhrs13	dehydrogenase/reductase (SDR family) member 13	1.82	0.046	1.42	0.018
Ehhadh	enoyl-Coenzyme A, hydratase/3-hydroxyacyl Coenzyme A dehydrogenase	1.64	0.025	1.93	0.014
Elovl6	ELOVL family member 6, elongation of long chain fatty acids (yeast)	−24.79	0.021	−11.11	0.000
Fasn	fatty acid synthase	−7.21	0.000	−6.69	0.000
Gpam	glycerol-3-phosphate acyltransferase, mitochondrial	−5.70	0.000	−2.26	0.000
Gpi1	glucose phosphate isomerase 1	−2.49	0.001	−2.16	0.000
Gpr146	G protein-coupled receptor 146	2.03	0.003	2.17	0.000
Gstm2	glutathione S-transferase, mu 2	−2.33	0.002	−1.76	0.000
Macrod2	MACRO domain containing 2	−1.97	0.005	−1.11	0.444
Mod1/Me1	malic enzyme 1, NADP(+)-dependent, cytosolic	−5.81	0.025	−5.35	0.000
Nars	asparaginyl-tRNA synthetase	−1.65	0.025	−1.49	0.133
Pdhb	pyruvate dehydrogenase (lipoamide) beta	−1.83	0.015	−1.58	0.007
Pdk1	pyruvate dehydrogenase kinase, isoenzyme 1	−1.72	0.004	−1.54	0.307
Pdk4	pyruvate dehydrogenase kinase, isoenzyme 4	−3.98	0.018	−2.00	0.004
Pklr	pyruvate kinase liver and red blood cell	−5.28	0.000	−5.28	0.000
Rps6kl1	ribosomal protein S6 kinase-like 1	2.61	0.015	1.63	0.026
Scd1	stearoyl-Coenzyme A desaturase 1	−8.57	0.024	−19.17	0.000
Slc17a4	solute carrier family 17 (sodium phosphate), member 4	−2.74	0.009	−1.91	0.000
Slc27a5	solute carrier family 27 (fatty acid transporter), member 5	1.62	0.004	1.77	0.000
Sucnr1	succinate receptor 1	−2.33	0.033	−2.55	0.379
Uox	urate oxidase	−1.65	0.015	−1.33	0.039

Representative genes were selected to validate the microarray results in liver, using real-time RT-PCR. For the comparison of *Acads*−/− HF diet vs. LF diet, 27 genes are shown. There was strong concordance between the two platforms, i.e., 23 PCR assays reached statistical significance in a two-tailed Student's *t*-test performed on ΔCt values

SCAD deficiency on common partners of *Rxr*, we used quantitative RT-PCR to measure the expression of eleven nuclear receptor genes, as well as some glucose metabolism genes, in all four diet and genotype comparisons (total of 44 tests) (Table 2). Statistical significance for differential expression in microarray analysis was confirmed in 36/44 or 82 % of the tests. In addition to this validation study, we selected a set of 27 transcripts to represent metabolic processes and examined their expression as a function of diet in *Acads−/−* mice. The results showed significant ($P < 0.05$) differences between high- and low-fat diets in 23/27 or 85 % of the genes (Table 3). We observed 100 % agreement in the direction of expression changes between the two platforms, and thus have confidence that the qRT-PCR and microarray results are congruent, and that they reveal a predominant effect of diet, but not of genotype.

Summary of fatty acid and glucose metabolism genes altered by SCAD deficiency and high-fat diet

The transcriptional changes in hepatic fatty acid and glucose metabolism in *Acads−/−* mice fed HF or LF diet are summarized in Fig. 8, in a manner similar to that of Zhang et al. [47].

In general, fatty acids are catabolized in the mitochondria and/or peroxisomes to produce energy through beta oxidation while excess lipids are stored as triglycerides. We observed the increased expression of genes encoding enzymes involved in peroxisomal beta oxidation and in cytosolic hydrolysis of C12-C16 acyl-CoAs, as well as increased expression of genes involved in routing lipids for metabolism. These include FA transport genes (*Abcc3*, *Slc27a2*, *Slc27a5*) and peroxisomal *Eci2* (formerly *Peci*) localized in both mitochondria and peroxisomes. In addition, acyl-CoA synthetase gene expression was decreased (e.g., *Acsl5*), which may promote the induction

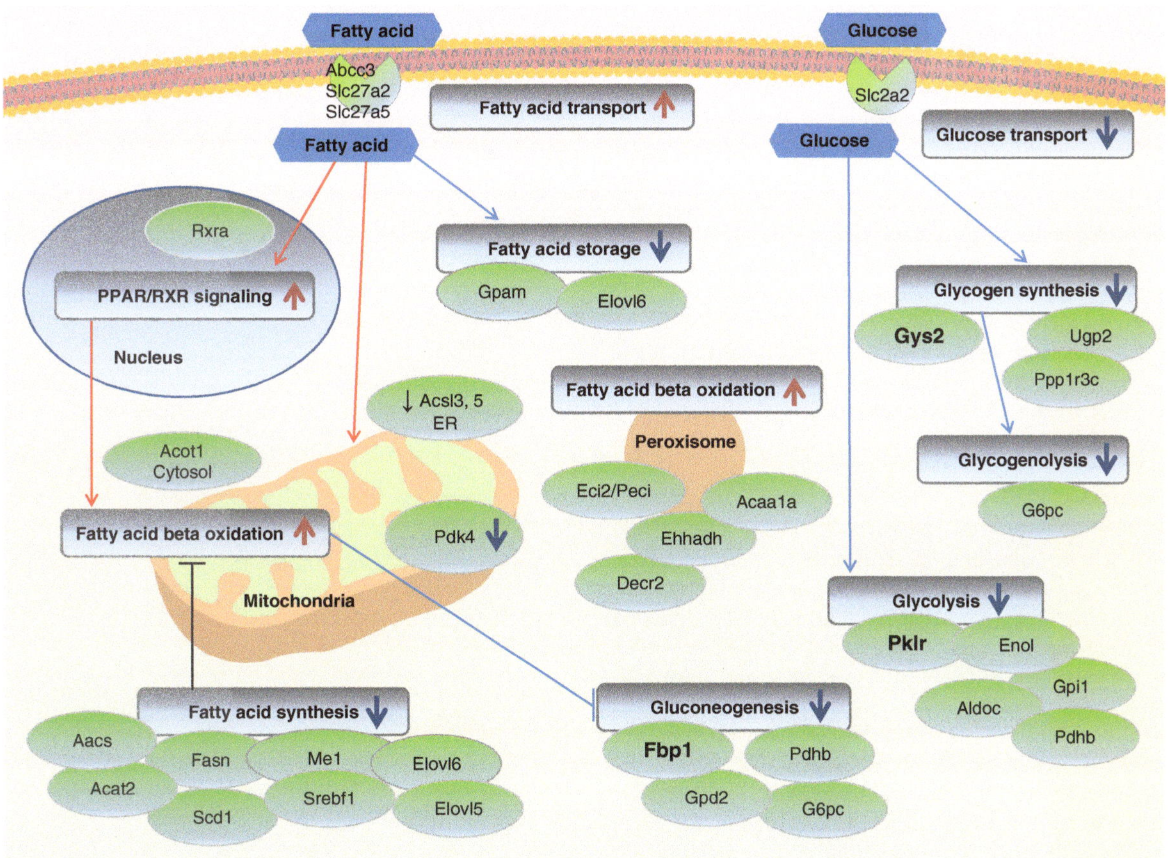

Fig. 8 Overview of differentially expressed genes in fatty acid and glucose metabolism in the liver of *Acads−/−* mice fed high- or low-fat diet. Legend: The gene nodes and their interactions are presented after the manner of Zhang et al. [47], based on significantly differentially expressed genes from the diet comparison in *Acads−/−* mice. Large arrows indicate the direction of gene expression (red, increased; blue, decreased) for the gene nodes associated with each pathway

of peroxisomes as an alternate route of lipid disposal [48]. The increased expression of *Rxra* indicates activation of the PPAR/RXR signaling pathway, as do the upstream regulator analyses, particularly the increased expression of PPARA-target gene *Cyp4a14* (Fig. 7b). The expression of genes encoding proteins involved in lipid biogenesis, as well fatty acid elongation and desaturation, was decreased in *Acads−/−* mice fed HF vs. LF diet, (Fig. 8).

The observed changes in gene expression are consistent with limited hepatic glucose utilization. For example, the expression of genes involved in glucose transport, as well as glycolysis and glycogen synthesis, including rate-limiting enzymes *Pklr* (−5.3-fold) and *Gys2*, respectively, was decreased. Furthermore, the expression of gluconeogenesis genes *G6pc* and *Gpd2*, together with rate-limiting enzyme fructose-1,6-bisphosphatase (*Fbp1*), was much lower in *Acads−/−* liver. Notably, we also observed a ~4-fold reduction in mitochondrial *Pdk4*, validated by qRT-PCR, along with a decrease in *Pdk1* (Table 3), suggesting increased pyruvate dehydrogenase complex (PDC) activity. This result appears paradoxical, based on what is known about the transcriptional regulation of pyruvate dehydrogenase kinase, and the prediction of an up-regulation of *Pdk4* in response to increased fat supply from the HF diet [49]. However, the decreased *Pdk4* gene expression may reflect the short-term nature of diet exposure (2 days), possibly indicating that the metabolically active liver tissue has not yet "switched" on its PDC activity to maintain ATP levels, i.e., by regulating entry of glycolytic products into the tricarboxylic acid cycle. These results suggest that the altered fuel utilization in *Acads−/−* animals differs from that of the classic fed-fasted cycle [49].

Conclusion

We identified altered acylcarnitine levels, enhanced pAMP-kinase signaling, and decreased mitochondrial oxidative function in the liver of *Acads−/−* animals fed high-fat diet for two days. Additionally, diet-induced liver transcriptomic responses in SCAD-deficient mice support increased RXR/PPARA signaling and upregulation of genes involved in multiple lipid handling pathways, including fatty acid oxidation. Nevertheless, the results of metabolite analyses suggest a substantial limitation in short-chain fatty acid oxidation, that may account for the activation of pAMPK, which is extremely sensitive to cellular energy levels. The indications of lower metabolic fuel utilization and ATP generation in *Acads−/−* animals, compared to wild type, correspond to previous observations of an energy deficient state [17] in this animal model.

Additional files

Additional file 1: Table S1. Body weight and energy intake for experimental animals used in microarray. (DOCX 14 kb)

Additional file 2: Table S2. Primers used for quantitative real-time PCR assays. (DOC 76 kb)

Additional file 3: Table S3. Two factor ANOVA table for liver acylcarnitines. (DOC 67 kb)

Additional file 4: Figure S1. Quantification of mtDNA in *Acads−/−* and *Acads+/+* liver. Legend: Relative amount of DNA from two mitochondrial markers, cytochrome B (*mt-Cytb*) and cyclo-oxygenase (*mtCo2*) vs. the nuclear markers hemoglobin beta chain complex (*Hbb*) and glucagon (*Gcg*) in *Acads−/−* and +/+ mice. Data are presented as mean ± S.E. ($n = 3$ per genotype). (PDF 35 kb)

Additional file 5: Table S4. Top 25 up- and down-regulated genes. (XLSX 423 kb)

Additional file 6: Table S5. Genotype-by-diet interactions affecting gene expression. (XLSX 23 kb)

Additional file 7: Table S6. IPA Pathways. (XLSX 15 kb)

Additional file 8: Table S7. Predicted activation/inhibition of upstream regulators all categories. (XLSX 18 kb)

Additional file 9: Figure S2. Average-linkage clustering of all categories (transcription factors, enzymes, chemokines, etc.) of candidate upstream regulators identified as significantly activated or inhibited in at least one of the four comparisons ($|z| \geq 2$). Clustering results are presented as a heat-map and are color coded according to the magnitude of the z-score. Positive z-scores are depicted in shades of red and negative z-scores in green. (PDF 262 kb)

Competing interests
The authors declare that they have no competing interests.

Authors' contributions
Conceived and designed the experiments: BR. Performed the experiments: SG, CK, SW, JS, GK, BR. Analyzed the data: SG, SW, WJ, BR. Wrote the paper: SG, SW, RN, BR. All authors read and approved the final manuscript.

Acknowledgments
This research was supported by NIH Grant DK-53113 to B. K. Smith Richards; NIH DK-088319, AHA 10SDG4230068, and support from the National Medical Research Council, Ministry of Health, Singapore, to S. Ghosh; NIH DK-103860 to R. C. Noland; NIH DK-089641 to R. L. Mynatt; T32 AT004094 to S. E. Wicks; as well as partial support from the NORC Center Grant P30 DK072476, COBRE Center Grant NIH 8 P20 GM103528, and NIH U54 GM104940 which funds the Louisiana Clinical and Translational Science Center (LA CaTS). This research used the Metabolomics Core Services supported by grant U24 DK097153 of NIH Common Funds Project to the University of Michigan. We acknowledge the expert technical assistance of Lisa M. DiCarlo and Ginger Robertson. We thank Dr. Krisztian Stadler for assistance with the Seahorse experiments and Dr. Claudia Kappen for valuable comments on the manuscript.

Author details
[1]Pennington Biomedical Research Center, Louisiana State University System, 6400 Perkins Road, Baton Rouge, LA 70808-4124, USA. [2]Duke-NUS Graduate Medical School, Singapore 169857, Singapore. [3]Present Address: Taconic Biosciences, Inc., Germantown, NY, USA.

References
1. Smith Richards BK, Belton BN, York B, Volaufova J. Mice bearing Acads mutation display altered postingestive but not 5-s orosensory response to dietary fat. Am J Physiol Regul Integr Comp Physiol. 2004;286:R311–9.
2. Langhans W, Geary N. Overview of the physiological control of eating. Forum Nutr. 2010;63:9–53.

3. Friedman MI, Horn CC, Ji H. Peripheral signals in the control of feeding behavior. Chem Senses. 2005;30 Suppl 1:i182–3.
4. Langhans W, Egli G, Scharrer E. Regulation of food intake by hepatic oxidative metabolism. Brain Res Bull. 1985;15:425–8.
5. Friedman MI. Control of energy intake by energy metabolism. Am J Clin Nutr. 1995;62:1096S–100.
6. Hinsdale ME, Kelly CL, Wood PA. Null allele at Bcd-1 locus in BALB/cByJ mice is due to a deletion in the short-chain acyl-CoA dehydrogenase gene and results in missplicing of mRNA. Genomics. 1993;16:605–11.
7. Kelly CL, Wood PA. Cloning and characterization of the mouse short-chain acyl-CoA dehydrogenase gene. Mamm Genome. 1996;7:262–4.
8. Wood PA, Amendt BA, Rhead WJ, Millington DS, Inoue F, Armstrong D. Short-chain acyl-coenzyme A dehydrogenase deficiency in mice. Pediatr Res. 1989;25:38–43.
9. Reue K, Cohen RD. Acads gene deletion in BALB/cByJ mouse strain occurred after 1981 and is not present in BALB/cByJ-fld mutant mice. Mamm Genome. 1996;7:694–5.
10. Armstrong DL, Masiowski ML, Wood PA. Pathologic characterization of short-chain acyl-CoA dehydrogenase deficiency in BALB/cByJ mice. Am J Med Genet. 1993;47:884–92.
11. Wood PA, Kelly-Kurtz CL, Hinsdale ME, Hamm DA, Rhead WJ. Lessons learned from the mouse model of short-chain acyl-CoA dehydrogenase deficiency. Adv Exp Med Biol. 1999;466:395–402.
12. Abramoff MD, Magalhaes PJ, Ram SJ. Image Processing with Image J. Biophoton Int. 2004;11:36–42.
13. Frezza C, Cipolat S, Scorrano L. Organelle isolation: functional mitochondria from mouse liver, muscle and cultured fibroblasts. Nat Protoc. 2007;2:287–95.
14. Rogers GW, Brand MD, Petrosyan S, Ashok D, Elorza AA, Ferrick DA, et al. High throughput microplate respiratory measurements using minimal quantities of isolated mitochondria. PLoS ONE. 2011;6:e21746.
15. Rogers GW, Murphy AN, Elorza AA, Brand MD: Technical Brief: Analyzing microgram quantities of isolated mitochondria in the XF24 analyzer. In, Seahorse Bioscience, 2015
16. Cunningham JT, Rodgers JT, Arlow DH, Vazquez F, Mootha VK, Puigserver P. mTOR controls mitochondrial oxidative function through a YY1-PGC-1alpha transcriptional complex. Nature. 2007;450:736–40.
17. Kruger C, Kumar KG, Mynatt RL, Volaufova J, Richards BK. Brain transcriptional responses to high-fat diet in Acads-deficient mice reveal energy sensing pathways. PLoS ONE. 2012;7:e41709.
18. Simon R, Lam A, Li MC, Ngan M, Menenzes S, Zhao Y. Analysis of gene expression data using BRB-ArrayTools. Cancer Inform. 2007;3:11–7.
19. Baldi P, Long AD. A Bayesian framework for the analysis of microarray expression data: regularized t -test and statistical inferences of gene changes. Bioinformatics. 2001;17:509–19.
20. Benjamini Y, Hochberg Y. Controlling the False Discovery Rate: A Practical and Powerful Approach to Multiple Testing. J R Stat Soc Ser B. 1995;57:289–300.
21. Schmittgen TD, Livak KJ. Analyzing real-time PCR data by the comparative C(T) method. Nat Protoc. 2008;3:1101–8.
22. Suchankova G, Tekle M, Saha AK, Ruderman NB, Clarke SD, Gettys TW. Dietary polyunsaturated fatty acids enhance hepatic AMP-activated protein kinase activity in rats. Biochem Biophys Res Commun. 2005;326:851–8.
23. Viollet B, Guigas B, Leclerc J, Hebrard S, Lantier L, Mounier R, et al. AMP-activated protein kinase in the regulation of hepatic energy metabolism: from physiology to therapeutic perspectives. Acta Physiol (Oxf). 2009;196:81–98.
24. McBride HM, Neuspiel M, Wasiak S. Mitochondria: more than just a powerhouse. Curr Biol. 2006;16:R551–60.
25. Hill BG, Benavides GA, Lancaster Jr JR, Ballinger S, Dell'Italia L, Jianhua Z, et al. Integration of cellular bioenergetics with mitochondrial quality control and autophagy. Biol Chem. 2012;393:1485–512.
26. Souri M, Aoyama T, Yamaguchi S, Hashimoto T. Relationship between structure and substrate-chain-length specificity of mitochondrial very-long-chain acyl-coenzyme A dehydrogenase. Eur J Biochem. 1998;257:592–8.
27. van Maldegem BT, Duran M, Wanders RJ, Waterham HR, de Koning TJ, Rubio E, et al. Fasting and fat-loading tests provide pathophysiological insight into short-chain acyl-coenzyme a dehydrogenase deficiency. J Pediatr. 2010;156:121–7.
28. Wolfe L, Jethva R, Oglesbee D, Vockley J. Short-Chain Acyl-CoA Dehydrogenase Deficiency. in Pagon RA, Adam MP, Ardinger HH, et al. (eds): GeneReviews® [Internet]. University of Washington, Seattle (WA), 1993–2015.
29. Leslie ND, Valencia CA, Strauss AW, Connor J, Zhang K: Very Long-Chain Acyl-Coenzyme A Dehydrogenase Deficiency. in Pagon RA, Adam MP, Ardinger HH, et al. (eds): GeneReviews®. University of Washington, Seattle (WA), 1993.
30. Nadal-Casellas A, Amengual-Cladera E, Proenza AM, Llado I, Gianotti M. Long-term high-fat-diet feeding impairs mitochondrial biogenesis in liver of male and female rats. Cell Physiol Biochem. 2010;26:291–302.
31. Tafti M, Petit B, Chollet D, Neidhart E, de Bilbao F, Kiss JZ, et al. Deficiency in short-chain fatty acid beta-oxidation affects theta oscillations during sleep. Nat Genet. 2003;34:320–5.
32. Xue M, Rabbani N, Momiji H, Imbasi P, Anwar MM, Kitteringham N, et al. Transcriptional control of glyoxalase 1 by Nrf2 provides a stress-responsive defence against dicarbonyl glycation. Biochem J. 2012;443:213–22.
33. Wang W, Mohsen AW, Uechi G, Schreiber E, Balasubramani M, Day B, et al. Complex changes in the liver mitochondrial proteome of short chain acyl-CoA dehydrogenase deficient mice. Mol Genet Metab. 2014;112:30–9.
34. Mangelsdorf DJ, Evans RM. The RXR heterodimers and orphan receptors. Cell. 1995;83:841–50.
35. Jump DB. Fatty acid regulation of hepatic lipid metabolism. Curr Opin Clin Nutr Metab Care. 2011;14:115–20.
36. Schiffer SP, Prochazka M, Jezyk PF, Roderick TH, Yudkoff M, Patterson DF. Organic aciduria and butyryl CoA dehydrogenase deficiency in BALB/cByJ mice. Biochem Genet. 1989;27:47–58.
37. Reddy JK, Mannaerts GP. Peroxisomal lipid metabolism. Annu Rev Nutr. 1994;14:343–70.
38. Reddy JK, Hashimoto T. Peroxisomal beta-oxidation and peroxisome proliferator-activated receptor alpha: an adaptive metabolic system. Annu Rev Nutr. 2001;21:193–230.
39. Okita RT, Okita JR. Cytochrome P450 4A fatty acid omega hydroxylases. Curr Drug Metab. 2001;2:265–81.
40. Misra P, Reddy JK. Peroxisome proliferator-activated receptor-alpha activation and excess energy burning in hepatocarcinogenesis. Biochimie. 2014;98:63–74.
41. Wanders RJ, Komen J, Kemp S. Fatty acid omega-oxidation as a rescue pathway for fatty acid oxidation disorders in humans. FEBS J. 2011;278:182–94.
42. Ma Q. Role of Nrf2 in oxidative stress and toxicity. Annu Rev Pharmacol Toxicol. 2013;53:401–26.
43. Vomhof-Dekrey EE, Picklo Sr MJ. The Nrf2-antioxidant response element pathway: a target for regulating energy metabolism. J Nutr Biochem. 2012;23:1201–6.
44. Patsouris D, Reddy JK, Muller M, Kersten S. Peroxisome proliferator-activated receptor alpha mediates the effects of high-fat diet on hepatic gene expression. Endocrinology. 2006;147:1508–16.
45. Mandard S, Muller M, Kersten S. Peroxisome proliferator-activated receptor alpha target genes. Cell Mol Life Sci. 2004;61:393–416.
46. Goetzman ES, Tian L, Wood PA. Differential induction of genes in liver and brown adipose tissue regulated by peroxisome proliferator-activated receptor-alpha during fasting and cold exposure in acyl-CoA dehydrogenase-deficient mice. Mol Genet Metab. 2005;84:39–47.
47. Zhang F, Xu X, Zhang Y, Zhou B, He Z, Zhai Q. Gene expression profile analysis of type 2 diabetic mouse liver. PLoS ONE. 2013;8:e57766.
48. Bu SY, Mashek DG. Hepatic long-chain acyl-CoA synthetase 5 mediates fatty acid channeling between anabolic and catabolic pathways. J Lipid Res. 2010;51:3270–80.
49. Jeong JY, Jeoung NH, Park KG, Lee IK. Transcriptional regulation of pyruvate dehydrogenase kinase. Diabetes Metab J. 2012;36:328–35.

Heat-treated high-fat diet modifies gut microbiota and metabolic markers in apoe–/– mice

Nittaya Marungruang*, Frida Fåk and Eden Tareke

Abstract

Background: High-fat diet has been known to have adverse effects on metabolic markers, as well as the gut microbiota. However, the effect of heat processing of high-fat diet, which leads to formations of advanced glycation end products (AGEs) has not been clearly distinguished from the effect of unheated fat. This study compared the effect of high-fat diet with heat-treated high-fat diet on adiposity, atherosclerosis and gut microbiota composition in the caecum of *apoe*$^{-/-}$ mice.

Method: Male *apoe*$^{-/-}$ mice were fed either low-fat (LF) control diet, high-fat (40 E% saturated fat, HF) control diet, or heat-treated high-fat (200 °C for 10 min, HT) diet, for 8 weeks. The plasma samples were used in the analysis of Nε-carboxy-methyl-lysine (CML) and Nε-carboxy-ethyl-lysine (CEL). The heart samples were analysed for atherosclerotic plaques, and the DNA from caecum was extracted and analysed for microbiota composition using 16S rRNA gene sequencing on a Miseq instrument. Additionally, the functions of microbial communities were also predicted based on the bacterial 16S rRNA gene sequence using Phylogenetic Investigation of Communities by Reconstruction of Unobserved States (PICRUSt).

Results: Here we found that HT modifies gut microbiota composition and host adiposity. Prediction of bacterial gene functions based on 16S rRNA gene sequence revealed that HF increased bacterial genera enriched in lipid metabolism genes, while HT did not. Plasma CML and CEL increased 1.7 and 2.5 times, respectively, in mice fed HT as compared to mice fed HF. Despite lower adiposity, mice fed HT maintained atherosclerosis and displayed enlarged spleens.

Conclusions: The results suggested that heat processing of high-fat diet modifies the substrates reaching the lower gut of *apoe*$^{-/-}$ mice, resulting in different effects on gut microbiota composition. AGEs seem to maintain the effect on atherosclerosis, despite lower adiposity, and causing enlarged spleens, which possibly reflect elevated levels of inflammation in the body.

Keywords: High-fat diet, Heat-treated high-fat diet, Advanced Glycation End products (AGEs), Gut microbiota, Atherosclerosis

Background

Modern diet involves heat processing of food, which leads to formation of Maillard reaction products (MRPs). These products are responsible for the aroma, colour, flavour, and texture as well as deterioration of nutritional value in the processed food and adverse health implications [1, 2]. Recently, more attention has been paid to the health implication of Maillard reaction products, especially those that lead to irreversible modifications in amino acids, peptides and proteins; advanced glycation end products (AGEs) [3–6]. AGEs are suggested to be associated to risk markers for inflammation mediated pathological conditions; such as cardiovascular disease, Alzheimer's disease and diabetes-linked-complications [5, 7–12]. The mechanism for AGEs induced toxicity can be mediated through binding to AGE receptors (RAGE) and inducing pro-inflammatory cascade [8, 13, 14], and consequently associated pathological conditions. Cross link formation affecting the structure of the protein may also

* Correspondence: nittaya.marungruang@food-health-science.lu.se
Food for Health Science Centre, Lund University, Medicon Village, Scheelevägen 2, SE-223 81 Lund, Sweden

affect the digestibility and thus modified proteins may reach the lower gut where they can be fermented by gut microbiota [15].

The gut microbiota is intimately involved in numerous aspects of host physiology. The overall balance in the gut microbiota composition is an important key factor ensuring normal host functions [16]. Several studies have revealed that presence or absence of gut microbiota or some specific groups of bacteria have been found to contribute to development of many diseases such as type-2 diabetes [17, 18], artherosclerosis [19, 20] and systemic inflammatory response syndrome [21]. The composition of the gut microbiota is known to be affected by dietary components reaching the lower gut. So far, the role of process induced structure alteration in proteins on the digestibility and possible metabolism by gut microbiota is an area that is largely unexplored.

Atherosclerosis is one form of chronic inflammatory response to accumulation of fat in blood vessels. The apolipoprotein E knock out (*apoe*$^{-/-}$) mouse is an animal model used for assessing effects of nutritional agents on lipid metabolism, inflammation and atherosclerosis [22]. *Apoe-/-* mice have an impaired ability for clearance of plasma lipoprotein, leading to the development of atherosclerosis in a short time. Several studies have been focusing on the pathological effects of high-fat diet. High intake of dietary fat has been known to induce several dynamic metabolic alterations, especially atherosclerosis, as well as changes in gut microbiota composition [17]. However, the fact that intake of fat is usually accompanied by heat processing [23], the specific effect of high fat intake versus the effect of AGEs has not been clearly distinguished. In the present study, we aimed to compare the effect of high-fat diet (40 E% saturated fat) with heat-treated (200 °C for 10 min) high-fat diet on adiposity, atherosclerosis and gut microbiota composition in the caecum of *apoe*$^{-/-}$ mice. Moreover, the study compared the possible effect of intake of high-fat diet on the above mentioned end points by comparing with intake of low-fat diet. Additionally, the functions of microbial communities were also predicted based on the bacterial 16S rRNA gene sequence using a recently developed software, Phylogenetic Investigation of Communities by Reconstruction of Unobserved States (PICRUSt) [24].

Methods

Experimental design

Male *apoe*$^{-/-}$ mice (Scanbur AB, Karlslunde, Denmark), 6 weeks of age, were adapted to the environment at the animal facility for 2 weeks before starting the experiment. At the age of 8 weeks, the mice were randomly divided into three weight-matched groups ($n = 10$, five mice/cage). The mice were fed low-fat (LF) control diet, high-fat (HF) control diet, or heat-treated high-fat (HT) diet. A picture of HF and HT is available as Additional file 1: Figure S1. The mice were weighed every week. After 8 weeks, the mice were anesthetized with isofluorane (Abbott Scandinavia AB, Solna, Sweden) and terminated by heart puncture. The liver, spleen and epididymal fat pads were weighed. Blood plasma, heart, and caecum were collected and frozen at −40 °C until further analyses. The plasma samples were used in the analysis of CML and CEL. The heart samples were analysed for atherosclerotic plaques, and the DNA from caecum was extracted and analysed for microbiota composition using 16S rRNA gene sequencing on a Miseq instrument.

High performance liquid chromatography coupled to tandem mass spectrometry for determination of CML and CEL

Plasma samples (50 μL) were hydrolysed for 12 h at 110 °C using 6 M HCl, together with isotope labelled d4-CML and d4-CEL as internal standard (Larodan Fine Chemicals AB, Malmö Sweden), and analysed using high-pressure liquid chromatography mass spectrometry (HPLC-MS/MS). The chromatographic separation of CML and CEL in the hydrolysed samples was performed using Accela UHPLC pump with autoinjector. Detection was performed using a LTQ Velos-Pro Orbitrap massspectrometer (Thermo Scientific, Waltham, USA) run in positive electrospray ionization ion trap tandem mass spectrometry (MS/MS) mode, detecting two selective-reaction monitoring (SRM) transitions for each analyte, and internal standard. The Xcalibur software (Thermo Scientific) was used both for data acquisition and evaluation. Solid phase extraction, chromatographic parameters, ion source parameter and the SRM transitions are the same as described in Tareke E. et al. [25].

Quantification of atherosclerosis

Frozen 10 μm sections of the aortic root region of the heart were prepared using a cryostat (Leica CM 1950, Leica Biosystems, Nusslock, Germany) and stained with Oil Red O (Histolab, Gothenburg, Sweden) and haematoxylin (Mayer's HTX, Histolab, Gothenburg, Sweden). Amount of atherosclerotic plaques covering the vessel area was quantified by a blinded observer using Bio-PixQ 2.0 (Biopix software, Gothenburg, Sweden). Three sections/mouse, with well-oriented root regions and all three valve cusps present, were evaluated.

Caecal microbiota composition

A total of 22 caecal samples (LF ($n = 4$), HF ($n = 8$), HT ($n = 9$)) were used in the microbiota analysis. Caecal tissue and content were thawed on ice and DNA was extracted using the QIAamp DNA Stool Mini Kit (Qiagen), with an addition of a bead beating step. Sterile glass beads (1 mm) were added in combination with stool lysis buffer and cell disruption was performed for 2 × 2 min at 25 Hz using a TissueLyser (Qiagen), followed by a heating step at 95 °C for 5 min. After lysis, DNA-damaging substances and PCR inhibitors were removed using InhibitEX tablet (provided with the kit) and the DNA was purified on QIAamp Mini spin columns. A normalized input of 5 ng/μL of the DNA was used in PCR reactions where 16S rRNA genes were amplified prior to sequencing.

The V1-V3 regions of 16S rRNA genes were amplified using a limited cycle PCR with forward and reverse primers containing Illumina adapter sequences and dual-index barcodes used for tagging each sample, primer sequences are listed in Table 1. Paired-end sequencing with a read length of 2×300 bp was performed on a Miseq Instrument (Illumina, Inc, San Diego, California) using a Miseq v3 reagent kit (Illumina, Inc, San Diego, California). Sequences were analysed using Quantitative Insights into Microbial Ecology (QIIME), as previously described [26]. The Operational Taxonomic Units (OTUs) were picked using a closed-reference OTU picking with UCLUST [27] algorithm against the Greengenes [28] database (version 13_8), pre-clustered at 97 % identify. After quality filtering, a total of 2,280,567 reads were included for downstream analyses and an average of 103,662 sequences (SD: 18,962) were assigned to each sample (ranging from 67,817 to 145,015 sequences). The relative abundances of bacterial taxa at phylum and genus levels were thereafter compared between groups. To correct for sampling depth differences, 67,817 reads/sample were randomly selected and utilized for further calculation of alpha-diversity and weighted and unweighted Unifrac as well as correlations between the gut microbiota and different metabolic markers.

Prediction of bacterial metagenomes using PICRUSt

The bacterial metagenomes were reconstructed based on the bacterial 16S rRNA gene sequence using the open-source software, PICRUSt [24]. The OTU table generated in QIIME from the 16S sequencing data at 67,817 rarefied sequences per sample was used as an input. The copy number per OTU was normalized before the metagenome was predicted using Kyoto Encyclopedia of Genes and Genomes (KEGG) database [29]. The output from metagenome prediction was an annotated table of predicted gene family counts for each sample, where gene families were grouped by KEGG Orthology (KO) identifiers.

Table 1 Primer sequences for amplification of 16S rRNA genes, amplicon length 507 bp

16S Amplicon PCR Forward Primer	27F AGAGTTTGATCCTGGCTCAG
16S Amplicon PCR Reverse Primer	534R ATTACCGCGGCTGCTGG

Statistical analyses

One-way analysis of variance (ANOVA) was used to calculate the differences in metabolic markers in different groups of mice using Graphpad Prism 6. Differences in within-community richness (α-diversity) were calculated in QIIME using a non-parametric *t*-test and the *P*-values were corrected for multiple comparisons using False Discovery Rate (FDR) correction [30]. Differences in community composition among groups of samples (β-diversity) were analyzed using the non-parametric analysis of similarity (ANOSIM) [31] statistical test in QIIME on both unweighted- and weighted Unifrac phylogenetic metrics. Graphpad Prism 6 was also used to identify significant differences in taxonomic distributions at phylum and genus levels between the groups of mice using two-way ANOVA and the Holm-Sidak method of correction for multiple comparisons. All the differences were considered to be significant at $P < 0.05$. Moreover, linear discriminant analysis (LDA) effect size (LEfSe) analysis [32] was performed to identify differentially abundant bacterial taxa (from phylum to species level) as well as the predicted metagenomes in each group of mice. A strict version of LEfSe was used, the discovered bacterial taxa and predicted genes with LDA score higher than two were considered to be enriched in the respective group as compared to all other groups. Partial Least Squares (PLS) Regression analysis was performed using SIMCA14 (Umetrics, Umeå, Sweden) and PLS loading score scatter plots were plotted to illustrate the associations between the parameters. Pearson's correlation was calculated for each pairwise combination of bacterial genera versus relative spleen weight, plasma CEL and CML, and atherosclerosis plaque using Graphpad Prism 6 and the *P*-values were then corrected by Benjamini-Hochberg procedure for multiple comparisons [30, 33].

Results

Biomarkers

Considering no difference in food consumption of the mice in different groups (Fig. 1a), mice fed HF had significantly higher body weight at the end point as compared to mice fed LF ($P < 0.001$, Fig. 1b). The liver weight did not differ between groups (Fig. 1c), while the epididymal fat pad weight was significantly lower in the HT and LF groups compared to the HF group (Fig. 1d). Relative spleen weight was significantly higher in HT mice as compared to HF mice ($P < 0.05$, Fig. 1e). Atherosclerotic plaque size (% of vessel area) was higher in HF and HT as compared to LF (both $P < 0.05$, Fig. 1f). Analysis of Advanced glycation end products (CML and

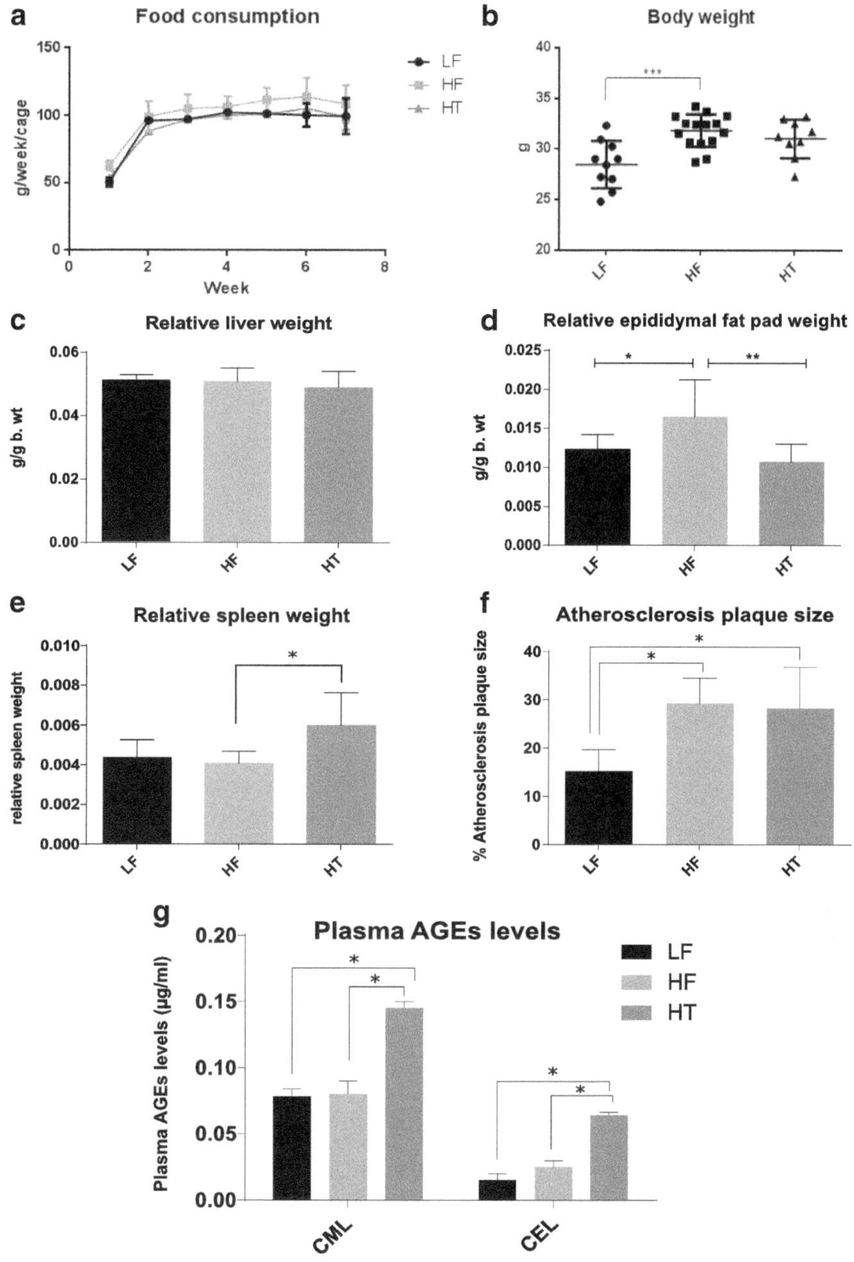

Fig. 1 Different biomarkers in mice fed LF, HF and HT. **a** Food consumption (g/week/cage). **b** Mice body weight at end point (g). **c** Relative liver weight (g/g body weight). **d** Relative epididymal fat pad weight (g/g body weight). **e** Relative spleen weight (g/g body weight). **f** Percentage of atherosclerotic plaque size (%). **g** Plasma levels of AGEs products, CML and CEL (µg/ml). One-way ANOVA was used to calculate significance among the different groups (*$P < 0.05$, **$P < 0.01$)

CEL levels) in plasma of mice revealed significant increases in levels of CML and CEL in plasma of HT mice as compared to LF and HF (all $P < 0.05$, Fig. 1g). CML increased 1.7 times in HT mice as compared to LF and HF, while CEL increased 3.5 and 2.5 times in HT as compared to LF and HF, respectively. There was no significant difference in plasma CML and CEL levels between HF and LF mice.

Microbial diversity indices

Estimation of α-diversity of bacterial 16S rRNA gene at the sequence number of 67,817 sequences/sample (Fig. 2a) demonstrated that HF had a tendency for decreased α-diversity as compared to LF. Moreover, HT lowered the α-diversity even more as the observed OTUs and phylogenetic diversity whole tree (PD whole-tree) indices showed significant differences between HT and LF ($P < 0.05$), although there was no significant difference with Chao1 index. ANOSIM analyses of both unweighted and weighted Unifrac revealed significant differences between the communities of the mice in the three treatment groups ($P < 0.01$ and $P < 0.05$, respectively). Principle coordinate analysis (PCoA) plots for unweighted and weighted Unifrac are shown in Fig. 2b and c, respectively.

Phylum-level taxonomic distributions

Relative abundance at phylum-level (Fig. 2d) revealed that Firmicutes was found to be the most dominant phylum in all groups and was followed by Bacteroidetes. The level of Firmicutes was significantly higher in HT than LF and HF (both $P < 0.01$), whereas the level of Bacteroidetes was significantly lower in HT than LF and HF ($P < 0.001$ and $P < 0.01$, respectively).

Genus-level taxonomic distributions

The most abundant genera presented in the mice (more than 5 % relative abundance) are shown in Fig. 2e. As compared to LF, HF significantly increased *Mucispirillum* ($P < 0.05$) and unclassified family of *Clostridiales* ($P < 0.05$) and reduced unclassified genus of *S24-7* ($P < 0.001$), while similar effects were observed in HT with significant increase in the relative abundance of unclassified family of *Clostridiales* ($P < 0.001$) and significant decrease in the relative abundance of unclassified genus of *S24-7* ($P < 0.01$). Moreover, a significant decrease of an unclassified genus of *Rikenellaceae* ($P < 0.001$) was also observed in HT, as compared to LF. In addition, HT was found to reduce the relative abundance of an unclassified genus of *Rikenellaceae* ($P < 0.001$) as well as to increase the relative abundance of *Allobaculum* ($P < 0.001$) and unclassified family of *Clostridiales* ($P < 0.001$) as compared to HF.

Differences in bacterial composition between groups of treatment using LEfSe

The strict version of LEfSe (all against all) detected 24 bacterial clades showing statistically significant differences between different groups of treatment with LDA scores higher than two (Fig. 3a). A Cladogram of these bacterial taxa is shown in Additional file 2: Figure S2. The most enriched bacteria in LF were *Sutterella* (from phylum to genus), *Anaeroplasma* (from phylum to genus), *Adlercreutzia* and *Lactobacillus. Mucispirillum schaedleri* (from phylum to species) and *Lactococcus* (from family to genus) were found to be the most enriched bacteria in HF while *Allobaculum* (from order to genus) was found to be enriched in HT.

Prediction of functional structure of genes based on 16S gene information using PICRUSt

By applying PICRUSt to the 16S sequencing data, a total of 328 genes were predicted to be involved in different functions (data not shown). Assigning the strict version (all against all) of LEfSe to the predicted genes from PICRUSt, detected a total of 11, 9 and 5 genes enriched in LF, HF and HT, respectively, with LDA scores higher than two (Fig. 3b). Of these, 7, 8 and 4 genes, enriched in LF, HF and HT, respectively, were involved in metabolism. Predicted metabolism genes enriched in LF encoded for metabolism of two amino acid groups; arginine and proline (KO00330), glycine, serine and threonine (KO00260), energy metabolism, particularly for methane metabolism (KO00680), enzyme families, especially for peptidases, and cofactors and vitamins, especially for vitamin B6 (KO00750). Predicted genes encoding for lipid metabolism, especially for lipid biosynthesis proteins (KO01004) and glycerophospholipid (KO00564) were enriched in HF. Moreover, metabolism of pyruvate (KO00620), lysine biosynthesis (KO00300), beta-alanine (KO00410), as well as pantothenate and CoA biosynthesis (KO00770) were also enriched in HF. These genes enriched in HF were shown to be involved in a cascade of the fatty acid biosynthesis KEGG pathway. Predicted genes encoding for carbohydrate metabolism; fructose and mannose metabolism (KO00051) and pentose and glucuronate interconversions (KO00040), energy metabolism encoding for photosynthesis proteins and an unclassified metabolism (no KO number) were enriched in HT.

Additionally, genes enriched in LF were involved in genetic information, especially for replication and repair of chromosome, ribosome biogenesis and an unclassified translation protein. A gene enriched in HF was involved in cellular processes, especially for cell growth and death and a gene enriched in HT was involved in an unclassified function (Fig. 3b).

Gut microbiota and metabolic biomarkers

Loading and score scatter (Fig. 4) PLS plots illustrated associations between the gut microbiota and different biomarkers as well as revealed separate clusters of the mice by different treatments (Fig. 4, small panel). The results supported the LEfSe results (Fig. 3a and Additional file 2: Figure S2) where those bacteria enriched in different groups of treatment were located in the corresponding area of the PLS plot (Fig. 4). *Sutterella, Anaeroplasma,*

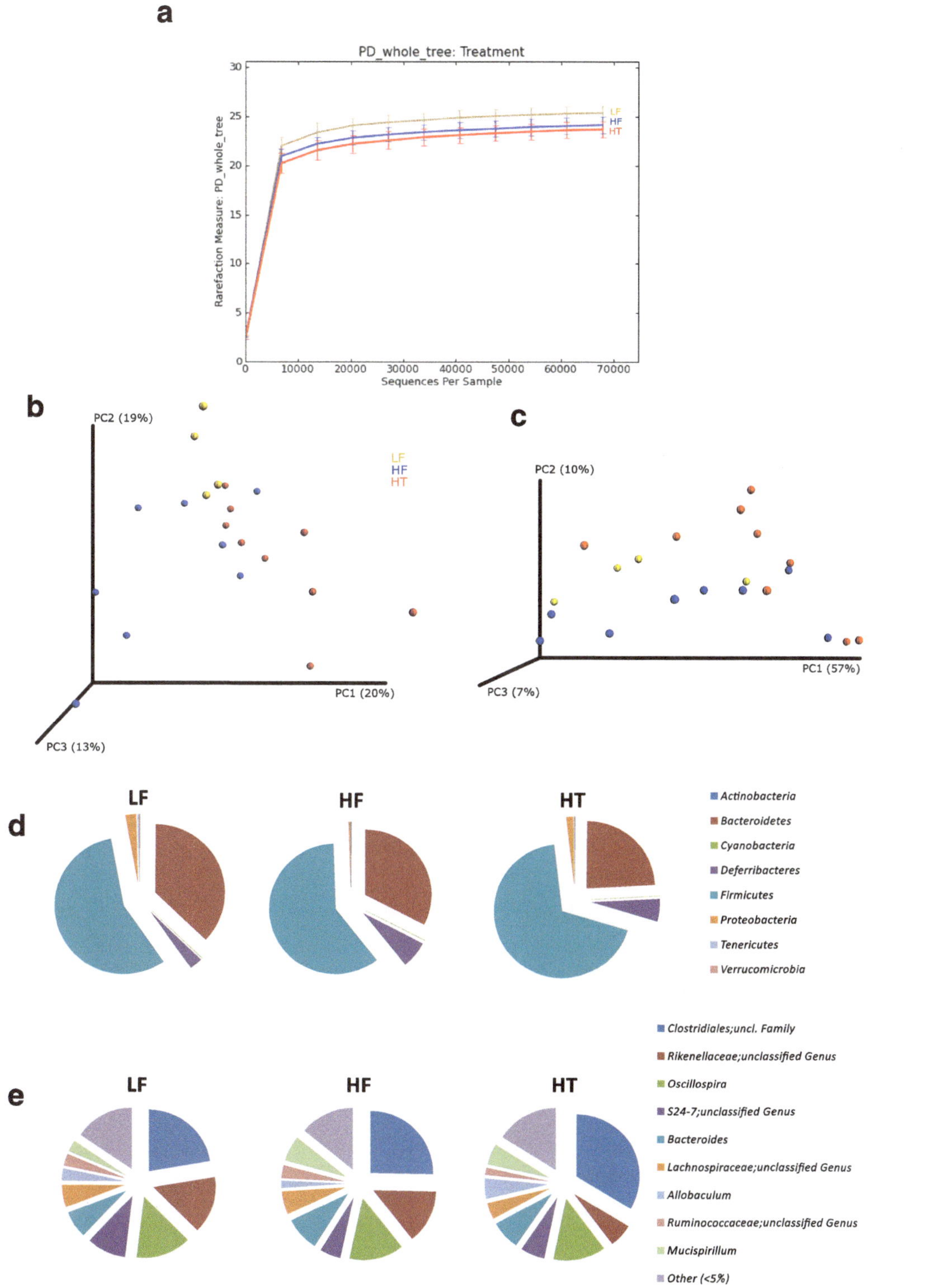

Fig. 2 (See legend on next page.)

(See figure on previous page.)
Fig. 2 Diversity indices and distributions at phylum and genus levels of the gut microbiota in mice fed LF, HF and HT. **a** Alpha rarefaction curve (whole-tree PD) showing differences in within-community richness (α-diversity). **b** Unweighted and **c** Weighted UniFrac PCoA plots showing differences in community composition among groups of mice (β-diversity). **d** Relative abundance of the gut microbiota at phylum. **e** Relative abundance of the most abundance genera (>5 % relative abundance). Reads normalized to 67,817 sequences/sample

Adlercreutzia and *Lactobacillus* which were found to be enriched in LF were located in the lower component of the PLS plot. *Mucispirillum* and *Lactococcus* enriched in HF were located in the upper right component, while *Allobaculum* was located in the upper left component of the PLS plot. Correlations between the gut microbiota and different biomarkers were also analyzed. Relative spleen weight was found to be positively correlated with *Dehalobacterium* ($P < 0.01$), *Clostridium* ($P < 0.05$), *Prevotella* ($P < 0.05$), unclassified family of *Clostridiales* ($P < 0.05$) and negatively correlated with unclassified genus of *Rikenellaceae* ($P < 0.05$) (Figs. 4 and 5). Plasma CEL and CML levels were located in the right component of and close to the relative spleen weight on the PLS plot. These suggested positive correlations between plasma CML and CEL versus relative spleen weight, and thus versus those bacterial genera that correlated with spleen weight, although the correlations were not statistically significant after correction for multiple corrections. No correlation was found between the gut microbiota and amount of atherosclerotic plaques.

Discussion

The findings from this study revealed that heat processing of fat led to changes in its effects on metabolic markers and the gut microbiota in *apoe*$^{-/-}$ mice as compared to unheated fat. Mice fed HT displayed elevated circulating levels of CML and CEL as well as enlarged spleens, to a higher extent than mice fed HF. Enlargement of the spleen has previously been observed even in healthy mice with intra-peritoneal administration of RAGE and this has been suggested to be exerted through stimulation of adaptive immune system in response to inflammation [34]. Interestingly, the amounts of atherosclerotic plaque were similar in HF and HT, which were both higher than LF. The amount of atherosclerotic plaques was anticipated to be higher in mice fed HT as heat processing of fat would add up the effect of AGEs to the effect of fat on atherosclerosis. The lower epididymal fat-pad weight observed in HT mice, to the same level as in LF mice, could possibly provide an explanation. Chemical modifications of fat by heat-treatment might abate the effect of unheated fat, leaving

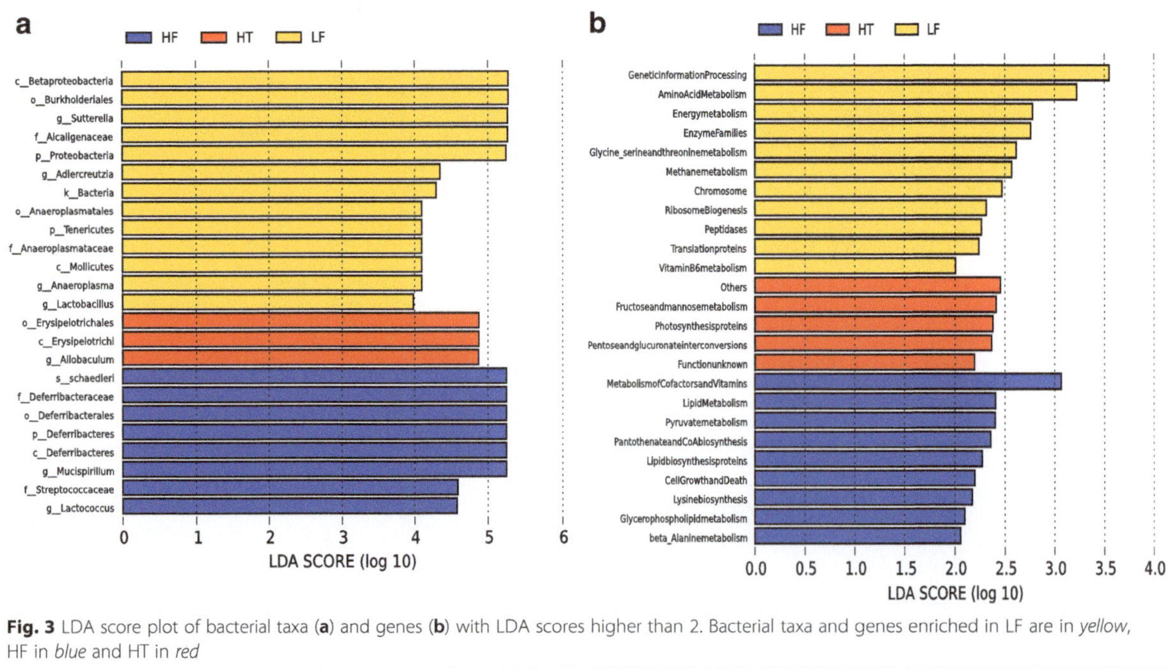

Fig. 3 LDA score plot of bacterial taxa (**a**) and genes (**b**) with LDA scores higher than 2. Bacterial taxa and genes enriched in LF are in *yellow*, HF in *blue* and HT in *red*

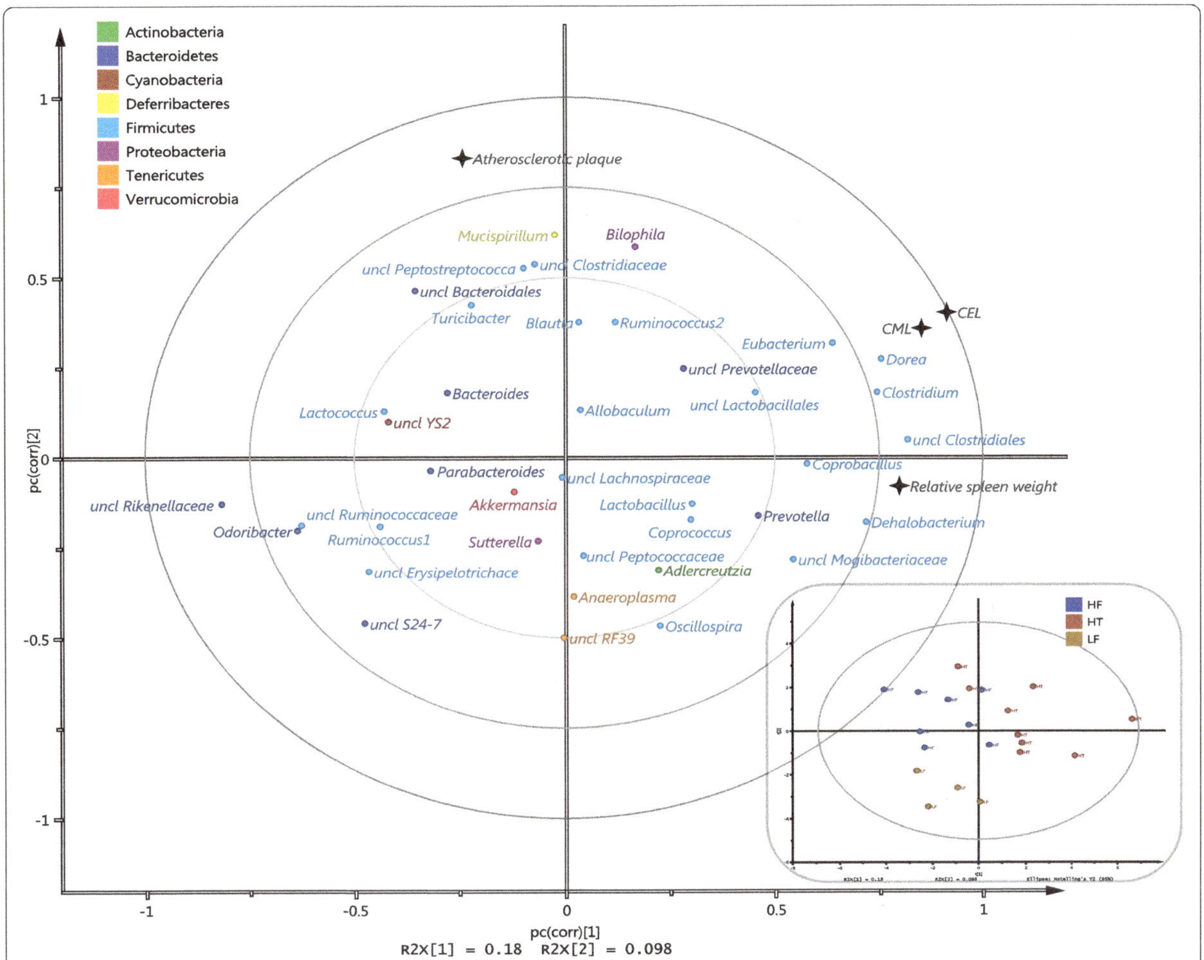

Fig. 4 Loading (*big panel*) and score scatter (*small panel*) PLS plots showing correlations between the gut microbiota and different biomarkers. Bacterial genera are shown in small circles and colored by the phylum they belong to (*green, Actinobacteria; dark blue, Bacteroidetes; red, Cyanobacteria; yellow, Deferribacteres; light blue, Firmicutes, purple, Proteobacteria; orange, Tenericutes; pink, Verrucomicrobia*). Metabolic biomarkers are shown in black stars. Each circle in score scatter plot (small panel) represents each mouse and is colored by the group they belong to (*yellow*, LF; *blue*, HF; *red*, HT)

only the effect of AGEs on atherosclerosis. Thus, HT mice reached similar levels of atherosclerosis as HF mice despite lower adiposity, which may suggest an additive effect of AGEs on atherosclerosis in the HT mice. Heat-treated LF has not been included in this study as the aim was only to compare the effects of fat and heat-treatment of HF (HT), using LF as a baseline control. However, heat-treatment of LF diet may provide more insight into the role of fat and AGEs on atherogenesis.

The results from 16S sequencing of caecal samples showed that HF and HT had an impact on the composition of the gut microbiota in the mice. Both HF and HT lowered the diversity of the gut microbiota, although the change was only significant with HT. The most dominant phyla in all groups were Firmicutes and Bacteroidetes, whose relative abundance were significantly altered with HT, as well as with HF but to a lesser extent. An imbalanced ratio of Firmicutes and Bacteroidetes has been found to be associated with risk factors of obesity in both animals and humans. High dimensional comparison using LEfSe analysis showed that both HF and HT mice differed in their gut microbiota composition and functions, as compared to each other and to LF mice. The LF group had a high diversity of bacterial genera from different phyla. Although most groups of bacteria found enriched in LF are not well known regarding their roles for the host, the predicted gene functions revealed increases of genes involved in a broad range of metabolism pathways including amino acids, enzymes, as well as cofactors and vitamins. *Mucispirillum* found enriched in the mice fed HF, is one of the putative mucin degraders [35] and has been

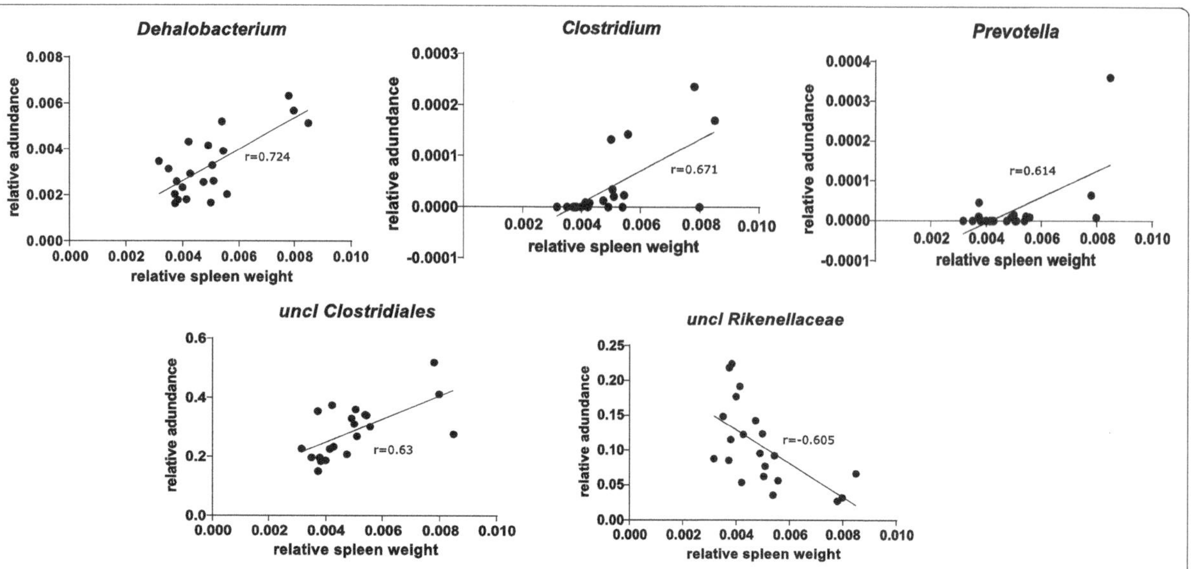

Fig. 5 Linear regression plots with Pearson's correlation coefficient (r) of bacterial genera significantly correlated with relative spleen weight. *Dehalobacterium, Clostridium, Prevotella,* unclassified family of *Clostridiales* and unclassified genus of *Rikenellaceae* were significantly correlated with relative spleen weight. Pearson's correlations with $P < 0.05$ after correction for multiple comparison using Benjamini-Hochberg procedure was considered to be significant

found in a study of Belzer et al., to be involved in the onset of symptomatic colitis in mice [36]. Interestingly, the lactic acid bacteria, *Lactococcus,* found enriched also in the mice fed HF, has been found in a study of Parks et al., to have positive correlation with body fat percentage gain in mice fed high-fat, high-sucrose diet [37]. Although genes enriched in HF mice were encoded for several metabolism pathways, it is remarkable that most of these were involved in a cascade of a fatty acid synthesis pathway. Some bacteria have been known to synthesize glycerophospholipid on the inner leaflet of the inner membrane and different lipid biosynthetic mechanisms have previously been defined [38]. These bacterial genera could therefore generate even more fat to the host's energy metabolism. In addition, the gut microbiota composition has also been shown to play a role in how much energy is harvested from the diet [39–41], and indeed, mice fed HF had significantly higher epididymal fat pad weight, as well as slightly higher body weight than mice fed HT. Interestingly, *Allobaculum* which has previously been found to be decreased in mice fed high-fat diet [37, 42], became enriched in HT mice in this study. Although these studies showed somewhat similar 16S gene results as observed in this current study, it is worth mentioning that some of them were performed on animal faeces as opposed to caecum and these two locations in the gut may harbour different bacterial species. Together with the finding that no bacterial genes encoding for lipid metabolism were enriched in mice fed HT, we hypothesize that heat processing of fat changed the chemical properties of the fat, allowing different substrates to reach the lower gut. However, the exact mechanism of how heat-treated fat appears to be less accessible to the gut microbiota than unheated fat needs further investigation.

Conclusions

In conclusion, intake of high-fat diet led to increased adiposity, decreased microbiota diversity and altered gut microbiota composition. Chemical modifications of high-fat diet by heat processing seemed to reduce the substrates available for members of the gut microbiota having lipid metabolism genes, resulting in lower adiposity. However, the overall alterations of the gut microbiota are still towards those associated with risk factors of obesity. Moreover, AGEs formed in HT could be a possible cause of spleen enlargement, which possibly reflect elevated levels of inflammation in the body. Lower intake of heat-processed food may need to be taken into consideration when developing a dietary preventative approach of the metabolic syndrome.

Ethics approval

The study was approved by the local ethical review committee for animal experiments in Lund, Sweden (approval number M-295-12).

Additional files

Additional file 1: Figure S1. Unheated (left) and heat-treated (200 °C for 10 min, right) high-fat diets. (PDF 241 kb)

Additional file 2: Figure S2. Cladogram plot showing bacterial taxa with LDA scores higher than two using strict version of LEfSe. Different colors represent the most abundant taxa in different groups of mice (yellow indicating LF, red indicating HF and blue indicating HT). Circles represent phylogenetic levels from phylum to genus. The sizes of the circle are proportional to the taxon's abundance. (PDF 436 kb)

Abbreviations

AGEs: Advanced Glycation End products; ANOSIM: analysis of similarity; ANOVA: analysis of variance; apoe−/−: apolipoprotein E knock out; CEL: Nε-carboxy-ethyl-lysine; CML: Nε-carboxy-methyl-lysine; DNA: deoxyribonucleic acid; HF: high-fat diet; HPLC-MS/MS: high-pressure liquid chromatography mass spectrometry; HT: heat-treated-high-fat diet; KEGG: Kyoto Encyclopedia of Genes and Genomes; KO: Kyoto Encyclopedia of Genes and Genomes Orthology; LDA: linear discriminant analysis; LEfSe: linear discriminant analysis effect size; LF: low-fat diet; MRPs: Maillard reaction products; MS/MS: tandem mass spectrometry; OTU: operational taxonomic unit; PCoA: principle coordinate analysis; PCR: polymerase chain reaction; PD: phylogenetic diversity; PICRUSt: Phylogenetic Investigation of Communities by Reconstruction of Unobserved States; PLS: Partial Least Squares; QIIME: Quantitative Insights into Microbial Ecology; RAGE: AGE receptor; rRNA: ribosomal ribonucleic acid; SRM: selective-reaction monitoring.

Competing interests

The authors declare that they have no competing interests.

Authors' contributions

ET designed the study, FF performed the animal study, NM performed gut microbiota analyses and ET performed AGEs analysis. All authors took part in writing the paper. All authors read and approved the final manuscript.

Acknowledgement

This research was funded by the Antidiabetic Food Center (AFC), a VINN Excellence Center funded by VINNOVA at Lund University, the Direktör Albert Påhlsson Foundation and the Per Håkansson Foundation. Chrysoula Matziouridou is greatly acknowledged for performing the atherosclerosis assessment.

References

1. Finot PA. Historical perspective of the Maillard reaction in food science. Ann N Y Acad Sci. 2005;1043:1–8.
2. Newton AE, Fairbanks AJ, Golding M, Andrewes P, Gerrard JA. The role of the Maillard reaction in the formation of flavour compounds in dairy products–not only a deleterious reaction but also a rich source of flavour compounds. Food Funct. 2012;3(12):1231–41.
3. Chuyen NV. Toxicity of the AGEs generated from the Maillard reaction: on the relationship of food-AGEs and biological-AGEs. Mol Nutr Food Res. 2006;50(12):1140–9.
4. Nemet I, Varga-Defterdarovic L, Turk Z. Methylglyoxal in food and living organisms. Mol Nutr Food Res. 2006;50(12):1105–17.
5. Vistoli G, De Maddis D, Cipak A, Zarkovic N, Carini M, Aldini G. Advanced glycoxidation and lipoxidation end products (AGEs and ALEs): an overview of their mechanisms of formation. Free Radic Res. 2013;47 Suppl 1:3–27.
6. Vlassara H, Striker GE. AGE restriction in diabetes mellitus: a paradigm shift. Nat Rev Endocrinol. 2011;7(9):526–39.
7. Alexiou P, Chatzopoulou M, Pegklidou K, Demopoulos VJ. RAGE: a multi-ligand receptor unveiling novel insights in health and disease. Curr Med Chem. 2010;17(21):2232–52.
8. Chuah YK, Basir R, Talib H, Tie TH, Nordin N. Receptor for advanced glycation end products and its involvement in inflammatory diseases. Int J Inflam. 2013;2013:403460.
9. Hegab Z, Gibbons S, Neyses L, Mamas MA. Role of advanced glycation end products in cardiovascular disease. World J Cardiol. 2012;4(4):90–102.
10. Pasinetti GM, Zhao Z, Qin W, Ho L, Shrishailam Y, Macgrogan D, Ressmann W, Humala N, Liu X, Romero C, et al. Caloric intake and Alzheimer's disease. Experimental approaches and therapeutic implications. Interdiscip Top Gerontol. 2007;35:159–75.
11. Baynes JW, Thorpe SR. Glycoxidation and lipoxidation in atherogenesis. Free Radic Biol Med. 2000;28(12):1708–16.
12. Miyazawa T, Nakagawa K, Shimasaki S, Nagai R. Lipid glycation and protein glycation in diabetes and atherosclerosis. Amino Acids. 2012;42(4):1163–70.
13. Poulsen MW, Hedegaard RV, Andersen JM, de Courten B, Bugel S, Nielsen J, Skibsted LH, Dragsted LO. Advanced glycation endproducts in food and their effects on health. Food Chem Toxicol. 2013;60:10–37.
14. Rojas A, Delgado-Lopez F, Gonzalez I, Perez-Castro R, Romero J, Rojas I. The receptor for advanced glycation end-products: a complex signaling scenario for a promiscuous receptor. Cell Signal. 2013;25(3):609–14.
15. Mills DJS, Tuohy KM, Booth J, Buck M, Crabbe MJC, Gibson GR, Ames JM. Dietary glycated protein modulates the colonic microbiota towards a more detrimental composition in ulcerative colitis patients and non-ulcerative colitis subjects. J Appl Microbiol. 2008;105(3):706–14.
16. Sekirov I, Russell SL, Antunes LC, Finlay BB. Gut microbiota in health and disease. Physiol Rev. 2010;90(3):859–904.
17. Cani PD, Bibiloni R, Knauf C, Waget A, Neyrinck AM, Delzenne NM, Burcelin R. Changes in gut microbiota control metabolic endotoxemia-induced inflammation in high-fat diet-induced obesity and diabetes in mice. Diabetes. 2008;57(6):1470–81.
18. Cani PD, Neyrinck AM, Fava F, Knauf C, Burcelin RG, Tuohy KM, Gibson GR, Delzenne NM. Selective increases of bifidobacteria in gut microflora improve high-fat-diet-induced diabetes in mice through a mechanism associated with endotoxaemia. Diabetologia. 2007;50(11):2374–83.
19. Bjorkbacka H, Kunjathoor VV, Moore KJ, Koehn S, Ordija CM, Lee MA, Means T, Halmen K, Luster AD, Golenbock DT, et al. Reduced atherosclerosis in MyD88-null mice links elevated serum cholesterol levels to activation of innate immunity signaling pathways. Nat Med. 2004;10(4):416–21.
20. Bukowska H, Pieczul-Mroz J, Jastrzebska M, Chelstowski K, Naruszewicz M. Decrease in fibrinogen and LDL-cholesterol levels upon supplementation of diet with Lactobacillus plantarum in subjects with moderately elevated cholesterol. Atherosclerosis. 1998;137(2):437–8.
21. Shimizu K, Ogura H, Goto M, Asahara T, Nomoto K, Morotomi M, Yoshiya K, Matsushima A, Sumi Y, Kuwagata Y, et al. Altered gut flora and environment in patients with severe SIRS. J Trauma. 2006;60(1):126–33.
22. Kolovou G, Anagnostopoulou K, Mikhailidis DP, Cokkinos DV. Apolipoprotein E knockout models. Curr Pharm Des. 2008;14(4):338–51.
23. Manzel A, Muller DN, Hafler DA, Erdman SE, Linker RA, Kleinewietfeld M. Role of "Western diet" in inflammatory autoimmune diseases. Curr Allergy Asthma Rep. 2014;14(1):404.
24. Langille MGI, Zaneveld J, Caporaso JG, McDonald D, Knights D, Reyes JA, Clemente JC, Burkepile DE, Vega Thurber RL, Knight R, et al. Predictive functional profiling of microbial communities using 16S rRNA marker gene sequences. Nat Biotech. 2013;31(9):814–21.
25. Tareke E, Forslund A, Lindh CH, Fahlgren C, Östman E. Isotope dilution ESI-LC-MS/MS for quantification of free and total Nε-(1-Carboxymethyl)-l-Lysine and free Nε-(1-Carboxyethyl)-l-Lysine: Comparison of total Nε-(1-Carboxymethyl)-l-Lysine levels measured with new method to ELISA assay in gruel samples. Food Chem. 2013;141(4):4253–9.
26. Caporaso J, Kuczynski J, Stombaugh J, Bittinger K, Bushman F, Costello E, Fierer N, Peña A, Goodrich J, Gordon J, et al. QIIME allows analysis of high-throughput community sequencing data. Nat Methods. 2010;7:335–6.
27. Edgar RC. Search and clustering orders of magnitude faster than BLAST. Bioinformatics. 2010;26(19):2460–1.
28. DeSantis T, Hugenholtz P, Larsen N, Rojas M, Brodie E, Keller K, Huber T, Dalevi D, Hu P, Andersen G. Greengenes, a chimera-checked 16S rRNA gene database and workbench compatible with ARB. Appl Environ Microbiol. 2006;72:5069–72.
29. Kanehisa M, Goto S, Sato Y, Furumichi M, Tanabe M. KEGG for integration and interpretation of large-scale molecular data sets. Nucleic Acids Res. 2012;40(Database issue):D109–14.
30. BaY HY. Controlling the False Discovery Rate: A Practical and Powerful Approach to Multiple Testing. J R Stat Soc Ser B Methodol. 1995;57(1):289–300.
31. Clarke KR. Non-parametric multivariate analyses of changes in community structure. Aust J Ecol. 1993;18(1):117–43.

32. Segata N, Izard J, Waldron L, Gevers D, Miropolsky L, Garrett WS, Huttenhower C. Metagenomic biomarker discovery and explanation. Genome Biol. 2011;12(6):R60.
33. McDonald JH. Multiple comparisons: Controlling the false discovery rate: Benjamini–Hochberg procedure. In: Handbook of Biological Statistics. Baltimore, Maryland: Sparkly House Publishing; 2014. p. 254–60.
34. Brisslert M, Amu S, Pullerits R. Intra-peritoneal sRAGE treatment induces alterations in cellular distribution of CD19+, CD3+ and Mac-1+ cells in lymphoid organs and peritoneal cavity. Cell Tissue Res. 2013;351(1):139–48.
35. Robertson BR, O'Rourke JL, Neilan BA, Vandamme P, On SL, Fox JG, Lee A. Mucispirillum schaedleri gen. nov., sp. nov., a spiral-shaped bacterium colonizing the mucus layer of the gastrointestinal tract of laboratory rodents. Int J Syst Evol Microbiol. 2005;55(Pt 3):1199–204.
36. Belzer C, Gerber GK, Roeselers G, Delaney M, DuBois A, Liu Q, Belavusava V, Yeliseyev V, Houseman A, Onderdonk A, et al. Dynamics of the Microbiota in Response to Host Infection. PLoS One. 2014;9(7), e95534.
37. Parks Brian W, Nam E, Org E, Kostem E, Norheim F, Hui Simon T, Pan C, Civelek M, Rau Christoph D, Bennett Brian J, et al. Genetic Control of Obesity and Gut Microbiota Composition in Response to High-Fat, High-Sucrose Diet in Mice. Cell Metab. 2013;17(1):141–52.
38. Parsons JB, Rock CO. Bacterial lipids: Metabolism and membrane homeostasis. Prog Lipid Res. 2013;52(3):249–76.
39. Velagapudi VR, Hezaveh R, Reigstad CS, Gopalacharyulu P, Yetukuri L, Islam S, Felin J, Perkins R, Borén J, Orešič M, et al. The gut microbiota modulates host energy and lipid metabolism in mice. J Lipid Res. 2010;51(5):1101–12.
40. Bäckhed F, Ding H, Wang T, Hooper LV, Koh GY, Nagy A, Semenkovich CF, Gordon JI. The gut microbiota as an environmental factor that regulates fat storage. Proc Natl Acad Sci U S A. 2004;101(44):15718–23.
41. Ley RE, Bäckhed F, Turnbaugh P, Lozupone CA, Knight RD, Gordon JI. Obesity alters gut microbial ecology. Proc Natl Acad Sci U S A. 2005;102(31):11070–5.
42. Ravussin Y, Koren O, Spor A, LeDuc C, Gutman R, Stombaugh J, Knight R, Ley RE, Leibel RL. Responses of Gut Microbiota to Diet Composition and Weight Loss in Lean and Obese Mice. Obesity (Silver Spring, Md). 2012;20(4). doi:10.1038/oby.2011.1111.

10

Multivitamins and minerals modulate whole-body energy metabolism and cerebral blood-flow during cognitive task performance: a double-blind, randomised, placebo-controlled trial

David O. Kennedy[1*], Emma J. Stevenson[1], Philippa A. Jackson[1], Sarah Dunn[1], Karl Wishart[2], Gregor Bieri[2], Luca Barella[2], Alexandra Carne[1], Fiona L. Dodd[1], Bernadette C. Robertson[1], Joanne Forster[1] and Crystal F. Haskell-Ramsay[1]

Abstract

Background: The brain is by far the most metabolically active organ in the body, with overall energy expenditure and local blood-supply closely related to neural activity. Both energy metabolism and cerebral vaso-dilation are dependent on adequate micronutrient status. This study investigated whether supplementation with ascending doses of multi-vitamin/minerals could modulate the metabolic and cerebral blood-flow consequences of performing cognitive tasks that varied in difficulty.

Methods: In this randomised, double-blind, placebo-controlled, parallel-groups study 97 healthy females (25–49 y), who were not selected on the basis of any nutritional parameters, received either placebo or one of two doses of multivitamins/minerals. Cerebral blood-flow (CBF) parameters in the frontal cortex, and total energy expenditure (TotalEnergy), carbohydrate and fat oxidation (CarbOxi/FatOxi), were measured during 5 tasks of graded cognitive difficulty and a control task (5 min per task) using Near-infrared spectroscopy (NIRS) and Indirect calorimetry of exhaled pulmonary gas (ICa) respectively. Assessments took place 60 min after the first dose and following eight weeks supplementation.

Results: During task performance supplementation with the first dose of micronutrients led to a dose-dependent increase in TotalEnergy and FatOxi throughout the post-dose assessment period following the higher dose, and increases in the total concentration of haemoglobin, a proxy measure for CBF, during task performance following the lower dose of vitamins/minerals (also containing coenzyme-Q10). Chronic supplementation over 8 weeks led to a dose-dependent increase in TotalEnergy during the task period. There were no interpretable effects on mood or cognitive performance.

(Continued on next page)

* Correspondence: david.kennedy@northumbria.ac.uk
[1]Brain, Performance and Nutrition Research Centre, Northumbria University, Newcastle-upon-Tyne NE1 8ST, UK
Full list of author information is available at the end of the article

(Continued from previous page)

Conclusions: These results show that acute supplementation with micronutrients in healthy adults can modulate metabolic parameters and cerebral blood flow during cognitive task performance, and that the metabolic consequences are sustained during chronic supplementation. These findings suggest that both brain function and metabolism are amenable to micronutrient supplementation, even in adults who are assumed to have nutritional status typical of the population.

Trial registration: ClinicalTrials.gov - NCT02381964.

Keywords: Cognitive, Metabolism, Indirect calorimetry, NIRS, Cerebral blood-flow, Vitamins, Minerals, Coenzyme Q10

Background

Whilst the brain represents only approximately 2 % of body weight, it receives 11 % of cardiac output and accounts for more than 20 % of the body's total energy expenditure [1]. Most of the brain's energy requirement is expended on neural signalling, with the high baseline levels of energy expenditure during resting wakefulness being augmented by comparatively small increases during focussed activity [1, 2]. During these periods of neural activity metabolic substrates (glucose/oxygen) cross the blood brain barrier and are delivered, on demand, to active brain areas via dilation of the local vasculature. Nitric oxide is a key mediator of this 'neurovascular coupling' between neuronal activity and increased blood supply in active tissue [3, 4] and is released from cortical neurons in an activity-dependent manner [5]. The direct local increases in blood flow or metabolic substrates during local activity provide the proxy markers of activity for brain imaging techniques such as functional magnetic resonance imaging (fMRI) and positron emission tomography (PET). Interestingly, several studies have used indirect calorimetry (ICa) of exhaled pulmonary air to investigate changes in whole-body metabolism during brain activity. These studies have demonstrated increased overall energy expenditure during the performance of cognitive tasks [6] and during rapid eye movement (REM) sleep, as compared to other sleep stages [7], and a shift towards fat oxidation during the middle and later stages of a chess game [8].

Vitamins and minerals play both direct roles in brain function (e.g. via neurotransmitter synthesis, receptor binding, membrane ion pump function) as well as indirect roles, for instance via their involvement in energy metabolism and the modulation of cerebral blood supply [9, 10]. With regards cellular energy production, most of the 13 vitamins and a number of minerals play direct or indirect roles in mitochondrial function [10–12]. As an example, the water-soluble B vitamins play ubiquitous and essential interacting roles as coenzymes and precursors in the majority of cellular functions. Of particular relevance here vitamins B_1, B_2, B_3, B_5 are essential cofactors in mitochondrial aerobic respiration and cellular energy production via their roles in the tricarboxylic acid cycle, the electron transport chain and the formation of adenosine triphosphate (ATP), the cell's energy currency; whereas vitamins B_6, B_9, and B_{12} play essential roles in all aspects of one-carbon metabolism [10, 12–14]. Similarly, coenzyme Q10 (CoQ10) is an essential coenzyme required alongside the vitamins for the mitochondrial production of ATP via oxidative phosphorylation. CoQ10, which is also a potent antioxidant, is synthesised endogenously at a low rate, and its level can be augmented from dietary sources. It has been noted that deficiencies in both the B vitamins and CoQ10 are associated with fatigue and a number of conditions related to compromised mitochondrial function [10, 13, 15]. The role of multiple vitamins in overall somatic energy production has been investigated directly in a single study conducted in 87 obese females which used ICa to assess the effects of 26 weeks supplementation with multivitamins/minerals or placebo on energy expenditure. The results showed that supplementation was associated with a significant increase in resting energy expenditure and fat oxidation [16].

As well as pivotal roles in mitochondrial energy production, both vitamins and CoQ10 are also associated with cardiovascular functioning, and therefore, by implication, the delivery of metabolic substrates to the brain. As an example, the status of vitamin C [17], vitamin D [18] and B vitamins [19] have all been shown to be related to peripheral blood flow as indicated by measures of endothelial function. Similarly, single doses of vitamins B_9, C, E and C/E combined have all been shown to increase vasodilation, as measured by flow mediated dilation, in groups with disease or dietary manipulation related endothelial dysfunction [20–23]. Similarly, there is evidence that longer term supplementation with vitamin C [24–26], vitamin B_{12} [27], vitamin B_9 [28] and vitamin D [29–31] can improve endothelial function in groups with poor endothelial function, cardio-metabolic disorders or a deficiency in the specific vitamin. In the case of CoQ10, a recent meta-analysis of the results of five methodologically adequate studies [32] suggested that supplementation with CoQ10 can also engender improvements in endothelial function and other cardiovascular parameters. The underlying hypothesis for the vasodilatory effects of these micronutrients typically relates to their antioxidant properties. However, in the case of vitamin C [24, 25], vitamin B_9 [28]. and CoQ10 [32], specific roles in the synthesis of nitric oxide or the activity of nitric oxide synthase have been identified.

The relationship between micronutrients and energy production/blood flow becomes most pertinent in light of evidence suggesting that a substantial proportion of the general population of developed countries are deficient in one or more vitamins and minerals [12, 33, 34]. The reversal of marginal insufficiencies/deficiencies may well underlie recent demonstrations of improved mood or cognitive performance following supplementation with multi-vitamins/minerals in healthy cohorts of children [35, 36] and adults [37, 38]. Given the above, the current study investigated whether supplementation with multi-vitamins/minerals (± CoQ10) could modulate the increases in energy expenditure and concentrations of haemoglobin, a proxy measure of local cerebral blood flow (CBF), associated with differing intensities of cognitive tasks, using ICa and near-infrared spectroscopy (NIRS) respectively. This randomised, double-blind, placebo-controlled, parallel-groups study therefore involved the monitoring of metabolic parameters and CBF parameters during five tasks that exerted varying levels of cognitive demand and a somatically matched control task.

Methods

Design

The study employed a randomised, double-blind, placebo-controlled, parallel groups design with energy metabolism, and cerebral hemodynamics during cognitive tasks being measured following a single dose (Day 1) and after eight weeks (Day 56) supplementation with one of two multivitamin/mineral supplements or placebo. In this exploratory study both the metabolic and CBF parameters were considered primary outcomes and all other measures secondary outcomes.

Treatments

The three treatment groups comprised:

- Supradyn® 1RDA + CoQ10, containing vitamins/minerals at levels up to 100 % of the 2008 European Union recommended dietary allowances (RDA), plus 4.5 mg CoQ10 (1RDA + Q10).
- Supradyn® 3RDA, containing vitamins and minerals at levels up to 300 % (water soluble vitamins only) of the 1990 European Union RDAs (3RDA).
- Placebo matched for appearance, taste, and odour (composed of excipients from the active formulae: talc, magnesium stearate, microcrystalline cellulose).

The active constituents of the multivitamin/mineral interventions are shown in Table 1.

The interventions were provided in a single bottle containing film coated tablets sufficient for a 63 day supplementation period. All treatments were prepared and bottled by the manufacturer in accordance with a computer-generated randomisation list and delivered to the investigational site identified only by their randomisation code. Participants were allocated sequentially to the randomisation code list. One dose of the intervention was taken orally, with water, once a day over a period of 56 days. Compliance was assessed with treatment diaries, pill counting, and an interim (~Day 28) phone conversation.

Participants

A total of 106 females in the age range 25 to 49 years were randomised. Following drop-outs and exclusions,

Table 1 Composition of the 1RDA + Q10 and 3RDA interventions

Active	Units	1RDA[1]+CoQ10	3RDA[2]
Vitamin A	μg	800	800
Vitamin B1	mg	1.1	4.2
Vitamin B2	mg	1.4	4.8
Vitamin B6	mg	1.4	6
Vitamin B12	μg	2.5	3
Vitamin C	mg	80	180
Vitamin D3	μg	5	5
Vitamin E	mg	12	10
Vitamin K1	μg	25	30
Biotin	μg	50	450
Folic acid	μg	200	600
Niacin	mg	16	54
Pantothenic acid	mg	6	18
Calcium	mg	120	120
Copper	mg	1	0.9
Iodine	μg	150	75
Iron	mg	14	8
Magnesium	mg	80	45
Manganese	mg	2	1.8
Molybdenum	μg	50	45
Selenium	μg	50	55
Zinc	mg	10	8
Coenzyme Q10	mg	4.5	
Phosphorus	mg		126.3
Chromium	μg		25
Fluoride	mg		1.5

[1]Up to 1 RDA as per EU directive 2008/100/EC (2008) [2] Up to 3 RDAs as per EU directive 90/496/EEC (1990)

as identified during a blind data-review meeting, a total of 87 participants who had provided a full set of data on Day and Day 56 were included in the statistical analyses. Participant demographics and dispositions are shown in Table 2/Fig. 1.

All participants had a body mass index (BMI) in the range of 18.50-34.99 kg/m^2 and they did not exhibit any clinically relevant deviations from normal blood pressure, pulse rate, respiratory rate and body temperature. All participants also self-reported that they were healthy, did not currently take any pharmaceutical treatments (with exception of oral contraceptives, or other routine medications to treat benign conditions) and did not have a history or current diagnosis of any relevant disease, including neurological or psychiatric diseases, significant head trauma, migraines within the last five years, or drug/alcohol abuse. Participants also self-reported that they were not pregnant or lactating and, if relevant, were using a medically acceptable form of birth control; that they did not smoke or consume excessive daily levels of caffeine (>500 mg caffeine per day); that they had not taken significant quantities of dietary supplements within the last 4 weeks. Participants agreed to abstain from alcohol for 24 h and to fast (with the exception of water) for 12 h before each visit, and to abstain throughout the trial from intake of any herbal extracts or dietary supplements. The participants' continued compliance with the inclusion/exclusion criteria was confirmed at the start of each visit to the laboratory.

This study was conducted according to the guidelines laid down in the Declaration of Helsinki and all procedures involving human subjects/patients were approved by the Northumbria University Faculty of Health and Life Sciences ethics committee. Written informed consent was obtained from all subjects. The trial was registered on ClinicalTrials.gov - Identifier: NCT02381964.

Measures

Energy metabolism - indirect calorimetry (ICa)

Oxygen uptake and carbon dioxide production were measured from expired pulmonary air using an on-line gas analysis system (Metalyzer 3B, Cortex, Leipzig, Germany). These data were used to calculate total energy expenditure (TotalEnergy), and fat and carbohydrate metabolism (FatOxi and CarbOxi respectively) using the standard formulae [39]. During the sampling period subjects breathed into a mask covering the nose and mouth; this was connected to the Metalyzer via falconia tubing. All subjects were familiarised with the procedure before commencing the trial. The Metalyzer 3B also collected heart rate data.

Cerebral blood-flow parameters - near- infrared spectroscopy (NIRS)

NIRS is non-invasive brain imaging technique predicated on the absorption by oxygenated (Oxy-Hb) and deoxygenated (Deoxy-Hb) hemoglobin of differing wavelengths of infra-red light, introduced through the intact scalp/skull. Continuous-wave NIRS (CW-NIRS) can be used to assess acute changes in local CBF, as indexed by concentration changes in total hemoglobin during a single continuous recording session. Given that CW-NIRS generates concentration change data that is intrinsically baseline-adjusted to the concentration immediately prior to the first data point in the recording session, it cannot

Table 2 Group demographics, including the results of one-way ANOVAs confirming equivalence on all parameters

	1RDA + Q10 *N* = 32		3RDA *N* = 31		Placebo *N* = 34			
Task period	Mean	SEM	Mean	SEM	Mean	SEM	F	p
Age (years)	32.97	1.26	33.65	1.26	33.38	1.32	0.07	0.93
Height (cm)	166.09	0.92	166.13	1.15	165.24	1.17	0.22	0.80
Weight (kg)	66.08	1.70	67.55	1.96	64.39	1.40	0.88	0.42
BMI (kg/m^2)	23.94	0.57	24.55	0.77	23.64	0.55	0.53	0.59
Fruit and veg (portions per day)	3.98	0.24	3.87	0.27	4.62	0.29	2.24	0.11
Physical activity (hours per week)	3.28	0.53	3.42	0.70	3.79	0.47	0.22	0.80
Weekly alcohol consumption (units)	6.5	0.81	5.29	0.82	6.47	0.98	0.6	0.55
Daily caffeine consumption (mg)	158.42	20.51	167.59	20.92	169.21	19.14	0.08	0.92
Systolic blood pressure (mm/Hg)	114.47	1.57	117.55	1.74	116.47	1.53	0.92	0.40
Diastolic blood pressure (mm/Hg)	78.16	1.38	77.16	1.57	78.15	1.23	0.17	0.85
Heart rate (bpm)	68.63	1.87	66.16	1.95	69.56	2.09	0.78	0.46
Respiratory rate	15.44	0.51	14.55	0.66	14.38	0.50	1.03	0.36
Tympanic temperature	36.82	0.07	36.93	0.05	36.87	0.07	0.66	0.52

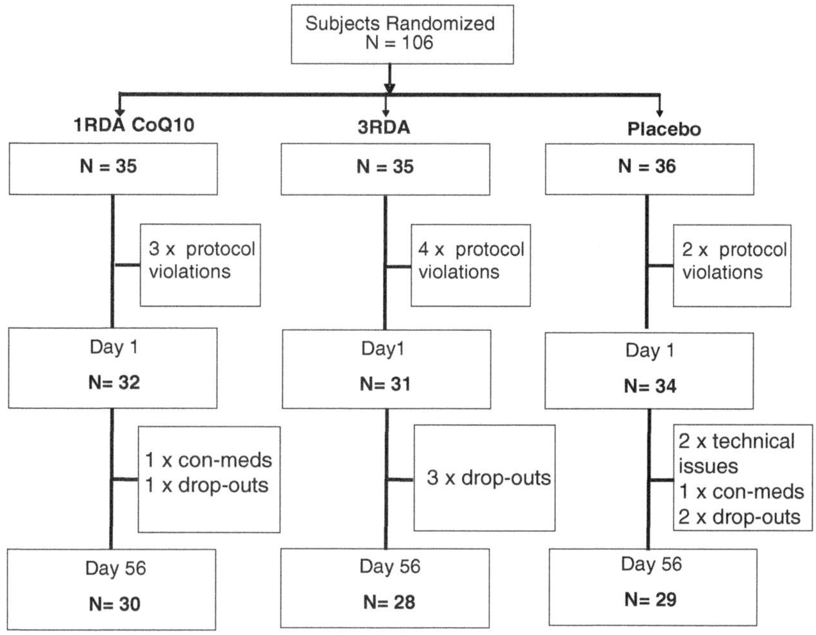

Fig. 1 Subject disposition flowchart

be used to quantify gross changes in CBF haemoglobin parameters that take place between two separate recording sessions. In this instance the change from baseline data generated by the NIRS system was subjected to a second baseline adjustment by creating 'change from baseline' data with respect to the 5 min of resting NIRS data collected immediately prior to consumption of the treatment on each day – this provided a more accurate baseline measure of immediately pre-treatment NIRS parameters.

When assessed by NIRS, the increase in cerebral blood flow (CBF) in the surface layers of the cortex during localized neural activity is typically seen as an increase in the concentration of Oxy-Hb and the total concentration of hemoglobin (Total-Hb) and comparative decrease in Deoxy-Hb [40] with both parameters suggested to correspond strongly with the functional magnetic resonance imaging (fMRI) blood oxygen level dependent (BOLD) signal [41, 42].

In this instance, relative changes in the absorption of near-infrared light were measured at a time resolution of 10Hz using a 12-channel Oxymon system (Artinis Medical Systems B.V.). The system emitted two nominal wavelengths of light (~765- and 855 nm) with an emitter/optode separation distance of 4 cm. The differential path-length factor was adjusted according to the age of the participant using the proprietorial software. Relative concentration changes in Oxy-Hb, Deoxy-Hb and Total-Hb were calculated by means of a modified Beer-Lambert law [43] using the proprietorial software. Given the extended recording period and the investigational aims, a simple two emitter/optode pair configuration was utilised (i.e. 2 channels). The emitter/optode pairs were positioned over the left and right frontal cortex using a standard optode holder headband, which separated the pairs from each other by 4 cm. Each pair therefore collected data from an area of prefrontal cortex that included the areas corresponding to the International 10–20 system Fp1 and Fp2 EEG positions. Prior to the primary analysis described below, ANOVAs including hemisphere (i.e. optode) as an additional factor (i.e. hemisphere x day x epoch x treatment) were carried out. In the absence of any treatment related interactions with 'hemisphere', data from the two optodes were simply averaged for all of the analyses reported in this paper. The methodology described above been used previously to demonstrate the effects of a number of nutritional interventions on cerebral cerebral blood-flow parameters [44–46].

Cognitive tasks

A range of cognitive tasks of varying levels of difficulty, plus a somatically matched control task, were delivered on laptop computers via the Computerised Mental Performance Assessment System (COMPASS) software (Northumbria University, UK). The order of the 5 cognitive tasks and the control task were counterbalanced across participants, with each individual participant completing the tasks in the same order during each assessment. Each task was of 5 min duration, with a two minute resting period between tasks. The selection of tasks comprised:

Serial subtractions (3 s, 7 s and 17 s) Serial subtraction tasks (Serial 3 s and Serial 7 s) have been used previously to elicit hemodynamic responses in the frontal cortex in a number of NIRS [45, 47] and fMRI [48] studies. In this instance modified, five minute versions of the Serial 3 s and Serial 7 s tasks, and a novel Serial 17 s task were employed. For each task a standard instruction screen informed the subject to count backwards in threes (sevens or seventeens) from a given randomly generated number between 800 and 999, as quickly and accurately as possible. Subjects were also instructed verbally that if they made a mistake they should carry on subtracting from the new incorrect number. Each three-digit response was entered via the linear number keys with each digit being represented on screen by an asterisk. Pressing the 'enter' key signalled the end of each response and cleared the three asterisks from the screen. The task was scored for total number of subtractions and number of errors. In the case of incorrect responses, subsequent responses were scored as positive if they were correct in relation to the new number.

3-back task N-Back tasks have been used widely in brain imaging studies probing brain activation, including in the frontal cortex, during working memory tasks [49]. Here the most difficult 3-back version was utilised. A continuous string of letters (upper and lower case; display time 500 msec; inter-stimulus interval of 2.5 s) was presented in the centre of the screen for 5 min. For each stimulus, subjects were instructed to indicate whether this was the same letter that appeared three letters before or not by pressing 'yes' and 'no' buttons on the response box as rapidly as possible. A third of all stimuli (40/120) represented target pairs. The task was scored for percentage of correct responses and reaction times to correct stimuli.

Stroop task The Stroop task is widely used as a measure of selective attention and executive function. Performance of the task activates multiple brain regions including the frontal cortex [50, 51]. In the five minute computerised version of the Stroop task employed here words describing colours (GREEN, BLUE, RED, YELLOW) were randomly presented in a congruent (e.g., GREEN presented in green text etc.) or incongruent coloured text (e.g., GREEN presented in blue text etc.). For each of the stimuli subjects were instructed to respond to the colour of the text the word was presented in, by pressing one of the four corresponding coloured buttons on the response pad. The task was scored for total % correct and reaction times to correct congruent and incongruent responses.

Key tapping control task A 5 min control task, somatically matched to the task that requires the most physical movement (Serial 3 s) was employed to control for the contribution of physical activity to the measures of metabolism and CBF. Subjects repeatedly made three keyboard key presses at the average rate of performance of the Serial 3 s task, plus 1 standard deviation, for 5 min. The rate of completion was controlled by a metronome tone.

Other measures

Subjective difficulty and mental fatigue ratings Visual analogue scales were used to assess the difficulty ("How difficult did you find the task that you have just completed?") and the subjects' subjective levels of mental fatigue ("How mentally fatigued do you feel right now?") following completion of each task. Participants indicated their answer to the question by positioning an 'x' on a line anchored "Not at all" and "Extremely" with the mouse/cursor. Each VAS was scored as % along the line towards "Extremely".

Bond-lader mood scales [52] Prior to and following the cognitive tasks, mood was assessed using 'Alert', 'Content' and 'Calm' factors derived from the Bond-Lader visual analogue mood scales.

Energy visual analogue scales (Energy VAS) Prior to and following the cognitive task period, visual analogue scales were completed which assessed (from 'very low' to 'very high') the subjects' self-ratings of 'concentration', 'mental stamina' and 'physical stamina'. Scales anchored at either end by 'not at all' and 'extremely' also assessed the subjects' self-rated levels of being 'mentally tired' and 'physically tired'. All VAS were scored as % along the line towards 'very high'/'extremely'.

Nutritional status

Nutritional status was assessed before and after the supplementation period with reference to serum/plasma concentrations of homocysteine, vitamin C, vitamin E, vitamin D (25-hydroxy vitamin D_3), iron, zinc and coenzyme Q10. A total of 18 ml whole blood was collected from each participant in 3 x 6 ml ethylenediaminetetraacetic acid (EDTA). Analysis of the plasma for vitamin E (alpha-tocopherol), coenzyme Q10 (ubichinone-10) and vitamin C (ascorbic acid) was then undertaken using high-performance liquid chromatography (HPLC); homocysteine levels were analysed using chemiluminescence immunoassay

(CLIA); and vitamin D (25-hydroxy Vitamin D3) levels were assessed using liquid chromatography-tandem mass spectrometry (LC-MS/MS). A further 4 ml whole blood was collected in 4 ml vacutainer serum tubes for the analysis of iron and zinc levels using photometry. All analyses were undertaken by Labor Dr. Limbach und Kollegen (Heidelberg, Germany).

Procedure

Participants attended the Brain, Performance and Nutrition Research Centre laboratory (Northumbria University), having fasted for 12 h, on three separate mornings. The practice visit comprised the obtaining of informed consent, the collection of demographic and medical history information and review of conformity to the inclusion and exclusion criteria. Vital signs, height, weight (plus calculation of BMI) were measured, and, where applicable, a confirmatory pregnancy test was carried out. Following screening, participants were instructed in the completion of the cognitive tasks, and were allocated their counterbalanced cognitive task order. They then underwent a full ICa/NIRS/cognitive assessment, as described below for Day 1 and Day 56, with the exception that the ICa and NIRS recording started 10 min before the cognitive task period rather than 70 min before (to allow for treatment absorption) on the subsequent days.

Within 28 days of the practice day participants attended the laboratory for the Day 1 assessment. Following confirmation of compliance with all inclusion/exclusion criteria, and the measurement of vital signs, participants were randomized to their treatment group, after which a venous blood sample was collected. Once the ICa mask and NIRS were in place, and the proper functioning of the equipment had been confirmed, the participant sat for a 10 min resting ICa and NIRS measurement, the last 5 min of which was used as the pre-dose baseline measure for the CBF parameters. Once the participant had consumed their day's treatment they sat quietly for 60 min, the last 5 min of this period was used to calculate the pre-task, resting-period ICa parameters. Participants then completed the Bond-Lader mood scales and 'energy' visual analogue scales. The six x five minute tasks were then completed in the counterbalancing order allocated to the participant, with a two minute rest period between each task. Finally, the participant completed the Bond-Lader mood scales and Energy VAS. NIRS data was collected continuously throughout the entire assessment. The Day 56 assessment was identical to that on Day 1. The running order of the Day 1/56 assessments are shown in Fig. 2.

Statistical analyses

Prior to commencement the sample size required for the study was calculated using G*Power 3 with respect to the medium effect size (f = 0.24) seen with similar nutritional interventions (e.g. polyphenols) using similar aspects of methodology. In order to exceed power of 0.8 for the measures which were repeated six times per assessment (e.g. ICa) a sample size of 30 participants per group was required, with measures that exceeded this number of repetitions having greater power.

Metabolic and CBF parameter data

Data from the metabolic parameters (FatOxi, CarbOxi, TotalEnergy) were collapsed into scores representing the average during 8 separate five minute epochs: comprising, pre-dose baseline, pre-task resting period, control task, and the five cognitive tasks.

The NIRS data, averaged across the left and right optodes, was baseline adjusted with regards the 5 min pre-dose baseline measure for the respective day. Data collected following consumption of the treatment was collapsed (i.e. the mean score was calculated) into: 11 x five minute epochs spanning the 60 min resting absorption period (data collected during completion of the mood scales was discarded), 6 x five minute epochs for the control task and each of the cognitive tasks, and 5 x two minute epochs for each of the rest periods between tasks (see Fig. 4).

Prior to the main analysis. in order to simply confirm that increasing task demands were associated with significant changes in metabolic and NIRS parameters irrespective of treatment, change from resting pre-task baseline data collected on Day 1 and Day 56 were analysed by two-way ANOVA (Day 1/56 x task). These data and results are presented in Additional file 1: Table S1 and Figure S1 in the online materials.

Given the exploratory nature of this study, in order to protect against potential Type II errors, no correction was made for the number of separate linear-mixed models (metabolic data - 3 in total) and ANOVA (NIRS data – 3 in total) analyses described below.

Effects of multivitamins/minerals on metabolic parameters The data for each individual metabolic parameter (FatOxi, CarbOxi, and TotalEnergy) from Day 1 and Day 56 were analysed separately using the linear mixed-effects models (MIXED) procedure in SPSS 21.0. This analysis is appropriate in repeated measures designs that include a baseline covariate as it accounts for the correlation between data points taken from the same subject and allows for missing data across time points (using maximum likelihood to estimate missing data to produce unbiased full datasets with no loss of power). In each of the separate models subject was entered as a random effect and condition, day, task period and their interactions entered as fixed factors. The resting baseline data collected prior to taking the treatment on Day 1

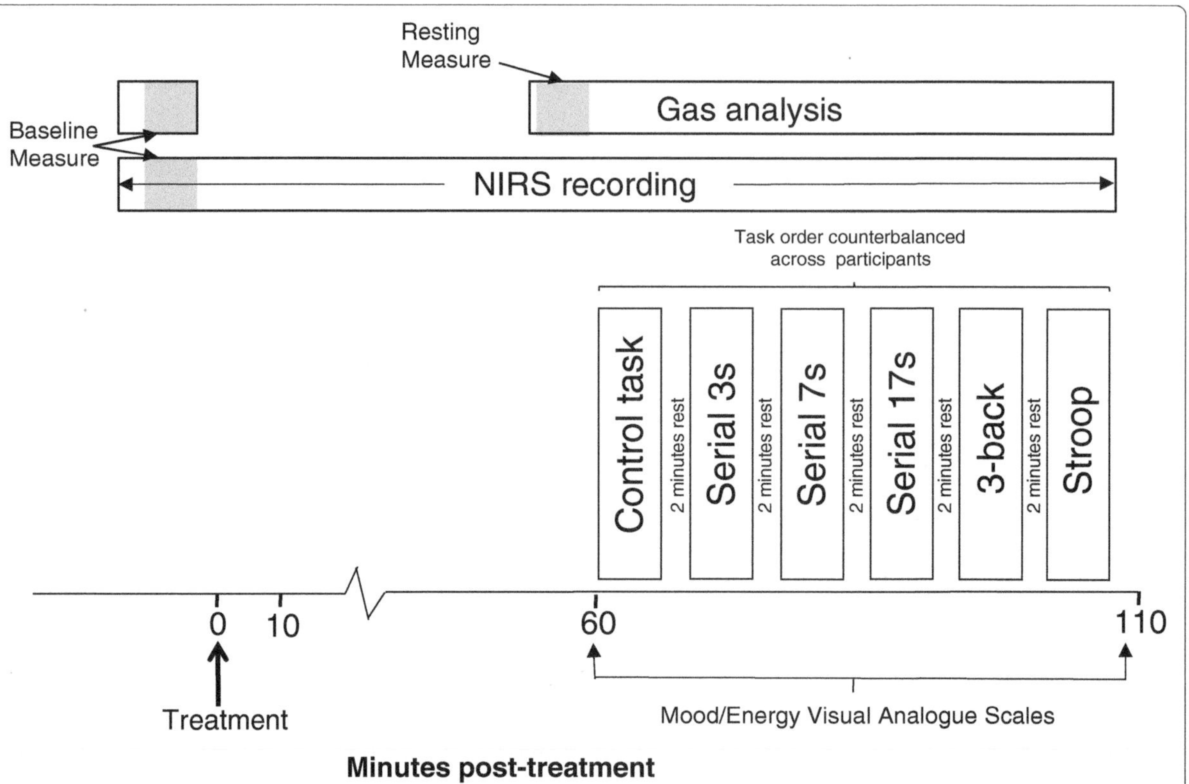

Fig. 2 Assessment schedule on Days 1 and 56. Both ICa and NIRS data-collection started with a 10 min pre-dose recording period, the last five minutes of which was used as the baseline measurement. NIRS data was then collected continuously throughout. Following consumption of the day's treatment participants sat quietly for 60 minutes, with data from the last five minutes of this period used as the ICa resting measurement. Participants then completed the control task, and the five cognitive tasks, in counterbalanced order, with a two minute resting period between each five minute task period

was entered as a covariate in the analysis of each outcome. Post-hoc, Bonferroni adjusted comparisons between the means from each of the multivitamin conditions and the placebo condition were carried out to explore any significant main or interaction effects from the primary analysis.

NIRS parameters (Day 1 and Day 56) The NIRS system utilised here generates 'change in concentration' data during a given recording session, rather than quantitative data, and therefore does not generate data that can be meaningfully used as a pre-treatment covariate. The analysis adopted here for each individual NIRS parameter (Oxy-Hb, Deoxy-Hb, Total-Hb) was therefore via separate three-way ANOVAs (Dayl/56 x treatment x epoch) of change from baseline (calculated from the relevant day's immediately pre-treatment rest period) data from each of the 22 epochs spanning the absorption and task periods (see above and Fig. 2.). The primary analysis was via planned comparisons, carried out using t tests calculated with MSError from the ANOVA, which were conducted between placebo and the two multivitamin treatments on means from each epoch. These comparisons were Bonferroni-adjusted to allow for any inflation of Type I errors due to violations of the sphericity assumption [53]. Only those planned comparisons associated with a significant effect on the relevant ANOVA are reported.

A further similar secondary analysis of data solely from the six task periods was conducted to identify any effects of the treatment related to increasing task demands.

Cognitive, mental fatigue, task difficulty and mood/energy outcomes

The cognitive outcome data (accuracy and speed of performance from each of five tasks – i.e. 10 outcomes in total) from Day 1 and Day 56 were explored with individual two-way (treatment x day) ANOVAs. Subjective mental fatigue and difficulty ratings acquired after performance of the tasks were explored with two-way (treatment x task) mixed ANOVAs of data from the individual day. Mood/energy outcome data were analysed with two-way (treatment x before/after tasks) mixed ANOVAs of data from the individual days. Post-hoc comparisons (Bonferroni adjusted) were conducted on data from each day for those measures that reached significance.

Nutritional parameters

Analysis of the nutritional blood analyte parameters was primarily by one-way ANCOVA of Day 56 data, using the corresponding Day 1 (pre-treatment) data as covariate. Separate one-way ANOVAs of Day 1 and Day 56 data were also conducted to confirm the equivalence of the groups pre-treatment, and post-treatment group differences on any measure.

Results

Data and results with regards the effects of differing task demands on all subjective, metabolic and CBF outcomes, irrespective of treatment, are presented in the online materials in Additional file 1: Figure S1 and Table S1.

Effects of multivitamins/minerals on metabolic parameters

Fat oxidation – there was a significant interaction between treatment and Day 1/56 [$F (2, 270) = 6.393$, $P < 0.05$]. Reference to the post-hoc comparisons between means showed that Fatoxi was significantly increased following a single dose of the 3RDA treatment on Day 1 ($p < 0.01$), with no significant differences evident after 8 weeks administration (Day 56).

Carbohydrate oxidation – there was a significant interaction between treatment and Day 1/56 [$F (2, 276) = 9.9$, $P < 0.01$]. However, this effect represented opposite, non-significant patterns on the two days, and reference to the post-hoc comparisons showed that there were no significant differences between the active treatment and placebo means on either day (all, $P > 0.1$).

Total energy - there was a significant main effect of treatment with regards Total Energy [F (2, 82 = 4.354, $P < 0.05$] with consumption of the 3RDA treatment resulting in increased energy expenditure during task performance both after a single dose and 8 weeks supplementation [Day 1 ($P < 0.05$), Day 56 ($P < 0.01$)].

Significant effects on the ICa measures are presented graphically in Fig. 3, with an additional illustrative graphic representation of the data for each task period. Data are presented in online Additional file 1: Table S2.

Effects of multivitamins/minerals on CBF parameters

Reference to the ANOVA of the combined Day 1/Day 56 NIRS data showed that there was a significant interaction between epoch, day and treatment for Total-Hb [$F (42,1617) = 1.521$, $P < 0.05$]. Reference to the Bonferroni adjusted planned comparisons of data from each of the 22 epochs showed that CBF, as indexed by Total-Hb concentrations, was significantly increased during the 2nd, 3rd , 5th and 6th task periods (all $P < 0.01$) on the 1st day of treatment following the 1RDA + Q10 treatment. There were no significant differences associated with the 3RDA treatment or during any epoch following either treatment on Day 56.

The pattern of effects in terms of Oxy-Hb was largely the same (epoch x day x treatment interaction, [$F(42,1617) = 1.396$, $P < 0.05$]). Following a single dose of the 1RDA + Q10 treatment, concentrations of Oxy-Hb were increased during the 2nd, 3rd, 5th and 6th task periods (all $P < 0.01$) on Day 1. Additionally Oxy-Hb was also elevated during the rest period between the 5th and 6th task periods following 1RDA + Q10 ($P < 0.05$) and during a single task period following the 3RDA treatment (1st Day, 6th task period - $P < 0.01$). There were no significant differences during any epoch following either treatment on Day 56.

There were no significant effects either with regards Deoxy-Hb. Mean data (+ SEM) for each epoch on both days for Total-Hb, Oxy-Hb and Deoxy-Hb are shown in Fig. 4.

Effects of multivitamins/minerals on cognitive performance, mood and VAS

There were no significant differences in task performance following either acute or chronic administration of the treatments with the exception of a main effect on 3-Back Correct across both days [$F (2,81) = 4.21$, $P < 0.05$]. Reference to the comparisons between placebo and treatment means showed that this effect represented more correct responses following placebo in comparison to the 1RDA + Q10 treatment (both days, $P < 0.05$). The cognitive data are presented in Additional file 1: Table S3 in the online materials.

There were no significant effects of treatment on ratings of either mental fatigue or task difficulty following a single dose (Day 1) or mental fatigue following 8 weeks administration. However, there was a significant difference evinced in terms of perceived difficulty ratings on Day 56 (treatment x task interaction, [$F (10,365) = 2.31$, $P < 0.05$]), with both multivitamin treatment groups ($P < 0.01$) rating the 3-Back task as having been more difficult in comparison to the placebo group. However, it may be notable that this finding was as a result of a sharp drop in difficulty ratings (as compared to other tasks and data from Day 1) restricted to this one task in the placebo condition. Subjective difficulty and mental fatigue outcome data (+SEM) for Day 1 and Day 56 are presented in Additional file 1: Table S4 in the online materials.

There were no significant effects on the Bond-Lader mood scales or Energy VAS.

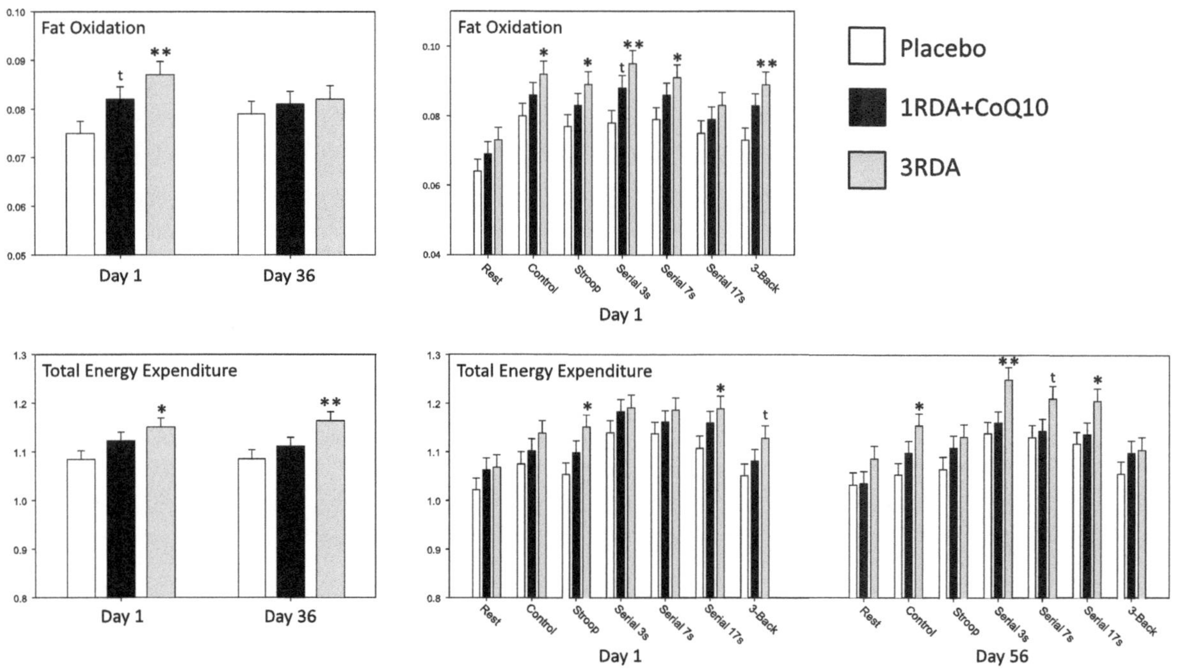

Fig. 3 Acute and chronic effects of the multivitamin treatments on metabolism. with Bonferroni corrected post-hoc comparisons to placebo. The graphs on the left show the treatment x day interaction with regards FatOxi and the main effect of treatment on TotalEnergy. The graphs on the right show the data broken down by task for illustrative purposes. All data are adjusted means (+SEM), derived from the linear mixed-effects models analysis incorporating the Day 1, pre-treatment baseline measure as a covariate. t, p <0.1; *, $p < 0.05$; **, $p < 0.01$; ***, $p < 0.001$ from the post-hoc comparisons between the two active treatments and placebo

Nutritional status parameters

ANOVA of baseline data (Day 1 pre-dose) showed that the groups did not differ significantly in terms of any nutritional status parameter at the outset of the study. However, there was a trend towards such an effect with regards CoQ10 levels, with inspection of the groups means suggesting that this was as a consequence of numerically higher levels in the 1RDA + Q10 group than the other two groups prior to treatment. The primary analysis (ANCOVA of Day 56 data using Day 1 as covariate) showed that by Day 56 both vitamin D3 and homocysteine levels were significantly modulated by treatment (vitamin D3 [F (2,75) = 4.13, $P < 0.05$], homocysteine [F (2,75) = 8.3, $p < 0.001$]). Both multivitamin treatments resulted in elevated vitamin D3 levels (1RDA + CoQ10, $P < 0.05$ – 3RDA, $P < 0.01$]) and reduced homocysteine levels (1RDA + CoQ10, $P < 0.05$ – 3RDA, $P < 0.001$]). A confirmatory analysis of micronutrient levels using data solely from Day 56 showed that, as well as significantly higher levels of vitamin D3 and lower levels of homocysteine in both multivitamin groups, CoQ10 levels were also significantly higher in the 1RDA + Q10 group post-treatment ($P < 0.05$). Data for the nutritional parameters from Day 1 and Day 56 (+SEM) are shown in Table 3.

Discussion

The results of the current study demonstrate that the administration of single doses of vitamins and minerals (± CoQ10) can modulate whole-body metabolic parameters and frontal cortex CBF hemodynamic responses during the performance of cognitive tasks of graded difficulty. The modulation of metabolic parameters was also seen following 8 weeks administration.

With regards to the metabolic parameters, the multivitamin/mineral treatment had a dose dependent effect, with significant modulation only achieved following the treatment containing the higher (3RDA) of two doses of water soluble vitamins. This treatment resulted in both increased fat oxidation (FatOxi) and increased total energy expenditure (TotalEnergy), as assessed using indirect calorimetry of exhaled pulmonary gas. These effects were seen throughout the cognitive task period which commenced 60 min post-dose. The increase in total energy expenditure was also sustained, and consolidated, at the end of the 8 week treatment period. Whilst not having a significant impact on metabolism, the lower dose of vitamins/minerals with added coenzyme Q10 (1RDA + Q10) increased the CBF hemodynamic response in the frontal cortex during tasks that activate this brain area following a single dose. In this case both

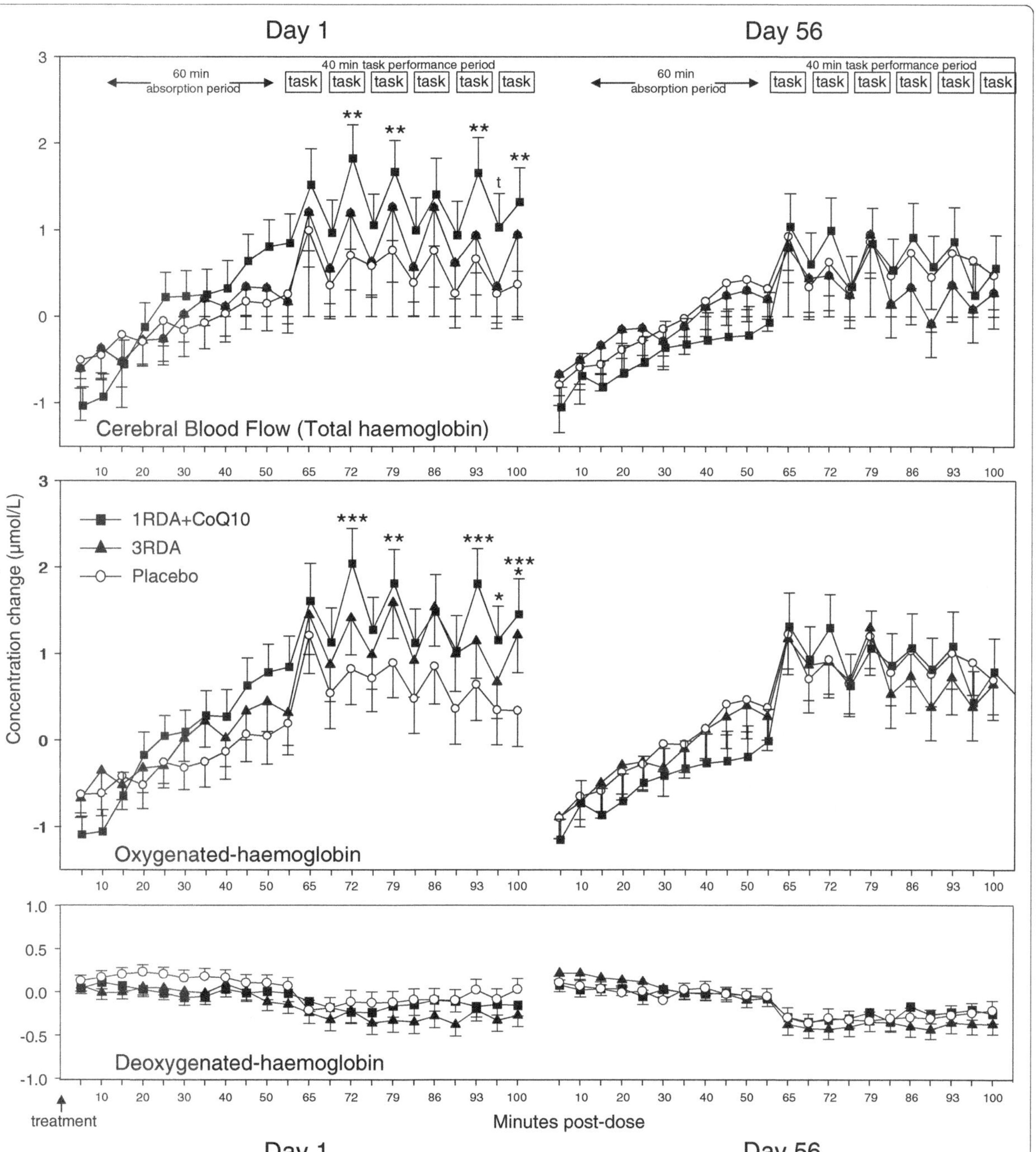

Fig. 4 Mean (+SEM) Total-Hb, Oxy-Hb and Deoxy-Hb data from each NIRS recording epoch on Day 1 and Day 56 baseline adjusted to a pre-treatment resting period. Following a 60 minute absorption period participants completed a control key-tapping task and 5 cognitive tasks (all 5 min duration) in counterbalanced order with a 2 min resting period between each task. t, $p < 0.1$; *, $p < 0.05$; **, $p < 0.01$; ***, $p < 0.001$, from Bonferroni adjusted comparisons between placebo and the two multivitamin treatments during each epoch

Total-Hb, a measure of overall local CBF, and Oxy-Hb were increased, with no significant effect on concentrations of Deoxy-Hb. Interestingly, the pattern of hemodynamic responses was similar, if less striking, in the 3RDA group (and reached statistical significance during several tasks prior to the Bonferroni corrections).

Table 3 Mean nutritional parameter data (+SEM) from Day 1 and Day 56

			Day 1		Day 56		Day 56 ANCOVA	
	Treatment	N	Mean	SEM	Mean	SEM	Adjusted mean	SEM
Vitamin C (mg/L)	1RDA + Q10	24	5.30	0.51	6.02	1.23	6.23	0.62
	3RDA	26	6.87	1.04	6.42	1.26	6.30	0.59
	Placebo	29	6.62	0.61	5.21	0.97	5.14	0.56
Vitamin D (mg/L)	1RDA + Q10	24	25.41	2.40	30.5[a]	6.22	28.73*	1.51
	3RDA	26	24.27	2.19	30.1[a]	5.90	29.23*	1.45
	Placebo	29	20.22	2.22	21.76	4.04	23.97	1.39
Vitamin E (mg/L)	1RDA + Q10	24	11.61	0.56	12.1	2.47	12.00	0.40
	3RDA	26	11.73	0.55	12.55	2.46	12.36	0.39
	Placebo	29	11.12	0.44	11.36	2.11	11.62	0.37
CoQ10 (μg/L)	1RDA + Q10	24	562.3	46.0	586.3[a]	119.7	541.8	36.64
	3RDA	26	473.1	33.3	452.5	88.8	463.4	34.41
	Placebo	29	447.1	26.3	437.8	81.3	464.8	32.89
Iron (μmol/L)	1RDA + Q10	24	1010.7	75.8	951.0	194.1	954.2	75.41
	3RDA	26	1064.4	100.1	1054.9	206.9	1042.4	72.55
	Placebo	29	992.9	89.6	985.2	183.0	993.7	68.65
Zinc (μmol/L)	1RDA + Q10	24	13.16	0.52	13.65	2.79	13.66	0.31
	3RDA	26	13.13	0.28	13.34	2.62	13.35	0.30
	Placebo	29	13.26	0.22	13.23	2.46	13.22	0.28
Homocysteine (μmol/L)	1RDA + Q10	24	11.79	0.61	10.54	2.15	10.35*	0.45
	3RDA	26	11.83	0.75	9.5[a]	1.86	9.30*	0.43
	Placebo	29	10.76	0.41	11.36	2.11	11.71	0.41

Footnote: a = $p < 0.05$ from t test comparing means for measures that evinced a significant difference on one way ANOVA of data from the individual day. * = $p < 0.05$ from t test comparing means for measures that evinced a significant difference on one way ANCOVA of data from Day 56 using Day 1 data as covariate

There was no evidence of acute modulation of hemodynamic parameters as a consequence of the day's dose of the treatment after 8 weeks administration of either treatment. However, as noted above, CW-NIRS generates concentration change, rather than quantitative data, and therefore only provides a measure of acute changes in CBF hemodynamics during each discrete recording session. It therefore provides no direct measure of any changes that have taken place between recording sessions, in this case as a consequence of chronic supplementation with micronutrients. The lack of a chronic effect may therefore reflect a simple attenuation of the acute effects seen following the first dose of 1RDA + Q10 on Day 1. However, this could equally, in turn, reflect either increased circulating levels of micronutrients as a consequence of 8 weeks administration, which may have precluded a further acute effect of an additional dose of micronutrients on Day 56; or it may indicate that a gross, undetectable change in CBF parameters had already taken place, attenuating the possibility of any additional acute effects of Day 56's treatment.

Whilst this study also provides the first demonstration that simply increasing the demands of cognitive tasks significantly modulates whole-body metabolic parameters, there was no significant interaction between treatment and specific tasks for either the metabolic or CBF parameters.

In general, the results with regards the effects of micronutrients on energy metabolism are broadly in line with those of Li et al. [16], who examined the effect of 26 weeks supplementation with multivitamin/minerals on overall resting metabolism in obese females using ICa, and found that micronutrient supplementation was associated with a significant increase in resting energy expenditure and fat oxidation. The specific acute, dose-related increase in fat oxidation seen here is also consistent with previous ICa studies that have demonstrated an increase in fat oxidation as a consequence of acute and chronic administration of calcium [54], acute supplementation with calcium and vitamin D [55] and chronic vitamin C supplementation [56]. In terms of the mechanisms underlying the effects on overall energy expenditure it is notable that vitamins as a group are directly involved in every aspect of mitochondrial function including aerobic respiration and cellular energy production [10–14]. With regards fat oxidation, the effects of calcium have been attributed in part to modulation of lipolysis and lipogenesis driven by modulation of levels of circulating 1,25-$(OH)_2D_3$ and parathyroid hormone [57], whereas vitamin C is theorised to have its effect via its role as a cofactor for the biosynthesis of carnitine, an essential molecule in the oxidation of fatty acids [56]. Whilst the effects on fat metabolism here may be predicated simply on the inclusion of calcium, and vitamins C and D in the micronutrient preparations, it is not possible to preclude modulation of a multitude of metabolic parameters by the other vitamin and mineral components. It is also worth noting that whereas the chronic effects of supplementation on fat oxidation were not significant, the numeric pattern of the data was consistent with the acute results.

The pattern of CBF parameter effects seen here was for a treatment related augmentation of the hemodynamic responses seen during the performance of the active cognitive tasks, with significant increases in total-haemoglobin, a proxy measure of CBF, seen during four of the five active task periods. In this instance, due to the counterbalancing of the order of task performance, the benefits could not be attributed to specific task demands, and a secondary task x treatment analysis did not demonstrate an interaction between the two factors. The modulation of CBF parameters seen here may reflect the requirement to deliver more metabolic substrates to active neural tissue to support the increased energy metabolism during task performance, although the lack of the linear dose–response that was seen with regards the fat/energy metabolism measures (for which the 3RDA elicited greater modulation) with respect to the NIRS measures argues against this. Rather, the increased hemodynamic response may well be driven by direct modulation of the neurovascular coupling of local blood flow to activity. In line with this, the cardiovascular/vasodilatory properties of several micronutrient components of the interventions here, including vitamin C [24, 25], vitamin B_9 [28] and CoQ10 [32], have previously been attributed to their roles in the synthesis of nitric oxide, the ubiquitous signalling molecule that mediates both peripheral vasodilation and neurovascular coupling [3, 4]. The results here certainly find support from those previous studies that demonstrated improved peripheral vasodilation (as assessed by flow mediated dilatation), following single doses of vitamins B_9, C and E [20–23]. Naturally, the question arises as to why the CBF effects were greater in the treatment containing lower levels of water soluble vitamins. The obvious answer is that the 1RDA treatment also contained CoQ10, which is intricately intertwined with the working of the vitamins with respect to mitochondrial function [15], and which may also exert an independent effect in terms of NO synthesis [32]. Supplementation with CoQ10 has been shown to consistently engender improvements in peripheral endothelial function and other cardiovascular parameters [32], which would be expected to co-vary with modified brain vasodilation. Having said this, the dose administered here was comparatively small; 4.5 mg as opposed to 150 mg + in most of the previous cardiovascular studies. This suggests that the doses administered in the cardiovascular studies are unnecessarily large, or that co-administration with vitamins relevant to CoQ10 function engenders a synergistic effect. Either way, reference to the nutritional parameter data showed that the 1RDA + Q10 group had significantly greater plasma levels of CoQ10 than the other treatment groups after 56 days supplementation, suggesting that this dose was adequate to augment the levels of CoQ10 that were being synthesised endogenously by individuals during the supplementation period.

It is also noteworthy that single doses of multivitamin/minerals have previously been shown to modulate regional brain activity during a task measuring focussed attention as measured with functional magnetic resonance spectroscopy (fMRI) [58], and cerebro-electrical activity during an attention task as measured by electroencephalography (EEG) [59].

It is also worth noting that, in this instance, visual inspection of the data in Fig. 4 shows that the pattern of concentration change in haemoglobin concentrations was for a gradual increase during the absorption period following all treatments. However, this pattern represents concentrations simply returning to approximately zero over this period i.e. reverting to the resting baseline values. We surmise that the initial reductions in haemoglobin concentrations immediately after the treatments reflect the break in 'quiet' sitting and the consumption of the treatment capsules plus water at this point. Given that all of the reported significant effects of treatment are directly in comparison to placebo, and that these are seen only during task completion, it seems unlikely that any underlying pattern of gradual modulation during the absorption period could have influenced the results reported here.

In terms of cognitive function, there was no interpretable evidence of modulated performance. Whilst a single measure evinced an isolated statistical difference, there was no evidence of similar effects from any other measure, so it seems likely this was just a chance finding. The lack of cognitive effects may be attributable to several factors; this was a comparatively small study with less than 30 participants per group (as opposed to over 100 per group in previous cognitive studies showing benefits of multivitamins/minerals [37, 38]; the participants were fitted with restrictive head gear and a face mask, potentially introducing physical or psychological noise into the data; and the cognitive outcomes did not have a baseline that could be used as a covariate, greatly reducing the sensitivity of the assessment.

With regards the nutritional parameters, Vitamin D was raised following 56 days supplementation with both multivitamin interventions, and plasma levels of CoQ10 were significantly higher in the 1RDA + Q10 group on Day 56 (although this did not represent a significant increase on the ANCOVA, possibly due to a trend towards higher pre-treatment levels in this group on Day 1). Homocysteine levels were also reduced by both treatments. This is of particular interest as this potentially neurotoxic amino acid, levels of which correlate positively with cardiovascular disease, age-associated cognitive decline and dementia [34], can be seen as a marker of low endogenous levels of a number of B vitamins. The mean pre-treatment homocysteine levels in this study were ~11.5 μmol/L on Day 1, a figure that is close to the 11.7 μmol/L reported as the average in the UK's Low Income Diet and Nutrition Survey [57]. The cut-off point in homocysteine levels associated with greater cardiovascular disease risk is typically taken as 12 μmol/L. Some 35 % of the current study's sample exceeded this cut-off. These figures, and the fact that supplementation with simple multi-vitamins significantly reduced homocysteine levels in a dose-related manner (to 10.5 and 9.5 μmol/L respectively for the 1RDA + Q10 and 3RDA treatments), suggest strongly that the cohort here, who were not selected on the basis of any nutritional parameters, did not have optimal, or even adequate, nutritional status as a group at the study outset. Similarly, pre-treatment vitamin D levels in the cohort of ~20–25 mg/L would be regarded as insufficient by some established cut-off parameters, suggesting that a dose of 200 IU is adequate to rectify this insufficiency.

With regards the limitations of the study, the most obvious is that one of the working hypotheses here was that the treatments might have a greater effect on CBF parameters and metabolism during the more difficult tasks. The individual tasks impacted on CBF parameters and metabolism depending on their cognitive demands, but the effects of the micronutrients were seen as main effects or interaction effects of treatment, with no task interactions. In hindsight a more comprehensive assessment of simple resting metabolism would have been informative. Having said this, the study provides a very useful starting point for future studies looking at the metabolic effects of micronutrients, and in particular it demonstrates that ICa is a sensitive measure of the somatic metabolic effects of brain activity. A second limitation of the study was the inability of the NIRS equipment utilised here to measure quantitative changes over time. This makes the absence of acute effects on Day 56 difficult to interpret, but again, suggests that research using the more recently introduced quantitative NIRS systems, which can be used to measure changes over time, would be informative.

Conclusions

In summary, the results of the current study suggest that simple supplementation with micronutrients, many of which are implicated in fat oxidation, mitochondrial metabolism and vasodilation, can increase fat oxidation, total somatic energy expenditure and cerebral blood-flow during task performance following a single dose, and increase energy expenditure following 8 weeks supplementation. These results suggest several conclusions. The first is that single doses of multi-vitamins/minerals are capable of modulating metabolic parameters, and that, furthermore, a single dose of multi-vitamins/minerals with added CoQ10 can increase the CBF response to task performance in the frontal cortex, thereby increasing the delivery of metabolic substrates to active neural tissue. Given that the higher 3RDA dose of water soluble vitamins failed to elicit significant modulation of oxygenated and total-haemoglobin these results suggest that the dosage of CoQ10 (4.5 mg) administered here was sufficient to act either additively or synergistically with the co-administered vitamins/minerals in terms of promoting cerebral vasodilation. Second, the results suggest that multivitamin/mineral supplementation over a longer period of time (in this case 56 days) is capable of significantly increasing overall energy metabolism/expenditure. Given that there was no interaction between task demands and treatment related effects, it is possible that these effects could also be seen at rest, and likely that they would be evident during physical exercise. These possibilities deserve further research attention.

Finally, the logical conclusion that can be garnered from the results here is that, if it is possible to beneficially modulate core physiological processes such as energy metabolism and cerebral blood-flow by simply administering vitamins and other micronutrients to healthy members of the population, then it must be the case that the nutritional status of the sample, and by implication the general population, is inadequate. This suggestion is supported by the comparatively high pre-treatment levels of homocysteine seen across the cohort here. If it is the case that our results reflect wide-spread nutritional insufficiency, and given the challenge that shifting the general population's dietary patterns poses, then, in the absence of a healthy diet, supplementation with vitamins and other micronutrients may prove a useful method of recharging nutritional status for a section of the population.

Additional file

Additional file 1: Figure S1. Exploratory analysis of the effects of differing task demands on ratings of mental fatigue/difficulty and all physiological variables, irrespective of treatment. **Table S1.** Mean scores (+SEM) averaged across Day 1 and Day 56 from the exploratory analysis of the effects of differing task demands on ratings of mental fatigue/difficulty and all physiological variables, irrespective of treatment. **Table S2.** Means (+SEM) of ICa data obtained during the 5 min pre-task resting period, the control tapping task and 5 task periods on Day 1 and Day 56. **Table S3.** Cognitive task performance scores (mean plus SEM) on Day 1 and Day 56. **Table S4.** Subjective difficulty and mental fatigue data (+SEM) from Day 1 and Day 56. (DOC 328 kb)

Abbreviations

BMI: body mass index; BOLD: blood oxygen level dependent; CarbOxi: carbohydrate oxidation; CBF: cerebral blood-flow; CLIA: chemiluminescence immunoassay; CoQ10: coenzyme Q10; Deoxy-Hb: deoxygenated hemoglobin; EDTA: ethylenediaminetetraacetic acid; FatOxi: fat oxidation; HPLC: high-performance liquid chromatography; ICa: indirect calorimetry; LC-MS/MS: liquid chromatography-tandem mass spectrometry; NIRS: near-infrared spectroscopy; Oxy-Hb: oxygenated hemoglobin; RDA: recommended dietary allowances; TotalEnergy: total energy expenditure; Total-Hb: total hemoglobin; VAS: visual analogue scales.

Competing interests

This study was supported financially by Bayer HealthCare – Consumer Care, Basel, Switzerland. Co-authors LB, KW and GB are employees of Bayer Healthcare. Co-authors LB and KW contributed to discussions about the design of the study, GB organized external auditing during the trial and LB, GB and KW reviewed and commented on the manuscript. Bayer HealthCare provided the study interventions labelled according to a computer-generated, double-blind randomisation schedule. The co-authors from the sponsoring organisation did not play any role in data collection, and did not have any input into the analysis or interpretation of the results. Otherwise the authors have no further competing interests to declare.

Authors' contributions

DK, ES, CHR, KW, and GB formulated the research question and designed the study. PJ, SD, AC, FD, BR, and JF carried out the study and contributed to the methods and results sections. GB organised external auditing of the study. PJ, CHR and DK analysed the data. DK co-ordinated the writing of the manuscript, with input from CHR, PJ, SD, AC, FD, BR, and JF. All co-authors reviewed and commented on the final manuscript. All authors read and approved the final manuscript.

Author details

[1]Brain, Performance and Nutrition Research Centre, Northumbria University, Newcastle-upon-Tyne NE1 8ST, UK. [2]Bayer HealthCare – Consumer Care, Peter Merian Strasse 84, P.O. Box 4002, Basel, Switzerland.

References

1. Raichle ME. Two views of brain function. Trends Cogn Sci. 2010;14(4):180–90.
2. Shulman RG, Rothman DL, Behar KL, Hyder F. Energetic basis of brain activity: implications for neuroimaging. Trends Neurosci. 2004;27(8):489–95.
3. Gally JA, Montague PR, Reeke GN, Edelman GM. The No Hypothesis - Possible Effects of a Short-Lived, Rapidly Diffusible Signal in the Development and Function of the Nervous-System. Proc Natl Acad Sci U S A. 1990;87(9):3547–51.
4. Kitaura H, Uozumi N, Tohmi M, Yamazaki M, Sakimura K, Kudoh M, et al. Roles of nitric oxide as a vasodilator in neurovascular coupling of mouse somatosensory cortex. Neurosci Res. 2007;59(2):160–71. doi:10.1016/j.neures.2007.06.1469.
5. Buerk DG, Ances BM, Greenberg JH, Detre JA. Temporal dynamics of brain tissue nitric oxide during functional forepaw stimulation in rats. Neuroimage. 2003;18(1):1–9. doi:10.1006/nimg.2002.1314.
6. Seematter G, Guenat E, Schneiter P, Cayeux C, Jequier E, Tappy L. Effects of mental stress on insulin-mediated glucose metabolism and energy expenditure in lean and obese women. Am J Physiol Endocrinol Metab. 2000;279(4):E799–805.
7. Katayose Y, Tasaki M, Ogata H, Nakata Y, Tokuyama K, Satoh M. Metabolic rate and fuel utilization during sleep assessed by whole-body indirect calorimetry. Metabolism. 2009;58(7):920–6.
8. Troubat N, Fargeas-Gluck M-A, Tulppo M, Dugué B. The stress of chess players as a model to study the effects of psychological stimuli on physiological responses: an example of substrate oxidation and heart rate variability in man. Eur J Appl Physiol. 2009;105(3):343–9.
9. Haller J. Vitamins and brain function. In: Lieberman HR, Kanarek RB, Prasad C, editors. Nutritional Neuroscience. Boca Raton, FL: CRC Press; 2005. p. 207–33.
10. Huskisson E, Maggini S, Ruf M. The role of vitamins and minerals in energy metabolism and well-being. J Int Med Res. 2007;35(3):277–89.
11. Yuen AW, Sander JW. Impaired mitochondrial energy production: The basis of pharmacoresistance in epilepsy. Med Hypotheses. 2011;77(4):536–40.
12. Kennedy DO. B vitamins and the brain: mechanisms, dose and efficacy – a review. Nutrients. 2016;8:68. doi:10.3390/nu8020068.
13. Depeint F, Bruce WR, Shangari N, Mehta R, O'Brien PJ. Mitochondrial function and toxicity: role of B vitamins on the one-carbon transfer pathways. Chem-Biol Interact. 2006;163(1):113–32.
14. Depeint F, Bruce WR, Shangari N, Mehta R, O'Brien PJ. Mitochondrial function and toxicity: role of the B vitamin family on mitochondrial energy metabolism. Chem-Biol Interact. 2006;163(1):94–112.
15. Dai Y-L, Luk T-H, Yiu K-H, Wang M, Yip P, Lee SW, et al. Reversal of mitochondrial dysfunction by coenzyme Q10 supplement improves endothelial function in patients with ischaemic left ventricular systolic dysfunction: a randomized controlled trial. Atherosclerosis. 2011;216(2):395–401.
16. Li Y, Wang C, Zhu K, Feng R, Sun C. Effects of multivitamin and mineral supplementation on adiposity, energy expenditure and lipid profiles in obese Chinese women. Int J Obes. 2010;34(6):1070–7.
17. Mah E, Matos MD, Kawiecki D, Ballard K, Guo Y, Volek JS, et al. Vitamin C status is related to proinflammatory responses and impaired vascular endothelial function in healthy, college-aged lean and obese men. J Am Diet Assoc. 2011;111(5):737–43.
18. Yiu Y-F, Chan Y-H, Yiu K-H, Siu C-W, Li S-W, Wong L-Y, et al. Vitamin D deficiency is associated with depletion of circulating endothelial progenitor cells and endothelial dysfunction in patients with type 2 diabetes. J Clin Endocrinol Metab. 2011;96(5):E830–5.
19. Kaplon RE, Gano LB, Seals DR. Vascular endothelial function and oxidative stress are related to dietary niacin intake among healthy middle-aged and older adults. J Appl Physiol. 2014;116(2):156–63.
20. Doshi SN, McDowell IFW, Moat SJ, Payne N, Durrant HJ, Lewis MJ, et al. Folic acid improves endothelial function in coronary artery disease via mechanisms largely independent of homocysteine lowering. Circulation. 2002;105(1):22–6.
21. Obad A, Palada I, Valic Z, Ivancev V, Bakovic D, Wisloff U, et al. The effects of acute oral antioxidants on diving-induced alterations in human cardiovascular function. Journal of Physiology-London. 2007;578(3):859–70. doi:10.1113/jphysiol.2006.122218.
22. Katz DL, Nawaz H, Boukhalil J, Giannamore V, Chan W, Ahmadi R, et al. Acute effects of oats and vitamin E on endothelial responses to ingested fat. Am J Prev Med. 2001;20(2):124–9.
23. Title LM, Cummings PM, Giddens K, Nassar BA. Oral glucose loading acutely attenuates endothelium-dependent vasodilation in healthy adults without diabetes: An effect prevented by vitamins C and E. J Am Coll Cardiol. 2000;36(7):2185–91.
24. Traber MG, Stevens JF. Vitamins C and E: beneficial effects from a mechanistic perspective. Free Radic Biol Med. 2011;51(5):1000–13.
25. Ladurner A, Schmitt CA, Schachner D, Atanasov AG, Werner ER, Dirsch VM, et al. Ascorbate stimulates endothelial nitric oxide synthase enzyme activity

by rapid modulation of its phosphorylation status. Free Radic Biol Med. 2012;52(10):2082–90.
26. Ashor AW, Lara J, Mathers JC, Siervo M. Effect of vitamin C on endothelial function in health and disease: A systematic review and meta-analysis of randomised controlled trials. Atherosclerosis. 2014;235(1):9–20.
27. Kwok T, Chook P, Qiao M, Tam L, Poon Y, Ahuja A, et al. Vitamin B-12 supplementation improves arterial function in vegetarians with subnormal vitamin B-12 status. J Nutr Health Aging. 2012;16(6):569–73.
28. Zhang Y, Janssens SP, Wingler K, Schmidt HH, Moens AL. Modulating endothelial nitric oxide synthase: a new cardiovascular therapeutic strategy. Am J Physiol Heart Circ Physiol. 2011;301(3):H634–46.
29. Witham M, Dove F, Sugden J, Doney A, Struthers A. The effect of vitamin D replacement on markers of vascular health in stroke patients–A randomised controlled trial. Nutr Metab Cardiovasc Dis. 2012;22(10):864–70.
30. Sugden J, Davies J, Witham M, Morris A, Struthers A. Vitamin D improves endothelial function in patients with Type 2 diabetes mellitus and low vitamin D levels. Diabet Med. 2008;25(3):320–5.
31. Harris RA, Pedersen-White J, Guo D-H, Stallmann-Jorgensen IS, Keeton D, Huang Y, et al. Vitamin D3 supplementation for 16 weeks improves flow-mediated dilation in overweight African-American adults. Am J Hypertens. 2011;24(5):557–62.
32. Gao L, Mao Q, Cao J, Wang Y, Zhou X, Fan L. Effects of coenzyme Q10 on vascular endothelial function in humans: A meta-analysis of randomized controlled trials. Atherosclerosis. 2012;221(2):311–6.
33. Ruston D, Hoare J, Henderson L, Gregory J, Bates C, Prentice A, et al. National Diet and Nutrition Survey: adults aged 19–64 years. Volume 4: Nutritional Status (anthropometry and blood analytes), blood pressure and physical activity. London: TSO; 2004.
34. Kennedy DO, Haskell CF. Vitamins and cognition: what is the evidence? Drugs. 2011;71(15):1957–71.
35. NEMO Study Group. Effect of a 12-mo micronutrient intervention on learning and memory in well-nourished and marginally nourished school-aged children: 2 parallel, randomized, placebo-controlled studies in Australia and Indonesia. Am J Clin Nutr. 2007;86(4):1082–93.
36. Haskell CF, Scholey AB, Jackson PA, Elliott JM, Defeyter MA, Greer J, et al. Cognitive and mood effects in healthy children during 12 weeks' supplementation with multi-vitamin/minerals. Br J Nutr. 2008;100(5):1086–96. doi:10.1017/s0007114508959213.
37. Kennedy DO, Veasey R, Watson A, Dodd F, Jones E, Maggini S, et al. Effects of high-dose B vitamin complex with vitamin C and minerals on subjective mood and performance in healthy males. Psychopharmacology. 2010;211(1):55–68. doi:10.1007/s00213-010-1870-3.
38. Haskell CF, Robertson B, Jones E, Forster J, Jones R, Wilde A, et al. Effects of a multi-vitamin/mineral supplement on cognitive function and fatigue during extended multi-tasking. Hum Psychopharmacol-Clin Exp. 2010;25(6):448–61. doi:10.1002/hup.1144.
39. Frayn K. Calculation of substrate oxidation rates in vivo from gaseous exchange. J Appl Physiol. 1983;55(2):628–34.
40. Steinbrink J, Villringer A, Kempf F, Haux D, Boden S, Obrig H. Illuminating the BOLD signal: combined fMRI-fNIRS studies. International School on Magnetic Resonance and Brain Function. Italy: Erice; 2005.
41. Chul J, Tak S, Jang KE, Jung J, Jang J. NIRS-SPM: Statistical parametric mapping for near-infrared spectroscopy. Neuroimage. 2009;44(2):428–47. doi:10.1016/j.neuroimage.2008.08.036.
42. Huppert TJ, Hoge RD, Diamond SG, Franceschini MA, Boas DA. A temporal comparison of BOLD, ASL, and NIRS hemodynamic responses to motor stimuli in adult humans. Neuroimage. 2006;29(2):368–82. doi:10.1016/j.neuroimage.2005.08.065.
43. Obrig H, Villringer A. Beyond the visible—imaging the human brain with light. J Cereb Blood Flow Metab. 2003;23(1):1–18.
44. Jackson PA, Reay JL, Scholey AB, Kennedy DO. DHA-rich oil modulates the cerebral haemodynamic response to cognitive tasks in healthy young adults: a near IR spectroscopy pilot study. Br J Nutr. 2011;1(1):1–6.
45. Kennedy DO, Wightman EL, Reay JL, Lietz G, Okello EJ, Wilde A, et al. Effects of resveratrol on cerebral blood flow variables and cognitive performance in humans: a double-blind, placebo-controlled, crossover investigation. Am J Clin Nutr. 2010;91(6):1590–7. doi:10.3945/ajcn.2009.28641.
46. Kennedy DO, Haskell CF. Cerebral blood flow and behavioural effects of caffeine in habitual and non-habitual consumers of caffeine: A Near Infrared Spectroscopy study. Biol Psychol. 2011;86(3):298–306.
47. Wightman EL, Reay JL, Haskell CF, Williamson G, Dew TP, Kennedy DO. Effects of resveratrol alone or in combination with piperine on cerebral blood flow parameters and cognitive performance in human subjects: a randomised, double-blind, placebo-controlled, cross-over investigation. Br J Nutr. 2014;112:203–13.
48. Drummond SPA, Brown GG, Stricker JL, Buxton RB, Wong EC, Gillin JC. Sleep deprivation-induced reduction in cortical functional response to serial subtraction. Neuroreport. 1999;10(18):3745–8.
49. Owen AM, McMillan KM, Laird AR, Bullmore E. N-back working memory paradigm: A meta-analysis of normative functional neuroimaging. Hum Brain Mapp. 2005;25(1):46–59. doi:10.1002/hbm.20131.
50. Adleman NE, Menon V, Blasey CM, White CD, Warsofsky IS, Glover GH, et al. A developmental fMRI study of the Stroop color-word task. Neuroimage. 2002;16(1):61–75.
51. Vanderhasselt M-A, De Raedt R, Baeken C. Dorsolateral prefrontal cortex and Stroop performance: Tackling the lateralization. Psychon Bull Rev. 2009;16(3):609–12.
52. Bond A, Lader M. Use of analog scales in rating subjective feelings. Br J Med Psychol. 1974;47(SEP):211–8.
53. Field A. A bluffer's guide to… sphericity. Brit Psychol Soc. 1998;6:13–22.
54. Gonzalez J, Rumbold P, Stevenson E. Effect of calcium intake on fat oxidation in adults: a meta-analysis of randomized, controlled trials. Obes Rev. 2012;13(10):848–57.
55. Chan She Ping-Delfos W, Soares M. Diet induced thermogenesis, fat oxidation and food intake following sequential meals: influence of calcium and vitamin D. Clin Nutr. 2011;30(3):376–83.
56. Johnston CS, Corte C, Swan PD. Marginal vitamin C status is associated with reduced fat oxidation during submaximal exercise in young adults. Nutr Metab (Lond). 2006;3:35.
57. Melanson E, Sharp T, Schneider J, Donahoo W, Grunwald G, Hill J. Relation between calcium intake and fat oxidation in adult humans. Int J Obes. 2003;27(2):196–203.
58. Scholey A, Bauer I, Neale C, Savage K, Camfield D, White D, et al. Acute Effects of Different Multivitamin Mineral Preparations with and without Guaraná on Mood, Cognitive Performance and Functional Brain Activation. Nutrients. 2013;5(9):3589–604.
59. White DJ, Camfield DA, Maggini S, Pipingas A, Silberstein R, Stough C, et al. The effect of a single dose of multivitamin and mineral combinations with and without guaraná on functional brain activity during a continuous performance task. Nutr Neurosci. 2014.

11

Mice subjected to *aP2-Cre* mediated ablation of microsomal triglyceride transfer protein are resistant to high fat diet induced obesity

Ahmed Bakillah[1,2*] and M. Mahmood Hussain[1,2,3]

Abstract

Background: Microsomal triglyceride transfer protein (MTP) is essential for the assembly of lipoproteins. MTP has been shown on the surface of lipid droplets of adipocytes; however its function in adipose tissue is not well defined. We hypothesized that MTP may play critical role in adipose lipid droplet formation and expansion.

Methods: Plasmids mediated overexpression and siRNA mediated knockdown of *Mttp* gene were performed in 3T3-L1 pre-adipocytes to evaluate the effects of MTP on cell differentiation and triglyceride accumulation. Adipose-specific knockdown of MTP was achieved in mice bybreeding MTP floxed ($Mttp^{fl/fl}$) mice with aP2-Cre recombinase transgenic mice. Adipose-specific MTP deficient ($A\text{-}Mttp^{-/-}$) mice were fed 60 % high-fat diet (HFD), and the effects of MTP knockdown on body weight, body fat composition, plasma and tissues lipid composition, glucose metabolism, lipogenesis and intestinal absorption was studied. Lipids were measured in total fasting plasma and size fractionated plasma using colorimetric assays. Gene expression was investigated by Real-Time quantitative PCR. All data was assessed using t-test, ANOVA.

Results: MTP expression increased during early differentiation in 3T3-L1 cells, and declined later. The increases in MTP expression preceded PPARγ expression. MTP overexpression enhanced lipid droplets formation, and knockdown attenuated cellular lipid accumulation. These studies indicated that MTP positively affects adipogenesis. The ablation of the Mttp gene using aP2-Cre ($A\text{-}Mttp^{-/-}$) in mice resulted in a lean phenotype when fed a HFD. These mice had reduced white adipose tissue compared with wild-type $Mttp^{fl/fl}$ mice. The adipose tissue of $A\text{-}Mttp^{-/-}$ mice had increased number of smaller size adipocytes and less macrophage infiltration. Further, these mice were protected from HFD-induced fatty liver. The $A\text{-}Mttp^{-/-}$ mice had moderate increase in plasma triglyceride, but normal cholesterol, glucose and insulin levels. Gene expression analysis showed that the adipose tissue of the $A\text{-}Mttp^{-/-}$ mice had significantly lower mRNA levels of PPARγ and its downstream targets.

Conclusion: These data suggest that MTP might modulate adipogenesis by influencing PPARγ expression, and play a role in the accretion of lipids to form larger lipid droplets. Thus, agents that inactivate adipose MTP may be useful anti-obesity drugs.

Keywords: Adipose, Lipoproteins, Lipid droplets, Inflammation, Macrophages, Obesity, Microsomal triglyceride transfer protein, High fat diet

* Correspondence: Ahmed.Bakillah@downstate.edu
[1]Department of Cell Biology, SUNY Downstate Medical Center, 450 Clarkson Avenue, Brooklyn, NY 11203, USA
[2]Department of Pediatrics, SUNY Downstate Medical Center, 450 Clarkson Avenue, Brooklyn, NY 11203, USA
Full list of author information is available at the end of the article

Background

The prevalence of obesity has steadily increased over the past three decades both in the United States and Worldwide, and it is associated with many diseases such as diabetes, dyslipidemia, cardiovascular disease and certain types of cancer [1–5]. Adipocytes are highly specialized cells that play an important role in the storage and utilization of fat as an energy source [6, 7]. Their main function is to synthesize and store triglycerides when there are excess calories, and mobilize this fat to other organs when caloric intake is low. Tremendous efforts with a focus on energy metabolism and lipid homeostasis have been made to obtain information about different proteins that contribute to obesity and its related complications [3, 8, 9].

Microsomal triglyceride transfer protein (MTP) assists in the assembly of triglyceride-rich lipoproteins in hepatic, intestinal, cardiac, embryonic yolk sac and glomeruli [10–13]. Besides these cells, MTP activity has been documented in adipocytes [14, 15] and macrophages [16] that do not synthesize lipoproteins. In adipose tissue, the amounts of MTP are ~ 1 % of the liver [14]. Similar low levels are also seen in macrophages suggesting that MTP expression is significantly lower in cells that do not assemble lipoproteins. In macrophages, MTP is involved in the biosynthesis of CD1 proteins that present glycolipid antigens to natural killer T (NKT) cells [12, 15, 16]. In apoB-producing cells, MTP physically interacts with apoB [10, 17, 18], whereas in macrophages it interacts with CD1d [16]. In both cases, these proteins are loaded with lipids. In case of apoB, several hundred lipid molecules are added to generate lipoproteins. By contrast, one phospholipid molecule is added to the nascent CD1 proteins in the endoplasmic reticulum (ER) [12, 19, 20]. MTP could play a similar role in adipocytes. In fact, a recent study revealed that MTP might play a role in the presentation of endogenous lipid antigens to NKT cells in adipocytes [21].

In mice, two MTP isoforms have been identified [14–16]. These two isoforms differ by two amino acids at the N-terminus and show no differences in their lipid transfer activity. MTP B is the major isoform in adipocytes [14, 15]. In enterocytes, hepatocytes and macrophages, MTP A is mainly present in the ER [16, 22, 23]. By contrast, MTP B has been suggested to be mainly present in the Golgi of non-differentiated 3T3-L1 cells [14, 15]. After differentiation, MTP was also seen on the surface of small lipid droplets [14]. Thus, there are significant differences about the subcellular localization of MTP in adipocytes as opposed to enterocytes and hepatocytes. The present study was designed to investigate potential role of MTP in adipocyte differentiation and lipid droplet formation. We hypothesized that adipose tissue MTP might participate in lipid droplet expansion by assisting in the fusion process of smaller lipid droplets and increasing their size. To test this, we used preadipocytes, 3T3-L1, and ablated the *Mttp* gene by breeding *Mttp*-floxed mice (*Mttp*$^{fl/fl}$) with *aP2-Cre* mice. Our studies demonstrate, for the first time, that MTP contributes to the biogenesis of larger lipid droplets in the adipose tissue.

Methods

Cell culture and induction of differentiation of 3T3-L1 pre-adipocytes

Extensive information has been obtained using cell culture models such as 3T3-L1 cells to study adipocyte differentiation [8, 24]. Culture and differentiation of 3T3-L1 preadipocytes were performed as described in previous studies [25–27]. Briefly, 3T3-L1 cells, kindly provided by Dr. Brasaemle of the Rutgers University, were seeded at 2×10^5/well of 6-well plates and cultured in DMEM medium supplemented with 10 % FBS, 30 μM biotin, 20 mM of glutamine, 1U/ml of penicillin/streptomycin. After confluence was reached, cell differentiation was induced by culturing in DMEM containing 1 μM insulin, 1 μM dexamethasone, and 0.5 mM of 3-isobutyl-1-methylxanthine (IBMX). After 48 h, induction media was removed and replaced with DMEM containing 10 % FBS, 1 μM insulin, 20 mM of glutamine and 1U/ml of penicillin/streptomycin, and renewed every 2 days. Lipid droplets in differentiated adipocytes (day 6 to day 10) were identified under microscope and after Oil Red O staining. In subsequent experiments, MTP inhibitors (MTPi), kindly provided by Dr. David Gordon of Bristol-Myers Squibb, were added to the media after cell induction. Fresh doses of MTPi were renewed every 2 days (D0-D10).

Animals and diets

Transgenic mice expressing Cre recombinase under the control of rat *aP2* promoter (Tg (Fabp4-cre)1Rev or *aP2-Cre* mice) were purchased from The Jackson Laboratory. In these mice, the expression of Cre was driven by the adipocyte protein 2 (aP2)-fatty acid binding protein 4 (FABP4) promoter. The C57/BL6J mice containing the floxed MTP allele *Mttp*$^{fl/fl(\text{exon}5,6)}$ [28] were bred with *aP2-Cre* mice to generate *aP2-Cre*$^{+}$/*Mttp*$^{fl/fl(\text{exon}5,6)}$ mice, thereafter referred to as *A-Mttp*$^{-/-}$ mice. Due to the deletion of exons 5 and 6 these mice are deficient in both the A and B MTP isoforms that arise due to alternate splicing of the exon 1 [15, 16]. Age and sex matched eight-weeks old female and male wild type (WT) *Mttp*$^{fl/fl(\text{exon}5,6)}$ and *A-Mttp*$^{-/-}$ mice were fed a high fat diet (Rodent Diet with 60 % kcal% fat., catalog #D12492, Research Diets, Inc., New Brunswick-NJ) for 15 and 24 weeks. All studies were approved by the Institutional Animal Care and

Use Committee of State University of New York Downstate Medical Center.

Measurements of plasma lipids and transaminases (ALT/AST)

Total cholesterol and triglyceride (Thermo-Fisher Scientific), free cholesterol and free fatty acids (Wako Chemicals), and glycerol (Sigma) levels were measured in the plasma and tissues using commercial kits. Glycerol levels were subtracted from triglyceride levels. Plasma lipoproteins were separated by gel filtration (flow rate of 0.2 ml/min) using a superpose-6-column, and 200-μl fractions were collected. Fractions were used to measure cholesterol and triglycerides. To measure plasma transaminases, 2–5 μl of plasma from $Mttp^{fl/fl}$ and $A\text{-}Mttp^{-/-}$ mice were used for aspartate aminotransferase (AST) and alanine aminotransferase (ALT) assays using specific kits from BioTron Diagnostics (Hemet, CA) according to the manufacturer's guidelines.

Determination of MTP activity

Cells and small pieces (100 mg) of white adipose, liver and proximal intestine (~1 cm) were homogenized in low salt buffer (1 mM Tris–HCl, pH 7.6, 1 mM EGTA, and 1 mM $MgCl_2$) and centrifuged, and supernatants were used for protein determination and the MTP assay [29, 30] using a commercial kit (Chylos, Inc.).

Cell transfection with plasmid DNA or siRNA

Plasmids pCMV6 (empty vector), pRcMTP expressing full length MTP, and MTP-FLAG have been previously described [30, 31]. SiRNA directed against mouse MTP (Sc-45276, MTP-siRNA) and nonspecific control siRNA (Sc-37007, Control) were obtained from Santa Cruz Biotechnology. Adipocytes were transfected in suspension as described by Kilroy et al. [32]. Briefly, 3T3-L1 cells were induced for 2 days and partially differentiated until day 4. At day 4, cells were trypsinized, resuspended in DMEM-high glucose containing 10 % FBS and gently centrifuged. Cell pellets were resuspended in 200 μl of OptiMEM (Gibco, Life Technologies) and incubated at 37 °C with equal volume of lipofectamine complexes (RNAiMax; Life Technologies) containing siRNA (100 nM) or plasmid DNA (1 μg/ml). After 20 min incubation, the mixtures were plated in 6-well plates and incubated at 37 °C in 95 % O_2 and 5 % CO_2 atmosphere. After 24 h-72 h post-transfection, cells were harvested to measure protein, lipid, and MTP activity.

Tissue histology and immunohistochemistry

Samples of white adipose tissue and liver were fixed by overnight immersion in 4 % paraformaldehyde in 0.1 M phosphate buffer, dehydrated in 30 % sucrose, embedded in M1 cryo-preservation media at −20 °C, and stored at −80 °C. To assess adipose tissue and liver morphology, sections (5–7 μm) were placed on Tissue-Tack (Polysciences) slides and stained with hematoxylin and eosin (H & E) [33, 34]. To assess fat cell number, white adipose tissue was incubated with 1 mg/ml of type I collagenase (Worthington Biochemical) for 1 h at 37 °C in Krebs buffer solution containing 1 % BSA and 200 nM adenosine and 50 μg/ml glucose and filtered through cheesecloth [35, 36]. Methylene blue was added to cell suspension and an aliquot was counted under microscope using a hemocytometer. To determine adipocyte size and number, stained samples were photographed using spot digital camera interfaced to an Olympus microscope and a Macintosh computer. Images of 100 adipocytes from each fat sample were converted into a binary format with public domain National Institutes of Health Image Program (Image J Basics, version 1.38). The data were averaged per section and then per animal. Other sections were used for immunostaining of adipose tissue macrophages using specific marker F4/80 [37–39]. Briefly, sections were incubated for 2 h at 25 °C with anti-mouse F4/80 primary antibody (1:100 in 1 % BSA/PBS; Abcam #ab6640) followed by the application of HRP-conjugated rabbit anti-goat IgG secondary antibody (Thermo Scientific, Pierce antibodies #31433). Histochemical reactions were performed using the EnVision™ Doublestain System (Dako) and counterstained with Hematoxylin. Sections were examined with a light microscopy, and digital images were taken to evaluate macrophage contents.

Oil Red O staining and measurement of cellular lipid accumulation

3T3-L1 cells were cultured and differentiated on sterile cover slips placed in 6-well plates. Differentiated cells were washed with PBS, fixed in 4 % formaldehyde solution for 15 min, washed with PBS and then stained for 1 h with Oil Red-O (Sigma-Aldrich Chemical) stain solution 0.5 % in isopropanol:water (60:40) filtered through a 0.2 μm filter. After several washes with water, pictures of samples were taken using a microscope [40]. Adipocyte differentiation was monitored by measuring cellular lipid accumulation using the same Oil Red-O staining method [40, 41]. Briefly, differentiated cells on 6-well plates were fixed with 10 % ice-cold formalin in PBS for 2 h and stained by adding Oil Red-O working solution for 10 min. Cells were thoroughly rinsed with water and the red dye retained by cells was eluted by adding isopropanol for 1 h. Aliquots were transferred to wells of a 96-well plate and optical density was measured at 500 nm wavelength. Blank samples (with no cells) were treated similarly and background values were subtracted. In subsequent experiments when the Oil Red

O stain is not used, cells were washed with PBS, lysed by polytron homogenizer in low salt buffer (1 mm Tris–HCl, pH 7.6, 1 mm EGTA, and 1 mm $MgCl_2$), and cellular lipids content were measured using commercial kits (Waco Chemicals; Thermo-Fisher Scientific).

Glucose and insulin tolerance tests

Whole body plasma glucose and insulin levels were measured after overnight fasting. For glucose tolerance test (GTT), mice were fasted overnight (~16 h) with full access of water, and injected intraperitoneally with 2 mg of glucose in saline solution/g of body weight. Blood glucose levels were measured at the indicated time points before and after glucose challenge. For insulin tolerance test (ITT), mice were fasted for 4 h prior to intraperitoneal injection of insulin (Novolin R, Novo Nordisk, Denmark; 0.75 U/kg body weight). Tail vein blood glucose was collected at the indicated times using a One-Touch basic glucometer (Bayer).

Fatty acid oxidation and de novo lipogenesis

For fatty acid oxidation measurements, 100 mg of tissues (sliced in small pieces) were incubated with [^{14}C]-Oleic acid (0.3 μCi) for 2 h at 37 °C, and the radiolabeled CO_2 was captured with filter paper soaked with phenylethylamine [42]. Radiolabel was quantified using a scintillation counter (Beckman LS 6000TA). Oxidation was presented per mg of protein. For de novo lipogenesis, 50 mg of tissue slices were placed in 1 ml Krebs-Ringer-Bicarbonate Hepes buffer containing 4 % (wt/vol) fatty acid-free BSA fraction V (Sigma), 3 mM glucose, 0.5 mM acetate and 1 μCi [1-^{14}C]-Acetate (56 mCi/mmol) at 37 °C for 2 h under 95 % O_2 – 5 % CO_2. The reaction was terminated by the addition of 40 μl 10 N H_2SO_4, and radiolabel incorporation into lipids was determined [43].

Postprandial triglyceridemic response and intestinal triglyceride secretion

Mice were fasted for 4 h prior to the fat challenge. To study postprandial response, mice were administered with 200 μl olive oil (via oral gavage). Plasma triglyceride concentration was determined at baseline (time 0) and at 2 h and 4 h. To assess intestinal triglyceride production, fasted mice (4 h) were injected with P407 (i.p.) to block lipase activity in the circulation. After 30 min, mice were orally administered with 200 μl olive oil, and plasma triglycerides were measured before and at 2 h and 4 h post fat load challenge.

Gene expression and qPCR

Total RNA from cells and tissues were isolated using TRIzol™ (Invitrogen). The purity of RNA was assessed by the A_{260}/A_{280} ratio. RNA preparations with A_{260}/A_{280} ratios more than 1.7 were used for cDNA synthesis. The first strand cDNA was synthesized using Omniscript RT (Qiagen) kit. Each reaction of quantitative PCR was carried out in a volume of 20 μl, consisting of 5 μl of cDNA sample (1:100 dilution of the first strand cDNA sample) and 15 μl of PCR master mix solution containing 1× PCR buffer (qPCR™ core kit for SYBR Green I, Eurogentec). The PCR was carried out by incubating the reaction mixture first for 10 min at 95 °C followed by 40 cycles of 15 s incubation at 95 °C and 1 min at 60 °C in an ABI 7000 SDS PCR machine. Data were analyzed using $\Delta\Delta C_T$ method, according to the manufacturer's instructions using the following equation: $2^{[CT\ \text{house keeping gene}\ -\ CT\ \text{target gene}]}$. Final results are presented as arbitrary units that were normalized to 18S mRNA.

Statistical analyses

Data are presented as mean ± S.D. Statistical significance ($p < 0.05$) was determined using Student's t test or one-way analysis of variance (GraphPad Prism 5).

Results

MTP activity changes during differentiation of 3T3-L1 cells do not correlate with adipogenesis

To understand how adipose tissue MTP might play a role in adipogenesis, we used 3T3-L1 cells that are routinely used to study adipocyte differentiation and adipogenesis. We studied changes in MTP activity during differentiation of these cells into adipocytes. Cells were treated with inducers of differentiation for 2 days and then cultured for 10 days. MTP activity increased in control cells (DMSO only) by ~ 50-100 % until day 4, stayed high till day 6, and then progressively declined until day 10 (Fig. 1a). We then measured changes in cellular lipids and droplet formation during this period. Intracellular cholesterol and fatty acids did not change significantly (data not shown). However, cellular triglyceride levels increased progressively during differentiation of control cells (Fig. 1b). Oil Red O staining also suggested higher amounts of lipids in differentiated cells (data not shown). These data suggest that MTP activity transiently increases during early differentiation and then declines later.

Lipid transfer activity is not required for triglyceride accumulation during differentiation of 3T3 L1 cells

Next, we sought to test the hypothesis that chemical inhibition of MTP lipid transfer activity in adipocytes would interfere with cell differentiation and/or adipogenesis. To test this, we treated 3T3-L1 cells with a potent pharmacological MTPi during differentiation. Supplementation of MTPi significantly reduced MTP activity during differentiation (Fig. 1a). MTPi did not affect intracellular triglyceride accumulation (Fig. 1b). No intracellular accumulation of cholesterol or free fatty acids was observed after MTPi treatment (Data not shown). These studies indicate that inhibition of MTP

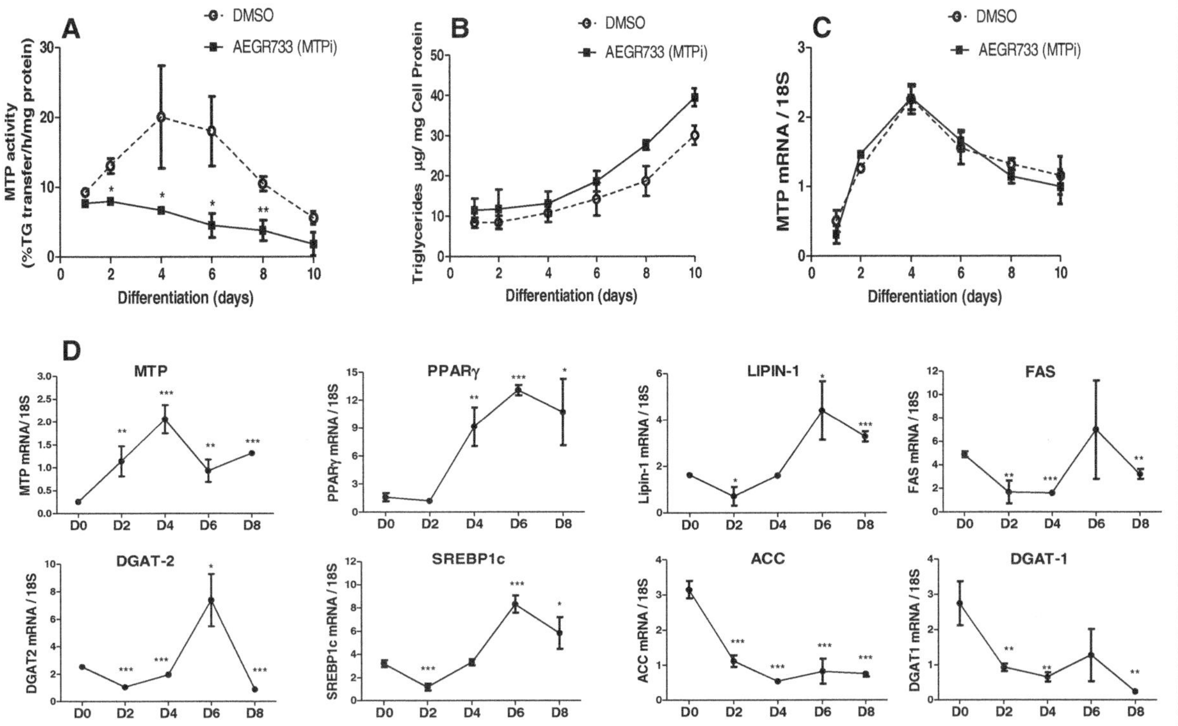

Fig. 1 Changes in MTP activity and lipid droplets formation during differentiation of 3T3-L1 preadipocytes into mature adipocytes. Cells were first induced with INS/DEX/IBMX for 2 days and then differentiated in 10 % FBS media containing insulin for 10 days. Following induction, differentiated cells were treated either with DMSO (*dotted lines*) or in the presence of 1 μM of MTPi [Lomitapide (AEGR-733); *solid lines*] and collected every 2 days until adipocytes full maturation (*D10*). Cells were homogenized and assayed for MTP activity (**a**), triglycerides content (**b**), and Mttp gene expression (**c**). In subsequent experiment, expression profiles of different genes were analyzed on different days (**d**). Relative mRNA levels were measured by qPCR and normalized to 18S RNA. Results are mean of triplicates ± SD. Significance is represented by *, $p < 0.05$ and **, $p < 0.01$. Data are representative of two independent experiments

lipid transfer activity does not affect triglyceride accumulation during differentiation of 3T3-L1 cells.

MTP expression is induced early during differentiation

To understand reasons for increased MTP activity during early differentiation, we measured MTP mRNA levels (Fig. 1c). MTP mRNA levels increased by two-fold, early during differentiation, and peaked at day four. In addition, MTPi had no effect on *Mttp* gene expression. The increases in MTP mRNA preceded increases in other adipocyte genes such as PPARγ, Lipin and Fas (Fig. 1d). Thus, MTP appears to be an early response gene induced during preadipocyte differentiation.

Knockdown and overexpression of MTP reduces and increases cellular triglyceride during differentiation of 3T3-L1 preadipocytes

To address whether early induction of MTP is important for preadipocyte differentiation, we reduced and increased MTP expression using siRNA and expression plasmids, respectively. siMTP significantly reduced MTP expression (Fig. 2a) and activity (Fig. 2b) by 82 % to 80 %, respectively, without altering total cell protein (Fig. 2c). Reductions in MTP were associated with 47 % decrease in lipid accumulation after Oil Red O staining (Fig. 2d). We also transfected differentiated 3T3-L1 cells with two different plasmids expressing human MTP cDNA resulting in significant increases in MTP activity (Fig. 2e) and cellular triglyceride after 48 h of transfection (Fig. 2f) with no effect on cellular protein levels (Fig. 2g). These studies indicated that changes in MTP levels directly correlate with changes in cellular triglyceride levels.

AP2-Cre-mediated ablation of the Mttp gene in the adipose tissue results in lean mouse phenotype

To study the role of MTP, we crossed $Mttp^{fl/fl}$ mice with *aP2-Cre* mice and generated *A-Mttp*$^{-/-}$ mice deficient in both the MTP isoforms. *A-Mttp*$^{-/-}$ mice had 50 % to 80 % less MTP mRNA levels in the adipose tissue compared to controls (Fig. 3a). However, MTP mRNA levels were not different in the liver and intestine of WT and *A-Mttp*$^{-/-}$ mice. Next, we measured MTP activity in

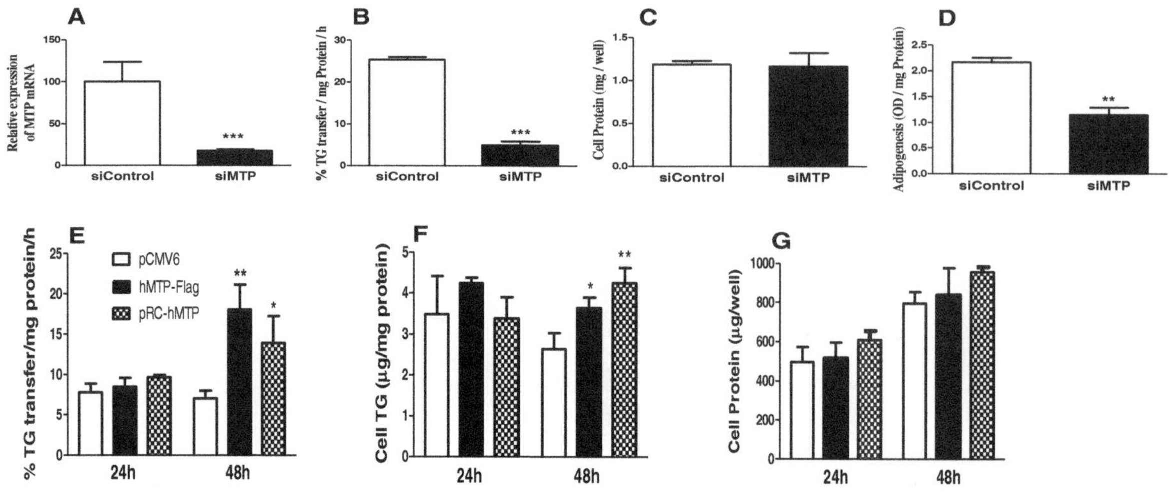

Fig. 2 RNAi-based MTP gene silencing and MTP overexpression in differentiated 3T3-L1 cells modulates adipogenesis. Cells were partially differentiated in DMEM containing 10 % FBS until D4. On day 4, cells were transfected with scrambled siRNA or siRNA for MTP and replated. Three days postransfection (day 7), cells were collected and assessed for MTP expression (**a**), MTP activity (**b**), total cell protein content (**c**), and lipid droplet formation (**d**). In a different experiment, cells were transfected using lipofectamine reagent and 1 µg of cDNA of empty vector (*pCMV6*) or human MTP (hMTP-Flag or pRC-hMTP) for 24 h and 48 h transfection. Cells were harvested in homogenization buffer to determine MTP activity (**e**), intracellular triglycerides (**f**), and total cell protein (**g**). Results shown are representative of two independent experiments. Values are mean of triplicates ± SD. *, $p < 0.05$ and **, $p < 0.01$

different tissues (Fig. 3b). AP2 is known to be expressed in the brain and spleen (rich in macrophages), but MTP activity was not reduced in these tissues in *A-Mttp*$^{-/-}$ mice compared to WT (Fig. 3b). However, > 50 % reduction in MTP activity was found in inguinal fat pads. Thus, *A-Mttp*$^{-/-}$ mice have significant MTP deficiency in the adipose tissue.

On a chow diet, *Mttp*$^{fl/fl}$ and *A-Mttp*$^{-/-}$ mice gained similar weight (not shown). Next, we studied the development of obesity in *Mttp*$^{fl/fl}$ and *A-Mttp*$^{-/-}$ mice. *A-Mttp*$^{-/-}$ mice appeared smaller in size and were leaner mainly due to significant absence of abdominal fat compared with control mice (Fig. 3c). Consistent with this, weights of inguinal and gonadal fat depots were ~50 % less in *A-Mttp*$^{-/-}$ mice (Fig. 3d). Female and male *Mttp*$^{fl/fl}$ control mice gained significant weight when fed HFD (Fig. 3e-f), but *A-Mttp*$^{-/-}$ mice did not despite similar amounts of food consumption and body temperature (Fig. 3g-h). These studies indicated that *A-Mttp*$^{-/-}$ mice are resistant to diet-induced obesity and accumulate less fat in their adipose tissue.

We then characterized the adipose tissue in these mice. *A-Mttp*$^{-/-}$ mice had smaller size adipocytes (Fig. 4a). Adipocytes isolated from inguinal and gonadal fat of *A-Mttp*$^{-/-}$ mice had an average size of 2585 μm^2 as compared to 4500 μm^2 of the control mice (Fig. 4b). Further, the number of adipocytes obtained from *A-Mttp*$^{-/-}$ inguinal fat was greater than the number obtained from WT mice (Fig. 4c). Thus, MTP deficiency increases the number of smaller adipocytes.

Increased macrophage infiltration in the adipose tissue is a common feature of obesity. Hence, we assessed whether adipose tissue macrophage infiltration was altered in *A-Mttp*$^{-/-}$ mice. WT adipose tissue showed significant staining for macrophage specific-antigen F4/80 after 15 weeks and 24 weeks of HFD feeding (Fig. 4d). In contrast, the adipose tissue from the *A-Mttp*$^{-/-}$ mice stained less for the macrophage antigen. These studies indicated that the adipose tissue of the *A-Mttp*$^{-/-}$ mice had less macrophage infiltration.

In short, these studies suggested that *aP2-Cre* mediated MTP ablation results in a leaner phenotype secondary to the presence of greater number of smaller size adipocytes with less number of macrophages in HFD fed mice.

Ablation of MTP reduces PPARγ expression and its downstream target genes

To understand reasons for the lean phenotype, we measured mRNA levels of different genes that play a role in adipocyte differentiation (Fig. 5). As anticipated, MTP mRNA levels were significantly lower in the adipose tissue of *A-Mttp*$^{-/-}$ mice. We also found significant reductions in PPARγ, FABP4, FAS and lipins; other mRNA levels did not differ in two groups. This suggests that MTP deficiency might reduce PPARγ expression resulting in reduced differentiation and lower fat storage in the adipose tissue.

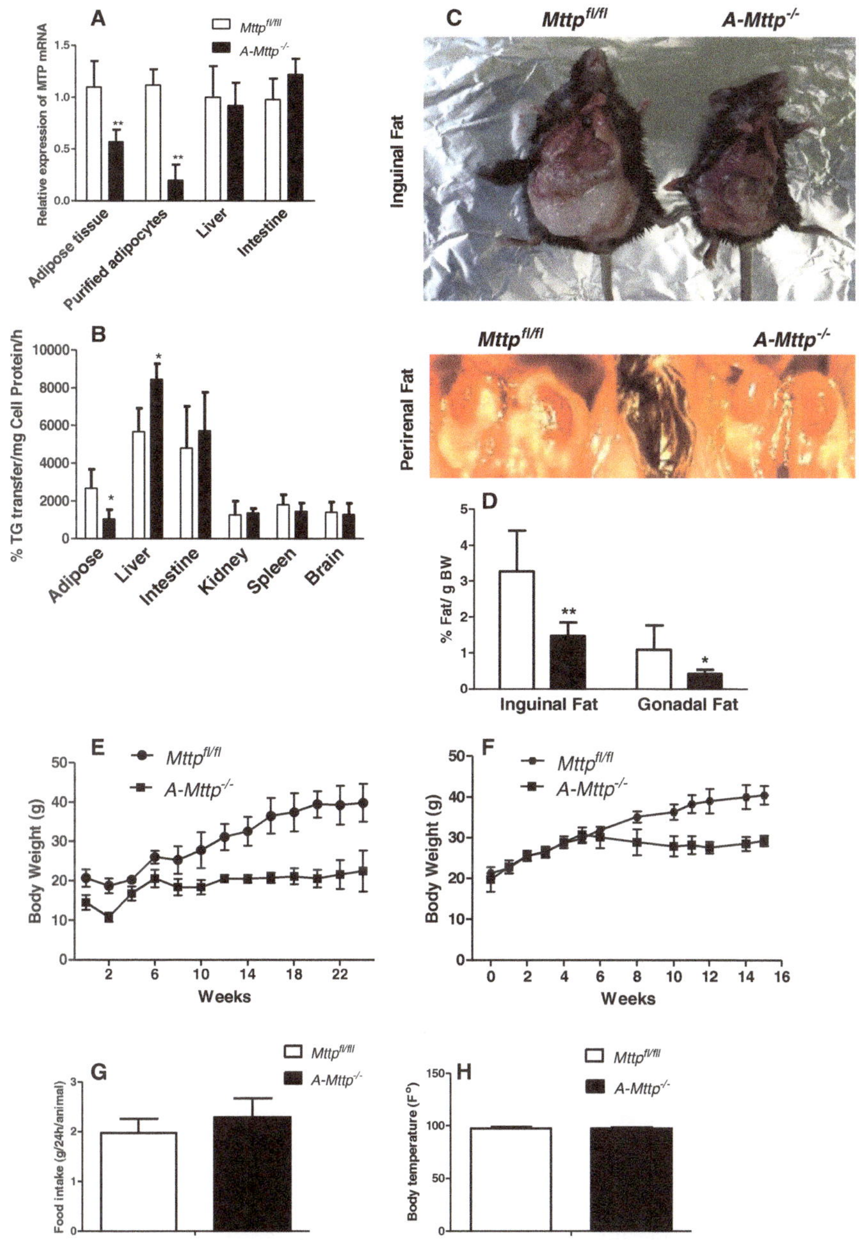

Fig. 3 *aP2-Cre* mediated MTP ablation reduces body weight and lipid accumulation in the adipose tissue. $Mttp^{fl/fl}$ and $A\text{-}Mttp^{-/-}$ mice were fed a HFD for 24 weeks. At the end of the experiment, control and $A\text{-}Mttp^{-/-}$ mice were sacrificed and organs collected for MTP mRNA measurement (**a**) and MTP activity (**b**). Representative pictures of visceral fat pads and animal morphology are shown in panel (**c**). Percentages of fat in different adipose tissues by gram body weight are plotted in (**d**). Body weights were recorded every 2 weeks during the experiment using female (**e**) and male mice (**f**). Data for food consumption and body temperature are represented in (**g & h**). Values are mean of 5–7 mice ± SD from each group. *, $p < 0.05$; **, $p < 0.01$; and ***, $p < 0.001$

We then measured F4/80, a macrophage marker, and found to be significantly less in $A\text{-}Mttp^{-/-}$ mice indicating less macrophage infiltration (Fig. 5). These studies indicate that $A\text{-}Mttp^{-/-}$ mice were deficient in adipocyte differentiation and macrophage markers.

$A\text{-}Mttp^{-/-}$ mice show normal blood glucose and insulin levels

Next, we concentrated on glucose metabolism in $A\text{-}Mttp^{-/-}$ mice. Fasting glucose and insulin levels did not differ significantly between WT and $A\text{-}Mttp^{-/-}$ mice (Fig. 6a-b). In addition, there were no significant

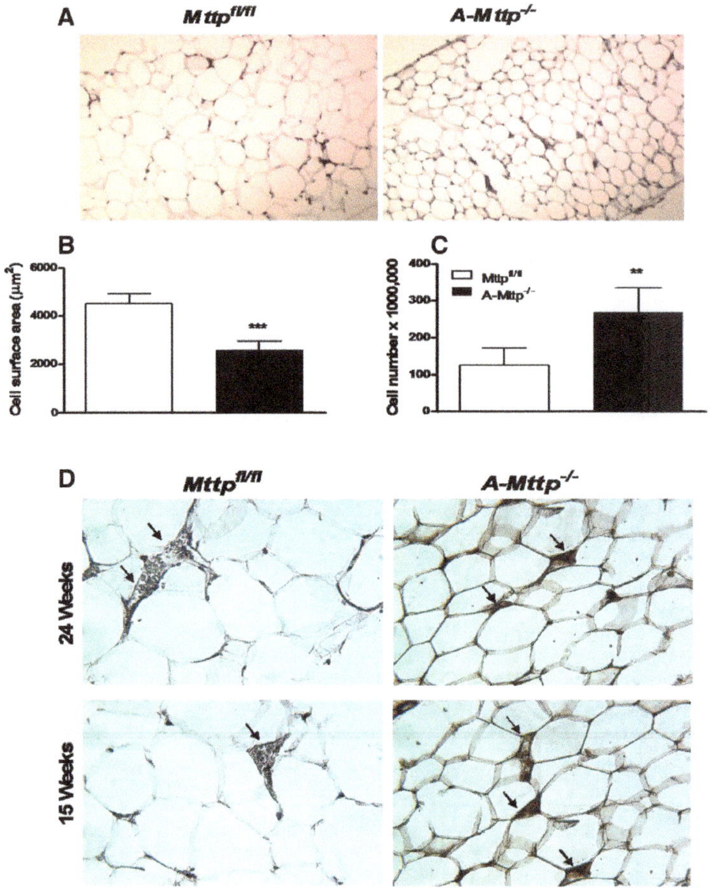

Fig. 4 *A-Mttp*$^{-/-}$ mice have smaller size adipocytes and less macrophages infiltration in the adipose tissue. Control *Mttp*$^{fl/fl}$ and *A-Mttp*$^{-/-}$ mice were fed 60 % high fat diet for 15 and 24 weeks. At the end of experiment, adipose tissue was collected for H & E staining (**a**), adipocyte size determination (**b**), and cell number quantification (**c**). Adipose tissue was isolated after collagenase treatment and counted under microscope. Immunohistochemical detection of cells expressing the macrophage-specific antigen F4/80 (arrows) was performed on paraffin section of adipose tissue in control *Mttp*$^{fl/fl}$ and *A-Mttp*$^{-/-}$ mice (**d**)

differences in the plasma glucose levels between WT and *A-Mttp*$^{-/-}$ mice following glucose and insulin tolerance tests (Fig. 6c-d). Thus, *A-Mttp*$^{-/-}$ mice showed no abnormality in glucose metabolism.

A-Mttp$^{-/-}$ mice have higher levels of plasma triglyceride and normal levels of cholesterol

HFD significantly increased fasting plasma triglyceride by week 18 and this increase continued until week 24 in *A-Mttp*$^{-/-}$ mice (Fig. 7a). Fasting plasma cholesterol (Fig. 7b) and free fatty acids levels were similar in these two groups (not shown). Gel filtration analysis of fasting plasma pools from the two groups revealed an increase of triglyceride in the VLDL/LDL fraction of *A-Mttp*$^{-/-}$ mice (Fig. 7c) with no significant effect on cholesterol in both VLDL/LDL and HDL fractions (Fig. 7d). These studies suggest that *aP2-Cre* mediated ablation of MTP increases plasma triglyceride-rich lipoproteins.

A-Mttp$^{-/-}$ mice have increased adipose lipogenesis with no effect on β-oxidation

We next studied the rate of *de novo* lipogenesis (DNL) and fatty acid oxidation by measuring incorporation of radiolabeled acetate and release of CO_2, respectively. Adipose tissues from *A-Mttp*$^{-/-}$ mice incorporated significantly higher amounts of acetate in newly synthesized fatty acids as compared to control *Mttp*$^{fl/fl}$ mice (Fig. 8a). In contrast, hepatic DNL was significantly decreased in *A-Mttp*$^{-/-}$ mice as compared to control mice. Fatty acid oxidation in adipose tissue and the liver was unchanged in *A-Mttp*$^{-/-}$ mice as compared to control mice (Fig. 8b). These studies suggest that *aP2-Cre* mediated adipose

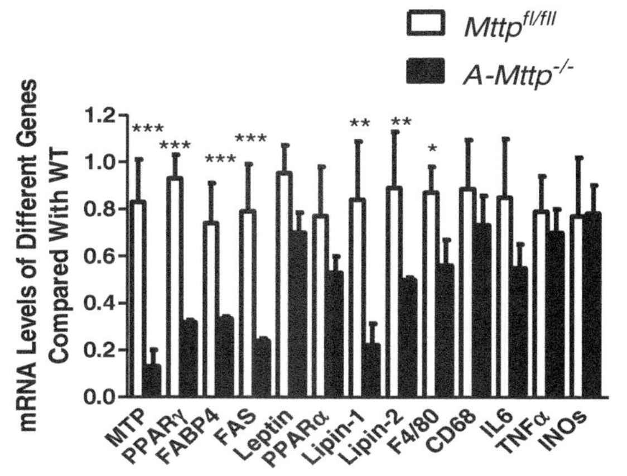

Fig. 5 *aP2-Cre* mediated MTP ablation reduces expression of genes involved in adipogenesis. Gene expression in the adipose tissue of *Mttp*$^{fl/fl}$ and *A-Mttp*$^{-/-}$ mice was quantified by qPCR and levels were normalized to 18S RNA. Mice were fed HFD for 24 weeks. After overnight fasting, animals were sacrificed, adipose tissues collected, and isolated inguinal fat adipocytes were used for total RNA extraction using Trizol reagent. cDNA was synthesized and levels of RNA were determined by qPCR. Data are represented as mean ± SD ($N = 4$). *, $p < 0.05$; **, $p < 0.01$ and ***, $p < 0.001$

MTP deficiency induces DNL in the adipose tissue but not in the liver.

A-Mttp$^{-/-}$ mice have lower intestinal triglyceride secretion after an acute dietary fat challenge

To determine whether postprandial triglyceridemic response was altered in lean *A-Mttp*$^{-/-}$ mice compared to *Mttp*$^{fl/fl}$ control mice, we measured plasma triglycerides concentration before and after 2 h and 4 h post olive oil bolus. At baseline, levels of plasma triglycerides were higher in lean *A-Mttp*$^{-/-}$ mice compared to *Mttp*$^{fl/fl}$ control mice as expected, and remained high at 2 h then dropped at 4 h post olive oil gavage (Fig. 9a). Percent increase in plasma triglyceride in the two groups were similar at 2 h (*A-Mttp*$^{-/-}$: 109.20 % ± 8.33 % vs. *Mttp*$^{fl/fl}$: 128.75 % ± 14.25 %; $p = 0.1109$) but decreased significantly after 4 h in *A-Mttp*$^{-/-}$ mice (*A-Mttp*$^{-/-}$: 51.76 % ± 8.45 % vs. *Mttp*$^{fl/fl}$: 98.16 % ± 18.71 %; $p = 0.0173$). To determine whether these changes are secondary to lipoprotein production, we repeated the same experiment in mice injected with P407 to inhibit lipoprotein lipase. As expected, basal plasma triglycerides were higher in *A-Mttp*$^{-/-}$ mice compared to *Mttp*$^{fl/fl}$ control mice at baseline. *A-Mttp*$^{-/-}$ mice had significantly lower amounts of triglycerides at 2 h and 4 h as compared to *Mttp*$^{fl/fl}$ control mice (Fig. 9b). The percent increase in plasma circulating triglycerides was significantly lower at 2 h (*A-Mttp*$^{-/-}$: 2084.79 % ± 139.75 % vs. *Mttp*$^{fl/fl}$: 6326.82 % ± 705.39 %; $p < 0.0001$) and 4 h (*A-Mttp*$^{-/-}$: 2019.56 % ± 284.54 % vs. *Mttp*$^{fl/fl}$: 5388.21 % ± 940.34 %; $p = 0.0004$) in *A-Mttp*$^{-/-}$ mice. We calculated the areas under the curves (AUC) and found that in the absence of P407, *Mttp*$^{fl/fl}$ control mice had lower AUC value ($AUC_{0-4} = 276.09 \pm 39.46$) as compared to *A-Mttp*$^{-/-}$ mice ($AUC_{0-4} = 464.13 \pm 49.50$). In contrast, after blocking the lipase activity in the circulation, the AUC value of *Mttp*$^{fl/fl}$ control mice was elevated ($AUC_{0-4} = 11587.17 \pm 1001.84$) compared to *A-Mttp*$^{-/-}$ mice ($AUC_{0-4} = 8397.79 \pm$

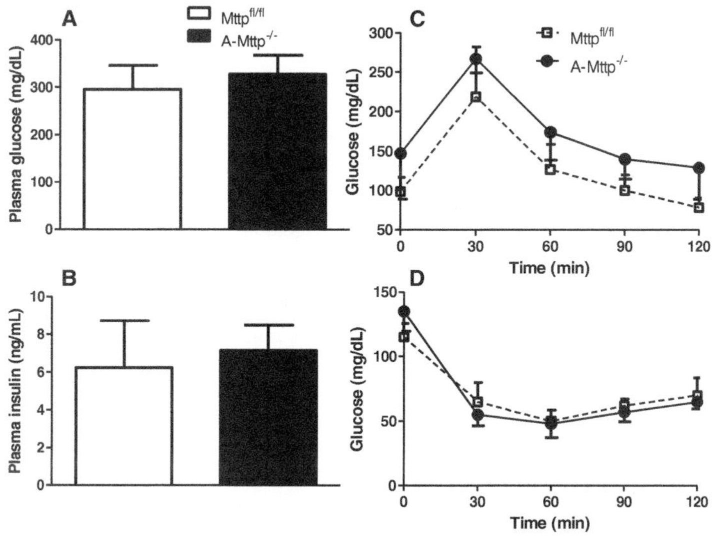

Fig. 6 *A-Mttp*$^{-/-}$ mice show normal glucose metabolism. Plasma glucose (**a**) and insulin (**b**) levels were measured in overnight fasted HFD fed animals. Glucose (**c**) and Insulin (**d**) tolerance tests were performed in *Mttp*$^{fl/fl}$ and *A-Mttp*$^{-/-}$ mice fed a HFD for 15 weeks. For glucose tolerance test, mice were fasted overnight (16 h) before glucose challenge (2 mg/kg body weight, i.p.). For insulin sensitivity test, mice were fasted for 4 h before ip insulin injection. Tail blood was collected before injection and after each 30 min up to 2 h. Data are represented as mean ± SD ($N = 4$). *, $p < 0.05$

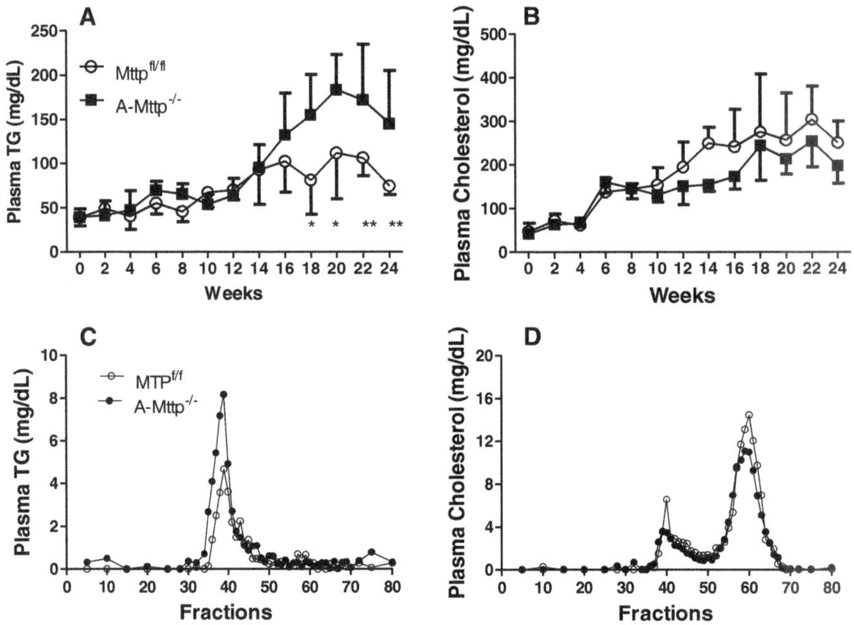

Fig. 7 Increased plasma triglycerides in *A-Mttp*$^{-/-}$ mice. Control *Mttp*$^{fl/fl}$ and *A-Mttp*$^{-/-}$ mice were fed 60 % HFD for 24 weeks. Blood samples were collected every 2 weeks and assessed for plasma triglycerides (**a**) and cholesterol (**b**) levels. Data are represented as mean ($N = 5$). Statistical differences between the two groups were obtained by one-way ANOVA analysis. ***, $p < 0.05$; **, $p < 0.01$ and ***, $p < 0.001$. Fasting plasma pool was obtained from five mice in each group and applied to FPLC column for lipoprotein separation. Triglycerides (**c**) and cholesterol (**d**) were measured in each fraction

723.81). These studies indicate that *A-Mttp*$^{-/-}$ mice absorb lower amounts of triglyceride suggesting that enhanced plasma triglycerides in lean *A-Mttp*$^{-/-}$ mice under HFD is not due to alterations in triglycerides secretion by intestine.

A-Mttp$^{-/-}$ mice are protected from HFD induced hepatic steatosis

As expected, livers of WT mice fed a HFD were pale indicating fat accumulation (Fig. 10a). In contrast, livers of *A-Mttp*$^{-/-}$ mice appeared normal. Consistent with this observation, livers from the WT mice weighed more than those from the *A-Mttp*$^{-/-}$ mice (Fig. 10b). Hematoxylin and eosin staining showed more vacuoles in the livers of WT mice (Fig. 10c). Further, lipid analysis revealed that livers obtained from WT mice had higher amounts of triglyceride compared with *A-Mttp*$^{-/-}$ mice (Fig. 10d). In contrast to the liver, accretions of triglyceride in the intestine were not different in these two groups. Hepatic cholesterol and free fatty acid contents were not different in these two groups of mice (Fig. 10e-f). Plasma transaminases are used to ascertain liver damage and function (34, 42). Interestingly, protection from hepatic steatosis in the *A-Mttp*$^{-/-}$ mice was associated with significant decrease of plasma AST and ALT (Fig. 10g-h). These studies showed that *A-Mttp*$^{-/-}$ mice exhibit less hepatosteatosis compared to WT mice on a HFD.

Discussion

In this study, we asked whether MTP plays a role in adipocyte biology. Our studies showed that MTP is induced early during differentiation of 3T3-L1 cells before the induction of PPARγ, a critical transcription factor for the differentiation of adipocytes. Further, we show for the first time that *A-Mttp*$^{-/-}$ mice are lean and resistant to diet-induced obesity when fed a high fat diet. The adipose tissue in these mice contained more number of smaller size adipocytes and had less macrophage infiltration. These studies suggest that MTP plays a role in determining size, number, and triglyceride content of adipocyte most likely by assisting in greater accretion of triglyceride and enhancing the size of adipocyte in high fat fed mice.

MTP expression changes during differentiation of 3T3-L1 preadipocytes into adipocytes. Undifferentiated 3T3-L1 preadipocytes had lipid transfer activity suggesting for the presence of pre-existing pools of MTP. *Mttp* gene was induced early during differentiation that preceded transcriptional regulation of key markers of differentiation such as PPARγ consistent with other studies [21]. Mechanistic studies by other investigators

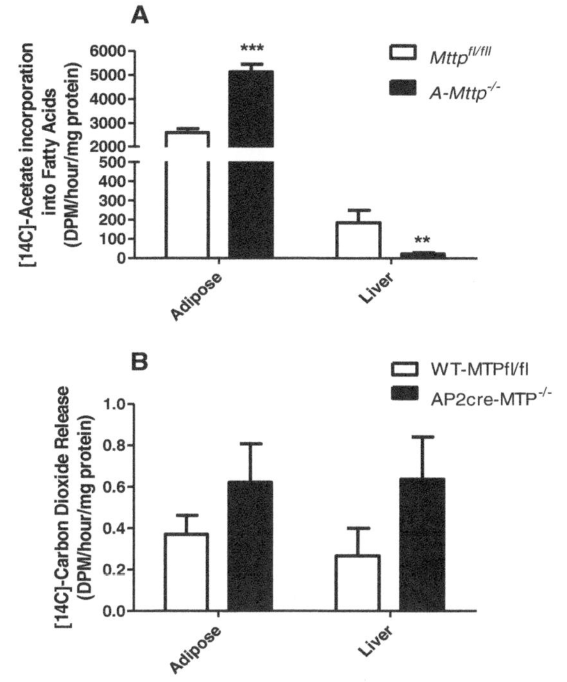

Fig. 8 *A-Mttp*$^{-/-}$ mice show enhanced adipose lipogenesis and reduced hepatic lipogenesis without any effect on β-oxidation. *De novo* lipogenesis (**a**) and Fatty acid β-oxidation (**b**) were performed in Control *Mttp*$^{fl/fl}$ and *A-Mttp*$^{-/-}$ mice after a 15 weeks HFD treatment. Adipose tissue and liver were collected from overnight fasted mice (~15 h) and rate of lipogenesis and fatty oxidation were measured. *, $p < 0.05$; **, $p < 0.01$ and ***, $p < 0.001$; and data are mean ± SD ($N = 4$)

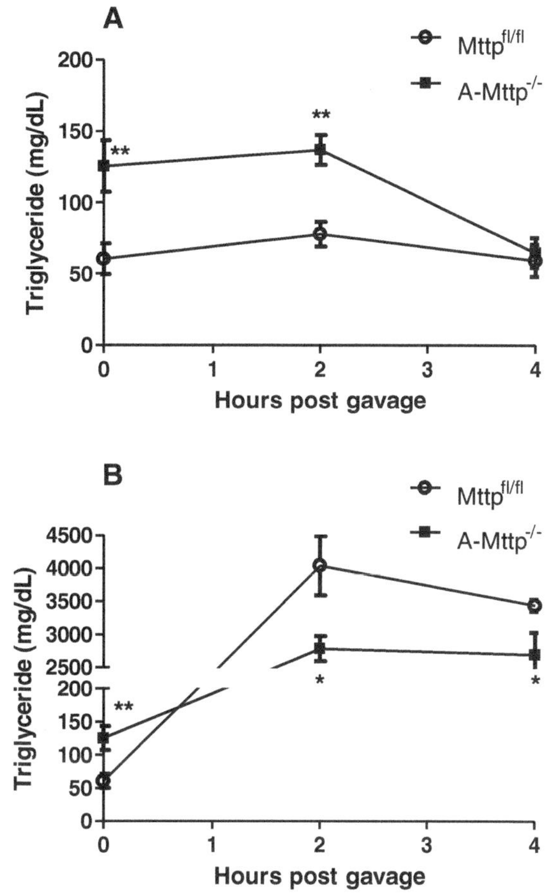

Fig. 9 *A-Mttp*$^{-/-}$ mice absorb fewer lipids after a fat tolerance test. Control *Mttp*$^{fl/fl}$ and *A-Mttp*$^{-/-}$ mice were fed 60 % HFD for 15 weeks. (**a**) Postprandial triglyceridemic response was measured in control *Mttp*$^{fl/fl}$ and *A-Mttp*$^{-/-}$ mice. Plasma triglyceride concentration was measured at baseline (4 h fasting) and at 2 h and 4 h following oral challenge of 200 μl olive oil. Data are represented as mean ± SD ($N = 3$). (**b**) After 4 h fasting, mice were injected with P407 in the intraperitoneal cavity to block lipase activity in the circulation. After 30 min, mice were administered 200 μl olive oil (oral gavage) and plasma triglycerides were measured before and at 2 h and 4 h post oil bolus. Data are represented as mean ± SD ($N = 4$). *, $p < 0.05$ and **, $p < 0.01$

have suggested that the induction of MTP in early differentiation might be due to the binding of C/EBPβ and C/EBPδ transcription factors to a specific region in the exon 1 of the *MTTP* gene [21]. Thus, MTP is an early response gene involved in adipocyte differentiation.

Our study shows that early expression of MTP during differentiation is critical for optimal lipid storage. Molecular approaches using siRNA-mediated knockdown of MTP and overexpression of MTP demonstrated that changes in MTP affect intracellular lipid storage and droplet formation (Fig. 2). Overexpression of MTP increases the accretion of triglyceride in differentiated 3T3-L1 cells, whereas knockdown reduces their accumulation. These data are consistent with those of Rakhshandehroo et al. [21] who reported that MTP depletion (stable shRNA knockdown of MTP) does not influence the differentiation of 3T3-L1 preadipocytes, as assessed by FABP4 expression. These data suggest that MTP plays a role in promoting adipogenesis and determines the amounts of lipids accreted by differentiated adipocytes. In contrast to these studies, MTPi did not interfere with triglyceride accumulation. Thus MTP protein, not its lipid transfer activity, might play a role during adipocyte differentiation by assisting in the fusion of small droplets into larger droplets.

Surprisingly, treatment of cells with MTPi did not affect adipocyte differentiation and adipogenesis (Fig. 1). This is consistent with a recent finding demonstrating that the lipid transfer activity of MTP is neither critical for the mobilization of fatty acids from adipocytes nor for cell differentiation as assessed by the number of intracellular lipid droplets [44]. Our findings are also in agreement with another study dealing with the CD1d-mediated lipid self-antigen presentation in adipocytes

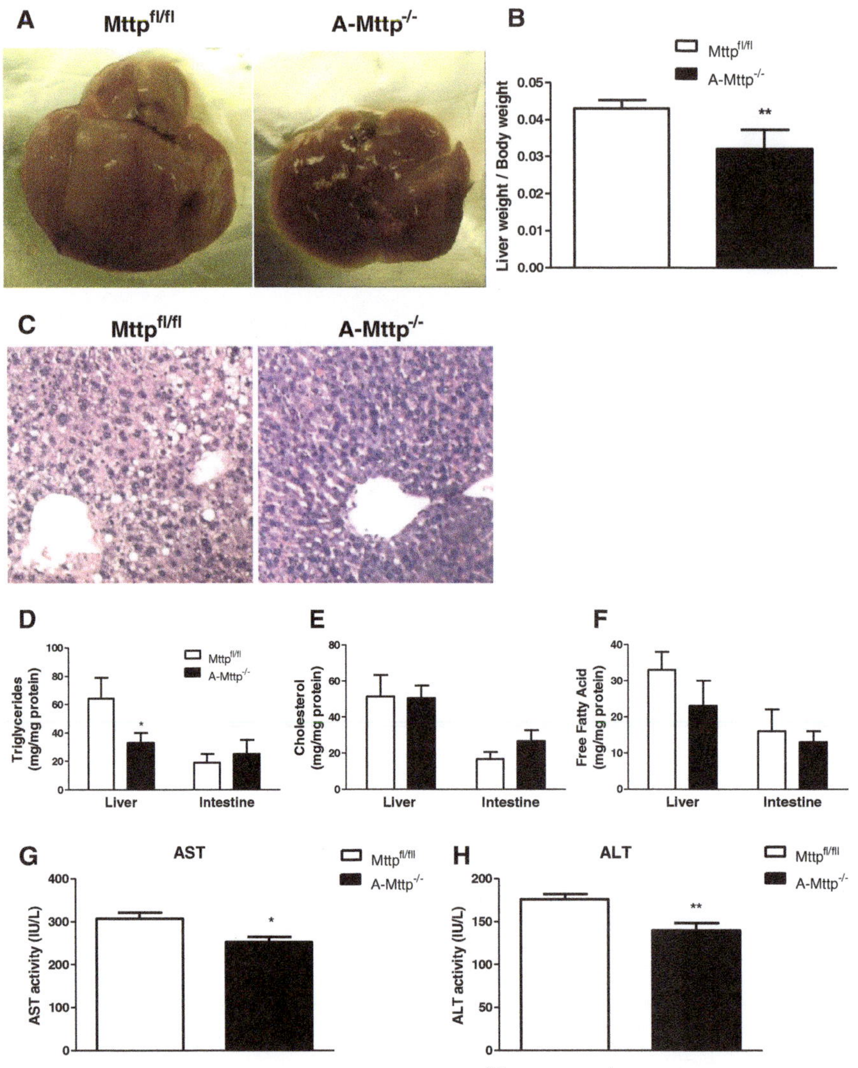

Fig. 10 *A-Mttp*$^{-/-}$ mice are protected from HFD induced fatty liver. Control *Mttp*$^{fl/fl}$ and *A-Mttp*$^{-/-}$ mice were fed 60 % HFD for 24 weeks. At the end of an experiment, overnight fasted animals were scarified and livers were collected (**a**), weighed (**b**) and fixed in paraffin and stored at −80 °C until use for H & E staining (**c**). Liver and intestine were homogenized and analyzed for triglyceride (**d**), cholesterol (**e**), and free fatty acid (**f**). Transaminase activities were measured on fasting plasma from five mice (**g & h**). ***, $p < 0.05$; **, $p < 0.01$ and ***, $p < 0.001$; and data are mean ± SD ($N = 7$)

showing that treatment of adipocytes with BMS-212122 at high dose (13 μM) for 24 h did not influence the differentiation potential of the preadipocytes [21]. Taken together, our results and observations from others suggest that MTP protein, but not its lipid transfer activity, may play a pivotal role in adipocyte lipid droplet formation and maturation. It is possible that MTP protein might be involved in the fusion of smaller lipid droplets to from larger droplets during adipocyte differentiation.

Understanding the precise function of MTP during adipocyte differentiation is critical in delineating its role in larger lipid droplet formation. MTP might participate in lipid accumulation via other mechanisms. Analysis of the expression pattern of relevant genes controlling adipocyte differentiation and adipogenesis identified that the induction of PPARγ was reduced in *A-Mttp*$^{-/-}$ mice and the maximum expression of MTP occurs prior to the maximum expression of PPARγ in 3T3-L1 cells. PPARγ is known to activate nearly all of the genes required for the formation of larger droplets, including FABP4 which is required for the transport of free fatty acids, and perilipin which is on the surface of mature lipid droplets. Thus, it is possible that reduced expression of PPARγ might be one mechanism contributing to reduced fat accumulation in MTP deficient adipocytes.

Another possibility is that MTP might interact with lipid droplet associated proteins, such as perilipin, and assist in droplet formation and/or stabilization of larger droplets. Immunohistochemical studies have shown that MTP surrounds small lipid droplets in 3T3-L1 adipocytes as well as in white and brown fat in mice [14, 15]. MTP has been found to physically interact with apoB in lipoprotein producing cells [10, 18]. Therefore, it is possible that MTP may interact with another protein(s) in adipocytes and act as a chaperone. For example, MTP could interact with one or more structural proteins on the surface of lipid droplets such as perilipin, adipophilin, TIP47, OXPAT/MLDP, and S3-12 [45–47], and assist in droplet fusion process by providing close access to triglycerides for smaller droplets, promoting lipid droplet growth and expansion. In fact, Love et al. demonstrated that MTP and perilipin-2 were associated with the same isolated lipid droplets from adipocytes, but they concluded that these proteins do not interact with each other [44]. More studies are needed to explore possible physical interactions between MTP and lipid droplet-coating proteins.

Our finding of lean phenotype associated with reduced fat pad weight and lack of an increase of adipocyte size in HFD fed *A-Mttp*$^{-/-}$ mice hints at a role of MTP in modulating adipocytes differentiation. Interestingly, reduction of fat mass in *A-Mttp*$^{-/-}$ mice was accompanied with increased number of smaller adipocytes (Figs. 3 and 4). Thus, it is likely that basal cellular levels of triglycerides are unaffected by MTP. However, increased accumulation of fat during diet-induced obesity may require MTP. This is supported by the observation that *A-Mttp*$^{-/-}$ mice on chow do not show any difference in body weight compared to controls.

Metabolic defects that alter adipose tissue fat accumulation are frequently associated with changes in glucose homeostasis. Unexpectedly, plasma glucose and insulin levels in the fasted HFD-fed animals did not differ between the *A-Mttp*$^{-/-}$ and WT mice. Further, despite marked reduction in body weight and adiposity, *A-Mttp*$^{-/-}$ mice did not exhibit any changes in whole-body glucose homeostasis and insulin sensitivity (Fig. 6). The reasons for no effect on glucose metabolism are not clear.

Using 1-^{14}C acetate as substrate, we observed that the adipose tissue and liver accounted for about 93 % and 7 % of DNL in WT mice. This in agreement with previous studies suggesting that adipose tissue DNL is a major site of lipogenesis in rodents [48–50]. In *A-Mttp*$^{-/-}$ mice, we found that DNL was significantly higher in the adipose tissue and was lower in the liver (Fig. 8). This is in good agreement with study showing significant elevation of adipose DNL in ob/ob mice in comparison with control mice [51]. Numerous studies indicated that enhanced adipose DNL, in contrast to the liver DNL, may be beneficial for whole-body metabolism. For example, liver-specific deletion of SCAP, a protein required for the cleavage of SREBP1c to its active form, has been shown to reduce hepatic lipogenesis and enhance adipose DNL by four-fold resulting in improved glucose homeostasis [52]. In another study, ablation of adipocyte/macrophage lipid chaperones *aP2* (FABP4) and *mal1* (FABP5) increased adipose DNL which protected mice from diet-induced obesity, fatty liver disease and insulin resistance [53]. The ob/ob mice that were rendered LPL deficient in adipose tissue also demonstrated increased DNL and diminished weight and fat mass [54]. Similar to these models, our finding suggest that increased DNL in adipocytes is associated with lean phenotype. The fact that DNL is upregulated while β-oxidation is decreased indicates for a possible higher rate of intracellular lipolysis and secretion of fatty acid from adipose tissue of lean *A-Mttp*$^{-/-}$ mice. More experiments are needed to illustrate potential impact of relevant lipases on the release of fatty acids and glycerol by adipose tissues.

Accumulation of adipose tissue macrophages has been well described in obese conditions in mice and humans [37, 55–57]. This process of macrophage infiltration is associated with adipocyte hypertrophy and metabolic dysfunction. In addition to the smaller size of adipocytes, we observed lesser macrophage infiltration in the adipose tissue of *A-Mttp*$^{-/-}$ mice (Fig. 4). Thus, MTP deficiency in *A-Mttp*$^{-/-}$ mice protects adipose tissue from HFD-induced macrophage infiltration.

Our studies also provide evidence that MTP deficiency in *A-Mttp*$^{-/-}$ mice modulates the expression of genes involved in adipocyte differentiation and lipid formation and storage. The expression of PPARγ and its downstream targets FAS, lipins and FABP4 were significantly reduced (55 %-75 %) in the adipose tissue of *A-Mttp*$^{-/-}$ mice. PPARγ is essential for adipocyte viability and regulates a number of genes involved in lipid uptake and storage [35, 58, 59]. Down regulation of PPARγ could provide protection from HFD induced inflammation and obesity [60–65]. It remains unclear how ablation of MTP in *A-Mttp*$^{-/-}$ mice impacts transcription of PPARγ and protects mice from HFD induced inflammation and obesity.

Although *A-Mttp*$^{-/-}$ mice consumed similar amounts of food, they did not accumulate fat in the adipose tissue and the liver compared with WT mice. Further, we did not find differences in rectal temperatures of these mice (Fig. 3). Thus, the physiologic reason for the leaner phenotype in these mice is not clear. It is possible that the *A-Mttp*$^{-/-}$ mice oxidize fat more efficiently and have higher metabolic rates than the WT mice. Future studies may identify the physiologic reasons for the leaner phenotype in *A-Mttp*$^{-/-}$ mice when challenged with a high fat diet.

A-Mttp$^{-/-}$ mice have higher plasma triglyceride (Fig. 7). These mice showed modest increase (~28 %) in hepatic MTP activity but mRNA levels did not change (Fig. 3). Thus, changes in hepatic MTP do not explain increases in plasma triglyceride in *A-Mttp*$^{-/-}$ mice. Further, intestinal lipoprotein assembly and secretion was reduced, not increased. Therefore, increased lipoprotein production is unlikely to be responsible for higher plasma triglyceride in these mice. In addition, postprandial secretion of triglycerides in response to acute fat challenge was significantly decreased in *A-Mttp*$^{-/-}$ mice after a 4 h oral fat tolerance test. These mice absorbed lesser amounts of fat than control. Further, we observed reduced lipid absorption in lipase inhibited *A-Mttp*$^{-/-}$ mice (Fig. 9). It is plausible that triglyceride elevations might be secondary to reduced amounts of lipoprotein lipase. This is based on several studies that show that adipocyte lipoprotein lipase is reduced in high fat fed animals. In fact, in recent study [66], mice lacking prostaglandin E receptor subtype 4 (EP4) manifested disrupted lipid metabolism associated with a 69 % reduction in weight gain and fat mass following HFD feeding. Plasma triglycerides in these mice were elevated by 245 %. Authors found that these mice had reduced lipoprotein lipase activity, the key enzyme responsible for trafficking of plasma triglycerides into peripheral tissues.

The data obtained with 3T3-L1 cells and high fat fed *A-Mttp*$^{-/-}$ mice appear to provide different results. If we assume that 3T3 cell culture studies are comparable to chow fed mice, then results in cells and mice are the same. Both cells and mice do not show any significant difference in fat accumulation during MTP deficiency. We only saw the effect of MTP deficiency when mice were fed a high fat diet. We did not do similar fat challenge studies in cells. Thus, adipose MTP might be more critical when cells are exposed to high lipids.

We are aware that adipocytes express two MTP isoforms, A and B. Dr. Swift's laboratory was the first to establish the presence of MTP in adipose tissue as well as in the pre-adipocyte cell line, 3T3-L1 [14]. The group has previously generated anti-MTP antibodies from a 19-amino acid peptide representing residues 843 through 861 in the MTP protein. In a recent report [44], they were able to monitor mRNA and protein levels of both the MTP isoforms in adipocytes. They showed that adipocytes predominantly (>95 %) express MTP B isoform and demonstrated that MTP protein expression increased linearly over the 8-day period of differentiation, but mRNA levels for MTP-A and MTP-B did not change significantly. In another study, MTP-B mRNA levels increased significantly within the first two days of differentiation and decreased slightly afterwards [21]. This later report is in good agreement with our observation for the decline of MTP expression at late stages of differentiation. Therefore, it is likely that MTP-B is the major isoform in adipocyte. Further, it should be pointed that no functional differences between these two isoforms have been reported. Therefore, expressions of these two different isoforms as determined by mRNA or protein levels do not appear to have any functional consequences.

In this study, we used *aP2-Cre* to ablate the *Mttp* gene. In these mice, MTP expression was greatly diminished in isolated adipocytes (>80 %) and decreased by ~ 50 % in adipose tissue which also includes non-adipocyte cell types. We are aware that *aP2-Cre* is expressed in adipocytes and macrophage. Therefore, the observed effects might be due to the deletion of MTP in both the adipose tissue and macrophages. In our study, we found significant reductions in the adipose tissue MTP but not in the spleen, a tissue rich in macrophages. Thus, it is likely that the observed effects are due to MTP deficiency in the adipose tissues. It is unlikely that reduction in T-cell mediated immune response due to possible deletion of MTP in macrophages could account for the lean phenotype and metabolic changes observed in *A-Mttp*$^{-/-}$ mice for the following reasons: (1) iNKT cell population and CD1d expression is reduced in the adipose tissue of obese mice and humans compared to those of lean subjects [67]; (2) iNKT cell-specific Jα18 knockout mice are obese and exhibit increased adipose tissue inflammation at the early stage of obesity [68]; (3) CD1d-deficient mice fed a high-fat diet show insulin resistance and hepatic steatosis [69–71]. Future studies may dissect the role of MTP in the adipose tissue and macrophages using cell-specific deletion of the gene.

Conclusion

In short, our study provides the first evidence of the role played by MTP in adipocyte differentiation and fat storage in mice. Ablation of the *Mttp* gene using *aP2-Cre* has no effect on glucose homeostasis but it prevents HFD induced hepatosteatosis. We present evidence that MTP protein plays a role in the accumulation of larger lipid droplets in the adipose tissue. We speculate that MTP may (1) activate expression of PPARγ and amplify expression of genes critical for adipocyte maturation and lipid storage, (2) interact with lipid droplet associated proteins, and/or (3) assist in the fusion of smaller lipid droplets. Future investigation of how MTP ablation could repress PPARγ transcriptional activity should provide additional insights into the role of MTP in adipocyte maturation and physiology. It is possible that down regulation of adipose MTP might avoid complications associated with obesity.

Abbreviations
ALT: alanine aminotransferase; AP2: adipocyte protein 2; ApoB: apolipoprotein B; AST: aspartate aminotransferase; CD1: cluster of differentiation 1; DNL: de novo lipogenesis; ER: endoplasmic reticulum; FABP4: fatty acid binding protein 4; FAS: fatty acid synthase; FBS: fetal bovine serum; GTT: glucose tolerance test; HFD: high-fat diet; IBMX: 3-isobutyl-1-methylxanthine; ITT: insulin tolerance test; MTP: Microsomal triglyceride transfer protein; NKT: natural killer T cells; PPARγ: peroxisome proliferator-activated receptor gamma; TG: triglycerides.

Competing interests
The authors declare that they have no competing interests.

Authors' contributions
AB and MMH conceived and designed the experiments. AB conducted the experiments and wrote the paper. AB analyzed the data and performed statistical analysis. MMH involved in critical editing of manuscript. All authors read and approved the final manuscript.

Acknowledgement
This work was supported in part by US National Institutes of Health grants HL-95924 and VA Merit Award (BX001728) to MMH. AB was recipient of a NIH/NHLBI Diversity Supplement Award (HL09524-03S1). Part of this work was presented at the Arteriosclerosis Thrombosis and Vascular Biology/ Peripheral Vascular Disease 2015 Scientific sessions meeting, May 7–9; San Francisco-California, USA.

Author details
[1]Department of Cell Biology, SUNY Downstate Medical Center, 450 Clarkson Avenue, Brooklyn, NY 11203, USA. [2]Department of Pediatrics, SUNY Downstate Medical Center, 450 Clarkson Avenue, Brooklyn, NY 11203, USA. [3]VA New York Harbor Healthcare System, Brooklyn, NY 11209, USA.

References
1. Karpe F, Dickmann JR, Frayn KN. Fatty acids, obesity, and insulin resistance: time for a reevaluation. Diabetes. 2011;60:2441–9.
2. Greenberg AS, Coleman RA, Kraemer FB, McManaman JL, Obin MS, Puri V, et al. The role of lipid droplets in metabolic disease in rodents and humans. J Clin Invest. 2011;121:2102–10.
3. Krahmer N, Farese Jr RV, Walther TC. Balancing the fat: lipid droplets and human disease. EMBO Mol Med. 2013;5:905–15.
4. Wagner M, Samdal Steinskog ES, Wiig H. Adipose tissue macrophages: the inflammatory link between obesity and cancer? Expert Opin Ther Targets. 2015;19:527–38.
5. Lavie CJ, McAuley PA, Church TS, Milani RV, Blair SN. Obesity and cardiovascular diseases: implications regarding fitness, fatness, and severity in the obesity paradox. J Am Coll Cardiol. 2014;63:1345–54.
6. Gesta S, Tseng YH, Kahn CR. Developmental origin of fat: tracking obesity to its source. Cell. 2007;131:242–56.
7. Frayn KN, Tan GD, Karpe F. Adipose tissue: a key target for diabetes pathophysiology and treatment? Horm Metab Res. 2007;39:739–42.
8. Gregoire FM, Smas CM, Sul HS. Understanding adipocyte differentiation. Physiol Rev. 1998;78:783–809.
9. Walther TC, Farese Jr RV. Lipid droplets and cellular lipid metabolism. Annu Rev Biochem. 2012;81:687–714.
10. Hussain MM, Bakillah A. New approaches to target microsomal triglyceride transfer protein. Curr Opin Lipidol. 2008;19:572–8.
11. Bartels ED, Nielsen JM, Hellgren LI, Ploug T, Nielsen LB. Cardiac expression of microsomal triglyceride transfer protein is increased in obesity and serves to attenuate cardiac triglyceride accumulation. PLoS One. 2009;4:e5300.
12. Hussain MM, Rava P, Walsh M, Rana M, Iqbal J. Multiple functions of microsomal triglyceride transfer protein. Nutr Metab (Lond). 2012;9:14.
13. Eresheim C, Plieschnig J, Ivessa NE, Schneider WJ, Hermann M. Expression of microsomal triglyceride transfer protein in lipoprotein-synthesizing tissues of the developing chicken embryo. Biochimie. 2014;101:67–74.
14. Swift LL, Kakkad B, Boone C, Jovanovska A, Jerome WG, Mohler PJ, et al. Microsomal triglyceride transfer protein expression in adipocytes: a new component in fat metabolism. FEBS Lett. 2005;579:3183–9.
15. Mohler PJ, Zhu MY, Blade AM, Ham AJ, Shelness GS, Swift LL. Identification of a novel isoform of microsomal triglyceride transfer protein. J Biol Chem. 2007;282:26981–8.
16. Dougan SK, Salas A, Rava P, Agyemang A, Kaser A, Morrison J, et al. Microsomal triglyceride transfer protein lipidation and control of CD1d on antigen-presenting cells. J Exp Med. 2005;202:529–39.
17. Bradbury P, Mann CJ, Kochl S, Anderson TA, Chester SA, Hancock JM, et al. A common binding site on the microsomal triglyceride transfer protein for apolipoprotein B and protein disulfide isomerase. J Biol Chem. 1999;274:3159–64.
18. Bakillah A, Nayak N, Saxena U, Medford RM, Hussain MM. Decreased secretion of ApoB follows inhibition of ApoB-MTP binding by a novel antagonist. Biochemistry. 2000;39:4892–9.
19. Sagiv Y, Bai L, Wei DG, Agami R, Savage PB, Teyton L, et al. A distal effect of microsomal triglyceride transfer protein deficiency on the lysosomal recycling of CD1d. J Exp Med. 2007;204:921–8.
20. Kaser A, Hava DL, Dougan SK, Chen Z, Zeissig S, Brenner MB, et al. Microsomal triglyceride transfer protein regulates endogenous and exogenous antigen presentation by group 1 CD1 molecules. Eur J Immunol. 2008;38:2351–9.
21. Rakhshandehroo M, Gijzel SM, Siersbaek R, Broekema MF, de Haar C, Schipper HS, et al. CD1d-mediated presentation of endogenous lipid antigens by adipocytes requires microsomal triglyceride transfer protein. J Biol Chem. 2014;289:22128–39.
22. Dougan SK, Rava P, Hussain MM, Blumberg RS. MTP regulated by an alternate promoter is essential for NKT cell development. J Exp Med. 2007;204:533–45.
23. Iqbal J, Hussain MM. Intestinal lipid absorption. Am J Physiol Endocrinol Metab. 2009;296:e1183–94.
24. Prokesch A, Hackl H, Hakim-Weber R, Bornstein SR, Trajanoski Z. Novel insights into adipogenesis from omics data. Curr Med Chem. 2009;16:2952–64.
25. Brasaemle DL, Dolios G, Shapiro L, Wang R. Proteomic analysis of proteins associated with lipid droplets of basal and lipolytically stimulated 3T3-L1 adipocytes. J Biol Chem. 2004;279:46835–42.
26. Scott MA, Nguyen VT, Levi B, James AW. Current methods of adipogenic differentiation of mesenchymal stem cells. Stem Cells Dev. 2011;20:1793–804.
27. Poulos SP, Dodson MV, Hausman GJ. Cell line models for differentiation: preadipocytes and adipocytes. Exp Biol Med (Maywood). 2010;235:1185–93.
28. Chang BH, Liao W, Li L, Nakamuta M, Mack D, Chan L. Liver-specific inactivation of the abetalipoproteinemia gene completely abrogates very low density lipoprotein/low density lipoprotein production in a viable conditional knockout mouse. J Biol Chem. 1999;274:6051–5.
29. Athar H, Iqbal J, Jiang XC, Hussain MM. A simple, rapid, and sensitive fluorescence assay for microsomal triglyceride transfer protein. J Lipid Res. 2004;45:764–72.
30. Rava P, Ojakian GK, Shelness GS, Hussain MM. Phospholipid transfer activity of microsomal triacylglycerol transfer protein is sufficient for the assembly and secretion of apolipoprotein B lipoproteins. J Biol Chem. 2006;281:11019–27.
31. Khatun I, Walsh MT, Hussain MM. Loss of both phospholipid and triglyceride transfer activities of microsomal triglyceride transfer protein in abetalipoproteinemia. J Lipid Res. 2013;54:1541–9.
32. Kilroy G, Burk DH, Floyd ZE. High efficiency lipid-based siRNA transfection of adipocytes in suspension. PLoS One. 2009;4:e6940.
33. Galarraga M, Campion J, Munoz-Barrutia A, Boque N, Moreno H, Martinez JA, et al. Adiposoft: automated software for the analysis of white adipose tissue cellularity in histological sections. J Lipid Res. 2012;53:2791–6.
34. Josekutty J, Iqbal J, Iwawaki T, Kohno K, Hussain MM. Microsomal triglyceride transfer protein inhibition induces endoplasmic reticulum stress and increases gene transcription via Ire1alpha/cJun to enhance plasma ALT/AST. J Biol Chem. 2013;288:14372–83.
35. Sugii S, Olson P, Sears DD, Saberi M, Atkins AR, Barish GD, et al. PPARgamma activation in adipocytes is sufficient for systemic insulin sensitization. Proc Natl Acad Sci U S A. 2009;106:22504–9.
36. Majka SM, Miller HL, Helm KM, Acosta AS, Childs CR, Kong R, et al. Analysis and isolation of adipocytes by flow cytometry. Methods Enzymol. 2014;537:281–96.

37. Weisberg SP, McCann D, Desai M, Rosenbaum M, Leibel RL, Ferrante Jr AW. Obesity is associated with macrophage accumulation in adipose tissue. J Clin Invest. 2003;112:1796–808.
38. Zhang L, Sugiyama T, Murabayashi N, Umekawa T, Ma N, Kamimoto Y, et al. The inflammatory changes of adipose tissue in late pregnant mice. J Mol Endocrinol. 2011;47:157–65.
39. Cao Q, Wang Y, Wang XM, Lu J, Lee VW, Ye Q, et al. Renal F4/80+ CD11c + mononuclear phagocytes display phenotypic and functional characteristics of macrophages in health and in adriamycin nephropathy. J Am Soc Nephrol. 2015;26:349–63.
40. Mehlem A, Hagberg CE, Muhl L, Eriksson U, Falkevall A. Imaging of neutral lipids by oil red O for analyzing the metabolic status in health and disease. Nat Protoc. 2013;8:1149–54.
41. Sung HY, Kang SW, Kim JL, Li J, Lee ES, Gong JH, et al. Oleanolic acid reduces markers of differentiation in 3T3-L1 adipocytes. Nutr Res. 2010;30:831–9.
42. Ibrahimi A, Bonen A, Blinn WD, Hajri T, Li X, Zhong K, et al. Muscle-specific overexpression of FAT/CD36 enhances fatty acid oxidation by contracting muscle, reduces plasma triglycerides and fatty acids, and increases plasma glucose and insulin. J Biol Chem. 1999;274:26761–6.
43. Harada N, Oda Z, Hara Y, Fujinami K, Okawa M, Ohbuchi K, et al. Hepatic de novo lipogenesis is present in liver-specific ACC1-deficient mice. Mol Cell Biol. 2007;27:1881–8.
44. Love JD, Suzuki T, Robinson DB, Harris CM, Johnson JE, Mohler PJ, et al. Microsomal Triglyceride Transfer Protein (MTP) Associates with Cytosolic Lipid Droplets in 3T3-L1 Adipocytes. PLoS One. 2015;10:e0135598.
45. Wolins NE, Rubin B, Brasaemle DL. TIP47 associates with lipid droplets. J Biol Chem. 2001;276:5101–8.
46. Brasaemle DL, Subramanian V, Garcia A, Marcinkiewicz A, Rothenberg A. Perilipin A and the control of triacylglycerol metabolism. Mol Cell Biochem. 2009;326:15–21.
47. Konige M, Wang H, Sztalryd C. Role of adipose specific lipid droplet proteins in maintaining whole body energy homeostasis. Biochim Biophys Acta. 2014;1842:393–401.
48. Jansen GR, Zanetti ME, Hutchison CF. Studies in lipogenesis in vivo: Fatty acid and cholesterol synthesis during starvation and re-feeding. Biochem J. 1966;101:811–8.
49. O'Hea EK, Leveille GA. Influence of fasting and refeeding on lipogenesis and enzymatic activity of pig adipose tissue. J Nutr. 1969;99:345–52.
50. Hems DA, Rath EA, Verrinder TR. Fatty acid synthesis in liver and adipose tissue of normal and genetically obese (ob/ob) mice during the 24-hour cycle. Biochem J. 1975;150:167–73.
51. Wiegman CH, Bandsma RH, Ouwens M, van der Sluijs FH, Havinga R, Boer T, et al. Hepatic VLDL production in ob/ob mice is not stimulated by massive de novo lipogenesis but is less sensitive to the suppressive effects of insulin. Diabetes. 2003;52:1081–9.
52. Kuriyama H, Liang G, Engelking LJ, Horton JD, Goldstein JL, Brown MS. Compensatory increase in fatty acid synthesis in adipose tissue of mice with conditional deficiency of SCAP in liver. Cell Metab. 2005;1:41–51.
53. Cao H, Gerhold K, Mayers JR, Wiest MM, Watkins SM, Hotamisligil GS. Identification of a lipokine, a lipid hormone linking adipose tissue to systemic metabolism. Cell. 2008;134:933–44.
54. Weinstock PH, Levak-Frank S, Hudgins LC, Radner H, Friedman JM, Zechner R, et al. Lipoprotein lipase controls fatty acid entry into adipose tissue, but fat mass is preserved by endogenous synthesis in mice deficient in adipose tissue lipoprotein lipase. Proc Natl Acad Sci U S A. 1997;94:10261–6.
55. Curat CA, Miranville A, Sengenes C, Diehl M, Tonus C, Busse R, et al. From blood monocytes to adipose tissue-resident macrophages: induction of diapedesis by human mature adipocytes. Diabetes. 2004;53:1285–92.
56. Bluher M. The distinction of metabolically 'healthy' from 'unhealthy' obese individuals. Curr Opin Lipidol. 2010;21:38–43.
57. Sorisky A, Molgat AS, Gagnon A. Macrophage-induced adipose tissue dysfunction and the preadipocyte: should I stay (and differentiate) or should I go? Adv Nutr. 2013;4:67–75.
58. Whitehead JP. Diabetes: New conductors for the peroxisome proliferator-activated receptor gamma (PPARgamma) orchestra. Int J Biochem Cell Biol. 2011;43:1071–4.
59. Janani C, Ranjitha Kumari BD. PPAR gamma gene — a review. Diabetes Metab Syndr. 2015;9:46–50.
60. Kadowaki T, Hara K, Kubota N, Tobe K, Terauchi Y, Yamauchi T, et al. The role of PPARgamma in high-fat diet-induced obesity and insulin resistance. J Diabetes Complications. 2002;16:41–5.
61. Arimura N, Horiba T, Imagawa M, Shimizu M, Sato R. The peroxisome proliferator-activated receptor gamma regulates expression of the perilipin gene in adipocytes. J Biol Chem. 2004;279:10070–6.
62. Phan J, Peterfy M, Reue K. Lipin expression preceding peroxisome proliferator-activated receptor-gamma is critical for adipogenesis in vivo and in vitro. J Biol Chem. 2004;279:29558–64.
63. Jones JR, Barrick C, Kim KA, Lindner J, Blondeau B, Fujimoto Y, et al. Deletion of PPARgamma in adipose tissues of mice protects against high fat diet-induced obesity and insulin resistance. Proc Natl Acad Sci U S A. 2005;102:6207–12.
64. Adida A, Spener F. Adipocyte-type fatty acid-binding protein as inter-compartmental shuttle for peroxisome proliferator activated receptor gamma agonists in cultured cell. Biochim Biophys Acta. 2006;1761:172–81.
65. Lefterova MI, Zhang Y, Steger DJ, Schupp M, Schug J, Cristancho A, et al. PPARgamma and C/EBP factors orchestrate adipocyte biology via adjacent binding on a genome-wide scale. Genes Dev. 2008;22:2941–52.
66. Cai Y, Ying F, Song E, Wang Y, Xu A, Vanhoutte PM, et al. Mice lacking prostaglandin E receptor subtype 4 manifest disrupted lipid metabolism attributable to impaired triglyceride clearance. FASEB J. 2015;29(12):4924–36.
67. Huh JY, Kim JI, Park YJ, Hwang IJ, Lee YS, Sohn JH, et al. A novel function of adipocytes in lipid antigen presentation to iNKT cells. Mol Cell Biol. 2013;33:328–39.
68. Huh JY, Park YJ, Ham M, Kim JB. Crosstalk between adipocytes and immune cells in adipose tissue inflammation and metabolic dysregulation in obesity. Mol Cells. 2014;37:365–71.
69. Kotas ME, Lee HY, Gillum MP, Annicelli C, Guigni BA, Shulman GI, et al. Impact of CD1d deficiency on metabolism. PLoS One. 2011;6:e25478.
70. Tajiri K, Shimizu Y. Role of NKT Cells in the Pathogenesis of NAFLD. Int J Hepatol. 2012;2012:850836.
71. Martin-Murphy BV, You Q, Wang H, De La Houssaye BA, Reilly TP, Friedman JE, et al. Mice lacking natural killer T cells are more susceptible to metabolic alterations following high fat diet feeding. PLoS One. 2014;9:e80949.

Rubus crataegifolius Bunge regulates adipogenesis through Akt and inhibits high-fat diet-induced obesity in rats

Min-Sup Jung[1†], Soo-Jung Lee[2†], Yuno Song[1], Sun-Hee Jang[1], Wongi Min[1], Chung-Kil Won[1], Hong-Duck Kim[3], Tae Hoon Kim[4] and Jae-Hyeon Cho[1,5*]

Abstract

Background: Obesity is one of the greatest public health problems and major risk factors for serious metabolic diseases and significantly increases the risk of premature death. The aim of this study was to determine the inhibitory effects of Rubus crataegifolius Bunge (RCB) on adipocyte differentiation in 3 T3-L1 cells and its anti-obesity properties in high fat diet (HFD)-induced obese rats.

Methods: 3 T3-L1 adipocytes and HFD-induced obese rats were treated with RCB, and its effect on gene expression was analyzed using RT-PCR and Western blotting experiments.

Results: RCB treatment significantly inhibited adipocyte differentiation by suppressing the expression of C/EBPβ, C/EBPα, and PPARγ in the 3 T3-L1 adipocytes. Subsequently, the expression of the PPARγ target genes aP2 and fatty acid synthase (FAS) decreased following RCB treatment during adipocyte differentiation. In uncovering the specific mechanism that mediates the effects of RCB, we demonstrated that the insulin-stimulated phosphorylation of Akt strongly decreased and that its downstream substrate phospho-GSK3β was downregulated following RCB treatment in the 3 T3-L1 adipocytes. Moreover, LY294002, an inhibitor of Akt phosphorylation, exerted stronger inhibitory effects on RCB-mediated suppression of adipocyte differentiation, leading to the inhibition of adipocyte differentiation through the downregulation of Akt signaling. An HFD-induced obesity rat model was used to determine the inhibitory effects of RCB on obesity. Body weight gain and fat accumulation in adipose tissue were significantly reduced by the supplementation of RCB. Moreover, RCB treatment caused a significant decrease in adipocyte size, associated with a decrease in epididymal fat weight. The serum total cholesterol (TC) and triglyceride (TG) levels decreased in response to RCB treatment, whereas HDL cholesterol (HDL-C) increased, indicating that RCB attenuated lipid accumulation in adipose tissue in HFD-induced obese rats.

Conclusion: Our results demonstrate an inhibitory effect of RCB on adipogenesis through the reduction of the adipogenic factors PPARγ, C/EBPα, and phospho-Akt. RCB had a potent anti-obesity effect, reducing body weight gain in HFD-induced obese rats.

Keywords: Rubus crataegifolius Bunge (RCB), 3 T3-L1 adipocyte, Adipogenesis, Akt, High fat diet, Obesity

* Correspondence: jaehcho@gnu.ac.kr
†Equal contributors
[1]Institute of Animal Medicine, College of Veterinary Medicine, Gyeongsang National University, Jinju 660-701, Korea
[5]College of Veterinary Medicine, Gyeongsang National University, Jiju Daero 501, Jinju-city, Gyeongsangnamdo 660-701, Korea
Full list of author information is available at the end of the article

Background

Obesity arises from adipocyte hyperplasia and hypertrophy caused by the intake of excess energy [1]. Excess fat accumulates in adipocytes as excessive amounts of lipids (triglycerides), resulting in elevated triglyceride levels in plasma and in tissues such as liver and muscle, which leads to pathological dysfunction in these tissues [2, 3]. Thus, adipocyte hyperplasia may be an important factor in the development of obesity. To prevent obesity, it is important to maintain an adequate balance between energy accumulation and energy consumption.

The excessive accumulation of adipose tissue is caused by increased adipogenesis accompanied by adipocyte differentiation, which converts immature pre-adipocytes into adipocytes. Abnormal fat accumulation and adipocyte differentiation in adipose tissue are associated with the development of obesity [4]. Adipogenesis, the process of adipose cell development, is associated with multiple steps in the regulation of several transcription factors. During the differentiation process, many key transcriptional factors are involved, such as CCAAT-enhancer-binding protein (C/EBP)-δ and C/EBPβ, which can collectively induce the expression of peroxisome proliferator-activated receptor (PPAR)-γ and C/EBPα [5, 6]. PPARγ and C/EBPα also play important roles as major transcription factors in adipogenesis [5]. In addition, these transcription factors are involved in the acceleration of lipogenesis and lipid homeostasis by modulating the expression of target genes, such as adipocyte fatty acid-binding protein 2 (aP2) and fatty acid synthase (FAS) [7].

The intracellular signaling cascade involving insulin/phosphoinositide 3-kinase (PI3K)/Akt plays a major role in adipocyte differentiation. Akt phosphorylates and regulates a number of substrates that are involved in a diverse array of biological processes [8], and it is essential in the induction of PPARγ expression [9]. Pharmacological inhibition of the PI3K/Akt signaling pathway [10, 11] and dominant negative mutations [12] can abolish adipocyte differentiation by inhibiting PI3K/Akt activity. Moreover, the overexpression of constitutively active Akt increases glucose uptake and adipocyte differentiation in 3 T3-L1 adipocytes [13].

Rubus crataegifolius Bunge (RCB) is a type of red raspberry and is a member of the Rosaceae family. Rubus is one of the most diverse and largest genera in the Rosaceae family and is comprised of approximately 600 to 800 species, including blackberries, raspberries and their hybrids [14, 15]. Traditionally, Rubi coreanus (Rubi Fructus) fruit has been used as a medicinal agent for the treatment of impotence, spermatorrhea, enuresis, and asthma [16]. Rubi crataegifolius has also been used for treatment of rheumatic arthritis, hepatitis and lung cancer in China [17]. Traditional herbal medicines may have some potential to prevent obesity. Although the use of these fruits in fresh and processed food items, such as jams, jellies and juices, represents a multimillion dollar industry [18], their medicinal properties—including their anti-inflammatory effects on ulcers and their capacity to reduce blood cholesterol levels [19] and cell proliferation [20] in animal models—have recently attracted the attention of the international market. However, no reports documenting the anti-obesity effects of RCB have been published.

In this study, we hypothesized that RCB could exert the inhibitory effect on the differentiation of 3 T3-L1 preadipocytes and its in vivo inhibition of high fat diet (HFD)-induced obesity in rats. To study this possibility, the inhibitory effects of RCB on differentiation of 3 T3-L1 preadipocytes into adipocytes was examined by measuring triglyceride accumulation levels and expression levels of genes involved in adipogenesis and lipogenesis in adipocytes. We also investigated the underlying mechanism whether Akt signaling is critical for the anti-obesity function of RCB. Moreover, we examined the effects of RCB on body weight, adipose tissue mass, and lipid metabolism in HFD-induced obese rats.

Methods

Preparation of Rubus crataegifolius Bunge (RCB) extracts

The fresh fruits of *Rubus crataegifolius Bunge* (RCB) were collected in Gyeongsan-si, Gyeongsangbuk-do, Korea in September 2013. A voucher specimen representing this collection was identified by Prof. Gon-Sup Kim and deposited at the Animal Bio Resources Bank of Gyeongsang National University. The fresh fruits of RCB were prepared by alcohol extraction. The fruit bodies were peeled off and air-dried in an oven at an initial temperature of 30 °C, which was increased by 5 °C every 3 h until it reached 40 °C. The dried fruit bodies of RCB were milled into a powder (40 mesh). Fifteen grams of RCB powder were then suspended in an 80 % (v/v) ethanol solution using a mixer, followed by the extraction of the samples for 3 days with vigorous shaking at room temperature and filtering through Whatman No. 1 filter paper. The 80 % ethanol extracts of RCB were concentrated using rotary-vacuum evaporation at 50 °C and then freeze-dried. The RCB extract was stored in the freezer until it was used for experiments.

Measurement of total phenolic content using folin-ciocalteu assay

The total phenolic content of RCB was measured using a spectrophotometer according to the Folin-Ciocalteu colorimetric method as previously described [21, 22]. Because quercetin is one of the polyphenol compounds found in RCB, the total phenolic content of the ethanol extract of RCB was expressed as mg catechin equivalents (QE)/g. Catechin was purchased from Sigma-Aldrich (St.

Louis, MO. USA). The measurements were performed four times.

Measurement of total flavonoids

Total flavonoid content was determined as previously described [23] with slight modifications. Briefly, 0.25 mL of RCB (100 μg/mL) was added to a tube containing 1 mL of double-distilled water. Following this, 0.075 mL of 5 % $NaNO_2$, 0.075 mL of 10 % $AlCl_3$ and 0.5 mL of 1 M NaOH were added sequentially at 0, 5 and 6 min. Finally, the volume of the reacting solution was adjusted to 2.5 mL with double-distilled water. The 410 nm absorbance of the solution was detected using an Ultrospec 2100 Pro Spectrophotometer (Section 3.3). The results are expressed in mg quercetin equivalents (QE)/g. The experiments were carried out in quadruplicate.

Measurement of free radical scavenging activity using a 2,2-diphenyl-1-picrylhydrazyl (DPPH) assay

The free radical scavenging activity of RCB (100 μg/mL in DW) was measured using a method created by Brand-Williams [24] with slight modifications. The inhibition percentage was calculated using the following equation: Inhibition % = [(absorbance of control - absorbance of sample)/absorbance of control] × 100. The absorbance was measured using a spectrophotometer (Ultrospec 2100 pro; Amersham Pharmacia Biotech Co., Piscataway, NJ, USA). The experiments were carried out in quadruplicate.

Measurement of superoxide anion ($O2^{\bullet-}$) radical scavenging and hydroxyl ($OH^{\bullet}$) radical scavenging activity

Superoxide radicals were generated according to a method described in a previous paper [25]. The samples (100 μg/mL in DMSO) were added to a reaction solution containing 100 μL of 30 mM EDTA (pH 7.4), 10 μL of 30 mM hypoxanthine in 50 mM NaOH, and 200 μL of 1.42 mM nitroblue tetrazolium (NBT). After the solution was preincubated at room temperature for 3 min, 100 μL of 0.5 U/mL xanthine oxidase was added to the mixture, and the volume was brought up to 3 mL with 50 mM phosphate buffer (pH 7.4). After the solution was incubated at room temperature for 20 min, absorbance was measured at 560 nm. The reaction mixture without xanthine oxidase was used as a blank (A1). The samples (A2) were added to the reaction mixture, in which $O2^{\bullet-}$ was scavenged and thereby inhibited the reduction of NBT. The absorbance was measured, and a decrease in $O2^{\bullet-}$ was represented by A2-A1. The scavenging activity of the superoxide anion radical (SRSA) was calculated using the following equation: SRSA % = (A2 – A1/A1) × 100. The scavenging activity of the samples (100 μg/mL) in DMSO on the hydroxyl radical ($OH^{\bullet}$) was measured using the deoxyribose method [26] with slight modifications. The deoxyribose assay was performed in 10 mM phosphate buffer (pH 7.4) containing 2.5 mM deoxyribose, 1.5 mM H_2O_2, 100 μM $FeCl_3$, 104 μM EDTA, and a test sample (0.5 mg/mL). The reaction was initiated by adding ascorbic acid to a final concentration of 100 μM. The reaction mixture was incubated for 1 h at 37 °C in a water bath. After incubation, the color was developed by the addition of 0.5 % thiobarbituric acid followed by an addition of ice-cold 2.8 % trichloroacetic acid in 25 mM NaOH and incubation for 30 min at 80 °C. A control experiment was performed without the samples (A1). The samples (A2) were cooled on ice, and the absorbance was measured at 532 nm. The hydroxyl radical scavenging activity (HRSA) was calculated using the following equation: HRSA% = (A1− A2/A1) × 100. The measurements were performed four times.

Cell culture

Murine 3 T3-L1 fibroblasts as preadipocytes were maintained in Dulbecco's modified Eagle's high-glucose medium (DMEM) containing 10 % calf serum, 100 units/mL penicillin, and 100 μg/mL streptomycin. Two-day post-confluent 3 T3-L1 cells, designated as day 0, were differentiated with complete DMEM containing 10 % FBS by adding a mixture (DMI) of 0.5 mM 3-isobutyl-1-methylxanthine, 100 μM indomethacin, 0.25 μM dexamethasone (DEX), and 167 nM insulin. The 3-isobutyl-1-methylxanthine, DEX, indomethacin, and Oil red O were purchased from Sigma-Aldrich (St. Louis, MO, USA). The medium was changed every 2 days. RCBs were added to the culture medium of the adipocytes on day 0. The cells were treated with 0, 50, or 150 μg/mL RCB extracts every day. After treatment with RCB on day 4 and day 7, the 3 T3-L1 adipocytes were harvested and lysed for Western blot analysis as described in section 2.12. To analyze cell viability, the cytotoxicity of the RCB was evaluated using 3-(4, 5-demethylthiazol-2-yl)-2, 5-diphenyltetrazolium bromide (MTT) according to the manufacturer's instructions.

Oil red O staining and triglyceride assay

Lipid accumulated within cells was visualized by Oil red O staining as described previously [27]. Oil red O staining was performed on day 7 of differentiation to stain accumulated lipid droplets in 3 T3-L1 adipocytes. The cells were gently washed with phosphate-buffered saline (PBS) and stained with filtered Oil red O solution (60 % isopropanol and 40 % water) for 30 min. After staining the lipid droplets red, the Oil Red O staining solution was removed, and the plates were rinsed with water and dried. The photographs were taken using an Olympus microscope (Tokyo, Japan). To analyze the content of cellular triglycerides, the cells were washed with PBS, scraped into 200 μL of PBS and sonicated for 1 min. The 3 T3-L1 cells were incubated with or without the selective PI3K inhibitor LY294002, which was purchased from Sigma-Aldrich (St. Louis, MO, USA) at a concentration of 10 μM in the presence or absence of RCB for 7 days. Total triglyceride content was measured in cell lysates using an assay kit, and cellular protein was measured using a Bio-Rad protein assay kit (Hercules, CA, USA). The results are expressed as percentage changes. All the experiments were carried out in triplicate.

RT-PCR

Total RNA was isolated from the 3 T3-L1 adipocytes using Trizol reagent (Invitrogen, CA, USA) according to the manufacturer's protocol. The total RNA (1 μg) was reverse-transcribed to cDNA using a reverse transcription system (Invitrogen, CA, USA) according to the manufacturer's protocol. The mRNA expression of adipocyte differentiation-related genes was examined using cDNA and the following gene-specific primers: C/EBPβ, 5′-GACTACGCAACACACGTGTAACT-3′ and 5′-CA AAACCAAAAACATCAACAACCC-3′; PPARγ, 5′-TT TTCAAGGGTGCCAGTTTC-3′ and 5′-AATCCTTG GCCCTCTGAGAT-3′; C/EBPα, 5′-TTACAACAGGC-CAGGTTTCC-3′ and 5′-GGCTGGCGACATACAGA TCA-3′; β-actin (control), 5′-GACAACGGCTCCGG CATGTGCAAAG-3′ and 5′-TTCACGGTTGGCCTT AGGGTTCAG-3′.

Western blot analysis

Western blotting was performed according to standard procedures [6] with slight modifications. Briefly, whole cells were lysed in lysis buffer containing 50 mM Tris–HCl (pH 8.0), 0.4 % Nonidet P-40, 120 mM NaCl, 1.5 mM $MgCl_2$, 0.1 % SDS, 2 mM phenylmethylsulfonyl fluoride, 80 μg/ml leupeptin, 3 mM NaF and 1 mM DTT. Cell lysates were separated by 10 % SDS-polyacrylamide gel electrophoresis, transferred onto a polyvinylidene fluoride membrane (Amersham Pharmacia, England, UK), blocked with 5 % skim milk and hybridized with primary antibodies. The following antibodies were purchased from Cell Signaling technology (Danvers, MA USA): PPARγ, C/EBPβ, C/EBPα, aP2, FAS, Akt, and GSK3β; the monoclonal β-actin antibody was purchased from Chemicon (Millipore Inc., Billerica, MA USA). HRP-labeled mouse anti-rabbit IgG was obtained from Jackson ImmunoResearch. The Chemiluminescence kit was from Pierce (Rockford, IL). After incubation with horseradish-peroxidase-conjugated secondary antibody at room temperature, immunoreactive proteins were detected using a chemiluminescent ECL assay kit (Amersham Pharmacia, UK) according to the manufacturer's instructions.

Measurement of glucose uptake

Glucose uptake in the 3 T3-L1 cells was measured using the fluorescent D-glucose analogue 2-[N-(7-nitrobenz-2-oxa-1,3-diazol-4-yl)amino]-2-deoxy-D-glucose (2-NBDG) (Invitrogen, Carlsbad, USA) with slight modifications to a previously reported protocol [28]. Briefly, 3 T3-L1 pre-adipocytes were differentiated in various concentrations (0, 50, and 150 μg/ml) of RCB or DMSO for 7 days in 6-well plates. After washing, the differentiated 3 T3-L1 cells were treated with or without the indicated concentrations of RCB and insulin in the absence or presence of 10 μM 2-NBDG. After incubation for 2 h, the cells were washed three times with PBS, and the resulting fluorescence was measured (excitation at 485 nm and emission at 530 nm) using a fluorescent microplate reader (Molecular Devices, USA). All the experiments were carried out in triplicate.

Animal experiments

Five-week-old Sprague–Dawley male rats were obtained from Central Lab Animal Inc. (Seoul, Korea). All animal experiments were conducted in accordance with the National Institutes of Health (NIH) guidelines and with the approval of the Animal Care and Use committee of Gyeongsang National University (Approval Number: GNU-140513-R0049). The rats were housed in polycarbonate cages in a room maintained at 22 °C with 55 % relative humidity on a 12 h dark/light cycle. All of the rats were allowed free access to food and water for five weeks. The rats were randomly divided into three groups that were fed a normal diet (ND, $n = 10$), a high-fat diet (HFD, $n = 10$), or a HFD supplemented with RCB (HFD + RCB, $n = 10$) for 5 weeks. The ND group was maintained on a normal diet based on a commercial diet (#55VXT0038, Samyang Co, Korea). The HFD group was fed an HFD based on a commercial diet (rodent diet with 60 % kcal fat, Research Diet, Korea). To test the anti-obesity activity of RCB extracts (200 mg/kg BW) orally administered to the HFD-fed rats for five weeks. Food intake was measured daily, and body weight was measured every two days. Rats were food deprived overnight prior to blood collection and euthanized by ketamine (40 mg/kg) plus xylazine (2 mg/kg).

Group 1: Normal diet group (ND)
Group 2: High-fat diet group (HFD)
Group 3: HFD + RCB 200 mg/kg BW (HFD + RCB)

Biochemical and histological analysis

Body weight and fatty tissue mass ($n = 10$ rats/group) were measured with sensitivity limits of 0.1 g and 0.01 g, respectively. Blood samples were collected and centrifuged 1000 x g for 15 min at 4 °C, and serum was separated to analyze plasma biomarkers. Epididymal fat pads were excised, weighed and stored at −20 °C until they were assayed. Concentrations of plasma triglyceride (TG), total cholesterol (TC), and high-density lipoprotein-cholesterol (HDL-C) were assayed enzymatically using commercial kits (Asan phams, Co., Korea) as previously described [27]. There were 10 animals per group in all experiments. Epididymal adipose tissue samples were dehydrated, embedded in paraffin, cut into 5-µm sections and stained with hematoxylin-eosin for microscopic assessment (Olympus, Tokyo, Japan). For quantification analysis, adipocyte dimensions were measured using MetaMorph image analysis software (Molecular devices, CA, USA) equipped for the automation and programmable distance and color segmentation ($n = 5$ rats/group).

Statistical analysis

Data were analyzed using SPSS version 12.0 software (SPSS Inc., Chicago, IL, USA). Each experiment was performed in at least triplicate. The data are expressed as the mean ± SD. Differences among multiple groups were analyzed by conducting one-way analysis of variance (ANOVA) followed by Duncan's multiple range test, and differences between 2 groups were identified using Student's t test. $P < 0.05$ was considered statistically significant and extremely significant between groups.

Results

Total phenol content (TPC) and total flavonoid content (TFC) of RCB

The antioxidant properties of RCB extracts are summarized in Table 1. The TPC and TFC content of RCB extract was found to be 125.3 ± 17.56 catechin equivalents/g and 35.45 ± 3.65 quercetin equivalents/g of extract, respectively (Table 1). RCB showed strong DPPH radical scavenging activity. The hydroxyl radical scavenging activity of RCB was measured by the inhibition of nitroblue tetrazolium and by RCB's reduction of hydroxyl radical generation. The RCB extract also exhibited a potent scavenging effect on superoxide radicals.

Inhibitory effect of RCB on 3 T3-L1 pre-adipocyte differentiation

To examine the effects of RCB on the differentiation of pre-adipocytes into adipocytes, confluent 3 T3-L1 pre-adipocytes were treated with various concentrations (0, 50, and 150 µg/ml) of RCB extract in the presence or absence of a DMI mixture. The cell culture media was supplemented with RCB extract from day 0 to day 7, and the fully differentiated cells exhibited numerous lipid droplets, indicating lipid accumulation. On the seventh day of incubation, lipid accumulation was examined as a marker of differentiation by Oil red O staining. RCB extract showed anti-adipogenic properties, as indicated by the decreased levels of Oil red O staining on differentiation day 7 in Fig. 1a. To further investigate whether RCB had an effect on adipocyte differentiation, lipid accumulation was quantified by measuring triglyceride content during 3 T3-L1 differentiation. The triglyceride content of the cells increased during 3 T3-L1 differentiation over the course of 7 days, whereas the addition of RCB extract into the differentiation media strongly blocked triglyceride accumulation (Fig. 1b). These results showed that treatment with 50 or 150 µg/ml RCB extract resulted in a 17 % or 28 % decrease, respectively, in triglyceride accumulation in the 3 T3-L1 adipocytes.

Cytotoxic effects of RCB on 3 T3-L1 cells

The toxic concentration of the RCB extract was assessed via an MTT viability assay using thiazoyl blue tetrazolium bromide. 3 T3-L1 cells were treated with different concentrations of RCB (0, 50, and 150 µg/ml) in combination with a DMI mixture for either 4 or 7 days. There were no significant differences in 3 T3-L1 cell viability at concentrations of up to 150 µg/ml of RCB extract compared to the control (Fig. 1c). These results demonstrated that RCB strongly blocks adipocyte differentiation in 3 T3-L1 cells.

Inhibitory effect of RCB on adipogenic-specific gene and lipogenic gene expression

Adipocyte differentiation is accompanied by changes in the expression of various adipogenesis- and lipogenesis-related genes. C/EBPs and PPARγ are known adipogenic genes that have roles in transforming pre-adipocytes into mature adipocytes [5]. To investigate the anti-adipogenic mechanism of RCB, its effects on both mRNA and protein levels of C/EBPα, C/EBPβ, and PPARγ were elucidated. After inducing differentiation, 3 T3-L1 cells were exposed for 4 or 7 days to a concentration of 50 and 150 µg/ml RCB. As shown in Fig. 2a, the mRNA level of

Table 1 Radical scavenging activities, total phenolic and flavonoid contents of RCB extract

	DRSA	HRSA	SRSA	TP (mgCE/g)	Flavonoids (mgQE/g)
RCB	28.24 ± 2.05^a	13.38 ± 1.47^a	32.43 ± 2.40^b	125.30 ± 17.56	35.45 ± 3.65
BHT	42.73 ± 0.50^b	13.76 ± 2.01^a	26.48 ± 1.95^a	-	-
Ascorbic acid	75.42 ± 3.33^c	18.14 ± 1.73^b	24.27 ± 2.17^a	-	-

DRSA, DPPH (2,2-diphenyl-1-picrylhydrazyl) radical scavenging activity; HRSA, hydroxyl radial scavenging activity; SRSA, superoxide anion radical scavenging activity; TPC, total phenolic acid. Total phenolic acid is expressed as milligrams of catechin equivalents (CE)/g of extract, and total flavonoid content is expressed as milligrams of quercetin equivalents (QE)/g of extract. Butylated hydroxytoluene (BHT) and ascorbic acid at the concentration of 100 µg/mL were used as positive control. Each value represents mean ± SD ($n = 4$). $^{a-c}$Means with different superscript letters in the same column were significantly different by Duncan's multiple range test ($p < 0.05$)

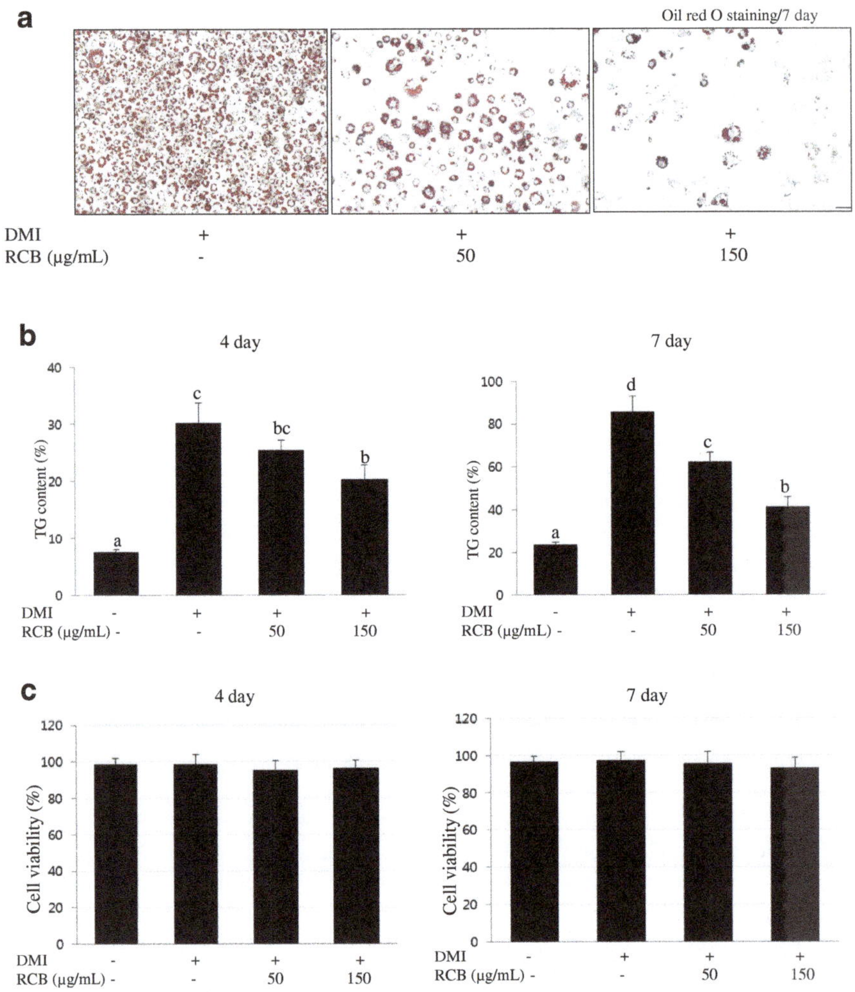

Fig. 1 Effect of RCB on adipocyte differentiation in 3 T3-L1 cells. **a** Lipid accumulation in 3 T3-L1 adipocytes assessed by Oil red O staining. 3 T3-L1 pre-adipocytes were differentiated into mature adipocytes and then treated with RCB for 7 days. At day 7 post-induction, the cells were fixed, and neutral lipids were stained with Oil red O. DMI, fully differentiated adipocytes (0.5 mM 3 IBMX, 100 μM indomethason, 0.25 μM dexamethasone and 167 nM insulin); 50, fully differentiated adipocytes (DMI + 50 μg/ml RCB); 150, fully differentiated adipocytes (DMI + 150 μg/ml RCB). RCB represents *Rubus crataegifolius Bunge* extracts. The scale bar is 50 μm. **b** Effect of RCB on TG accumulation in differentiating 3 T3-L1 cells. Triglyceride content was measured using a triglyceride assay kit. The results shown are representative of at least three independent experiments. The values are presented as the means ± SD. Different letters on the each bar graph indicate that the differences were statically significant (I 0.05) according to Duncan's multiple range test. **c** Effect of RCB on cytotoxicity during 3T3L1 pre-adipocyte differentiation into adipocytes. 3 T3-L1 cells were treated with RCB at various concentrations (0, 50, or 150 μg/ml) in a DMI mixture for 4 or 7 days. Cell viability after treatment with RCB was determined with an MTT assay

C/EBPβ was significantly lower in cells treated with 150 μg/ml RCB extract during adipocyte differentiation than that in the cells treated with DMI alone. The expression of C/EBPα and PPARγ mRNA was also significantly reduced following treatment with RCB extract (Fig. 2a). Furthermore, the protein levels of C/EBPβ, C/EBPα, and PPARγ were reduced in a dose-dependent manner after RCB treatment for 4 or 7 days (Fig. 2b). The activation of C/EBPα and PPARγ induces the expression of lipogenesis-related genes, including aP2 and FAS [5]. Thus, we examined whether the above-detailed down-regulation was related to decreased C/EBPα and PPARγ target gene expression levels. Consistent with the above observations, RCB suppressed the expression levels of C/EBPα and PPARγ target genes, such as aP2 and FAS (Fig. 2b). We also found that RCB extract treatment resulted in a dose-dependent suppression of aP2 and FAS at the protein level. Taken together, these results suggest that the activation of C/EBPα and PPARγ plays a critical role in the regulation of adipogenesis by RCB.

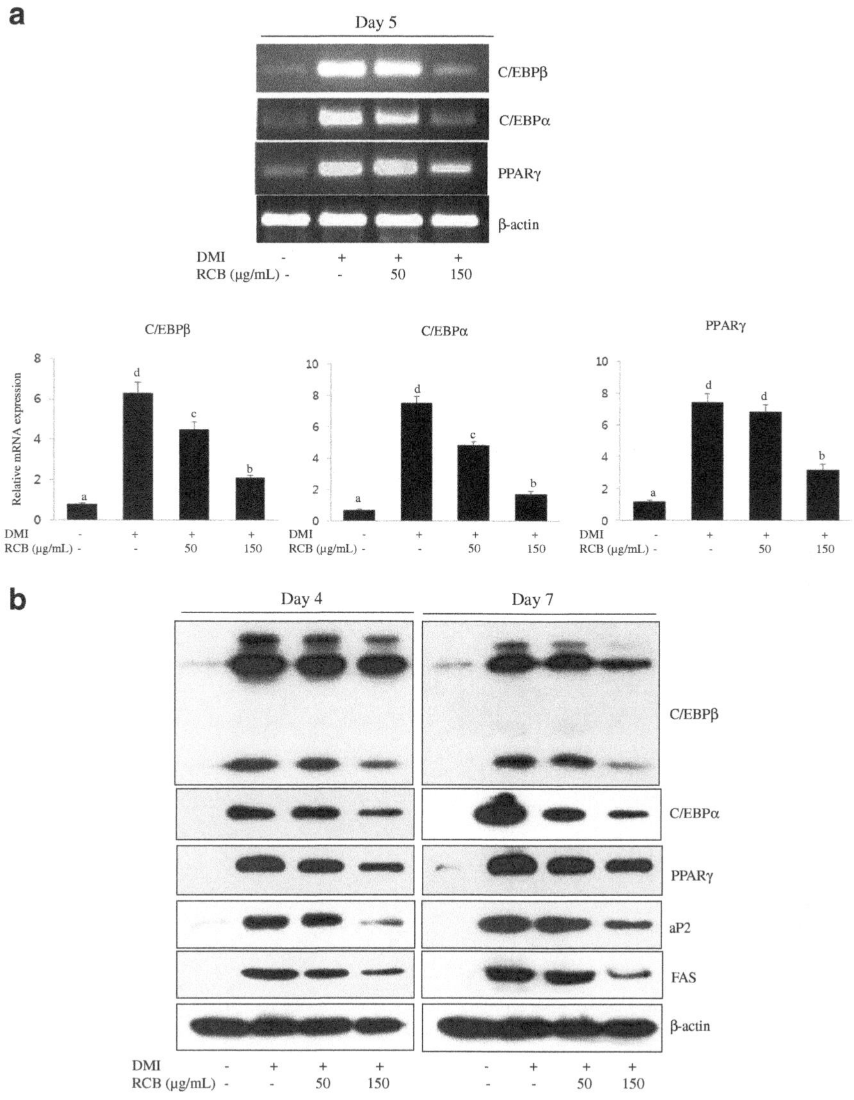

Fig. 2 Effects of RCB on the mRNA and protein expression of genes related to adipogenesis. **a** RCB inhibited the mRNA expression of adipocyte-specific factors during 3 T3-L1 adipocyte differentiation. Differentiation of 3 T3-L1 pre-adipocytes into adipocytes was induced using DMI media in the absence or presence of RCB (50 μg/mL or 150 μg/mL) for 5 days. β-actin expression in each sample was used as an internal control to normalize expression. The results shown are representative of at least three independent experiments. The different letters on each bar graph indicate significant differences ($p < 0.05$), as determined by Duncan's multiple range test. **b** RCB inhibited the protein expression of adipocyte-related factors in 3 T3-L1 adipocytes. Cell lysates from the 3 T3-L1 cells were prepared at day 4 or day 7 after the induction of differentiation. Western blotting analysis was described in detail in the *Materials and Methods* section

Effect of RCB on the phosphorylation of Akt and GSK3β during adipocyte differentiation

To investigate whether Akt, a major factor in adipocyte differentiation, is regulated by RCB during 3 T3-L1 differentiation, levels of phosphorylated Akt and GSK3β were analyzed and compared with total levels of Akt. Our results showed that DMI-stimulated 3 T3-L1 adipocytes exhibited strongly increased phosphorylation levels of Akt (Ser473) and GSK3β (Ser9). The phosphorylation of Akt was significantly decreased in the RCB-treated groups compared to the differentiated 3 T3-L1 adipocytes (Fig. 3a). Likewise, the expression of phospho-GSK3β was also substantially decreased following treatment with RCB during 3 T3-L1 cell differentiation (Fig. 3b). These results suggest that RCB extract treatment decreases Akt phosphorylation and down-regulates the phosphorylation of

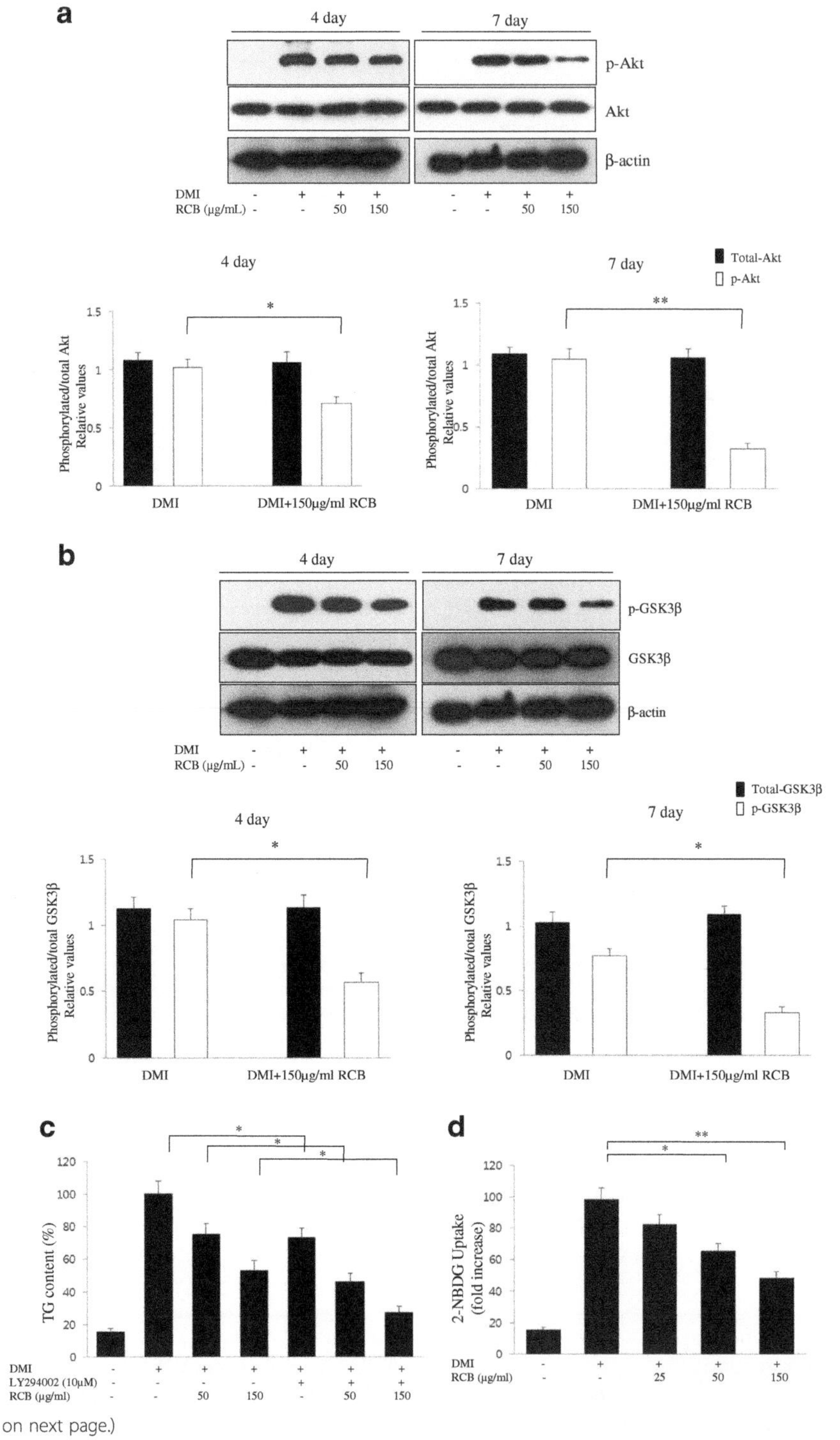

Fig. 3 (See legend on next page.)

(See figure on previous page.)
Fig. 3 Effect of RCB on Akt and GSK3β phosphorylation during 3 T3-L1 adipogenesis. **a** RCB downregulated Akt phosphorylation induced by DMI in 3 T3-L1 adipocytes. The 3 T3-L1 pre-adipocytes were induced to differentiate with DMI media in the absence or presence of RCB for 4 or 7 days, and the phosphorylation levels of Akt were detected with its specific antibody. The results are reported as the means ± SD of three independent experiments. **P* < 0.05. ***P* < 0.01. **b** Effect of RCB on GSK3β phosphorylation during 3 T3-L1 adipogenesis. The phosphorylation levels of GSK3β were determined using a specific antibody. The results are reported as the means ± SD of three independent experiments. **P* < 0.05. **c** Inhibitory effects of LY294002 on 3 T3-L1 adipocyte differentiation. 3 T3-L1 cells were incubated with or without RCB at a concentration of 50 or 150 μg/ml during differentiation in the presence or absence of LY294002 (10 μM). After differentiation, the TG contents in the 3 T3-L1 adipocytes were determined by a triglyceride assay. The data presented are the mean ± SD from three independent experiments. **P* < 0.05. **d** RCB inhibited DMI-stimulated glucose uptake in 3 T3-L1 adipocytes. Glucose uptake activity in differentiated 3 T3-L1 cells was analyzed by measuring the fluorescence intensity of the cells after incubation with 10 μM 2-NBDG for 2 h. The results are reported as the mean ± SD of three independent experiments. **P* < 0.05. ***P* < 0.01

GSK3β, a substrate kinase of Akt, leading to the inhibition of the adipogenesis pathway.

RCB inhibited 3 T3-L1 adipocyte differentiation through the Akt signaling pathway

To further understand the underlying mechanism of the inhibitory effects of RCB on adipocyte differentiation, we performed an experiment with LY294002, a chemical inhibitor of the Akt pathway. After treatment with DMI for 7 days, differentiated 3 T3-L1 cells showed increased accumulation of triglyceride droplets compared to undifferentiated 3 T3-L1 cells (Fig. 3c). Interestingly, treatment with 10 μM LY294002 resulted in a decrease in intracellular triglyceride accumulation in the differentiated 3 T3-L1 cells. Moreover, we found that the inhibitory effects of RCB on the formation of lipid droplets were more enhanced by the combined treatment of LY29400 and RCB than by treatment with RCB alone (Fig. 3c). These results indicate that the role of Akt signaling is significantly associated with the functional modulation of the RCB, which reduces adipogenesis in 3 T3-L1 cells.

RCB reduced glucose uptake in 3 T3-L1 adipocytes

To examine the effects of RCB on glucose uptake in 3 T3-L1 adipocytes, a fluorescent deoxyglucose analog (2-NBDG) was used to calculate glucose uptake rates. 3 T3-L1 cells were exposed to 0, 10, 50, and 150 μg/ml concentrations of RCB extract in differentiation media for 7 days. The RCB treatment led to a significant dose-dependent decrease in glucose uptake compared to cells treated with DMI alone; glucose uptake in the 50 and 150 μg/ml RCB-treated groups showed decreases of 27 % and 38 %, respectively, compared to the DMI alone group (Fig. 3d).

RCB induced decreases in body weight and adipose tissue weight in HFD-induced obese rats

We further evaluated whether RCB possessed anti-obesity effects in rats fed a HFD for 5 weeks. At the end of the experiment, the body weights of the HFD group were 39 % greater than those of the ND control group, demonstrating that HFD-fed rats developed obesity (Additional file 1 and Fig. 4a). The weight gain observed for the group of rats that were administered RCB extract (200 mg/kg/daily) was markedly decreased compared to the HFD only group. We did not observe any significant changes in food intake in any of the treatment groups compared to the HFD-fed group and the HFD-fed plus RCB extract treatment group (data not shown). Thus, these data indicate that the reduction in body weight gain in the RCB-treated rats was not mediated by a reduction of food and water intake in the HFD rats. To investigate whether the reduction in body weight gain in the RCB-treated group was related to decreased fat accumulation, epididymal and perirenal adipose tissues were weighed. Supplementation with RCB significantly reduced epididymal fat (25 %) and perirenal fat (22 %) mass compared to the untreated HFD group (Fig. 4b and c). Histological examination of the epididymal adipose tissue revealed that adipocyte size was significantly smaller in the epididymal adipose tissue of the RCB-treated group than in that of the HFD only group (Fig. 4d), further demonstrating that the reduction in body weight gain primarily arose because of decreased fat accumulation and adipocyte size.

RCB changed serum triglyceride (TG), total cholesterol and HDL cholesterol levels in HFD-induced obese rats

To support biochemical evidence underlying changes in epididymal and perirenal adipose tissues following treatment with RCB extract, we further investigated the effects of RCB on the serum levels of TG, total cholesterol (TC), and HDL-cholesterol (HDL-C) in HFD-induced obese rats. The serum levels of TG and TC were significantly reduced in the RCB extract-treated obese rats. Compared to the ND group, the serum levels of TG and TC in the HFD group increased, whereas the serum levels of TG and TC were significantly reduced by 29 % and 26 %, respectively, in the RCB extract-treated obese rats compared to the levels observed in the HFD only group (Fig. 5a and b). The serum HDL-C level was significantly higher in the HFD + RCB group compared to the HFD group (Fig. 5c).

Discussion

Metabolic syndrome has become a major public health problem throughout the world. It is characterized by a

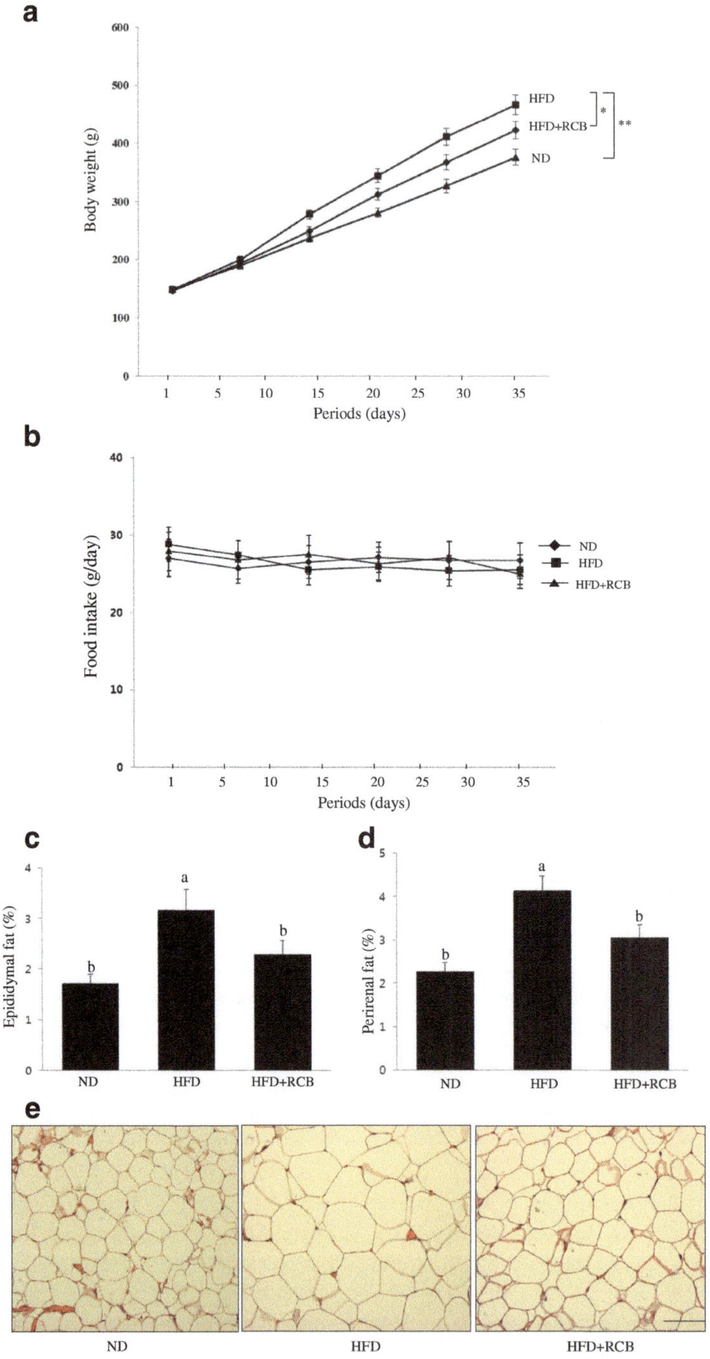

Fig. 4 (See legend on next page.)

(See figure on previous page.)

Fig. 4 Effects of RCB extracts on body weight in HFD-induced obese rats. **a** Body weight gain. The rats were divided into three groups ($n = 10$): an ND group given a normal diet (ND), an HFD group fed an HFD, and an HFD + RCB group fed an HFD in addition to treatment with RCB (200 mg/kg BW) orally by gavage once a day for 5 weeks. There were significant differences between the body weights of the HFD and ND (**$P < 0.01$) and HFD and HFD + RCB groups (*$P < 0.05$) at the end of the experimental period. **b** Food intake. The mean daily food consumption was 26.7 g and no significant differences were found in food intake between ND and HFD groups. **c** Adipose tissue mass. The weight of the epididymal adipose tissue was measured by dividing fatty tissue weight by body weight (fatty tissue/body weight x 100). Values represent the means ± SD; $P < 0.05$, as shown by ANOVA. Bars labeled with different letters indicate significant differences at according to Duncan's multiple range test. **d** The weight of the perirenal adipose tissue was measured by dividing fatty tissue weight by body weight (fatty tissue/body weight x 100). The data presented are the mean ± SD from three independent experiments. Values represent the means ± SD; $P < 0.05$ as shown by ANOVA. Different letters (**a** and **b**) mean that values are significantly different among groups. **e** Representative hematoxylin and eosin-stained sections of epididymal adipose tissue. The adipocyte sizes from the HFD + RCB group were smaller than those from the HFD only group. The scale bar is 100 μm

cluster of risk factors that occur simultaneously, including insulin resistance, obesity, hypertension, and dyslipidemia, all of which considerably increase the risk of developing cardiovascular disease and type 2 diabetes mellitus [29]. Among these risk factors, obesity correlates most strongly with the prevalence of metabolic syndrome [30]. Due to the severe side effects of anti-obesity drugs, natural products for treating obesity have been recognized to be beneficial as an alternative.

In the present study, we investigated the anti-adipogenic effects of RCB in 3 T3-L1 adipocytes and evaluated its anti-obesity properties in HFD-induced obese rats. RCB extract treatment decreased lipid droplet formation in 3 T3-L1 adipocytes and reduced triglyceride accumulation in RCB-treated 3 T3-L1 adipocytes when used at a concentration of 150 μg/ml; these effects were not due to cellular cytotoxicity. These results demonstrate that RCB inhibits the differentiation of 3 T3-L1 preadipocytes into adipocytes as well as the accumulation of lipid droplets in cytoplasm, which is an adipocyte phenotype that occurs following differentiation based on lipid accumulation.

Differentiation-associated lipid accumulation was accompanied by induction of the adipogenic transcription factors C/EBPα and PPARγ, which are active during the early stages of adipocyte differentiation and stimulate the expression of numerous metabolic genes to produce an adipocyte phenotype [31]. C/EBPα induces the autoactivation of its own transcription as well as PPARγ expression, and it maintains the expression levels of PPARγ and C/EBPα, which enables PPARγ to stimulate adipocyte differentiation. Rosen et al. [32] reported that C/EBPα supports adipocyte-specific gene expression in the presence of PPARγ in genes associated with cell morphology and lipid accumulation. In the present study, we found that treatment of 3 T3-L1 adipocytes with RCB extract exhibited decreased mRNA expression and protein expression of C/EBPα and PPARγ, which are master regulators of adipocyte differentiation. Moreover, our data indicated that the exposure of 3 T3-L1 adipocytes to RCB extract significantly decreased the expression levels of aP2 and FAS compared to differentiated 3 T3-L1 adipocyte cells. aP2, a member of the cytoplasmic fatty acid-binding protein family, has been detected in adipose tissue, and its expression is highly regulated during the differentiation of adipocytes [33]. FAS is a lipogenic enzyme that stimulates triglyceride synthesis and facilitates fatty acid storage in the cell cytoplasm [34]. PPARγ activation is required for proper functioning of the fat-selective enhancement of the aP2 and FAS genes in adipocytes [5]. Overall, we suggested that RCB inhibited adipocyte differentiation by reducing the expression of adipocyte-specific factors, including C/EBPβ, C/EBPα, and PPARγ, which leads to the downregulation of lipogenesis-related genes, such as aP2 and FAS.

Activation of the Akt pathway during adipogenesis has been shown to promote differentiation by activating factors that regulate the C/EBP family and PPARγ expression [9]. Insulin signaling activates Akt through PI3K and induces the serine/threonine phosphorylation of downstream targets, such as GSK3β [35]. Expression of a constitutively active variant of Akt kinase in 3 T3-L1 cells has been shown to result in the spontaneous differentiation of fibroblasts into adipocytes, which is associated with the increased accumulation of lipid droplets [13]. A previous study used LY294002 to demonstrate that the function of PI3-kinase was indispensable to lipid accumulation in 3 T3-L1 adipocytes. Thus, the PI3-kinase and Akt kinase pathways play pivotal roles in terminal adipocyte differentiation. Therefore, to explore the above-mentioned question, we examined whether RCB increased TG accumulation and the expression of adipocyte-related genes through the Akt signaling pathway.

In the present study, we showed that RCB caused a marked attenuation in Akt phosphorylation induced by insulin in a dose-dependent manner. RCB extract treatment also strongly suppressed insulin-induced GSK3β phosphorylation in 3 T3-L1 adipocytes. DMI induced a strong increase in the Akt phosphorylation in 3 T3-L1 cells, which is consistent with the observed enhancement in Akt activation. Moreover, treatment of 3 T3-L1 cells with a combination of LY294002 and RCB showed significantly stronger inhibitory effects on triglyceride

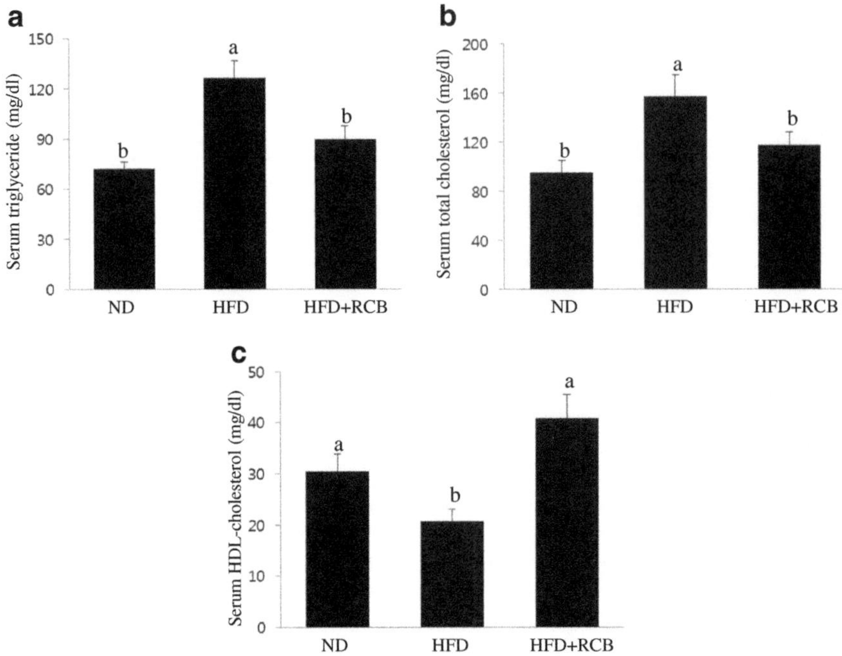

Fig. 5 Effect of RCB on lipid content in HFD-induced obese rats. **a** Serum triglyceride level. The RCB extract-administered group showed significantly lower levels of serum triglyceride compared with the HFD group. Data are expressed as the means ± SD. Differences among multiple groups were analyzed with ANOVA followed by Duncan's multiple range test. Different letters (**a** and **b**) indicate that the column means are significantly different at $P < 0.05$. **b** Total cholesterol level. Total cholesterol level decreased in the RCB-treated groups compared to the HFD only group. The results are presented as the means ± SD. Different letters (**a** and **b**) indicate that the column means are significantly different; $p < 0.05$ according to Duncan's multiple range test. **c** HDL cholesterol level. A significant difference was observed in HDL cholesterol levels between the HFD and HFD + RCB groups. The values are expressed as the means ± SD. Different letters (**a** and **b**) on the each bar graph mean that values are significantly different among groups; $p < 0.05$ according to Duncan's multiple range test

accumulation than treatment with RCB alone. In addition, our present results confirmed that the level of Akt phosphorylation decreased significantly after RCB extract treatment, which also significantly reduced insulin-stimulated glucose uptake, indicating that the Akt signaling pathway might be involved in the inhibitory effect of RCB on 3 T3-L1 adipocyte differentiation. Based on these findings, we concluded that RCB acts through Akt kinase pathways, resulting in decreased levels of TG accumulation and adipocyte-related gene expression. Therefore, our results suggest that the inhibition of Akt phosphorylation and activation via RCB blocked insulin-induced adipocyte differentiation in 3 T3-L1 pre-adipocytes.

Previous studies have revealed that the fruits of raspberry species have essential positive effects on the human diet and human health, which are likely mainly due to their medicinally active phytochemicals, such as polyphenols, various flavonoids (such as anthocyanins and flavanols), condensed and hydrolysable tannins and phenolic acid derivatives [36]. The major polyphenols in raspberries are anthocyanins and ellagitannins [37, 38], which comprise > 90 % of the total phenolic content of the fruit. Many studies have shown that the polyphenols present in green tea, Schisandra chinensis, blueberry peel, and grapefruit combat adipogenesis at the molecular level and also induce lipolysis [27, 39]. The administration of *Rubus coreanus* (RC) to HFD-fed mice combined with exercise has previously been shown to accelerate energy expenditure and protect against oxidative stress [40]. RC exerts an anti-obesity effect by upregulating Carnitine palmitoyl transferase I (CPT1) and elevating antioxidant levels [40]. In the present study, our data revealed that RCB exhibited free radical scavenging activity similar to DPPH, superoxide anion and hydroxyl radicals, and displayed potent antioxidant activity correlated with levels of strong phenols and flavonoids.

Adipose mass, which reflects the average adipocyte size and total adipocyte number, is increased in obese individuals. Adipogenesis occurs when extra fat mass is required for caloric gain or for cellular homeostasis [41]. Increased sizes (hypertrophy) and numbers (hyperplasia) of fat cells were present in the HFD-induced obese rats in the current study. Adipose tissue hyperplasia is a result of increased adipogenesis, which includes preadipocyte proliferation and adipocyte differentiation. We investigated whether RCB modulates obesity in HFD-induced obese rats. These results showed that the body weights of rats that were fed a HFD plus RCB extract were significantly reduced and comparable to those of rats that were fed a control HFD diet.

To examine whether the reduction in body weight gain exhibited by the RCB-treated group was related to decreased fat accumulation, epididymal and perirenal adipose tissues were weighed. The weights of both of these tissue types were significantly reduced in the RCB-treated group compared to the HFD group, indicating that the alleviation of obesity in the RCB-treated rats was due to reduced adiposity in adipose tissues. In addition to the effects of RCB on epididymal fat mass, histological examinations of the epididymal adipose tissues revealed that RCB extract greatly decreased the average size of adipocytes in the HFD-induced obese rats. The adipocyte size in epididymal adipose tissue was 26 % lower in the HFD-RCB group compared to the adipocyte size in the HFD group, which further demonstrated that the reduction in body weight gain was primarily due to decreased fat accumulation in adipocytes.

Excessive body weight gain causes obesity-related health problems and dyslipidemia, characterized by an increase in circulating triglycerides and a decrease in high-density lipoprotein cholesterol (HDL-C) [42, 43]. In particular, triglyceride accumulation is mainly responsible for weight gain or adiposity, accelerating the development of obesity and metabolic diseases. In parallel with its effect on body weight, we also found that RCB extract supplementation significantly decreased serum TG and TC levels and increased serum HDL-C level, indicating that RCB efficiently prevents abnormal metabolism of TC and cholesterol in HFD-induced obese rats. Therefore, our results demonstrate that the effects of RCB supplementation were much more evident with respect to reductions of adipose tissue mass compared to body weight gain. Overall, these results may shed light on the fact that RCB suppressed HFD-induced increases in adipose tissue mass and body weight gain, which may reflect the influence of adipose tissue metabolism, particularly by increasing lipid excretion.

Conclusion

In the present study, we investigated the anti-obesity effects of RCB on adipocyte differentiation and the associated mechanisms in 3 T3-L1 cells, and we confirmed our findings in a rat model of obesity that was induced with a HFD. Treatment with RCB extract significantly inhibited the expression of C/EBPβ and subsequently downregulated the activation of the key transcriptional regulators C/EBPα and PPARγ in 3 T3-L1 adipocytes. The phosphorylation levels of Akt and its substrate GSK3β were significantly reduced in response to RCB treatment, suggesting that RCB induced the inhibition of adipogenesis by regulating Akt phosphorylation and the upstream signaling of C/EBPα and PPARγ in 3 T3-L1 cells. Moreover, RCB significantly decreased body weight gain, body fat accumulation, and serum TG and TC levels in HFD-induced obese rats, which can prevent the development of HFD-induced obesity. Our results in cell lines and animal studies revealed that the anti-obesity effects of RCB were caused by decreased adipogenesis. It may be worthwhile to explore whether RCB could serve as a suitable candidate for enhancing anti-obesity activity or the development of therapeutic supplements for obesity.

Additional file

Additional file 1: Effects of supplementing RCB on body weight gain, and serum profiles in rats fed a high fat diet for two weeks. (A) Weight gain, (B) serum triglyceride level, and (C) total cholesterol level. The values are expressed as the mean ± SD. The bars showing different letters indicate significant differences among each group of bars, according to Duncan's test; $^*p < 0.05$. (ZIP 90 kb)

Abbreviations

RCB: rubus crataegifolius bunge; FAS: fatty acid synthase; HFD: high-fat diet; C/EBPδ: CCAAT/enhancer binding protein-δ; C/EBPα: CCAAT/enhancer binding protein-α; PPARγ: peroxisome proliferator-activated receptor-γ; HDL-C: high-density lipoprotein-cholesterol; PI3K: phosphoinositide 3-kinase; TG: triglyceride; aP2: adipocyte fatty acid-binding protein 2; DPPH: 2,2-diphenyl-1-picrylhydrazyl; HRSA: hydroxyl radial scavenging activity; SRSA: superoxide anion radical scavenging activity; TPC: total phenolic acid; MIX: 3-isobutyl-1-methylxanthine; DEX: dexamethasone; TC: total cholesterol; HDL-C: high-density lipoprotein-cholesterol; FAS: fatty acid synthase CE, catechin equivalents; QE: quercetin equivalents; HPLC: high-performance liquid chromatography; NBT: nitroblue tetrazolium; CPT1: Carnitine palmitoyl transferase I.

Competing interests

The authors declare that they have no competing interest.

Authors' contributions

MSJ, SJL, YS, SHJ, and WM performed the experiments. CKW, THK and HDK conceived the idea, designed the experiments, and interpreted the experimental results. JHC participated in the study design, data analyses and writing the manuscript. All authors read and approved the final manuscript.

Acknowledgement

This work was supported by the Ministry of Education, Basic Science Research Program, National Research Foundation, Korea (No. 2014045966).

Author details

[1]Institute of Animal Medicine, College of Veterinary Medicine, Gyeongsang National University, Jinju 660-701, Korea. [2]Department of Foods and Nutrition, Gyeongsang National University, Jinju 660-701, Korea. [3]Department of Environmental Health Science, New York Medical College, Valhalla, NY 10595, USA. [4]Department of Food Science and Biotechnology, Daegu University, Gyeongsan 38453, Korea. [5]College of Veterinary Medicine, Gyeongsang National University, Jiju Daero 501, Jinju-city, Gyeongsangnamdo 660-701, Korea.

References

1. Lee JY, Hashizaki H, Goto T, Sakamoto T, Takahashi N, Kawada T. Activation of peroxisome proliferator-activated receptor-a enhances fatty acid

oxidation in human adipocytes. Biochem Biophys Res Commun. 2011; 407(4):818–22.
2. Tang QQ, Jiang MS, Lane MD. Repressive effect of Sp1 on the C/EBPalpha gene promoter: role in adipocyte differentiation. Mol Cell Biol. 1999;19(7): 4855–65.
3. Frühbeck G, Gómez-Ambrosi J, Muruzábal FJ, Burrell MA. The adipocyte: a model for integration of endocrine and metabolic signaling in energy metabolism regulation. Am J Physiol Endocrinol Metab. 2001;280(6):E827–47.
4. Jeon T, Hwang SG, Hirai S, Matsui T, Yano H, Kawada T, et al. Red yeast rice extracts suppress adipogenesis by down-regulating adipogenic transcription factors and gene expression in 3 T3-L1 cells. Life Sci. 2004;12(26):3195–203.
5. Cristancho AG, Lazar MA. Forming functional fat: a growing understanding of adipocyte differentiation. Nat Rev Mol Cell Biol. 2011;28:722–34.
6. Tang QQ, Zhang JW, Daniel LM. Sequential gene promoter interactions of C/EBPb, C/EBPa, and PPARg during adipogenesis. Biochem Biophys Res Commun. 2004;319(1):235–9.
7. Jefcoate CR, Wang S, Liu X. Methods that resolve different contributions of clonal expansion to adipogenesis in 3 T3-L1 and C3H10T1/2 cells. Methods Mol Biol. 2008;456:173–93.
8. Green CJ, Göransson O, Kular GS, Leslie NR, Gray A, Alessi DR, et al. Use of Akt inhibitor and a drug-resistant mutant validates a critical role for protein kinase B/Akt in the insulin-dependent regulation of glucose and system a amino acid uptake. J Biol Chem. 2008;283(41):27653–67.
9. Peng XD, Xu PZ, Chen ML, Hahn-Windgassen A, Skeen J, Jacobs J, et al. Dwarfism, impaired skin development, skeletal muscle atrophy, delayed bone development, and impeded adipogenesis in mice lacking Akt1 and Akt2. Genes Dev. 2003;17(11):1352–65.
10. Xia X, Serrero G. Inhibition of adipose differentiation by phosphatidylinositol 3-kinase inhibitors. J Cell Physiol. 1999;178(1):9–16.
11. Tomiyama K, Nakata H, Sasa H, Arimura S, Nishio E, Watanabe Y. Wortmannin, a specific phosphatidylinositol 3-kinase inhibitor, inhibits adipocytic differentiation of 3 T3-L1 cells. Biochem Biophys Res Commun. 1995;212(1):263–9.
12. Sakaue H, Ogawa W, Matsumoto M, Kuroda S, Takata M, Sugimoto T, et al. Posttranscriptional control of adipocyte differentiation through activation of phosphoinositide 3-kinase. J Biol Chem. 1998;273(44):28945–52.
13. Xu J, Liao K. Protein kinase B/Akt 1 plays a pivotal role in insulin-like growth factor-1 receptor signaling induced 3 T3-L1 adipocyte differentiation. J Biol Chem. 2004;279(34):35914–22.
14. Bushakra JM, Stephens MJ, Atmadjaja AN, Lewers KS, Symonds W, Udall JA, et al. Construction of black (Rubus occidentalis) and red (R idaeus) raspberry linkage maps and their comparison to the genomes of strawberry, apple, and peach. Theor Appl Genet. 2012;125(2):311–27.
15. Hummer KE. Rubus pharmacology: antiquity to the present. Hortscience. 2010;45:1587–91.
16. Oh MS, Yang WM, Changa MS, Park W, Kim DR, Lee HK, et al. Effects of *Rubus coreanus* on sperm parameters and cAMP-responsive element modulator (CREM) expression in rat testes. J Ethnopharmacol. 2007; 114(3):463–7.
17. Du G, Lin H, Xu Q. J, China Pharm Univ. 2001;32:468–70.
18. Montrose DC, Horelik NA, Madigan JP, Stoner GD, Wang LS, Bruno RS, et al. Antiinflammatory effects of freeze-dried black raspberry powder in ulcerative colitis. Carcinogenesis. 2011;32(3):343–50.
19. Ash MM, Wolford KA, Carden TJ, Hwang KT, Carr TP. Unrefined and refined black raspberry seed oils significantly lower triglycerides and moderately affect cholesterol metabolism in male Syrian hamsters. J Med Food. 2011; 14(9):1032–8.
20. Chen HS, Liu M, Shi LJ, Zhao JL, Zhang CP, Lin LQ, et al. Effects of raspberry phytochemical extract on cell proliferation, apoptosis, and serum proteomics in a rat model. J Food Sci. 2011;76(8):T192–8.
21. Singleton VL, Rossi JR. Colorimetry of total phenolics with phosphomolybdic-phosphotungstic acid. Am J Enol Vitic. 1965;16:144–58.
22. Singleton VL, Orthofer R, Lamuela-Raventos RM. Analysis of total phenols and other oxidation substrates and antioxidants by means of Folin–Ciocalteu reagent. Methods Enzymol. 1999;299:152–78.
23. Meda A, Lamien CE, Romito M, Millogo J, Nacoulma OG. Determination of the total phenolic, flavonoid and proline contents in Burkina. Fasan honey, as well as their radical scavenging activity. Food Chem. 2005;91(3):571–7.
24. Brand-Williams W, Cuvelier ME, Berset C. Use of a free radical method to evaluate antioxidant activity. LWT-Food Sci Technol. 1995;28:25–30.
25. Liu F, Ooi VEC, Chang ST. Free radical scavenging activity of mushroom polysaccharide extracts. Life Sci. 1997;60(10):763–71.
26. Lopes GK, Schulman HM, Hermes-Lima M. Polyphenol tannic acid inhibits hydroxyl radical formation from Fenton reaction by complexing ferrous ions. Biochim Biophy Acta. 1999;1472(1–2):142–52.
27. Park HJ, Yun J, Jang SH, Kang SN, Jeon BS, Ko YG, et al. Coprinus comatus cap inhibits adipocyte differentiation via regulation of PPARγ and Akt signaling pathway. PLoS One. 2014;9(9):e105809.
28. Zou C, Wang Y, Shen Z. 2-NBDG as a fluorescent indicator for direct glucose uptake measurement. J Biochem Biophys Methods. 2005;64(3):207–15.
29. Plutzky J. Emerging concepts in metabolic abnormalities associated with coronary artery disease. Curr Opin Cardiol. 2000;15(6):416–21.
30. Weiss R, Dziura J, Burgert TS, Tamborlane WV, Taksali SE, Yeckel CW, et al. Obesity and the metabolic syndrome in children and adolescents. N Engl J Med. 2004;350(23):2362–74.
31. Gregoire FM, Smas CM, Sul HS. Understanding adipocyte differentiation. Physiol Rev. 1998;78(3):783–809.
32. Rosen ED, Hsu CH, Wang X, Sakai S, Freeman MW, Gonzalez FJ, et al. C/EBPalpha induces adipogenesis through PPARgamma: a unified pathway. Genes Dev. 2002;16(1):22–6.
33. Glatz JF, B¨orchers T, Spener F, Van Der Vusse GJ. Fatty acids in cell signalling: Modulation by lipid binding proteins. Prostaglandins Leukot Essent Fatty Acids. 1995;52(2–3):121–7.
34. Claycombe KJ, Jones BH, Standridge MK, Guo Y, Chun JT, et al. Insulin increases fatty acid synthase gene transcription in human adipocytes. Am J Physiol. 1998;274(5 Pt 2):1253–9.
35. Summers SA, Kao AW, Kohn AD, Backus GS, Roth RA, Pessin JE, et al. The role of glycogen Synthase Kinase 3β in Insulin-stimulated Glucose Metabolism. J Biol Chem. 1999;274(25):17934–40.
36. Kahkonen MP, Hopia AI, Heinonen M. Berry phenolics and their antioxidant activity. J Agric Food Chem. 2001;49(8):4076–82.
37. Dobson P, Graham J, Stewart D, Brennan R, Hackett CA, McDougall GJ. Over-seasons analysis of quantitative trait loci affecting phenolic content and antioxidant capacity in raspberry. J Agric Food Chem. 2012;60(21):5360–6.
38. Mullen W, McGinn J, Lean MEJ, MacLean MR, Gardner P, Duthie GG, et al. Ellagitannins, flavonoids, and other phenolics in red raspberries and their contribution to antioxidant capacity and vasorelaxation properties. J Agric Food Chem. 2002;50(18):5191–6.
39. Park HJ, Cho JY, Kim MK, Koh PO, Cho KW, Kim CH, et al. Anti-obesity effect of Schisandra chinensis in 3 T3-L1 cells and high fat diet-induced obese rats. Food Chem. 2012;134(2012):227–34.
40. Chung C, You Y, Yoon HG, Kim K, Lee YH, Lee J, et al. Alleviation of weight-gain in mice by an ethanolic extract from Rubus coreanus under conditions of a high-fat diet and exercise. Biosci Biotechnol Biochem. 2013;77(10):2148–50.
41. Rosen ED. The molecular control of adipogenesis, with special reference to lymphatic pathology. Ann N Y Acad Sci. 2002;979:143–58.
42. Paccaud F, Schlüter-Fasmeyer V, Wietlisbach V, Bovet P. Dyslipidemia and abdominal obesity: an assessment in three general populations. J Clin Epidemiol. 2000;53(4):393–400.
43. Modan M, Halkin H, Almog S, Lusky A, Eshkol A, Shefi M, et al. Hyperinsulinemia. A link between hypertension obesity and glucose intolerance. J Clin Invest. 1985;75(3):809–17.

13

Metabolism and bioavailability of newly developed dietary fiber materials, resistant glucan and hydrogenated resistant glucan, in rats and humans

Sadako Nakamura[1,2], Kenichi Tanabe[2,3], Shigeki Morita[2], Norihisa Hamaguchi[4], Fumio Shimura[1] and Tsuneyuki Oku[1,2*]

Abstract

Background: Resistant glucan (RG) and hydrogenated resistant glucan (HRG) are new dietary fiber materials developed to decrease the risk of metabolic syndrome and lifestyle-related diseases. We investigated the metabolism and bioavailability of RG and HRG using rats and humans.

Methods: Purified RG and HRG were used as test substances. After 25 Wistar male rats (270 g) were fed with an experimental diet (AIN93M diet with the cellulose replaced by β-corn starch) *ad libitum* for 1 week, they were used for the experiment involving blood collection and circulating air collection. Ten participants (5 males, 22.5 y, BMI 20.4 kg/m^2; 5 females, 25.8 y, BMI 20.9 kg/m^2) voluntarily participated in this study. The study was carried out using a within-subject, repeated measures design. Effects of RG and HRG on the response for blood glucose and insulin and hydrogen excretion were compared with those of glucose and a typical nondigestible and fermentable fructooligosaccharide (FOS) in rats and humans. Available energy was evaluated using the fermentability based on breath hydrogen excretion.

Results: When purified RG or HRG (400 mg) was administered orally to rats, blood glucose and insulin increased slightly, but less than when glucose was administration ($P < 0.05$). Hydrogen started to be excreted 120 min after administration of RG with negligibly small peak at 180 min, thereafter excreted scarcely until 1440 min. Hydrogen excretion after HRG administration showed a larger peak than RG at 180 min, but was markedly less than FOS. RG and HRG were excreted in feces, but not urine. When purified RG or HRG (30 g) were ingested by healthy humans, blood glucose and insulin levels increased scarcely. Breath hydrogen excretion increased slightly, but remarkably less than FOS. Ingestion of purified RG or HRG (5 g) to evaluate available energy, increased scarcely glucose and insulin levels and breath hydrogen excretion. Available energy was evaluated as 0 kcal/g for purified RG and 1 kcal/g for HRG.

Conclusion: The bioavailability was very low in both humans and rats, because oligosaccharide of minor component in purified RG and HRG was metabolized via intestinal microbes but major components with higher molecular weight were metabolized scarcely. Moreover, the ingestion of 30 g of RG or HRG did not induce apparent acute side effects in healthy adults. RG and HRG might potentially be used as new dietary fiber materials with low energy.

Keywords: Metabolism, Bioavailability, Available energy, Dietary fiber materials, Resistant glucan, Hydrogenated resistant glucan

* Correspondence: okutsune@sun.ac.jp
[1]Institute of Food, Nutrition and Health, Jumonji University, 2-1-28, Sugasawa, Niiza, Saitama 352-8510, Japan
[2]Graduate School of Human Health Science, University of Nagasaki Siebold, 1-1-1, Manabino, , Nagayo, Nagasaki 851-2195, Japan
Full list of author information is available at the end of the article

Background

Resistant glucan (RG) and hydrogenated resistant glucan (HRG) are new dietary fiber materials that have been developed to decrease the risk of metabolic syndrome and lifestyle-related diseases. RG is prepared by heating glucose at 180 °C in the presence of activated carbon [1], and is a mixture of monosaccharides, oligosaccharides and glucose polymers with an average molecular weight of approximately 2600. RG is a white odourless powder that is easily dissolved in cold water and can be widely used as a low energy bulking carbohydrate material. HRG is produced from RG by hydrogenation, and is more stable than RG toward degradation by the Maillard reaction [1].

In order to use widely RG and HRG as food materials, it is necessary to clarify the physiological effects of RG and HRG on the response for blood glucose and insulin, the occurrence of abdominal symptoms, the maximum non-effective dose for osmotic diarrhea, fermentability by intestinal microbes and metabolic fate. In addition, the available energy including nondigestible carbohydrates must be expressed as nutritional labeling in processed foods based on the Law of some countries [2, 3]. We have already proposed the indirect and simple method to evaluate the available energy of dietary fiber materials in healthy humans [4–6]. In accordance with our method, the digestibility is estimated based on the response of blood glucose and insulin and the fermentability is estimated by breath hydrogen excretion. In the present study, the metabolism and bioavailability of RG and HRG were investigated using rats and healthy human subjects and the available energy for purified RG and HRG was estimated by our proposed method.

In a previous study [7], it has been demonstrated that purified RG and HRG were consist of small amounts of glucose and digestible and fermentable oligosaccharides, and large amounts of nondigestible glucose polymers with high molecular weight. Purified RG and HRG are hydrolyzed to a limited extent by digestive enzymes, and did not inhibit small intestinal disaccharidases such as sucrase and maltase. These results agree roughly with the dietary fiber content of purified RG (99 %) and HRG (82 %), which have been measured by the enzymatic-high performance liquid chromatography (HPLC) method of the Association of Official Analytical Chemists (AOAC) 2001.03 method [8].

In rats, the ingestion of a diet containing 5 % of purified RG or HRG caused loose stools in consecutive feeding experiments. However, the growth and development of the rats were normal and no specific abnormal observations in the tissues and organs were inspected, except for a notable increase in the weight of cecal tissue and content. In addition, blood biochemical parameters such as glucose, insulin, total cholesterol, free fatty acid, total protein, AST and ALT *etc.* were normal in the RG, HRG, resistant maltodexitrin (RMD), fructoologosaccharide (FOS) and control groups and they were not significantly different among the five groups [7]. Furthermore, the abnormality is not detected in acute, subacute and chronic toxicity tests of RG [9]. Also, RG and HRG have been confirmed in the earlier work on the safety and stability of RG [1]. Therefore, RG and HRG seem to be safety as nondigestible carbohydrate materials.

RMD and polydextrose (PD) have been widely used in the processed foods and the health claim for its use in processed foods is potentially reduce the energy density [10–14]. The available energy is evaluated as 1 kcal/g for RMD and PD based on our proposed method [5]. Also, Auerbach, et al. [12] and Goda, et al. [14] report that the available energy is estimated as 1 kcal/g each for RMD and PD using different methods. The results obtained from in vitro and in vivo experiments for RG and HRG demonstrate that RG and HRG are notably resistant to hydrolysis by human α-amylase and small intestinal enzymes and are difficult to be fermented by intestinal microbes compared with RMD and PD [7]. Therefore, we hypothesize that the available energy of purified RG and HRG is less or at least the same than quality obtained from RMD and PD.

In the present study, prior to the human study, we performed a study using rats to investigate some physiological effects such as the response indicated by blood glucose and insulin, hydrogen excretion, and fecal and urinary excretion after single dose of the tested substances. Then, we carried out human experiments using a within-subject repeated measures design. The response of blood glucose and insulin, breath hydrogen excretion, the occurrence of abdominal symptoms, and fecal shape were investigated using healthy human subjects. In addition, the available energy of purified RG and HRG for human subjects was evaluated by an indirect and simple method based on fermentability using breath hydrogen excretion [4–6, 15, 16]. The results obtained will contribute to the practical application of RG and HRG for potentially decreasing the risk of metabolic syndrome and lifestyle-related diseases.

Methods

Ethical approval of the study protocol

All experiments complied with the code of ethics of the World Medical Association (Declaration of Helsinki, Oct. 2013). The study protocol involving human subjects was approved by the Ethical Committee of the University of Nagasaki (received No.184, approval No.177). All participants provided written informed consent to participate in the study.

The protocol for animal studies was approved by (approved No. 2011-15) the Committee on Animal

Experiments of the University of Nagasaki. These experiments were conducted according to the Guidelines on the Care and Use of Laboratory Animals (National Institutes of Health, MD, USA) and the standards relating to the Care and Management of Experimental Animals (Notification number 88, from the Prime Minister's Office). All experiments were carried out in the Public Health Nutrition Laboratory of the Graduate School of Human Health Science, University of Nagasaki Siebold.

Materials

Purified RG (Nihon Shokuhin Kako Co., Ltd., Tokyo, Japan) by removing mono- and di-saccharides from RG, was used to focus for the main components with degrees of polymerization (DP) of more than 2 in the present study, and HRG (Nihon Shokuhin Kako Co., Ltd.) was also used to compare with purified RG. RMD (Fibersol-2, dietary fiber content: 92 %, Matsutani Chemical Industry Co., Ltd., Hyogo, Japan), FOS (purity: > 99 %, Meiji Co., Ltd., formerly-Meiji Seika Kaisha Ltd., Tokyo, Japan) and glucose (Nihon Shokuhin Kako Co., Ltd.) were also used in the present study. Glucose was used as a reference of the response of blood glucose and insulin. RMD is a mixture of monosaccharides, oligosaccharides and glucose polymers with an average molecular weight of about 2000 [10, 11]. It was used as a reference of dietary fiber established already. FOS was used as a reference of a typical oligosaccharide that is not hydrolyzed by digestive enzymes and is fermented completely by intestinal microbes [17, 18] and consists of 1-kestose (39 %), nystose (53 %), and 1^F-β-fructofranosyl-nystose (7 %).

Animal experiments using rats

Animals and diets

To investigate the effect of RG and HRG on the response of blood glucose and insulin and the fermentability of RG and HRG by intestinal microbes, 25 Wistar male rats (270 g, Clea Japan Inc., Tokyo, Japan) as the previous studies [7, 17], were fed with an experimental diet *ad libitum* or 1 week. They were used twice: for the experiment involving blood collection and the experiment involving circulating air collection. The experimental diet was AIN93M diet [19] with the cellulose replaced by β-corn starch to exclude the effect of cellulose on the intestinal microflora. Rats were housed in individual stainless steel cages and kept at room temperature (22–24 °C). The relative humidity was maintained at 50–55 % with a 12-h light/dark cycle.

Experimental setup for determination of plasma glucose and insulin responses

The effects of glucose, RG, HRG and RMD on the response of blood glucose and insulin were investigated. Glucose was used as a control and RMD was used as a positive control, as it has been established previously as a dietary fiber material. The dose (400 mg) of test substance which does not cause loose stool in rat was dissolved in 2.5 ml of distilled water as the previous studies [18, 20]. The test solution was orally administered to a rat using a stomach tube after fasting for 16 h ($n = 5$ per group). Blood (120 μl) was collected from the rat's tail vein using heparinized hematocrit tubes at 30-min intervals until 180 min after administration of the test substance, and then the plasma was prepared by hematocrit centrifugation (3300, Kubota Co., Ltd., Tokyo, Japan) at 2000 × g, 20 °C for 5 min.

Glucose concentration was measured by the Trinder method using glucose oxidase [21]. After plasma (10 μl) was pipetted into a small test tube, glucose oxidase reagent (1.5 ml) was added and the test tube was incubated at 37 °C for 15 min. Then the test tube was steeped in boiling water for 150 s to stop the reaction. The absorbance was read immediately using a spectrophotometer (UVmini-1240, Shimadzu Corp., Kyoto, Japan) at a wavelength of 505 nm. The insulin concentration was measured immunologically by an ELISA kit (Morinaga Biochemical Institute Co., Kanagawa, Japan) using guinea pig-derived antibody [22].

Circulating air collection and analysis of hydrogen

The effects of FOS, RG, HRG and RMD on hydrogen excretion were also investigated using rats. FOS was used as a reference of typical nondigestible and fermentable oligosaccharide to compare fermentability. Each test solution was prepared as 400 mg in 2.5 ml distilled water. Five rats fed with the experimental diet and 15 rats fed with the experimental diet for 2 days after blood collection, were used in the experiment involving circulating air collection. Fifteen rats which had been used in the experiment of blood collection were administered with same test solution as the experiment of blood collection and five new rats were administered with FOS solution. The test solution (400 mg/2.5 ml) was orally administered to a rat ($n = 5$ per group) after fasting for 16 h. Then the rats were immediately moved to the Metabolica apparatus (5-gang, Sugiyamagen Co., Ltd., Tokyo, Japan) (Fig. 1) to collect the circulating air for hydrogen determination.

The flow rate of the circulating air in the apparatus was adjusted to 200 ± 30 ml/min. To obtain the initial value, 40 ml of circulating air was collected using a plastic syringe at 10 min after moving the rat into the apparatus. Then the circulating air was collected at 1-h intervals until 4 h, 2-h intervals from 4 h to 10 h, and at 24 h after administration of the test solution [23]. To avoid hunger, the experimental diet was fed to the rats at 4 h after administration of test solution. Five millilitres of the circulating

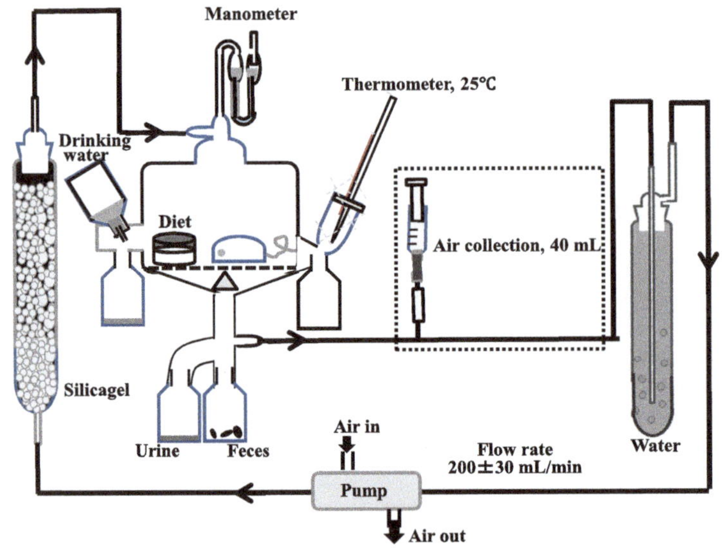

Fig. 1 Metabolica apparatus to collect the circulating air, urine and faeces of rats

air were loaded into a simple gas chromatograph (Breath Gas Analyzer BGA1000D, Laboratory for Expiration Biochemistry Nourishment Metabolism Co., Ltd., Nara, Japan) to measure the concentration of hydrogen.

Extraction of RG and HRG from feces and urine and analysis by HPLC

After RG or HRG (400 mg/2.5 ml) was orally administered to the rats, their urine and feces were collected separately using the Metabolica apparatus for 24 h. The collected feces were combined, stood for 10 min in boiling water to stop the reaction by microbes-derived enzymes and homogenized with 9 volumes of ice-cold 0.9 % NaCl using a homogenizer (Polytron; Kinematica Inc., Lucerne, Switzerland). Then the suspension was centrifuged under refrigeration (Himac CR22GII, Hitachikoki Co., Ltd., Tokyo, Japan) at 20,000 × g, 4 °C for 20 min. The precipitate was re-suspended with 4 volumes of 0.9 % NaCl and centrifuged again. The supernatants collected were combined and filtered through a membrane filter (0.22 μm × 13 mm; Millipore Corp., MA, USA) to remove bacteria and small pellets, then used in the HPLC analysis. The urine collected was measured the volume, and then was also filtered through a membrane filter (0.22 μm × 13 mm) to remove bacteria and small pellets.

The analysis of RG and HRG was carried out using an HPLC system (LC-20 AD; Shimadzu Corp.) using a refractive index detector (RID-10A; Shimadzu Corp.) and a Shodex SUGAR KS-802 column (8.0 ϕ × 300 mm; Showa Denko Co., Ltd., Tokyo, Japan). Analysis was performed at a column temperature of 70 °C. The sample (10 μl) was injected into the HPLC system and eluted with deionized distilled water at a flow rate of 0.5 ml/min [24]. The limit concentration of detection of glucose by HPLC analysis was 10 μg/ml.

Human experiments using healthy subjects

Participants

The present study involving human participants was carried out using a within-subject, repeated measures design. Each subject ingested repeatedly the test substance at intervals of 1-week or more. Ten healthy participants (5 males, 22.5 ± 1.7 year old, 59.7 ± 2.5 kg, BMI 20.4 ± 1.2 kg/m^2; 5 females, 25.8 ± 3.8 year old, 50.5 ± 4.0 kg, BMI 20.9 ± 1.1 kg/m^2) voluntarily participated in this study. The exclusion criteria were a history of gastrointestinal diseases, carbohydrate malabsorption, diabetes, obesity or pulmonary disease. The average value of fasting blood glucose concentration of the subjects was 4.6 ± 0.2 mmol/L and it was within normal range. Before the experiments, we ensured that all participants were hydrogen producers and not methane producers. The participants had not taken any antibiotics or laxatives in the 2 weeks before the experiments.

Preparation of test solutions

The effects of glucose, FOS, RG and HRG on blood glucose and insulin response and breath hydrogen excretion were investigated. Glucose was used as a control and FOS was used as a typical nondigestible and fermentable oligosaccharide. Thirty grams of glucose, RG or HRG were dissolved in 120 ml of warmed safety water as the previous studies [4, 5, 25–28]. The tolerance level of FOS, because of its osmotic effects in the large bowel, is 0.3 g/kg of body weight for Japanese normal people [6, 25]. Therefore, 5 g of FOS was dissolved in 120 ml of warmed safety water in accordance with our proposed method [4, 5, 25]. Five grams of RG or HRG were also dissolved in 120 ml of warmed safety water to evaluate available energy.

Special meals for experiments

The period during which the food intake of the subjects was restricted was very long. Hence, the experimental meals, from which hydrogen was not produced, were given to the subjects after the final blood collection, at 7 h and 11 h after ingestion of test substance. Canned tuna fish (Sea-chicken mild, 80 g, Hagoromo Food Co., Ltd., Shizuoka, Japan), boiled egg (50 g) and tea containing 10 g of table sugar were used as food materials for experimental meals. The energy supplied to the subjects on the experimental day was 895 ~ 970 kcal and protein was 58 ~ 65 g. If needed, tea containing sugars or boiled egg was given. In addition, each subject was given a multivitamin tablet containing mineral (Nature Made, Otsuka Pharmaceutical Co., Ltd., Tokyo, Japan) as a supplement every day during the experimental periods.

Experimental protocol

All test substances were given in a random order at intervals of 1-week or more. Experiments were carried out under the direction of a physician. The experimental protocol was carried out in accordance with the methods employed in our previous studies [4–6, 25–29].

After overnight fasting, the subjects came to our laboratory in the morning, their health status was examined and their blood pressure and pulse rate were measured. Then, 750 ml of end-expiratory gas were collected using a collection bag (Quin Tron Instrument Co., Inc., WI, USA) and 120 μl of blood from the fingertip using a heparinized hematocrit tube. After ingesting the test substance, the end-expiratory gas was collected at 1-h intervals until 14 h [4], and blood (120 μl) was collected at 30-min intervals until 180 min. Participants were prohibited from ingesting foods containing nondigestible carbohydrates for 3 days before each experimental day. During the experiment, they were also prohibited from ingesting foods or beverages except for warmed water and tea, as well as from sleeping and smoking. Subjects were required to sit on a chair and were prohibited from exercising with hyperventilation until the final collection of end-respiratory gas. Participants ingested an experimental meal that did not produce breath hydrogen, so that they would not feel hungry.

After ingesting the test substance, the type and onset time of abdominal symptoms, the frequency of defecation and the macroscopic observation of stool shape were recorded by the participants themselves using constructed format. The research supervisor explained to all participants the method for self-recording and classifying the stool shape and abdominal symptoms, and then confirmed their recordings, when they were received. The examination of stools used the following descriptors: stage 1, very hard; stage 2, hard; stage 3, normal; stage 4, soft; stage 5, very soft; and stage 6, watery [30]. The questionnaire on abdominal symptoms were asked to the subjects about their experience of upper and lower abdominal pain, vomiting, nausea, thirst, flatus, distension, and borborygmus for 14 h after ingesting the test substance.

Assay of plasma glucose and insulin and analysis of breath hydrogen

The plasma glucose and insulin concentrations and hydrogen in the end-expiratory gas were measured by the methods described above.

Evaluation of relative available energy of RG and HRG

An indication of energy content is an essential item for the nutritional labelling of processed foods [2, 3]. The available energy in dietary fiber materials and nondigestible oligosaccharides can be evaluated using an indirect and simple method based on the breath hydrogen excretion which reflects the fermentability of nondigestible carbohydrate [4–6, 25]. As energy production is dependent on the fermentability of nondigestible carbohydrates, the available energy can be categorized to 0 kcal/g, 1 kcal/g and 2 kcal/g. Available energy was calculated based on the ratio of fermentability versus FOS, which has 2 kcal/g of available energy, in the present study [15, 16].

To evaluate the available energy of RG and HRG using the indirect and simple method based on fermentability, 5 g of the test substance were ingested by a healthy subject as well as other dietary fiber materials. The end-respiratory gas was collected to measure hydrogen excretion for 14 h after ingestion. FOS (2 kcal/g) was used as a convenient reference to estimate the relative fermentability [4, 5, 25].

Calculations and Statistical analyses

We calculated the means and standard deviations in blood glucose, insulin and concentration of hydrogen excretion in rats and humans. Evaluation of the available energy in humans was calculated based on the ratio [4, 5]. The ratio was calculated based on the areas under the curve (AUC) of hydrogen excretion by the ingestion of test materials versus that of FOS. Thereafter, the available energy was classified into 0 kcal/g, 1 kcal/g and 2 kcal/g as described above. The normal distribution was tested, and the data with normal distribution were compared with control (reference) using ANOVA and Dunnett's *post hoc* test or Tukey's *post hoc* test, and non-normal distribution data were compared using non-parametric analysis by Steel or

Steel-Dwass method. A *P*-value less than 0.05 obtained two-sided analysis was considered as significant using SPSS for Windows 20.0 (SPSS Inc., Tokyo, Japan).

Results

Animal experiments using rats

The effects of RG and HRG administration on blood glucose and insulin levels

The plasma glucose and insulin concentrations increased spontaneously at 30 min after glucose (400 mg/2.5 ml) was administered orally to rats (Fig. 2a, b). The results show that the response of blood glucose and insulin is normal in rats. For RG administration, the plasma glucose level increased to 5.6 mmol/L and plasma insulin level reached at more than 450 pg/mL at 30 min after administration. The response of plasma glucose and insulin after administration of HRG and RMD was similar to that of RG and not significantly different among three test substances. Moreover, the response of plasma glucose and insulin after administration of RG, HRG and RMD were significantly lower than those of the administration of glucose ($P < 0.05$). These results suggest that when RG and HRG are given orally to rats, they are partially hydrolyzed by gastrointestinal enzymes and cause similar increases in blood glucose and insulin levels.

The effects of RG and HRG administration on hydrogen excretion

We considered that the excretion profile of hydrogen was normal, because when FOS (400 mg/2.5 ml) was given to rats, hydrogen which is produced only through fermentation by intestinal microbes, started to excrete about 120 min after administration and reached the maximum (80 ppm) at 480 min (8 h) (Fig. 3). For purified RG (400 mg/2.5 ml), hydrogen was excreted less than 10 ppm about 120 min after administration and then decreased to the basal level at 360 min. Hydrogen excretion after HRG administration (400 mg/2.5 ml) exhibited a similar behaviour to that of RG and was not significantly different. Hydrogen excretions of RG and HRG were significantly lower than that of FOS ($P < 0.05$). Hydrogen excretion after RMD administration showed a different pattern from that of RG and HRG, and it was significantly lower compared with that of FOS ($P < 0.05$).

Urinary and fecal excretion of RG and HRG administered to rats fed with control diet

After RG or HRG (400 mg/2.5 ml) was orally administered to rats fed with the experimental diet, urine and feces were separately collected with the Metabolica apparatus for 24 h. Neither RG nor HRG were detected in the urine, but 20.4 % of the RG and 23.2 % of the HRG administered were excreted into feces for 24 h.

Human experiments using healthy subjects

Subject participation

No participants dropped out of the study and experienced side effects. Their health status throughout the entire study period was well. The average intake of energy by a participant was 935 kcal/day and that of protein was 61 g/day.

The effects of ingestion of RG and HRG on blood glucose and insulin levels and breath hydrogen excretion

Figure 4 shows the changes in blood glucose and insulin levels after the ingestion of 30 g of glucose, purified RG or HRG by healthy participants. As the incremental blood glucose concentration was approximately 3.1 mmol/L at 30 min after the ingestion of glucose, the participants were

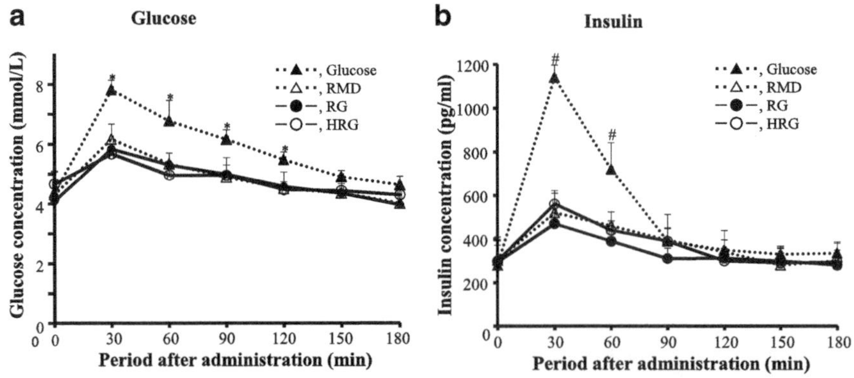

Fig. 2 Changes of blood glucose and insulin levels after oral administration of RG, HRG or RMD to rats fed with an experimental diet. RG, resistant glucan; HRG, hydrogenated resistant glucan; RMD, resistant maltodextrin. Test substance (400 mg/2.5 ml) was administered orally to each rat which was fed with an experimental diet (n = 5 per group) and blood was collected from the tail vein at indicated periods. Values were means ± SD. *,#, The elevation of glucose in RG, HRG, and RMD were significantly lower than that of glucose at each time point, at $P < 0.05$ by Dunnett's *post hoc* test. There was no significantly difference among RG, HRG, and RMD by Tukey's *post hoc* test

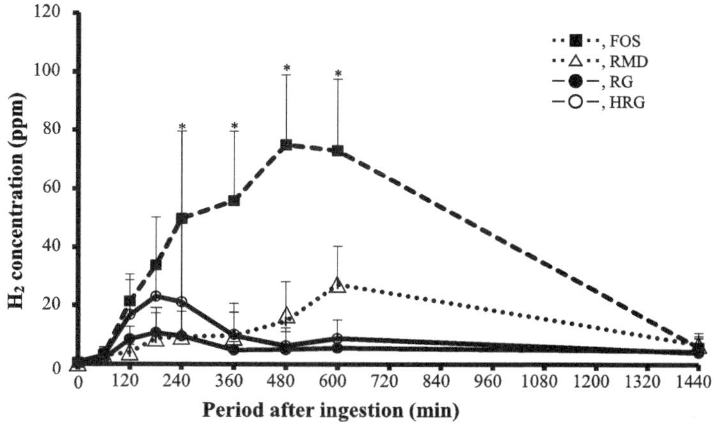

Fig. 3 Changes of hydrogen excretion after oral administration of RG HRG or RMD to rats fed with an experimental diet. FOS, fructooligosaccharide; RG, resistant glucan; HRG, hydrogenated resistant glucan; RMD, resistant maltodextrin. Immediately after test substance (400 mg/2.5 ml) was orally administered to each rat fed with an experimental diet ($n = 5$ per group), rats were moved to the Metabolica apparatus to collect circulating air. Values were means ± SD. *, The excretion of hydrogen was significantly lower in RG, HRG and RMD than in FOS at each peak point, at $P < 0.05$ by Steel method. There was no significant difference among RG, HRG, and RMD by Steel-Dwass method

normally tolerant of glucose. After ingestion of RG or HRG, both the blood glucose and insulin concentrations showed no incremental response. Blood glucose and insulin concentrations in RG ingestion were significantly lower than that of glucose administration at 30 min after ingestion ($P < 0.05$). Also, blood glucose and insulin concentrations in HRG ingestion were distinctly lower than that of glucose administration at 30 min as well as RG. These results which blood glucose and insulin concentrations increase scarcely after ingestion of RG or HRG are distinctly different from the results observed in rats.

The participants enrolled in the present study, were normal responders to breath gas test. When FOS (5 g), which is not digested by intestinal enzymes and is completely fermented by intestinal microbes, was ingested by healthy participants, no increasing on blood glucose and insulin concentration was observed (data not shown). The breath hydrogen started to excrete at 3 h after ingestion and showed a peak (23 ± 9 ppm) at 6 h after administration (Fig. 5a). Thereafter, it decreased gradually, but continued to excrete over 14 h until the end of the experiment. In the ingestion of purified RG (30 g), breath hydrogen started to excrete slightly at 1 h after ingestion, and then showed a flat without a clear peak during 2-4 h after ingestion. Thereafter, hydrogen was excreted scarcely up to the end of the experiment (Fig. 5a). Although breath hydrogen from ingesting HRG (30 g)

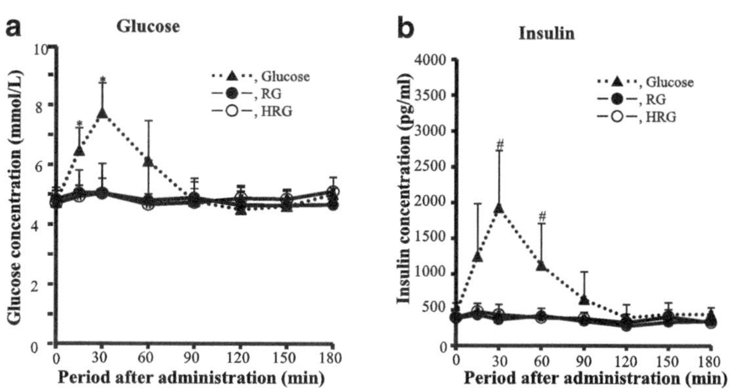

Fig. 4 Change of plasma glucose and insulin levels after ingestion of RG or HRG in healthy human subjects. RG, resistant glucan; HRG, hydrogenated resistant glucan. After overnight fasting, 30 g of test substance (glucose, Purified RG and HRG) were ingested by 10 healthy subjects and blood (120 μl) was collected from the tip of finger at 30 min-intervals for 180 min after ingestion. Values were means ± SD. *, #, Plasma glucose (**a**) and insulin (**b**) concentrations in RG or HRG administration were significantly lower than those in glucose administration at each peak point, at $P < 0.05$ by Dunnett's *post hoc* test for glucose (**a**) and by Steel method for insulin (**b**)

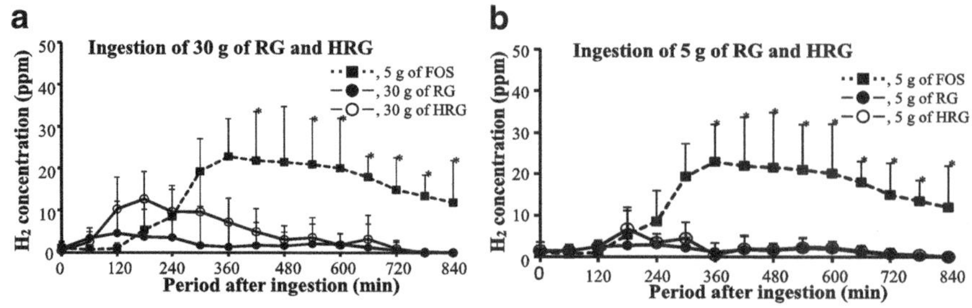

Fig. 5 Changes of breath hydrogen excretion after ingestion of RG or HRG in healthy human subjects. FOS, fructooligosaccharide; RG, resistant glucan; HRG, hydrogenated resistant glucan. Test solution containing 30 g of purified RG or HRG was ingested by 10 healthy subjects shown in Fig. 4 after overnight fasting, and end-respiratory gas (750 ml) was collected using collection bag at 1-h intervals for 14 h after ingestion (**a**). Furthermore, to evaluate the available energy test solution containing 5 g of purified RG or HRG was ingested by healthy subjects after overnight fasting (**b**). FOS (5 g) was used as a typical oligosaccharide which is nondigestible and completely fermentable. Figure 5-a shows the change of hydrogen excretion 14 h after ingestion of 30 g of test substance, and Fig. 5-b shows the change of hydrogen excretion 14 h after ingestion of 5 g of test substance. Values were means ± SD. *, The excretion of breath hydrogen in RG or HRG ingestion were significantly lower versus that in FOS ingestion, at $P < 0.05$ by Steel method. There was no significantly difference between RG and HRG by Steel-Dwass method

started to excrete clearly about 2 h later than that from RG, but it was not significantly different.

In the experiments to evaluate the available energy, hydrogen excretion after ingesting of RG (5 g) did not increase and showed a flat during the experiment. Also, hydrogen excretion after HRG ingestion (5 g) was less than 5 ppm at 3 h after ingestion and were markedly smaller compared with a peak value (23 ppm) at 6 h after FOS ingestion ($P < 0.05$) (Fig. 5b). Namely, hydrogen excretion after ingestion of RH or HRG (5 g) was very little and did not show a significant increment.

Table 1 shows a comparison of the AUC from the excretion curves of breath hydrogen for 14 h after ingestion of the test substances (5 g or 30 g). Although breath hydrogen excretion was not 0 ppm at 0 min after ingestion (5 g) of FOS, RG or HRG, the AUC from the curve of breath hydrogen excretion for 14 h after ingestion was calculated simply. AUC versus time (14 h) was 850 ppm after purified RG (5 g) ingestion, 1250 ppm after HRG (5 g) ingestion and 11,740 ppm after FOS (5 g) ingestion. AUC versus time (14 h) of high level dose (30 g) was 1320 ppm for purified RG and 3150 ppm for HRG, respectively, and the AUC values were clearly larger than that of lower level dose.

Evaluation trial of available energy of RG and HRG

To evaluate the available energy, 5 g of purified RG or HRG were ingested by healthy participants as well as the evaluation of other dietary fiber materials [4–6]. Blood glucose and insulin concentrations did not increase overall and breath hydrogen excretion was negligible after purified RG ingestion and increased very slightly after HRG ingestion (Fig. 5b). The AUC from the curve of breath hydrogen excretion for 14 h after ingestion was 11,740 ppm for FOS ingestion, 850 ppm for purified RG ingestion and 1250 ppm for HRG ingestion (Table 1). Based on the available energy of FOS is 2 kcal/g, that of RG was evaluated as 0.14 kcal/g ($850 \div 11,740 \times 2 = 0.14$) and that of HRG was evaluated as 0.21 kcal/g ($1250 \div 11,740 \times 2 = 0.21$). The content of dietary fiber, which is resistant for hydrolyzing enzymes in AOAC 2001.03 method, are 99 % for purified RG and 82 % for HRG, respectively. Thus, the content of digestible saccharide, which the available energy is 4 kcal/g, is 1 % (0.04 kcal/g) for purified RG and 18 % (0.72 kcal/g) for HRG. Therefore, the total available energy becomes to 0.18 kcal/g ($0.14 + 0.04 = 0.18$) for purified RG and 0.93 kcal/g ($0.21 + 0.72 = 0.93$) for HRG, respectively. Because numerical values to two

Table 1 Estimation of available energy of RG and HRG in healthy human

	Nondigestable fractions			Digestable fractions		Estimated available energy (kcal/g)
	AUC (ppm/14 h)	Ratio versus AUC of FOS (%)	Calculated energy (kcal/g)	Content (%)	Calculated energy (kcal/g)	Calculated actual
			(1)		(2)	(1) + (2)
FOS	10,200 (7,800–15,855)	100.0	2			2
RG	601 (120–1,151)	6.1	0.12	1	0.04	0.16 → 0
HRG	674 (467–2,500)	6.6	0.13	18	0.72	0.85 → 1

FOS fructooligosaccharide, *RG* resistant glucan, *HRG* hydrogenated resistant glucan, *AUC* area under the curve. Five grams of test substances were ingested by healthy subjects. Data were expressed as median and interquartile in 10 healthy subjects. AUCs versus time for 14 h after ingestion of test substance were calculated based on the date shown in Fig. 5. The available energy of digestable fractions was calculated by content (%) × 4 kcal/g. Available energy was calculated based on our proposed method [4–6]

decimal places are not practicable for use in nutrition education and nutritional labelling, the nearest whole numbers are used [15, 16]. Therefore, the relative available energy values were 0 kcal/g for purified RG and 1 kcal/g for HRG.

Discussion

In the present study we investigated the metabolism and bioavailability of RG and HRG using rats and healthy human subjects, thereafter we estimated that the available energy was 0 kcal/g for purified RG and 1 kcal/g for HRG in healthy humans, respectively. A small amount of oligosaccharides in RG and HRG were only digested and fermented slightly, while a large amount of high molecular weight carbohydrates were digested scarcely and fermented barely in healthy humans. These results demonstrate that the bioavailability of purified RG and HRG is very low in both humans and rats, although the response of blood glucose and insulin and the breath hydrogen excretion are different a little between rats and humans. Therefore, we discussed first in terms of rats, and next from the view point of the bioavailability in humans.

Animal experiments using rats

When purified RG or HRG (400 mg/2.5 ml) was orally administered to rats, the blood glucose and insulin concentrations showed a small but clear peak at 30 min after administration, although the elevation was clearly lower than that of glucose administration. Previous experiments have demonstrated that purified RG and HRG contain a small amount of glucose and a small amount of oligosaccharides which are hydrolyzed by the small intestinal enzymes [7]. Therefore, the elevation of blood glucose level after the administration of purified RG or HRG seems to depend on a small amount of glucose and digestible oligosaccharides. Although the contents of glucose and digestible oligosaccharide were higher in HRG than in purified RG, the elevation of blood glucose and insulin was not significantly different between purified RG and HRG in rats. The blood glucose and insulin levels might be unable to respond because the amount of glucose and digestible oligosaccharide in the purified RG and HRG administered was very little. The blood glucose level was elevated by the administration of RMD as well as RG and HRG. RMD also contains a small amount of glucose and digestible oligosaccharide [10]. Dietary fiber materials that are not natural and have an average molecular weight of 1500-3000 seem to elevate slightly blood glucose and insulin levels. Although it has been recognized that natural dietary fiber materials do not increase blood glucose and insulin levels, the newly developed materials which contain a small amount of glucose and digestible oligosaccharides seems to increase slightly blood glucose and insulin levels.

Hydrogen is a specific product of fermentation of nondigestible carbohydrate by intestinal microbes. The amount of hydrogen excretion fluctuates widely from rat to rat and among groups, and includes the greater error at the basal levels. In rats, a small peak of hydrogen excretion was observed at 2–3 h after administration of purified RG or HRG and the peak value was greater for HRG than for purified RG. The results demonstrate that hydrogen excretion depends on the content of nondigestible oligosaccharides, because nondigestible oligosaccharides are more abundant in HRG than in purified RG, from which mono- and di-saccharides have been removed. Furthermore, this suggests that the amount of nondigestible oligosaccharides is very little compared with the amount of carbohydrate of high molecular weight in purified RG and HRG. In contrast, the production of hydrogen was maintained for a long time, because FOS is readily and completely fermented by intestinal microbes existed abundantly in the gastrointestinal tract after the administration of FOS. If high molecular weight carbohydrates in RG and HRG are fermented spontaneously by intestinal microbes, hydrogen must be excreted actively as much as FOS and would not decrease within 6-8 h after administration. These results suggest that purified RG and HRG contain a small amount of fermentable oligosaccharides and a large amount of high molecular weight carbohydrates which are resistant to fermentation.

Purified RG and HRG are partially hydrolyzed by small intestinal enzymes and are lightly fermented by intestinal microbes in rats [7]. In particular, high molecular weight carbohydrates, which are the main component of RG and HRG, were hardly hydrolyzed by small intestinal enzyme and were scarcely fermented by intestinal microbes. Therefore, a large proportion of RG and HRG would be excreted in the feces. However, the recovery for 24 h after administration to rats was very low. They were 23.4 % for purified RG and 20.2 % for HRG. One reason for this is that the perfect recovery of feces is very difficult, because the stool becomes moistened with urine adhering to the Metabolica apparatus. Another reason is that a part of administered RG and HRG may remain in the gastrointestinal tract, because the collection period (24 h) for cecal and colonic contents and stools might have been too short. In addition, the extraction of RG and HRG from stools might not have been complete. However, it could be confirmed that RG and HRG are excreted into feces.

The results obtained from the experiments using rats have demonstrated that purified RG, which the content of dietary fiber is 99 %, is more resistant to digestion and fermentation than HRG, which the content of dietary fiber is 82 %. A part of oligosaccharide fractions, which are the minor components of RG and HRG, is digested by small intestinal enzymes, and other oligosaccharide fractions, which are not digested by small intestinal enzymes, are fermented by intestinal microbes. It has also shown that high molecular weight carbohydrates, which are the main component of RG and HRG, are difficult to be digested and fermented.

Human experiments using healthy subjects

The blood glucose and insulin levels increased slightly but obviously after oral administration of purified RG or HRG (400 mg) in rats (Fig. 2). However, they increased scarcely after ingestion of purified RG (30 g) or HRG (30 g) in the experiments using human participants (Fig. 4). This discrepancy could be explained partially by the observation that the hydrolysis of purified RG and HRG was slightly lower in humans than in rats in the previous experiments using small intestinal homogenates [7]. The similar phenomenon, which the hydrolyzing activity is lower in humans than in rats, has also been observed for highly cross-linked starch [31]. However, the hydrolyzing activity for sucrose and maltose, which are consisted of a simple structure, is similar between humans and rats [32]. The hydrolyzing activity for carbohydrates such as RG and HRG with a unique property may be different between humans and rats. The response of blood glucose and insulin by ingesting RG and HRG seem to be different in humans when composed to rats. In addition, since the dosage of the test substance per kg of body weight is calculated as 1333 mg for rats and 545-588 mg for humans, this difference may have also brought the low response of blood glucose in humans.

The content of dietary fiber, which is resistant to hydrolyzing enzymes in AOAC 2001.03 method [8], is 99 % for purified RG and 82 % for HRG. Thus, 1 % of purified RG and 18 % of HRG are digestible saccharides producing 4 kcal/g. A part of dietary fiber fraction in RG and HRG is fermented by intestinal microbes and hydrogen is produced. In humans, the breath hydrogen excretion after HRG ingestion was higher than that for purified RG, but not statistically significant. These results demonstrate that HRG contains more fermentable oligosaccharides compared with purified RG, although the dietary fiber content is less than purified RG. But, the excretion of breath hydrogen after HRG ingestion (30 g) was very low compared with that after ingesting of fermentable FOS (5 g). In addition, these results were similar to those observed in rats. If high molecular weight carbohydrates in RG and HRG are readily fermented by intestinal microbes, the excretion of breath hydrogen must be greatly enhanced and maintained the high level until the end of the experiment as well as FOS. Moreover, the hydrogen excretion by ingesting RG and HRG indicates that short chain fatty acids, which are further metabolized to energy in the host, are produced by intestinal microbes. Therefore, the available energy which is brought by the fermentation of RG and HRG is not 0 kcal/g. However, in the present study the available energy including that of digestible saccharides was evaluated as 0 kcal/g for purified RG and 1 kcal/g for HRG, respectively.

The available energy calculated from fermentation of nondigestible saccharide and available saccharide was 0.18 kcal/g ($0.14 + 0.04 = 0.18$) for purified RG, which the dietary fiber content is 99 %, and was 0.93 kcal/g ($0.21 + 0.72 = 0.93$) for HRG, which is more fermentable than purified RG and the dietary fiber content is 82 %. The hydrogen excretion showed only a small peak at 3 h after ingestion of purified RG or HRG (400 mg/2.5 ml) in rats. But, the pattern of hydrogen excretion after RMD administration (400 mg/2.5 ml) was clearly different from those after administration of RG and HRG. In other word, the hydrogen excretion of RMD showed a small shoulder at 3 h and a maximum excretion at 10 h after administration. Furthermore, in humans a peak of breath hydrogen is also showed at 6-10 h after ingestion of RMD as well as rats [5]. The high molecular weight carbohydrates, which are contained in RMD seem to be fermented more readily than those in RG and HRG in rats. Hence, the available energy of RMD, which the content of digestible oligosaccharides is less than HRG, is estimated as 1 kcal/g by our proposed method [5] and other different methods [14].

Extensive intake of nondigestible and/or non-absorbable mono- or oligo-saccharides such as FOS, 1-kestose, galactosylsucrose, lactulose, trehalose, cellobiose, lactitol, xylitol and D-tagatose induces essentially loose stool and abdominal symptoms such as thirst, flatus, distension or borborygmus in rats and humans, and each maximum non-effective dosage on them are evaluated using healthy human subjects [25–28, 33–35]. But, natural dietary fiber materials with high molecular weight do not cause osmotic loose stool. Abdominal symptoms and loose stool are influenced by the rate of digestibility and absorbability, molecular weight and habituation of sugar substitutes. The maximum non-effective dose of non-digestible oligosaccharides is 0.3-0.4 g/kg of body weight [6, 25]. Since RG and HRG contain the small amount of low molecular weight saccharides which are resistant for digestion, the extensive intake of them may induce abdominal symptoms and loose stool. But, none of the participants experienced loose stools and abdominal symptoms after ingesting 30 g of purified RG or HRG. However, two participants experienced light loose stools, flatus, and borborygmus in the preliminary experiment after ingesting 50 g of HRG (data not shown). These results suggest that ingesting 30 g of purified RG and HRG does not induce side effects in healthy adult.

On the other hand, FDA (Administration of Drug and Food) in USA does not decide the maximum non-effective dose of PD and RMD which are similar characteristics to RG and HRG and contain much small molecular nondigestible saccharides; in spite of they cause more readily loose stool than RG and HRG [36]. Side effects such as abdominal symptoms and loose stool may not be important to dietary fiber ingredient which the intake is much in quantity under the law. But, the maximum non-effective dose for abdominal symptoms and loose stool is essential for design of processed foods. Therefore, it is important knowledge that the non-effective dose of RG or HRG as ingredients is more than 30 g, which are not ingested once in the common living life. However, the ingestion of 30 g of purified RG and HRG may induce side effects in children and aged persons. Further studies are necessary for children, aged persons and pregnant women.

In previous experiment using rats, the body weight gain was normal in all groups given the test diet or the experimental diet, and the blood biochemical parameters were not significantly different among the control, RG and HRG groups in consecutive feeding of rats using diets containing purified RG or HRG [7]. Thus, RG and HRG did not harm the growth and development of rats. Furthermore, side effects such as loose stool and abdominal symptoms do not appear after ingestion of RG and HRG (30 g) in healthy adults. In addition, the abnormality was not detected in acute, subacute and chronic toxicity tests of RG [1, 9]. Therefore, RG and HRG can be used aggressively in processed foods as a dietary fiber supplement.

The indication of energy is an essential item in the nutritional labelling for processed foods. The available energy of purified RG and HRG was evaluated according to the indirect and simple method in the present study. This method has been proposed by the Japanese Society for Dietary Fiber Research, with the relative available energy of newly developed dietary fiber and nondigestible oligosaccharide materials being evaluated using FOS as a convenient reference [4, 5, 25]. The breath hydrogen excretion is used as an indicator of extent of fermentation in the proposed method to evaluate the available energy, and FOS, which the available energy is 2 kcal/g in practice, is used as a reference of typical nondigestible and fermentable oligosaccharide [4, 5]. The expiration to measure the hydrogen needs to collect for 14 h or longer after administration of test substances, because some test materials are slowly fermented by intestinal microbes in humans [5]. The collection period for more than 14 h is given more stress for subjects. The available energy is calculated from the AUC of breath hydrogen excretion for 14 h against that of FOS.

In this method, 5 g of the test substance was ingested by healthy participants, and the expiration was collected to measure the hydrogen excretion for 14 h after ingestion. The AUC of breath hydrogen excretion for 14 h after 5 g ingestion of test substances were 11,740 ppm for FOS, 850 ppm for purified RG and 1250 ppm for HRG, respectively. The available energy from fermentation is calculated as 0.14 kcal/g for purified RG and 0.21 kcal/g for HRG, because the value of FOS, which is fermented completely by intestinal microbes, is 2 kcal/g. The content of dietary fiber, which is resistant for hydrolyzing enzymes in AOAC 2003.01method, is 99 % for purified RG and 82 % for HRG, respectively. Since 1 % of purified RG and 18 % of HRG are digested and converted to energy production, the available energy becomes 0.04 kcal/g for purified RG and 0.72 kcal/g for HRG. Therefore, total available energy of digestible and nondigestible saccharides becomes to 0.18 ($0.14 + 0.04 = 0.18$) kcal/g for purified RG and 0.93 ($0.21 + 0.72 = 0.93$) kcal/g for HRG. The practical nearest whole number after rounding is 0 kcal/g for purified RG and 1 kcal/g for HRG. The difference of available energy is dependent on the difference of dietary fiber content in purified RG and HRG.

Conclusions

The ingestion of purified RG or HRG (30 g) increased scarcely blood glucose and insulin levels and excreted slightly hydrogen in healthy human subjects. A small amount of oligosaccharides in RG and HRG were only digested and fermented slightly, while a large amount of high molecular weight carbohydrates were digested scarcely and fermented barely in healthy humans. Therefore, the bioavailability of purified RG and HRG was very low in both humans and rats, although the response of blood glucose and insulin, and breath hydrogen excretion were slightly different between humans and rats. Moreover, the ingestion of 30 g of RG or HRG did not induce any apparent side effects in healthy adults. Available energy was evaluated as 0 kcal/g for purified RG and 1 kcal/g for HRG. Therefore, RG and HRG could be potentially used as new dietary fiber materials with low energy.

Abbreviations

RD: Resistant glucan; HRD: Hydrogenated resistant glucan; HPLC: High performance liquid chromatography; AOAC: The Association of Official Analytical Chemists; FOS: Fructooligosaccharide; AUC: Area under the curve; RMD: Resistant maltodextrin; PD: Polydextrose; AST: Aspartate transaminase; ALT: Alanine transaminase.

Competing of interests

The authors declared that they have no competing interest.

Authors' contributions

All authors read and approved the final manuscript.

Acknowledgements

We thank the Nihon Shokuhin Kako Co. Ltd. (Tokyo, Japan) for providing purified resistant glucan and hydrogenated resistant glucan. We also thank Matsutani Chemical Industry Co. Ltd. (Hyogo, Japan) for providing RMD and

Meiji Co. Ltd. (formerly-Meiji Seika Kaisha Ltd., Tokyo, Japan) for providing FOS. This study was supported in part by Grant-in-Aid for Scientific Research (B) (2) 22300263, 26350128, and university funding for research to T.O.

Author details
[1]Institute of Food, Nutrition and Health, Jumonji University, 2-1-28, Sugasawa, Niiza, Saitama 352-8510, Japan. [2]Graduate School of Human Health Science, University of Nagasaki Siebold, 1-1-1, Manabino, , Nagayo, Nagasaki 851-2195, Japan. [3]Department of Food Science and Nutrition, Nagoya Women's University, 3-40, Shioji, Mizuho-ku, Nagoya 467-8610, Japan. [4]Institute of Food Materials, Nippon Shokuhin Kako Co. Ltd., Tajima, Fuji 417-8530, Japan.

References

1. Hamaguchi N, Hirai H, Aizawa K, Takada M. Production of water-soluble indigestible polysaccharides using activated carbon. J Appl Glycosci. 2014; 61:100–15.
2. The Ministry of Health and Labour and welfare. Detailed enforcement regulations for the application of Japanese Health Promotion Law.1995. http://www.mhlw.go.jp/ to www.mhlw.go.jp/shingi/2004/12/dl/s1202-4g. pdf. Accessed 25 December, 2015.
3. U.S. Department of Health and Human Services, Food and Drug Administration, Center for Food Safety and Applied Nutrition. A Food Labeling Guide - Guidance for Industry. 2013.
4. Nakamura S, Oku T. Evaluation of available energy of several dietary fiber materials based on the fermentability from breath hydrogen excretion in healthy human subjects. J Jpn Assoc Dietary Fiber Res. 2005;9:34–46 (in Japanese).
5. Oku T, Nakamura S. Evaluation of the relative available energy of several dietary fiber preparations using breath hydrogen evolution in healthy humans. J Nutr Sci Vitaminol. 2014;60:246–54.
6. Oku T, Nakamura S. Digestion, absorption, fermentation and metabolism of functional sugar substitutes and their available energy. Pure ApplChem. 2002;74:1253–61.
7. Oku T, Tanabe K, Morita S, Hamaguchi N, Shimura F, Nakamura S. Digestibility of new dietary fiber materials, resistant glucan and hydrogenated resistant glucan, and physical effects by consecutive feeding in rats. Br J Nutr. 2015;114: 1550–59.
8. Joint FAO/WHO Food Standards Programme. Codex Committee on Nutrition and Foods for Special Dietary Uses 32th Session. Draft table of Conditions for Methods of Analysis for Dietary Fiber. 2010. REP11/NFSDU 2 and Appendix IV.
9. Bito H, Hamaguchi N, Hirai H, Ogawa K. Safety evaluation of newly-developed dietary fiber: resistant glucan mixture. J Toxicol Sci, 2016; 41 (in press).
10. Hashizume C, Kishimoto Y, Kanamori S, Yamamoto T, Okuma K, Yamamoto K. Improvement effect of resistant maltodextrin in humans with metabolic syndrome by continuous administration. J Nutr Sci Vitaminol. 2012;58:423–30.
11. Bear DJ, Stote KS, Henderson T, Paul DR, Okuma K, Tagami H. The metabolizable energy of dietary maltodextrin is variable and alters fecal microbiota composition in adult men. J Nutr. 2014;144:1023–29.
12. Auerbach MH, Craig SAS, Howlett JF, Hayes KC. Caloric availability of polydextrose. Nutr Rev. 2007;65:544–9.
13. Konings E, Schoffelen PF, Stegen J, Blaak EE. Effect of polydextrose and soluble maize fiber on energy metabolism, metabolic profile and appetite control in overweight men and women. Br J Nutr. 2013;107:1–11.
14. Goda T, Kajima Y, Suruga K, Tagami H, Livesey G. Availability, fermentability, and energy value of resistant maltodextrin: modelling of short-term indirect calorimetric measurements in healthy adults. Am J Clin Nutr. 2006;83:1321–30.
15. Oku T, Yamada K, Kanaya K. Estimation of available energy of dietary fiber in various food materials. J Jpn Assoc Dietary Fiber Res. 2002;6:81–6 (in Japanese).
16. Oku T, Aoe S, Kanaya K, Kurasawa S, Sanada H, Yamada K. Opinion of evaluation of available energy on Luminacoid (dietary fiber), and available energy of methylcellulose, hydrogenated resistant maltodextrin and high cross starch by the method. J Jpn Assoc Dietary Fiber Res. 2013;17:47–51. in Japanese.
17. Oku T, Tokunaga T, Hosoya N. Nondigestibility of a new sweetener, "Neosugar" in the rat. J Nutr. 1984;114:1574–81.
18. Tokunaga T, Oku T, Hosoya N. Utilization and excretion of a new sweetener, fructooligosaccharide (Neosugar), in rats. J Nutr. 1989;119:553–9.
19. Reeves PG, Nielsen FH, Fahey Jr GC. AIN-93 purified diets for laboratory rodents: final report of the American Institute of Nutrition ad hoc writing committee on the reformulation of the AIN-76A rodent diet. J Nutr. 1993; 123:1939–51.
20. Oku T, Murata-Takenosita Y, Yamazaki Y, Nakamura S. D-sorbose inhibits disaccharidaseactivity and demonstrates suppressive action on postprandial blood levels of glucose and insulin in the rat. Nutr Res. 2014;34:961–7.
21. Trinder P. Determination of blood glucose using an oxidase-peroxidase system with a non-carcinogenic chromogen. J Clin Pathol. 1969;22:158–61.
22. Liversy JH, Hodgkinson SC, Round HR, Donald RA. Effect of time, temperature and freezing on the stability of immunoreactive LH, FSH, TSH, growth hormone, prolactin and insulin in plasma. Clin Biochem. 1980;13:151–5.
23. Hongo R, Nakamura S, Oku T. Utilization of orally administered D-[^{14}C] mannitol via fermentation by intestinal microbes in rats. J Nutr Sci Vitaminol. 2010;56:387–95.
24. Tanabe K, Nakamura S, Oku T. Fatal imperfection of enzymatic-HPLC quantitative HPLC method for non-digestible oligosaccharides and its proposed solution strategy. Current Nutr Food Sci. 2011;7:209–15.
25. Oku T, Nakamura M, Hashiguchi-Ishiguro M, Tanabe K, Nakamura S. Bioavailability and laxative threshold of 1-kestose in human adults. Dynamic Biochem Process Biotech Mol Bio. 2009;3(S1):90–5.
26. Oku T, Okazaki M. Effect of single and divided ingestions of the nondigestible oligosaccharide "galactosylsucrose" on transit diarrhea and laxative threshold in normal female subjects. J Jpn Soc Nutr Food Sci. 1999;52:201–08 (in Japanese).
27. Oku T, Nakamura S, Ichinose M. Maximum permissive dosage of lactose and lactitol for transitory diarrhea, and utilizable capacity for lactose in Japanese female adults. J Nutr Sci Vitaminol. 2005;51:51–7.
28. Yamazaki Y, Nakamura S, Shimura F, Oku T. Maximum permissive dosage for transitory diarrhea, estimation of available energy, and fate of D-tagatose in healthy female subjects. J Jpn Soc Nutr Food Sci. 2011;64:403–13 (in Japanese).
29. Oku T, Nakamura S. Comparison of digestibility and breath hydrogen gas excretion of fructooligosaccharide, galactosylsucrose, and isomaltooligosaccharide in healthy human subjects. Eur J Clin Nutr. 2003;57:1150–6.
30. Nakamura S, Oku T. Replicability of the effect of galactosylsucrose-containing food for specified health uses on fecal improvement in the case of availableness on usual life. J Jpn Assoc Dietary Fiber Res. 2002;6:73–80 (in Japanese).
31. Tachibe M, Ohga H, Nishibata T, Ebihara K. Digestibility, fermentability, and energy value of highly cross-linked phosphate tapioca starch in men. J Food Sci. 2011;76:H152–5.
32. Oku T, Tanabe K, Ogawa S, Sadamori N, Nakamura S. Similarity of hydrolyzing activity of human and rat small intestinal disaccharidases. Clin Experi Gastroenterol. 2011;4:155–61.
33. Nakamura S, Ichinose M, Oku T. Bioavailability of cellobiose by tolerance test and breath hydrogen excretion in humans. Nutrition. 2004;20(11/12):979–83.
34. Oku T, Okazaki M. Transitory laxative threshold of trehalose and lactulose in healthy women. J Nutr Sci Vitaminol. 1998;44:787–98.
35. Oku T, Nakamura S. Threshold for transitory diarrhea induced by ingestion of xylitol and lactitol in young male and female adults. J Nutr Sci Vitaminol. 2006;53:13–20.
36. Oku T, Okamatsu H, Fujii Y. Effect of polydextrose on fecal weight and gastrointestinal transit time in beagle dogs. J Jpn Assoc Dietary fibre Res. 2000;4:29–35 [in Japanease].

14

Effects of selected bioactive food compounds on human white adipocyte function

Christel Björk[1,5*], Uta Wilhelm[1], Susanne Mandrup[2], Bjørk Ditlev Larsen[2], Alessandra Bordoni[3], Per Hedén[4], Mikael Rydén[1], Peter Arner[1] and Jurga Laurencikiene[1]

Abstract

Background: Previous studies suggest that intake of specific bioactive compounds may have beneficial clinical effects on adipose tissue partly due to their anti-inflammatory and insulin-sensitizing properties. With the overall aim to contribute to better understanding of the mechanisms of selected bioactive nutrients on fat metabolism, we investigated their role on human white adipocyte function.

Methods: The influence of the omega-3-fatty acid docosahexaenoic acid (DHA), the anthocyanin (AC) cyanidin-3-glucoside and its metabolite protocatechuic acid, and the beta-glucan metabolite propionic acid (PI) on adipokine secretion, fatty acid metabolism (lipolysis/lipogenesis) and adipocyte differentiation (lipid accumulation) was studied in human fat cells differentiated in vitro. To investigate possible synergistic, additive or antagonistic effects, DHA was also combined with AC or PI.

Results: Each compound, alone or together with DHA, suppressed basal adipocyte lipolysis compared to control treated cells. DHA alone attenuated the secretion of pro-inflammatory adipokines such as chemerin, interleukin-6 (IL-6) and monocyte chemoattractant protein-1 (MCP-1/*CCL2*), whereas AC suppressed only the latter two. Treatment with PI decreased IL-6, tumour necrosis factor alpha (TNFα) and adiponectin secretion. A combination of DHA and AC decreased TNFα secretion and increased insulin-stimulated lipogenesis. No effect was found on adipocyte differentiation. At the selected concentrations, none of the compounds was found to be cytotoxic.

Conclusion: The studied bioactive food compounds or their metabolites have beneficial effects in human primary fat cells measured as decreased basal lipolytic activity and secretion of inflammatory markers. A minor effect was also observed on insulin-stimulated glucose uptake albeit only with the combination of DHA and AC. Taken together, our results may link the reported health benefits of the selected bioactives on metabolic disorders such as insulin resistance, hypertension and dyslipidemia to effects on white adipocytes.

Keywords: Anthocyanin, Beta-glucan, Cyanidin-3-glucoside, Docosahexaenoic acid, Inflammation, Insulin sensitivity, Lipolysis, Propionic acid, Protocatechuic acid

* Correspondence: christel.bjork@ki.se
[1]Lipid Laboratory, Department of Medicine, Karolinska Institutet, Huddinge, Stockholm, Sweden
[5]Department of Medicine, Karolinska Institutet, Lipid Laboratory, Novum, NVS D4, Hälsovägen 7, 14186 Stockholm, Sweden
Full list of author information is available at the end of the article

Background

It is well established that white adipose tissue (WAT) metabolism and inflammatory status affect whole body homeostasis [1]. The major role of WAT is to store and release energy. Storing energy in the form of triacylglycerol (TAG) in adipocytes through lipogenesis has been shown to regulate systemic insulin sensitivity [2, 3]. Hydrolysis of TAGs into non-esterified fatty acids and glycerol is a tightly controlled enzymatic process denoted lipolysis. Basal (spontaneous) lipolytic activity is increased in obesity and may attenuate insulin sensitivity through increased delivery of FAs to skeletal muscle (reviewed in [4]). Another important aspect of WAT function is the secretion of a class of proteins called adipokines, several with pro- or anti-inflammatory properties (see [1] for review). An elevated release of monocyte chemoattractant protein-1 (MCP-1/ *CCL2*) produced by adipocytes [5, 6] recruits macrophages, which in turn promote a chronic low grade inflammation in WAT [7]. Release of other pro-inflammatory adipokines, such as interleukin-6 (IL-6), tumour necrosis factor-alpha (TNFα) and chemerin may also contribute to metabolic disorders such as insulin resistance, dyslipidemia, hypertension and cardiovascular disease [8–10], which are associated with the development of the metabolic syndrome [11]. The anti-inflammatory adipokine adiponectin has on the other hand been shown to correlate negatively with BMI (Body mass index, defined as body weight in kilograms divided by height in meters squared) and positively with insulin sensitivity [12, 13] and its high levels are associated with a lower risk for developing type 2 diabetes [14].

Diet composition can affect the metabolic and endocrine function of WAT as well as overall energy balance [15]. Certain diets that provide high amounts of bioactive components may have beneficial clinical effects partly due to their anti-inflammatory effects on adipose tissue (see [15, 16] for reviews). A number of natural bioactive compounds that can be added to the food or their metabolic derivatives have been tested for their action on fat cells. The omega-3 long-chain polyunsaturated fatty acid docosahexaenoic acid (DHA) can be synthesized from the essential alpha-linoleic acid. However, minor (clinically insufficient) amounts are synthesized endogenously and significant levels can only be provided exogenously through intake of fish and fish oil. A previous study using human adipocytes and WAT suggested an anti-inflammatory effect of DHA via decreased levels of IL-6 and MCP-1 [17]. In vitro studies regarding the regulation of DHA on adiponectin production have been performed both in mouse and human adipocytes, however the results are conflicting [18–20]. Anthocyanins (AC) are naturally occurring polyphenol compounds present in blue or purple berries, fruit and vegetables [21]. Cyanidin-3-glucoside (C3G) is the most studied anthocyanin that together with its main metabolite protocatechuic acid (PCA) has been shown to be protective against insulin resistance in both human adipocytes in vitro [22, 23] and an in vivo diabetic mouse model [24, 25] as well as having anti-inflammatory properties [22, 24–26]. Beta-glucan (BG) is a soluble dietary fiber present in oats and barley. However, BG is not absorbed in vivo, but its metabolism by the gut microbiota results in increased production an uptake of short-chain fatty acids (SCFA), such as propionic acid (PI), which has been shown to regulate adipokine production and enhance lipogenesis and glucose uptake in isolated human WAT [27, 28].

Most studies investigating effects of these compounds have been conducted in murine adipose cell lines or in vivo mouse or rat models [29–32], which display a number of species-specific differences concerning adipose tissue function [33–35]. Furthermore, in previous studies the compounds have been tested individually and the experimental conditions as well as fat cell model systems have varied markedly. In addition, in most cases a single metabolic or inflammatory aspect of adipocyte function has been investigated.

As a part of the pan-European study PATHWAY-27 (http://www.pathway27.eu/) with the overall aim to contribute to better understanding of the mechanisms of bioactive nutrients on metabolism in different food-environments and help to develop health-promoting food for the growing demand of the health-conscious consumer, we have investigated the role of selected bioactives or their main metabolites on adipocyte phenotypes linked to obesity and the metabolic syndrome.

Methods

Cell cultures of primary human adipocytes

Primary human pre-adipocytes for in vitro differentiation from 22 female subjects and 2 male subjects between 26-65 (mean 42) years of age with a BMI ranging from 21-31 kg/m^2 (mean 25) were isolated from the stromal vascular fraction of subcutaneous WAT, which was obtained as a waste product from cosmetic liposuction. Isolation, culture and differentiation into adipocytes were performed as previously described [36]. The subjects were healthy according to self-report and not selected for age, sex or BMI. Briefly, intact pieces of adipose tissue were cut into 3-4 mm pieces and digested with collagenase for 90 min at 37 °C, whereas material obtained from liposuctions was digested with collagenase for 45 min at 37 °C. Thereafter the cell suspension was filtered, centrifuged at 200 × g for 10 min. The remaining pre-adipocytes and mesenchymal stem cells in the stromal vascular fraction were then suspended in erythrocyte lysis buffer for 10 min and centrifuged. The supernatant was discarded, the cells suspended in proliferation medium containing Dulbecco's Modified Eagle Medium (DMEM)/F12 (Biochrome AG, Berlin, Germany/ Gibco, Life Technologies) supplemented with 10 % fetal bovine serum (Gibco, Life Technologies) and 2 % Pen-Strep (Gibco, Life Technologies) and subsequently filtered through a 70 µm cell strainer (BD BioSciences, Durham, NC) .

To study the effects of bioactives on fat cell metabolism and adipokine secretion, the cells were plated in proliferation medium at a density of 115 000 to 120 000 cells/well in 24-well plates. After 24 h, the medium was changed to DMEM/F12 supplemented with 15 mM HEPES (Gibco, Life Technologies), 100 µg/ml penicillin-streptomycin (Gibco, Life Technologies), 66 nM human insulin, 1 nM triiodo-L-thyronine, 10 µg/ml human transferrin, 33 µM biotin, 17 µM panthothenate, 100 nM cortisol (all from Sigma St. Louis, MO), 1.25 µg/ml amphotericin B (Gibco, Life Technologies) and 10 µM rosiglitazone (BRL49653) (GlaxoSmithKline, Durham, UK) to induce differentiation. Rosiglitazone was included during the first 3-4 days and then removed from the differentiation medium. Medium was changed every 2-3 days and the cells were kept until full differentiation (12-14 days). Forty-eight hours before full differentiation, the compounds were added in adipogenic medium.

To investigate the effects of bioactives on lipid accumulation, 20 000 cells/well were seeded in 96-well plates. Medium was supplemented with the compounds after 6 days in differentiation medium and treatment was performed for 6 days until day 12 of differentiation. Adipose tissue stromal vascular fraction, which we use to in vitro differentiate adipocytes, contains various cell types including immune cells. At day 6 of differentiation, immune cells are almost entirely washed away and absent and this is the earliest time point in differentiation, where effects unspecific for adipocytes could be excluded. Each experiment was repeated in cells isolated separately from at least three individuals in duplicates (lipid accumulation and lipogenesis) or quadruplicates (lipolysis and adipokine secretion). Cytotoxicity of compounds was measured for all treatment conditions. The grade of differentiation was determined under the microscope and cells with differentiation grade below 80 % were discarded. The study was approved by the Ethics Committee at Karolinska Institutet (Sweden). All subjects were informed about this study and provided their written informed consent.

Treatment with bioactive compounds

The cells were treated with DHA (D8768, sodium salt, Sigma, St. Louis, MO), C3G (1201-1, chloride salt, Polyphenols Laboratories AS, Sandes, Norway) together with its metabolite PCA (03930590, Sigma) or the BG metabolite PI (P1880, sodium salt, Sigma). To study possible synergistic, additive or antagonistic effects with DHA, the bioactive compound was also studied in combination with AC or PI. Compound concentrations were based on relevant literature [27, 37] and unpublished treatment optimizations in the human Simpson-Golabi-Behmel syndrome (SGBS) pre-adipocyte cell line or in a hepatocyte cell line by collaborators in the PATHWAY-27 consortium. DHA was coupled to bovine serum albumin (BSA; A6003, Fraction V, Sigma) in a 4:1 ratio. Firstly, BSA was dissolved in 150 mM NaCl in a 37 °C water bath and filtered via a sterile 0.2 µm polypropylene membrane (VWR International, USA). Shortly after, DHA was dissolved in water and heated to 70 °C in a water bath. The coupling was performed through mixing both heated solutions and stirring for 1 h at 37 °C (pH 7.4). The final DHA concentration in the cell culture medium was 0.5-60 µM. C3G was dissolved in phosphate-buffered saline (PBS, Gibco, Life Technologies) whereas its main metabolite PCA was diluted in 50 % v/v solution of ethanol in water. According to agreements within the PATHWAY-27 consortium, C3G and PCA were added together to represent AC in a final concentration of 130 nM and 13 µM, respectively. PI (P1880, sodium salt, Sigma) was dissolved in 50 % v/v solution of ethanol in water and added to the cells at a final concentration of 100 µM. Corresponding concentrations of BSA and EtOH were added the control samples. As higher concentrations of BSA has been reported to have stimulatory effect on inflammatory cytokine secretion [38], we have performed control experiments comparing BSA and EtOH (at concentrations used in all our treatments) to untreated cells. Such treatment did not affect release of IL-6 and glycerol (Additional file 1: Figure S1).

Cytotoxicity measured as lactate dehydrogenase (LDH) activity in conditioned medium

Medium from bioactive treated cells was collected when full differentiation was reached. LDH activity, as a measure of damaged cells, was quantified according to the manufacturer's instructions (Cat. No. 11 644 793 001, Roche Diagnostics GmbH, Mannheim, Germany).

Lipolysis assay

Conditioned medium was collected after 48 h of treatment with the bioactive compounds. Basal lipolytic activity was measured as glycerol release with a bioluminescence method using Free Glycerol determination kit from Sigma (FG100) in combination with the fluorescence probe Amplex ultra red reagent (Cat. No. A36006, Molecular Probes, Life Technologies) [39, 40]. Glycerol release was normalized to protein concentration in each cell culture well.

Lipogenesis

Determination of basal and insulin-stimulated glucose incorporation into lipids was made when cells reached full differentiation that is after 48 h of bioactive treatment. Cells were initially washed twice with insulin- and glucose free DMEM (BioChromeAG) and incubated in DMEM containing 1 μM glucose. After 3 h, 3-^{3}H glucose (37 MBq/ml; Perkin Elmer-Cetus, Norwalk, CT) diluted 1:1000 in DMEM containing 1 μM glucose with was added. For stimulated lipogenesis, insulin was added to a final concentration of 100 nM. After 2 h of incubation, the cells were washed three times with 4 °C PBS and thereafter lysed in aqueous 0.1 % SDS (sodium dodecyl sulfate, Sigma) solution. An aliquot was saved for protein determination and the rest of the lysate was transferred to scintillation tubes. Toluene scintillation liquid (toluene with 5 g/l 2,5-diphenyloxazol and 0.3 g/l 1,4-bis (4-methyl-5-phemyl-2-oxazolyl)-benzene; Sigma-Aldrich) was added and the samples were incubated overnight to extract the lipids. Glucose incorporation into lipids as a proxy of lipogenesis was quantified as 3-^{3}H counts per minute (CPM) using a LS 6500 Multi-Purpose scintillation counter (Beckman, USA).

Adipokine quantification by enzyme-linked immunosorbent assay (ELISA)

To quantify the secretion of pro- (IL-6, MCP-1, chemerin, and TNFα) and anti-inflammatory (adiponectin) adipokines, cells were treated with bioactive compounds for 48 h and conditioned medium was collected for adipokine quantification by ELISA according to the manufacturer's instructions. The samples were diluted 5-60 fold for IL-6 detection (Quantikine ELISA Human IL-6 Immunoassay; R&D Systems, Minneapolis, MN, Intra-assay precision: CV <5 %, Inter-assay precision: CV <4 %), 3-10 fold for MCP-1 (Quantikine ELISA Human CCL3/MCP-1 Immunoassay; R&D Systems, Intra- and Inter-assay precision: CV <6 %) and 2-10 fold for chemerin (Quantikine ELISA Human Chemerin Immunoassay; R&D Systems, Intra-assay precision: CV ≤3 %, Inter-assay precision: CV <6 %) to match the standard curve. Adiponectin (Mercodia Adiponectin ELISA; Mercodia AB, Uppsala, Sweden, Intra-assay precision: CV <5 %, Inter-assay precision: CV <8 %) and TNFα (Quantiglo ELISA Human TNFα Immunoassay; R&D Systems, Intra-assay precision: CV <6 %, Inter-assay precision: CV <9 %) secretion were measured in undiluted samples. Levels of TNFα were detectable in adipocyte cultures treated with AC from only two subjects.

Protein quantification

Protein amount was quantified in SDS lysates from the lipogenesis experiments using Pierce™ BCA Protein Assay Kit (Cat. No. 23225 Pierce, Rockford, IL) according to the manufacturer's instructions. The protein concentration for each well was used to normalize glucose incorporation into lipids as well as glycerol release, LDH activity and adipokine secretion for cell amount.

Neutral lipid and DNA staining

The cells were differentiated in 96-well plates and treated with the bioactive compounds for 6 days before full differentiation. Medium supplemented with the compounds was added to the cell cultures every second day. Before staining, the cells were washed with PBS and fixed with 4 % paraformaldehyde solution (PFA) containing 0.123 M $NaH_2PO_4xH_2O$, 0.1 M NaOH and 0.03 M glucose for 10 min at room temperature. Fixed cells were washed with PBS and stained with Hoechst 33342 (2 μg/ml; staining cell nuclei, Cat. No. H3570, Molecular probes) and Bodipy 493/503 (0.2 μg/ml; staining neutral lipids, Cat. No. D-3922, Molecular probes) diluted in PBS for 20 min at room temperature. After washing with PBS, accumulation of intracellular lipid droplets and cell number (stained nuclei) were quantified with Acumen eX3 imager (TTP Labtech, Hertfordshire, UK). Bodipy lipid droplet fluorescence was normalized to the amount of nuclei in each well (Hoechst).

Statistical analysis

The impact of DHA, AC and PI on cytotoxicity, lipid accumulation, adipokine secretion and metabolic outcomes (lipolysis/lipogenesis) was compared to control cells without bioactives. If statistical significance was reached, the effect was also compared with the other bioactives having significant outcomes. Additionally, to investigate possible combinatorial (synergistic, additive or antagonistic) effects of DHA exposure, the impact of DHA alone was compared to that obtained in combination with AC or PI. If a difference was found, AC and PI exposure alone was compared to the effect of the respective bioactive in combination with DHA. The data was tested for normal distribution with the Shapiro-Wilk test. If the criteria for normal distribution were fulfilled, one-way analysis of variance (ANOVA) with subsequent Tukey's HSD post-hoc test was utilized. When the criteria for normal distribution were not achieved, the non-parametric Kruskal-Wallis and Mann-Whitney pair-wise comparison tests were used. The level of statistical significance was set as 0.05 with $^*p < 0.05$, $^{**}p < 0.01$ and $^{***}p < 0.001$. Bars are shown as mean ± standard deviation.

Results

Titration of the in vitro conditions for DHA treatment of primary human adipocytes

DHA concentrations that have been used in other fat cell systems (10-60 μM) [18–20, 41] as well as in optimizations by PATHWAY-27 collaborators in SGBS cells, induced LDH activity in conditioned media (after 6 days of stimulation) and increased IL-6 secretion (after 48 h of stimulation), indicating both cytotoxic and pro-inflammatory effects (Additional file 2: Figure S2). These findings are difficult to reconcile with the reported physiological effects of omega-3-fatty acids in vivo [42]. Consequently, the DHA concentration was titrated down and 0.5 μM was selected as the highest non-toxic DHA concentration in our primary culture system.

Decreased basal adipocyte lipolysis after treatment with bioactive compounds

Glycerol release was significantly decreased after all treatments when compared to control, with the exception of AC (p = 0.056) (Fig. 1). Treatment with PI had the strongest attenuating effect on glycerol release compared to control-treated cells which was stronger than that of DHA (p = 0.009). None of the compounds induced cytotoxicity at the selected concentrations, but rather reduced LDH activity in cell cultures after 48 h of treatment (Additional file 3: Figure S3), except for AC in combination with DHA (p = 0.321, due to a large inter-individual variation of the response). LDH activity remained unaltered up after 6 days of treatment with the bioactive compounds.

Combined treatment with DHA and AC increased insulin-stimulated adipocyte lipogenesis

To determine the effects of the bioactive compounds or their metabolites on insulin-stimulated lipogenesis, relative glucose incorporation into lipids was measured in the in vitro differentiated primary adipocytes. Insulin induced lipogenesis in the control and all treatment conditions (Fig. 2). No effect on insulin-stimulated response was found after treatment with any of the compounds alone.

However, combined treatment with DHA and AC increased insulin-stimulated glucose uptake compared to the control.

Bioactives alter secretion of pro-inflammatory adipokines and adiponectin

To investigate the effect of the bioactive compounds or their metabolites on a panel of the most important pro- (IL-6, MCP-1, TNFα, chemerin) and anti-inflammatory (adiponectin) adipokines, conditioned media from the adipose cells were collected after 48 h of treatment and secretion was measured by ELISA. IL-6, MCP1 and chemerin secretion were suppressed by DHA (Fig. 3a, b and e). The effect of DHA on MCP-1 and chemerin secretion was also statistically significant in combination with PI (Fig. 3b and e). Additionally, DHA combined with PI impeded TNFα secretion, a

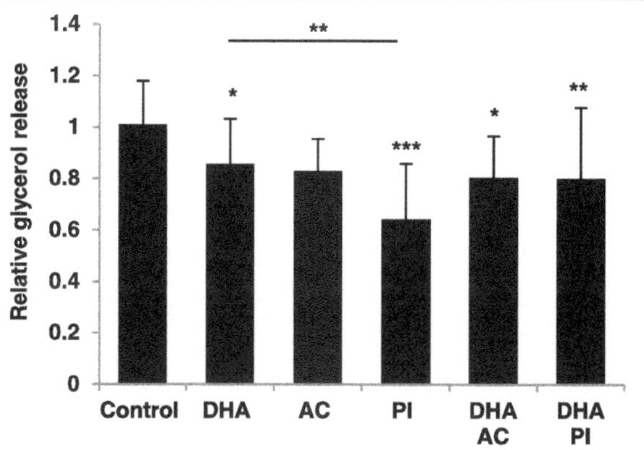

Fig. 1 Decreased basal adipocyte lipolysis after treatment with bioactive compounds or metabolites. Glycerol release after 48 h of treatment with 0.5 μM docosahexaenoic acid (DHA), anthocyanin (AC), that is 130 nM cyanidin-3-glucoside (C3G) and 13 μM protocatechuic acid (PCA), and 100 μM propionate (PI), relative to control, measured in conditioned medium from human in vitro differentiated adipocytes. Control, n = 9; 0.5 μM DHA, n = 6; AC alone and with DHA, n = 3; 100 μM PI alone and with DHA, n = 4 biological/independent experiments in quadruplicates. Normalized data is adjusted for protein amount and presented as means +/- standard deviation. *$p < 0.05$, **$p < 0.01$ and ***$p < 0.001$ versus control. Statistical significance was determined by one-way ANOVA with Tukey's multiple comparisons post hoc test

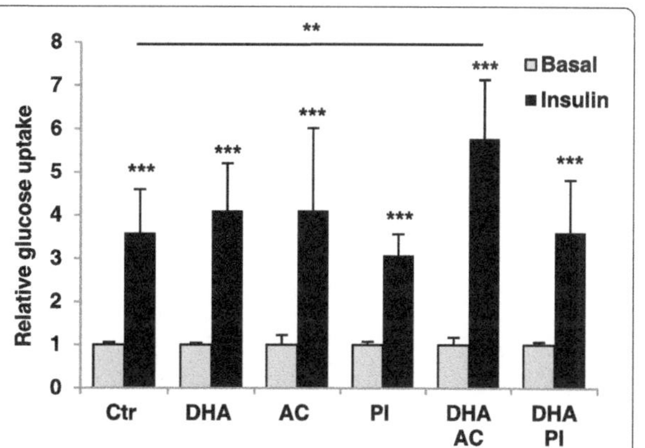

Fig. 2 Combined treatment with DHA and AC increased insulin-stimulated adipocyte lipogenesis. Basal and insulin-stimulated lipogenesis measured in cell lysates after 48 h of treatment with bioactive compounds. Control, n = 8; 0.5 μM DHA, n = 6; AC alone and with DHA, n = 3; 100 μM PI alone, n = 3 and with DHA, n = 4 biological/independent experiments in duplicates. Glucose incorporation into lipids (3-^{3}H counts per minute) is normalized for protein concentration in the cell lysates for each well. Normalized data is presented as means +/- standard deviation. *$p < 0.05$, **$p < 0.01$ and ***$p < 0.001$ counted against basal control with the same bioactive treatment or insulin-stimulated control compared with insulin-stimulated bioactive treated cells. Statistical significance was determined by the non-parametric Kruskal-Wallis test with subsequent Mann-Whitney multiple comparisons post hoc test

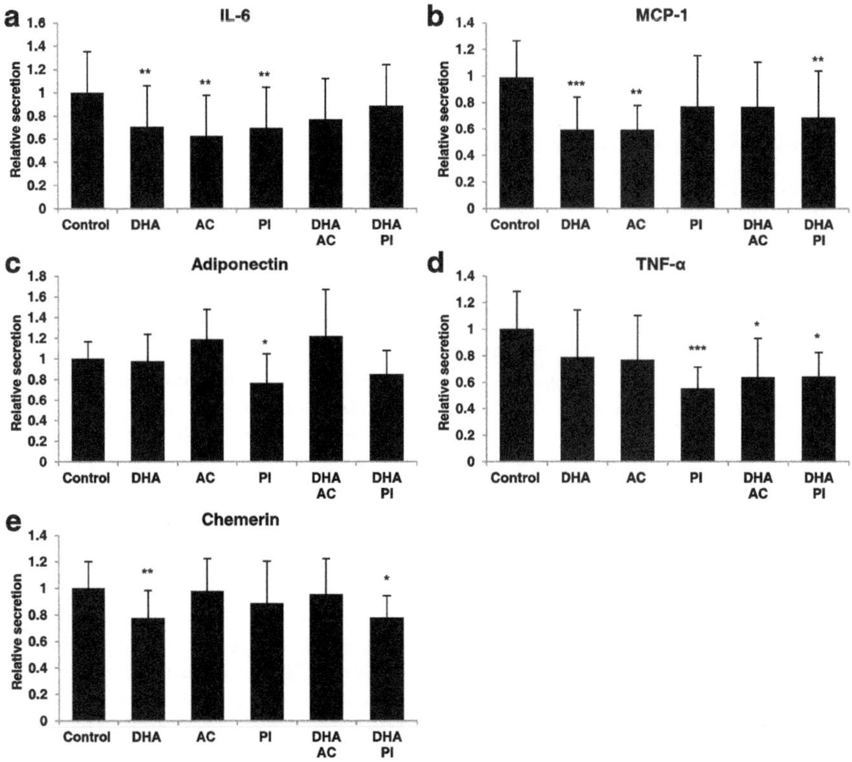

Fig. 3 Bioactives or metabolites alter secretion of pro-inflammatory adipokines and adiponectin. Secretion of adipokines; interleukin-6 (IL-6) (**a**), monocyte chemoattractant protein-1 (MCP-1) (**b**), adiponectin (**c**), tumour necrosis factor α (TNFα) (**d**) and chemerin (**e**); after 48 h of treatment with bioactive compounds relative to control in conditioned media. Control, n = 6-9; 0.5 μM DHA, n = 3-6; AC alone and with DHA, n = 3; 100 μM PI alone and with DHA, n = 3-4 in biological/independent experiments in quadruplicates, with the exception of TNFα where n = 2-6 due to levels below minimum detectable dose in four subjects. Normalized data is adjusted for protein amount and presented as means +/- standard deviation. $^{*}p < 0.05$, $^{**}p < 0.01$ and $^{***}p < 0.001$ versus control. Statistical significance was obtained by one-way ANOVA with Tukey's multiple comparisons post hoc test

result that was also obtained with PI alone (Fig. 3d). PI was the only compound that had an effect on adiponectin, contributing to a slightly decreased secretion (Fig. 3c). As the other two compounds, PI suppressed IL-6 secretion (Fig. 3a). AC alone attenuated IL-6 and MCP-1 secretion and in combination with DHA, demonstrated a suppressed secretion of TNFα (Fig. 3a, b and d).

No effects of bioactives on adipocyte differentiation

To measure possible effect of bioactives on adipocyte differentiation and lipid accumulation, cells were treated for 6 days and lipid content was measured by Bodipy staining and normalized per cell based on DNA staining by Hoechst (Fig. 4a). No effects were found of the selected compounds on lipid accumulation after 6 days of treatment (Fig. 4b).

Discussion

Using a systematic assessment of the effects of specific bioactive food compounds and their metabolites in human white fat cells, we found beneficial effects of DHA, AC and PI, either alone or in combination with DHA, on fat cell metabolism and inflammatory phenotype in vitro. The in vitro differentiated non-expanded human primary adipocytes used herein, is the closest model to human fat cells in vivo and enables longer treatments with the compounds. Treatments in in vitro systems always raise a question on the physiological concentrations of the stimuli applied and relevance of the resulting effects for the in vivo situation. We utilized lower concentrations of DHA than that measured in blood [43, 44]. However, higher concentrations of DHA induced cytotoxicity and pro-inflammatory response as in previous studies [20, 45]. Since the formation of reactive oxygen species (ROS) correlates with the number of double bonds in a polyunsaturated fatty acid, DHA is highly susceptible to spontaneous oxidation. ROS activate surface receptors such as Toll-like receptors which can trigger a downstream signalling cascade, leading to activation of the NF-kappaB pathway, which then turn

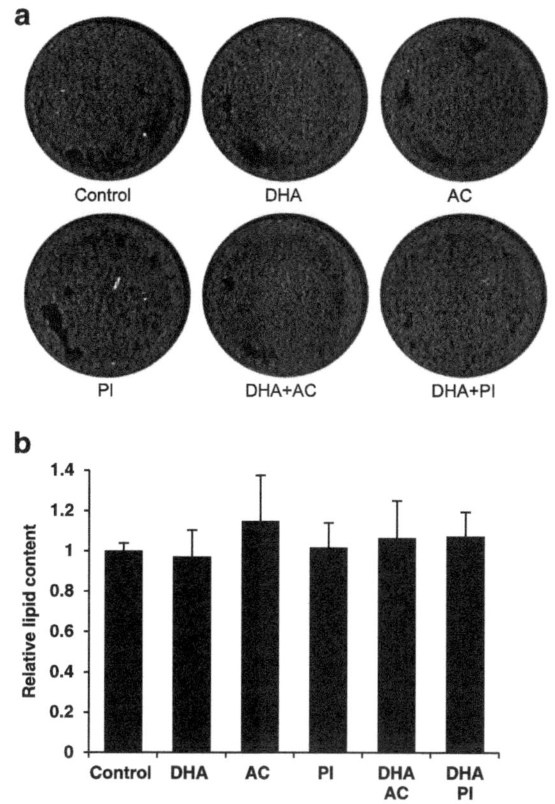

Fig. 4 No effects of bioactives or metabolites on lipid accumulation. Representative pictures of neutral lipid accumulation (green) and cell nuclei (blue) staining after 6 days of treatment with bioactive components (**a**). Quantified lipid accumulation adjusted for cell amount (control, n = 8; 0.5 μM DHA, n = 8; AC alone and with DHA, n = 4; 100 μM PI alone and with DHA, n = 6 biological/independent experiment in duplicates (**b**). Normalized data is presented as means +/- standard deviation versus control. The absence of statistical significance was determined by the non-parametric Kruskal-Wallis test

on the transcription of many pro-inflammatory genes [46, 47]. In the support of this hypothesis, ascorbic acid suppressed the pro-inflammatory effect in our primary human adipocyte culture (data not shown). Furthermore, total plasma levels of DHA should not be interpreted as equivalent to local extracellular or intracellular concentrations. To the best of our knowledge, there are no studies that have measured the actual concentration of DHA in adipose tissue. However, we cannot exclude that in the in vivo environment higher concentrations of DHA would be needed for optimal effects. Additionally, none of the other compounds displayed cytotoxicity in our cell cultures and the concentrations used for PI and AC were close to those reported in human blood [48, 49].

All three compounds suppressed basal adipocyte lipolysis, where the effect of PI was slightly more pronounced compared with DHA and AC. This could at least in part be due to a fact that PI also significantly attenuated the secretion of TNFα, a potent inducer of adipocyte lipolysis [33]. Our finding corroborate results from a study where healthy subjects were supplemented for 4 weeks with non-digestible starch and demonstrated decreased adipose tissue glycerol release as well as reduction in the activity of hormone-sensitive lipase, the rate-limiting enzyme responsible for mobilization of stored TAGs [49]. We therefore suggest that PI might exert its effects at least in part by altering adipocyte lipid metabolism via indirect (through TNFα) or direct mechanisms. In fact, although the latter mechanism has not been not studied in humans, in mice PI has been suggested to interact with the G-protein coupled receptor 43 [29], a receptor that is suggested to be involved in regulating inflammatory responses, and is also expressed in human WAT [28]. Regarding ACs, an anti-lipolytic effect has been observed in 3T3-L1 adipocytes during hyperglycemia, where C3G regulated FoxO1-mediated transcription of adipose triglyceride lipase resulting in decreased expression of this lipolytic enzyme [50]. Whether or not this also implies for human adipocytes remains to be investigated. The mechanism of lipolysis reduction by DHA is not known. However, no additive effects between compounds were observed, suggesting that they might act via similar mechanisms.

The synergistic effect between DHA and AC on insulin-induced lipogenesis might partly be explained by the activation of PPARγ by AC, which results in increased expression and translocation of GLUT4 [22]. In addition, the effect on lipogenesis could result from decreased TNFα secretion caused by combined DHA and AC treatment. We and others have shown that TNFα addition in cultures of primary human adipocytes causes insulin resistance [51, 52]. However, a combination of PI and DHA also lowered TNFα secretion but did not affect lipogenesis, which may suggest different mechanisms of action.

Earlier studies both in mice WAT and human adipocytes have shown suppression of pro-inflammatory cytokines by AC [24–26], DHA [17] and PI [27], effects that are generally corroborated in the current study. DHA appears to be the strongest anti-inflammatory compound among the tested ones as this fatty acid decreased expression of three out of four investigated pro-inflammatory cytokines. We also for the first time report effects of bioactive compounds on chemerin – an insulin resistance inducing cytokine [8], which is largely secreted by adipocytes. DHA was the only compound suppressing chemerin secretion, which was antagonized by AC. Admittedly, at present we do not know how the selected bioactives regulate adipokine secretion, a question which needs further investigations. The outcome of compound interaction could also depend on their concentrations, the effects might not be linear and additional experiments using a concentration-dependent response for each bioactive alone and in combination are warranted to better establish any possible additive/synergistic effects on human adipocytes. However, our data suggest interactions between bioactives on fat cell function, which is relevant for in vivo physiology and nutrition.

Publications from murine 3T3-F442A and -L1 fat cells as well as isolated primary human adipocytes have demonstrated increased adiponectin secretion after DHA treatment [18, 19, 53]. However, it should be noted that fetal bovine serum, an additive which may protect the cells from ROS exposure, was included in the cell culture medium in all these previous studies. This may explain why higher concentrations of DHA could be used in those experiments. Other possible reasons for the discrepancies may be treatment duration or delivery as in vitro cell systems seem to be sensitive to this compound. The effect of PI on adiponectin secretion was unexpected, but could be due to its effect on PPARγ reported previously [54]. On the other hand we did not observe any effects of the compounds on fat cell differentiation/lipid accumulation, which speaks against their possible role regulating important adipogenic factors at least in in vitro cell system.

Conclusions

Our systematic assessment of DHA, AC and PI, either alone or in combination with DHA, indicate a beneficial role on human fat cell function. The selected compounds decreased basal lipolytic activity and secretion of inflammatory markers in human fat cells which might explain some of the reported health benefits induced by bioactive compound-containing diets in humans, including reduced insulin resistance, hypertension and dyslipidemia [21, 42, 55]. To further elucidate this question, our in vitro results will be used to identify specific biomarkers to be measured in volunteers recruited in a clinical intervention study within the PATHWAY-27 project.

Additional files

Additional file 1: Figure S1. No effect of BSA and EtOH on glycerol release or IL-6 secretion. Glycerol release (a) and IL-6 secretion (b) after 48 h of treatment with 0.05 % Ethanol (EtOH) and 0.125 μM bovine serum albumin (BSA) relative to untreated cells in conditioned media (n = 2 biological/independent experiments in quintuplicates). Normalized data is adjusted for protein amount and presented as means +/- standard deviation. The absence of statistical significance was determined by Tukey's test. (PPTX 46 kb)

Additional file 2: Figure S2. Adverse effects of DHA on adipocyte cytotoxicity and IL-6 secretion. Cytotoxicity detection measured as lactate dehydrogenase (LDH) activity in conditioned media after 6 days of treatment with 0.5 μM, 10 μM or 60 μM DHA, relative to control (a). Control, n = 7; 0.5 μM DHA, n = 3; 10 μM and 60 μM DHA, n = 2 biological/independent experiments in at least duplicates. Secretion of IL-6 from human in vitro differentiated adipocytes after 48 h of treatment with 0.5 μM, 5 μM, 10 μM, 20 μM, 30 μM or 60 μM DHA compared to control (b). Control, n = 2 and DHA n = 1 biological/independent experiments in triplicates. Normalized data is adjusted for protein amount and presented as means +/- standard deviation. *$p < 0.05$, **$p < 0.01$ and ***$p < 0.001$ versus control. Statistical significance was obtained by one-way ANOVA with Tukey's multiple comparisons post hoc test. (PPTX 47 kb)

Additional file 3: Figure S3. Decreased cytotoxicity after treatment with bioactive compounds or metabolites. Lactate dehydrogenase (LDH) activity after 48 h or 6 days treatment with bioactive compounds relative to control in conditioned media. Forty-eight hours; control, n = 9; 0.5 μM DHA, n = 6; AC alone and with DHA, n = 3; 100 μM PI alone and with DHA, n = 4 biological/independent experiments in quadruplicates; 6 days; control, n = 7; 0.5 μM DHA, n = 7; AC alone and with DHA, n = 4; 100 μM PI alone and with DHA, n = 5 biological/independent experiments in duplicates. Normalized data is adjusted for protein amount in each well as a measure of cell amount and presented as means +/- standard deviation. *$p < 0.05$, **$p < 0.01$ and ***$p < 0.001$ versus control. Statistical significance was determined by one-way ANOVA with Tukey's multiple comparisons post hoc test. (PPTX 44 kb)

Abbreviations

AC: anthocyanin; BG: beta-glucan; BMI: body mass index; BSA: bovine serum albumin; C3G: cyanidin-3-glucoside; CPM: counts per minute; DHA: docosahexaenoic acid; ELISA: enzyme-linked immunosorbent assay; LDH: lactate dehydrogenase; IL-6: interleukin-6; MCP-1/ *CCL2*: monocyte chemoattractant protein-1; PCA: protocatechuic acid; PI: propionic acid; PFA: paraformaldehyde solution; PBS: phosphate-buffered saline; PPARγ: Peroxisome Proliferator-Activated Receptor Gamma; SCFA: short-chain fatty acid; SDS: sodium dodecyl sulfate; SGBS: Simpson-Golabi-Behmel syndrome; TAG: triacylglycerol; TNFα: tumour necrosis factor-alpha; WAT: white adipose tissue.

Competing interests

The authors declare that they have no conflict of interests.

Authors' contributions

Conception and design (CB, SM, AB, MR, PA, JL); acquisition, analysis and interpretation of data (all co-authors), drafting the article (CB, UW, MR, PA, JL); critical revising of the manuscript and final approval of the version to be published (all co-authors).

Acknowledgements

The research leading to these results has received funding from the European Union Seventh Framework Programme (FP7/2007-2013) under grant agreement n° 311876: Pathway-27, the Swedish Research Council and Karolinska Institutet. We thank Stefan Storcksdieck, Caroline Orfila and Samantha Sutulic from the PATHWAY-27 consortium (www.pathway27.eu) for assisting with preparation of the manuscript. The excellent technical assistance of Gaby Åström, Elisabeth Dungner and Kerstin Wåhlen is greatly appreciated.

Author details

[1]Lipid Laboratory, Department of Medicine, Karolinska Institutet, Huddinge, Stockholm, Sweden. [2]Department of Biochemistry and Molecular Biology, University of Southern Denmark, 5230 Odense M, Denmark. [3]Department of Agro-Food Sciences and Technologies, University of Bologna, Bologna, Italy. [4]Department of Plastic Surgery, Akademikliniken, Stockholm, Sweden. [5]Department of Medicine, Karolinska Institutet, Lipid Laboratory, Novum, NVS D4, Hälsovägen 7, 14186 Stockholm, Sweden.

References

1. Maury E, Brichard SM. Adipokine dysregulation, adipose tissue inflammation and metabolic syndrome. Mol Cell Endocrinol. 2010;314:1–16.
2. Bays H, Mandarino L, DeFronzo RA. Role of the adipocyte, free fatty acids, and ectopic fat in pathogenesis of type 2 diabetes mellitus: peroxisomal proliferator-activated receptor agonists provide a rational therapeutic approach. J Clin Endocrinol Metab. 2004;89:463–78.
3. Hoffstedt J, Forster D, Lofgren P. Impaired subcutaneous adipocyte lipogenesis is associated with systemic insulin resistance and increased apolipoprotein B/AI ratio in men and women. J Intern Med. 2007;262:131–9.
4. Arner P, Langin D. Lipolysis in lipid turnover, cancer cachexia, and obesity-induced insulin resistance. Trends Endocrinol Metab. 2014;25:255–62.
5. Christiansen T, Richelsen B, Bruun JM. Monocyte chemoattractant protein-1 is produced in isolated adipocytes, associated with adiposity and reduced after weight loss in morbid obese subjects. Int J Obes (Lond). 2005;29:146–50.
6. Dahlman I, Kaaman M, Olsson T, Tan GD, Bickerton AS, Wahlen K, et al. A unique role of monocyte chemoattractant protein 1 among chemokines in adipose tissue of obese subjects. J Clin Endocrinol Metab. 2005;90:5834–40.
7. Weisberg SP, McCann D, Desai M, Rosenbaum M, Leibel RL, Ferrante Jr AW. Obesity is associated with macrophage accumulation in adipose tissue. J Clin Invest. 2003;112:1796–808.
8. Bozaoglu K, Bolton K, McMillan J, Zimmet P, Jowett J, Collier G, et al. Chemerin is a novel adipokine associated with obesity and metabolic syndrome. Endocrinology. 2007;148:4687–94.
9. Fried SK, Bunkin DA, Greenberg AS. Omental and subcutaneous adipose tissues of obese subjects release interleukin-6: depot difference and regulation by glucocorticoid. J Clin Endocrinol Metab. 1998;83:847–50.
10. Sewter CP, Digby JE, Blows F, Prins J, O'Rahilly S. Regulation of tumour necrosis factor-alpha release from human adipose tissue in vitro. J Endocrinol. 1999;163:33–8.
11. Grundy SM, Brewer Jr HB, Cleeman JI, Smith Jr SC, Lenfant C. Definition of metabolic syndrome: Report of the National Heart, Lung, and Blood Institute/American Heart Association conference on scientific issues related to definition. Circulation. 2004;109:433–8.
12. Arita Y, Kihara S, Ouchi N, Takahashi M, Maeda K, Miyagawa J, et al. Paradoxical decrease of an adipose-specific protein, adiponectin, in obesity. Biochem Biophys Res Commun. 1999;257:79–83.
13. Hoffstedt J, Arvidsson E, Sjolin E, Wahlen K, Arner P. Adipose tissue adiponectin production and adiponectin serum concentration in human obesity and insulin resistance. J Clin Endocrinol Metab. 2004;89:1391–6.
14. Li S, Shin HJ, Ding EL, van Dam RM. Adiponectin levels and risk of type 2 diabetes: a systematic review and meta-analysis. JAMA. 2009;302:179–88.
15. Siriwardhana N, Kalupahana NS, Cekanova M, LeMieux M, Greer B, Moustaid-Moussa N. Modulation of adipose tissue inflammation by bioactive food compounds. J Nutr Biochem. 2013;24:613–23.
16. Rosa FT, Zulet MA, Marchini JS, Martinez JA. Bioactive compounds with effects on inflammation markers in humans. Int J Food Sci Nutr. 2012;63:749–65.
17. Murumalla RK, Gunasekaran MK, Padhan JK, Bencharif K, Gence L, Festy F, et al. Fatty acids do not pay the toll: effect of SFA and PUFA on human adipose tissue and mature adipocytes inflammation. Lipids Health Dis. 2012;11:175.
18. Banga A, Unal R, Tripathi P, Pokrovskaya I, Owens RJ, Kern PA, et al. Adiponectin translation is increased by the PPARgamma agonists pioglitazone and omega-3 fatty acids. Am J Physiol Endocrinol Metab. 2009;296:E480–489.
19. Tishinsky JM, Ma DW, Robinson LE. Eicosapentaenoic acid and rosiglitazone increase adiponectin in an additive and PPARgamma-dependent manner in human adipocytes. Obesity (Silver Spring). 2011;19:262–8.
20. Warnke I, Goralczyk R, Fuhrer E, Schwager J. Dietary constituents reduce lipid accumulation in murine C3H10 T1/2 adipocytes: A novel fluorescent method to quantify fat droplets. Nutr Metab (Lond). 2011;8:30.
21. He J, Giusti MM. Anthocyanins: natural colorants with health-promoting properties. Annu Rev Food Sci Technol. 2010;1:163–87.
22. Scazzocchio B, Vari R, Filesi C, D'Archivio M, Santangelo C, Giovannini C, et al. Cyanidin-3-O-beta-glucoside and protocatechuic acid exert insulin-like effects by upregulating PPARgamma activity in human omental adipocytes. Diabetes. 2011;60:2234–44.
23. Scazzocchio B, Vari R, Filesi C, Del Gaudio I, D'Archivio M, Santangelo C, et al. Protocatechuic acid activates key components of insulin signaling pathway mimicking insulin activity. Mol Nutr Food Res. 2015;59:1472–81.
24. Guo H, Xia M, Zou T, Ling W, Zhong R, Zhang W. Cyanidin 3-glucoside attenuates obesity-associated insulin resistance and hepatic steatosis in high-fat diet-fed and db/db mice via the transcription factor FoxO1. J Nutr Biochem. 2012;23:349–60.
25. Sasaki R, Nishimura N, Hoshino H, Isa Y, Kadowaki M, Ichi T, et al. Cyanidin 3-glucoside ameliorates hyperglycemia and insulin sensitivity due to downregulation of retinol binding protein 4 expression in diabetic mice. Biochem Pharmacol. 2007;74:1619–27.
26. Tsuda T, Ueno Y, Yoshikawa T, Kojo H, Osawa T. Microarray profiling of gene expression in human adipocytes in response to anthocyanins. Biochem Pharmacol. 2006;71:1184–97.
27. Al-Lahham S, Roelofsen H, Rezaee F, Weening D, Hoek A, Vonk R, et al. Propionic acid affects immune status and metabolism in adipose tissue from overweight subjects. Eur J Clin Invest. 2012;42:357–64.
28. Al-Lahham SH, Roelofsen H, Priebe M, Weening D, Dijkstra M, Hoek A, et al. Regulation of adipokine production in human adipose tissue by propionic acid. Eur J Clin Invest. 2010;40:401–7.
29. Ge H, Li X, Weiszmann J, Wang P, Baribault H, Chen JL, et al. Activation of G protein-coupled receptor 43 in adipocytes leads to inhibition of lipolysis and suppression of plasma free fatty acids. Endocrinology. 2008;149:4519–26.
30. Han JH, Kim IS, Jung SH, Lee SG, Son HY, Myung CS. The effects of propionate and valerate on insulin responsiveness for glucose uptake in 3 T3-L1 adipocytes and C2C12 myotubes via G protein-coupled receptor 41. PLoS One. 2014;9:e95268.
31. Heimann E, Nymann M, Degerman E. Propionic acid and butyric acid inhibit lipolysis and de novo lipogenesis and increase insulin-stimulated glucose uptake in primary rat adipocytes. Adipocyte. 2014;4:1–8.
32. Hong YH, Nishimura Y, Hishikawa D, Tsuzuki H, Miyahara H, Gotoh C, et al. Acetate and propionate short chain fatty acids stimulate adipogenesis via GPCR43. Endocrinology. 2005;146:5092–9.
33. Arner P. Human fat cell lipolysis: biochemistry, regulation and clinical role. Best Pract Res Clin Endocrinol Metab. 2005;19:471–82.
34. Mikkelsen TS, Xu Z, Zhang X, Wang L, Gimble JM, Lander ES, et al. Comparative epigenomic analysis of murine and human adipogenesis. Cell. 2010;143:156–69.
35. Rosen ED, Spiegelman BM. What we talk about when we talk about fat. Cell. 2014;156:20–44.
36. van Harmelen V, Skurk T, Hauner H. Primary culture and differentiation of human adipocyte precursor cells. Methods Mol Med. 2005;107:125–35.
37. Wang YC, Kuo WH, Chen CY, Lin HY, Wu HT, Liu BH, et al. Docosahexaenoic acid regulates serum amyloid A protein to promote lipolysis through down regulation of perilipin. J Nutr Biochem. 2010;21:317–24.
38. Schlesinger JB, van Harmelen V, Alberti-Huber CE, Hauner H. Albumin inhibits adipogenesis and stimulates cytokine release from human adipocytes. Am J Physiol Cell Physiol. 2006;291:C27–33.
39. Hellmer J, Arner P, Lundin A. Automatic luminometric kinetic assay of glycerol for lipolysis studies. Anal Biochem. 1989;177:132–7.
40. Stenson BM, Ryden M, Venteclef N, Dahlman I, Pettersson AM, Mairal A, et al. Liver X receptor (LXR) regulates human adipocyte lipolysis. J Biol Chem. 2011;286:370–9.
41. Murali G, Desouza CV, Clevenger ME, Ramalingam R, Saraswathi V. Differential effects of eicosapentaenoic acid and docosahexaenoic acid in promoting the differentiation of 3 T3-L1 preadipocytes. Prostaglandins Leukot Essent Fatty Acids. 2014;90:13–21.
42. Lorente-Cebrian S, Costa AG, Navas-Carretero S, Zabala M, Martinez JA, Moreno-Aliaga MJ. Role of omega-3 fatty acids in obesity, metabolic syndrome, and cardiovascular diseases: a review of the evidence. J Physiol Biochem. 2013;69:633–51.
43. Attar-Bashi NM, Weisinger RS, Begg DP, Li D, Sinclair AJ. Failure of conjugated linoleic acid supplementation to enhance biosynthesis of docosahexaenoic acid from alpha-linolenic acid in healthy human volunteers. Prostaglandins Leukot Essent Fatty Acids. 2007;76:121–30.
44. Pawlosky RJ, Hibbeln JR, Herion D, Kleiner DE, Salem Jr N. Compartmental analysis of plasma and liver n-3 essential fatty acids in alcohol-dependent men during withdrawal. J Lipid Res. 2009;50:154–61.
45. Kim HK, Della-Fera M, Lin J, Baile CA. Docosahexaenoic acid inhibits adipocyte differentiation and induces apoptosis in 3 T3-L1 preadipocytes. J Nutr. 2006;136:2965–9.

46. Shi H, Kokoeva MV, Inouye K, Tzameli I, Yin H, Flier JS. TLR4 links innate immunity and fatty acid-induced insulin resistance. J Clin Invest. 2006;116:3015–25.
47. Ruan H, Hacohen N, Golub TR, Van Parijs L, Lodish HF. Tumor necrosis factor-alpha suppresses adipocyte-specific genes and activates expression of preadipocyte genes in 3 T3-L1 adipocytes: nuclear factor-kappaB activation by TNF-alpha is obligatory. Diabetes. 2002;51:1319–36.
48. Czank C, Cassidy A, Zhang Q, Morrison DJ, Preston T, Kroon PA, et al. Human metabolism and elimination of the anthocyanin, cyanidin-3-glucoside: a (13)C-tracer study. Am J Clin Nutr. 2013;97:995–1003.
49. Robertson MD, Bickerton AS, Dennis AL, Vidal H, Frayn KN. Insulin-sensitizing effects of dietary resistant starch and effects on skeletal muscle and adipose tissue metabolism. Am J Clin Nutr. 2005;82:559–67.
50. Guo H, Guo J, Jiang X, Li Z, Ling W. Cyanidin-3-O-beta-glucoside, a typical anthocyanin, exhibits antilipolytic effects in 3 T3-L1 adipocytes during hyperglycemia: involvement of FoxO1-mediated transcription of adipose triglyceride lipase. Food Chem Toxicol. 2012;50:3040–7.
51. Chuang CC, Bumrungpert A, Kennedy A, Overman A, West T, Dawson B, et al. Grape powder extract attenuates tumor necrosis factor alpha-mediated inflammation and insulin resistance in primary cultures of human adipocytes. J Nutr Biochem. 2011;22:89–94.
52. Pettersson AM, Acosta JR, Bjork C, Kratzel J, Stenson B, Blomqvist L, et al. MAFB as a novel regulator of human adipose tissue inflammation. Diabetologia. 2015;58:2115–23.
53. Oster RT, Tishinsky JM, Yuan Z, Robinson LE. Docosahexaenoic acid increases cellular adiponectin mRNA and secreted adiponectin protein, as well as PPARgamma mRNA, in 3 T3-L1 adipocytes. Appl Physiol Nutr Metab. 2010;35:783–9.
54. Besten GD, Bleeker A, Gerding A, van Eunen K, Havinga R, van Dijk TH, et al. Short-chain fatty acids protect against high-fat diet-induced obesity via a PPARgamma-dependent switch from lipogenesis to fat oxidation. Diabetes. 2015;64:2398–408.
55. El Khoury D, Cuda C, Luhovyy BL, Anderson GH. Beta glucan: health benefits in obesity and metabolic syndrome. J Nutr Metab. 2012;2012:851362.

15

Weight restoration on a high carbohydrate refeeding diet promotes rapid weight regain and hepatic lipid accumulation in female anorexic rats

Erin D. Giles[1,2], Jennifer Hagman[3], Zhaoxing Pan[4], Paul S. MacLean[1,2] and Janine A. Higgins[1,5*]

Abstract

Background: There is currently no standard clinical refeeding diet for the treatment of anorexia nervosa (AN). To provide the most efficacious AN clinical care, it is necessary to define the metabolic effects of current refeeding diets.

Methods: An activity-based model of anorexia nervosa (AN) was used in female rats. AN was induced over 7d by timed access to low fat (LF) diet with free access to a running wheel. Plasma hormones/metabolites and body composition were assessed at baseline, AN diagnosis (day 0), and following 28d of refeeding on LF diet. Energy balance and expenditure were measured via continuous indirect calorimetry on days −3 to +3.

Results: AN induction caused stress as indicated by higher levels of corticosterone versus controls ($p < 0.0001$). The rate of weight gain during refeeding was higher in AN rats than controls ($p = 0.0188$), despite lower overall energy intake ($p < 0.0001$). This was possible due to lower total energy expenditure (TEE) at the time of AN diagnosis which remained significantly lower during the entire refeeding period, driven by markedly lower resting energy expenditure (REE). AN rats exhibited lower lipid accumulation in visceral adipose tissues (VAT) but much higher liver accumulation (62 % higher in AN than control; $p < 0.05$) while maintaining the same total body weight as controls. It is possible that liver lipid accumulation was caused by overfeeding of carbohydrate suggesting that a lower carbohydrate, higher fat diet may be beneficial during AN treatment. To test whether such a diet would be accepted clinically, we conducted a study in adolescent female AN patients which showed equivalent palatability and acceptability for LF and moderate fat diets. In addition, this diet was feasible to provide clinically during inpatient treatment in this population.

Conclusion: Refeeding a LF diet to restore body weight in female AN rats caused depressed TEE and REE which facilitated rapid regain. However, this weight gain was metabolically unhealthy as it resulted in elevated lipid accumulation in the liver. It is necessary to investigate the use of other diets, such as lower carbohydrate, moderate fat diets, in pre-clinical models to develop the optimal clinical refeeding diets for AN.

Keywords: Anorexia nervosa, Refeeding, Indirect calorimetry, Energy expenditure, Activity-based anorexia, Carbohydrate, Diet, Rat, Clinical

* Correspondence: Janine.Higgins@childrenscolorado.org
[1]Center for Human Nutrition, University of Colorado Anschutz Medical Campus, Aurora, CO, USA
[5]Department of Pediatrics, School of Medicine, University of Colorado Anschutz Medical Campus, Aurora, CO, USA
Full list of author information is available at the end of the article

Background

Anorexia nervosa (AN) is a psychiatric illness characterized by body dissatisfaction accompanied by restriction of energy intake leading to a significantly low body weight, and persistent behaviors, including high levels of physical activity, that interfere with weight gain [1]. Individuals with AN become severely malnourished and develop significant medical complications [2, 3]. Although weight restoration is a primary intervention for AN, along with psychotherapy and behavioral interventions, there has been little research on optimal refeeding strategies. There is currently no standard, evidence-based clinical refeeding diet for the treatment of anorexia nervosa (AN) and nutritional treatment is focused primarily on calories and less on diet composition [4]. However, studies in both rats and humans show that diet composition can affect the rate of weight regain following weight loss, impact the ability to maintain at a target weight, and dramatically alter metabolic health [5–7]. Therefore, in order to provide the most efficacious clinical care for AN patients, it is necessary to define the effect of current refeeding diets on markers of metabolic health and use this information to develop optimal AN refeeding diets. Our ultimate goal is to achieve metabolically healthy weight gain in this population.

Given the low overall prevalence of AN in the population and the challenges in treating the illness, it would be difficult to test multiple different refeeding diets in AN patients. However, there is an established rodent model of AN that can be used for this purpose. Activity-based anorexia (ABA) is a well-established paradigm in which restricted time with access to food combined with free access to exercise causes hyperactivity, reduced energy intake, and, ultimately, anorexia in rats [8] (reviewed in [9, 10]) and to a lesser extent mice (reviewed in [11]). Most early studies of the ABA model utilized male rats, provided access to food for 1–2 h per day, and defined anorexia as a body weight at 65–75 % of free feeding or initial body weight. However, because AN in humans is most common in females, there has been a shift towards the use of female rats in the ABA model, primarily to study brain structure and neuronal biology/signaling in AN [12–15]. We endeavored to use recently published data about the diet and physical activity characteristics of female adolescent AN patients [16] to refine the ABA model in pubertal female rats to more closely mimic the human condition.

The goals of this study were to: 1) define the metabolic effects of a clinical refeeding diet on markers of metabolic health in a modified rodent model of AN and, 2) to develop a rat model of AN that closely mimics the human condition which could be used to screen more effective refeeding diets in the future. We hypothesized that, during the refeeding phase, AN rats would exhibit "catch-up growth" with preferential deposition of ingested energy into adipose depots [17–19], especially visceral adipose, indicative of a higher metabolic risk for cardiovascular disease and associated co-morbidities.

Methods

Rat energy balance study

Animals and housing

Female Sprague–Dawley rats (104-140 g; 5 weeks of age) possessing a polygenic predisposition for leanness and increased physical activity (lean/activity-prone, LAP) were purchased from Taconic Farms Inc. (Hudson, New York). Rats were housed individually in suspended wire cages at the University of Colorado Anschutz Medical Campus. All rats had free access to water in a temperature (22–25 °C) and humidity (30–40 %) controlled room with a 12 h light–dark cycle (lights off at 1300). All procedures were approved by the institutional animal care and use committee. Rats were allowed to acclimatize for 5 days, during which they had free access to a moderate fat (MF) diet (25 % kcal fat, 21 % kcal protein, 54 % kcal carbohydrate; Research Diets #D07091301, New Brunswick, NJ).

Activity-based anorexia model

Anorexia nervosa induction Following acclimatization, rats were randomly assigned to either the anorexia nervosa (AN) or control groups. AN rats were moved to wire mesh cages (13 x 25 x 13 cm) attached to a running wheel of 1.1 m circumference, and were given free access to the wheel for 23 h per day. The door separating the cage and the running wheel was closed for 1 h each day (1400–1500 h), during which time animals were given *ad libitum* access to a low fat (LF) diet (12 % kcal fat, 20 % kcal protein, 68 % kcal carbohydrate; Research Diets #D11724, New Brunswick, NJ). Control rats had the same *ad libitum* access to the LF diet for 1 h per day, but remained in suspended wire cages without access to a running wheel for the entire study. Food intake and body weight were measured daily.

Anorexia Rats were identified as anorexic (day 0) when their body weight decreased to ≤75 % of initial weight. 75 % of initial body weight was chosen as the threshold for AN as we previously found that this was the mean percent ideal body weight of female adolescent AN patients who presented for inpatient medical care at Children's Hospital Colorado [16]. For control animals, day 0 was defined as the seventh day of timed feeding.

Weight regain Access to running wheels was blocked and refeeding began on day 1 in all animals. All rats were refed on LF diet (described above). This diet is similar in composition to the standard refeeding diet used in the treatment AN patients at the Children's Hospital Colorado Eating Disorders Program [16].

For the AN group, refeeding for the first 3 days was based on each animal's energy intake measured on day 0. On days 1 and 2, AN rats were given 200 % of their energy intake at day 0. This was increased to 300 % on day 3, followed by *ad libitum* feeding for the remainder of the study. This staged re-feeding protocol for the AN group was conducted to mimic the clinical dietary paradigm currently used in adolescent AN patients. In the clinical program, caloric intake is increased by 250 kcal/d until patients reach a weight gain of 1 kg/wk. This paradigm was accelerated in the rat model by increasing caloric intake more quickly for two reasons: 1) at AN diagnosis, rats were frail so we wanted provide an opportunity for rapid recovery, and 2) to measure the effect of this approach on energy balance while rats were undergoing indirect calorimetry.

Indirect calorimetry

A metabolic monitoring system (Columbus Instruments, Columbus, OH) was used to assess energy intake and total energy expenditure in a subset of rats from the third day of timed feeding (anorexia induction; d-3) through three days of refeeding (d + 1, +2, and +3). Rats were randomly chosen for calorimetry, as the metabolic monitoring system did not have space to accommodate all rats used in this study. The multi-chamber indirect calorimetry system allows for the continuous monitoring of up to eight rats, obtaining measurements of oxygen consumption (vO_2) and carbon dioxide production (vCO_2) from each chamber every 16 min [19–21]. The chambers also allow for the collection of daily urine, feces, and food spillage. Daily total energy expenditure (TEE) was calculated from gas exchange measurements acquired over the 24-h period using the Weir equation ($MR = 3.941 \cdot vO_2 + 1.106 \cdot vCO_2 - 2.17 \cdot N$, where N represents urinary nitrogen) [22]. All data is expressed as kcal/day.

Body composition analysis

Body composition was determined by quantitative magnetic resonance (qMR; Echo MRI Whole Body Composition Analyzer; Echo Medical Systems, Houston, TX). Measurements were obtained on the first day of the timed feeding protocol, day 0, day 7, and at the end of study (day 30). Liver qMR measurements were taken at end of study, and only livers with weights ≥5.5 g were used for analysis due to the limits of sensitivity of our instrumentation.

Plasma and urine analyses

Urine samples were taken from the experimental and control group rats every 48 h while they were in the metabolic monitoring system. Urine was assayed for corticosterone, creatinine, and urea using a commercially available ELISAs (Fisher Scientific, Lafayette, CO). Urinary nitrogen was estimated from measurements of urea and creatinine, as previously described [20, 23].

Tail vein blood was collected under isoflurane anesthesia (MWI Veterinary Supply, Meridian, ID) from the animals at baseline, day 0, and end of study (day 28). Blood draws were taken after the animals had been fasting for 16–19 h (2.5 to 5.5 h prior to the next feeding period). The plasma was assayed using commercially available ELISAs for insulin (Alpco, Salem, NH), glucose (Fisher Scientific, Lafayette, CO), and leptin (Millipore Corp. Billerica, MA).

Clinical feasibility and proof of concept study

To determine the feasibility of feeding a diet higher in fat to patients with AN, we conducted 1) a diet palatability and acceptance study, and 2) a proof of concept study. These studies were conducted according to Declaration of Helsinki guidelines and all procedures were approved by the University of Colorado Anschutz Medical Campus Combined Institutional Review Board (COMIRB). All participants provided written assent with the written informed consent of a parent or guardian. Female subjects 12–21 years of age with a diagnosis of AN (restricting or binge/purge type) were recruited. All subjects were required to be undergoing inpatient eating disorder treatment to ensure that the most severely affected individuals are capable of eating a modified diet. All subjects had to be able to read and comprehend English at a 4th grade level.

a) Diet Palatability and Acceptance in AN patients
   Eight female inpatients, aged 12 to 21 years, diagnosed with AN were asked to rate the taste and acceptability of two different diets presented in random order: 1) the current clinical AN refeeding diet based on a lower fat, moderate protein diet (15 % protein, 26 % fat, 59 % carbohydrate), or 2) a moderate fat, high protein test diet (20 % protein, 40 % fat, 40 % carbohydrate). The single, acute meal tests replaced the participant's normal lunch. The macronutrient content of the clinical diet was calculated based on analysis (Nutrition Data System for Research; NDSR, University of Minnesota, Nutrition Coordinating Center) of photographs of all breakfasts, lunches, and daytime snacks served on the EDU over two consecutive days. Subjects had free access to water during the meals. All portions were weighed before and after consumption to measure the amount of food eaten.
   The main endpoint was taste assessment, based on a validated five face scale [24]. Participants were asked to complete a Likert scale for 1) taste, and 2) "would

you eat this again?" after consuming both the LF and MF diets. Scores were analyzed in two ways: the raw distribution of the five faces, and a two-group score (very good + good + average representing satisfactory taste and bad + very bad, representing unsatisfactory taste). Percent distribution of taste satisfaction score was calculated with 95 % confidence interval estimates.

b) Proof of Concept Case Study
To test whether the MF diet (20 % protein, 40 % fat, 40 % carbohydrate) could logistically be provided by the food services department at the hospital, and that it could be consumed consistently on an inpatient basis, we also performed a proof of concept study in which one patient followed the test MF diet for 10 consecutive days. The MF diet utilized only foods available from the hospital food service department. The participant was a 13 year old female with a 9 month documented duration of AN. She was at 72 % of ideal body weight at the commencement of the study (BMI 12.4). The participant, working with a research nutritionist, self-selected daily menus from the complete option list according to the nutrition intervention utilized in the treatment program. The menu for this subject was altered to provide over 120 menu options that would fulfill the dietary requirements of the study. All menus met clinical care targets for daily caloric goal. All other aspects of standard psychiatric and medical care were provided during this study.

Statistical analysis

SAS 9.3 was used for all the analyses. Repeated measures ANOVA by linear mixed effects model was used to make with-group and between-group comparisons for energy expenditure, energy balance, hormone, metabolite and body composition data collected prior to and at diagnosis and during re-feeding phases. A quadratic linear mixed effects model with random intercept, linear and quadratic coefficients was used to model daily body weight of rats during the refeeding phase. Two sample t-test was used to compare two group for data at rat sacrifice. No adjustment for multiple comparisons was applied. A p-value less than 0.05 was deemed to be statistically significant.

Results

Rat energy balance study

EI, wheel use, and body weight

Energy intake (EI; kcal/d) in the AN group decreased by approximately 50 % from day −2 to diagnosis of AN (day 0), and AN rats were consuming significantly fewer calories on day 0 than controls ($p = 0.0002$; Fig. 1a). Wheel running increased significantly in the 4 days leading up to AN diagnosis (Fig. 1b). This combination of increased physical activity and decreased energy intake precipitated the decline to an anorexic body weight, defined as 75 % of initial weight (90.1 ± 2.8 g), in 4 to 7 days (Fig. 1c). 75 % of initial body weight was chosen as the threshold for AN because we previously found that this was the mean percent ideal body weight of female adolescent AN patients who presented for inpatient medical care [16]. When given the same timed access to food without running wheels, control animals remained weight stable over the 7 day lead-in period (Fig. 1c).

In the AN group, refeeding was modeled after the staged refeeding protocol currently used in adolescent AN patients at our hospital. Thus, on days 1 and 2 of refeeding, rats were provided 200 % of their intake on d0. This was increased to 300 % on d3, and ad libitum intake for the remainder of the study. Conversely, control rats were allowed ad libitum food access for the entire refeeding period. In a mixed model analysis, a model consisting of group indicator, linear, quadratic terms and linear by group interaction as fixed effects best described the weight regain (Fig. 1d). Both AN and control rats gained a significant amount of weight over the weight re-gain period, but the rate of weight gain was significantly greater in the AN rats than controls ($p = 0.0188$). By d19 of refeeding, the body weights of the AN rats (180.9 ± 6.0 g) were no longer statistically different from controls (194.3 ± 5.7 g; Fig. 1c).

Energy expenditure and energy balance

Total energy expenditure (TEE) gradually declined in the 5 days leading to the AN diagnosis (Fig. 2a), a result of a declining resting energy expenditure (REE, Fig. 2b). During this time, nonresting energy expenditure (NREE) increased (Fig. 2c) as physical activity increased (Fig. 1b), until energy intake precipitously declined (Fig. 1a). At the time of AN diagnosis, REE reached a distinct nadir, while NREE remained relatively high. AN rats were in a negative energy imbalance during the entire lead-in period. The adaptive response to decrease REE minimized the energy imbalance in AN rats to −10 kcal at the time of diagnosis. In addition, protein disappearance increased during the days leading up to AN diagnosis (Fig. 2e), implying that these animals are breaking down lean body mass in attempt to maintain body weight. In contrast, the control group were in relative energy balance throughout the entire lead-in period (Fig. 2d) with little variation in TEE, REE, and NREE, consistent with stable body weight (Fig. 1c).

Over the first 4 days of refeeding, TEE increased in both the AN and control groups, but TEE was lower in AN rats compared to controls (Fig. 2a). This decrease in TEE is explained primarily by the lower REE in the AN group (Fig. 2b). NREE did not change significantly in either the AN or control group during the first few days of refeeding, despite the fact that wheel running activity

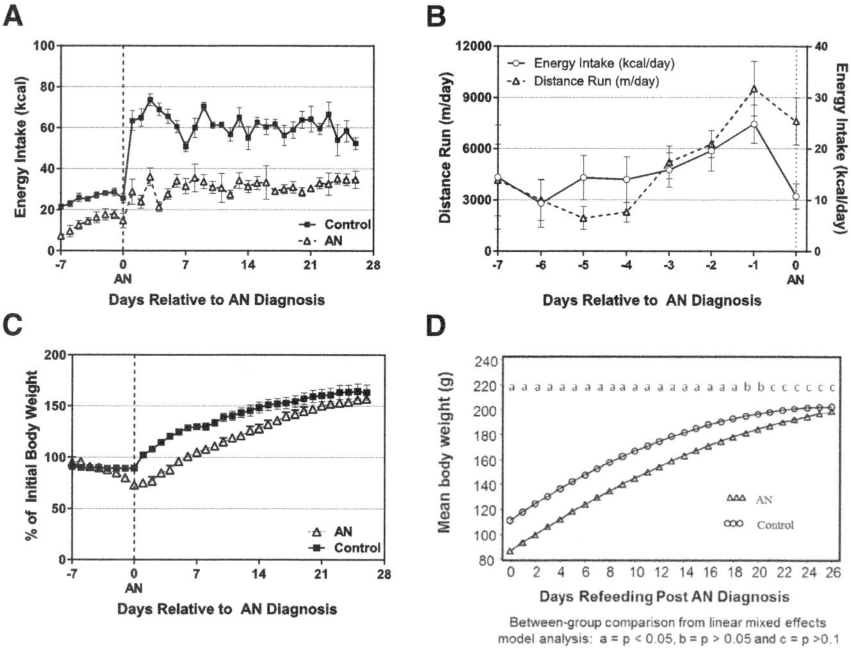

Fig. 1 Energy intake, running activity, and body weights for AN and control rats. **a** Energy Intake (EI) in control and AN rats for the duration of the study; **b** Distance run (left axis; m/d) and energy intake (right axis; kcal/d) during development of AN; **c** Body weights (expressed as % of initial body weight) for AN and control rats. **d** Body weights for AN and control rats with the results of mixed model analysis. For A-C, data shows group mean ± SEM

was stopped. This suggests that the increased food intake during this time, and the resulting increase in thermic effect of food (TEF), offset the decrease in activity thermogenesis, resulting in no change in NREE (Fig. 2c). As a result, EB increased in both the AN and control group during the refeeding period, with no difference between the groups (Fig. 2d).

EI was lower in AN than controls rats (EI = 33, 35, and 71 % of control on days 1, 2, and 3 of refeeding, respectively; $p < 0.0001$) resulting in lower thermic effect of food in the AN group during this time. Despite this lower EI in AN rats, TEE was so much lower that energy balance was the same for the AN and control groups on days 2 and 3 of refeeding (Fig. 2d). The differences in TEE between AN and control rats during refeeding was primarily due to suppression of REE (Fig. 2b) with a much lower contribution from NREE (Fig. 2c).

Hormone and metabolite responses

The ABA protocol induced a significant stress response, as demonstrated by significantly higher levels of urinary corticosterone in AN rats, compared to controls ($P < 0.0001$; Fig. 3a). Corticosterone levels began to decline immediately with the cessation of exercise and increased food intake, and were not significantly different than controls by d1 of refeeding (Fig. 3a).

Plasma glucose, insulin and leptin concentrations were measured in the fasted state at three time points: 1) at baseline, prior to the start of the AN protocol; 2) during the early refeeding period (d2 to 14 of refeeding); and 3) at end of the study. Blood draws were not performed at AN diagnosis (day 0) as the animals were too fragile. Glucose levels increased over time (Fig. 3b; $p < 0.001$), as was expected given that all rats were overfeeding and in a positive energy imbalance, but there were no differences between groups. Plasma insulin levels also increased over time in the control, but not AN rats, and, at the end of study, insulin levels were significantly lower in the AN group when compared to controls (Fig. 3c; $p < 0.05$).

As expected, leptin levels increased in the control animals (Fig. 3d) as body fat increased (Fig. 4a). AN rats, however, had lower leptin levels in the early refeeding phase, despite having the same body weight and fat mass as control rats. At the end of the study, leptin was 3.7 fold lower in the AN rats compared to control rats, which is lower than what would be expected based on the 1.6 fold lower body fat.

Body composition

At the time of AN diagnosis (day 0) there was no difference in body fat or lean body mass between the two groups (Fig. 4a-b) despite a significantly lower body

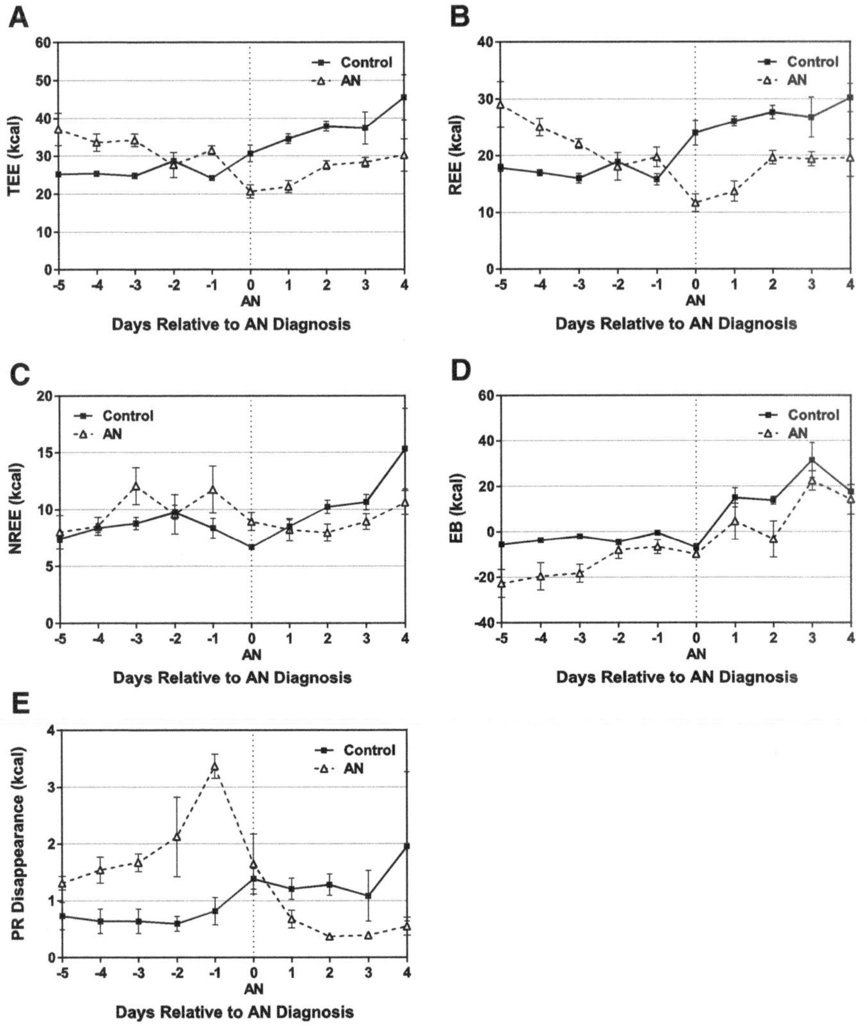

Fig. 2 Energy expenditure, energy balance, and protein disappearance during the development of AN and the early refeeding period. **a** Total Energy Expenditure (TEE), which was also divided into its **b** Non-resting (NREE) and **c** Resting (REE) components. **d** Energy Balance (EB) **e** Protein Disappearance. All data shows group mean ± SEM

mass in the AN animals. Thus, while both access to a running wheel and timed food access are required for the development of AN, timed food access alone (control rats) led to a decrease in body fat without a significant change in total body weight. During the weight regain period, body fat increased significantly in both the AN and control groups (Fig. 4a-b). However, fat gain plateaued in the AN group during the second week of refeeding, but continued to increase in the control animals. As a result, AN rats gained significantly less fat over the follow-up period (day 0 vs 28, $p < 0.001$), perhaps an indication that they are "defending" their lower body weight. At the time of sacrifice, the amount of subcutaneous fat was not different between control and AN rats but visceral fat was significantly lower in the AN rats relative to controls ($p = 0.02$, Fig. 4d), suggesting that a decrease in visceral fat was primarily responsible for the lower total body fat in the AN group. Refeeding increased liver fat by approximately 40 % in AN rats relative to controls (0.7 vs 1.9 g in AN and controls, respectively; $p < 0.05$, Fig. 4e).

Clinical feasibility and proof of concept study

Clinical acceptance of a diet higher in fat and protein

The average macronutrient content of the meal plan (selected by parents from a specialized menu, with dietician support and oversight) in the clinical program for adolescents with AN was 15 % protein, 26 % fat, and

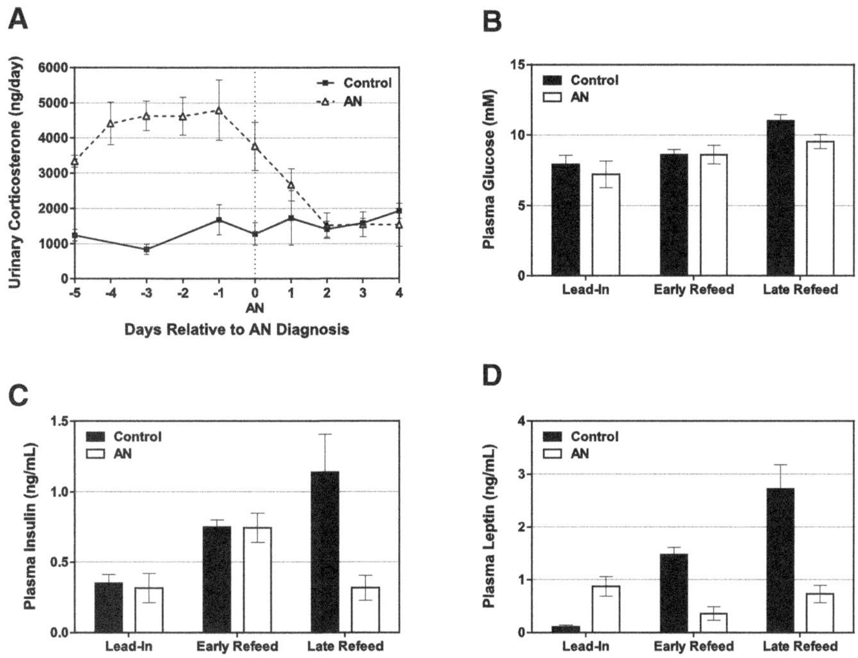

Fig. 3 Metabolite and hormone measurements. **a** Urinary corticosterone, **b** plasma glucose, **c** plasma insulin, and **d** plasma leptin concentrations during the development of AN and the refeeding period. All data shows group mean ± SEM

59 % carbohydrate. Meals accounted for 64 % of total calories (16 % protein, 31 % fat, and 53 % carbohydrate), while snacks accounted for the remaining 36 % of total calories (11 % protein, 21 % fat, and 68 % carbohydrate).

To follow up on the finding of increased liver fat observed during the rat refeeding model, and to explore the possibility of feeding a different "test diet" to patients with AN, which might decrease the risk of accumulation of liver fat during refeeding, we conducted feasibility studies utilizing a moderate fat (MF) diet. The current LF (15 % protein, 26 % fat, 59 % carbohydrate) and test MF (20 % protein, 40 % fat, 40 % carbohydrate) diets were ranked the same for both taste and palatability (Fig. 5a and b). There was no difference in the energy consumption between the two meals as participants consumed all food presented to them under both conditions. These data suggest that feeding a MF diet would be possible in this population. In addition, a single inpatient admitted to the clinical program was fed a dietician-directed, self-selected MF diet for 10 consecutive days proving that it is indeed possible to plan meals with a higher fat, higher protein and lower carbohydrates clinically in adolescents with AN during the refeeding period (Fig. 5c-d).

Discussion

The primary goal of this study was to develop a rat model that can be used to evaluate refeeding strategies and potentially improve the process of weight restoration during the treatment of AN. Specifically, it is likely that different dietary regimens could be used to strengthen the biological response to refeeding and potentially improve weight regain and maintenance in this population. Thus, developing a model that mirrors the human condition was of critical importance. Our model, which combined a classic exercise induced anorexia paradigm (free access to a running wheel with timed access to food; [12]) with the addition of using female adolescent rats genetically predisposed to leanness, led to the development of AN within 4–7 days and was characterized by a loss in both total body mass and body fat. Unlike data from Dixon et al. [12], rats in the AN group in this study ate significantly less food during the AN induction phase than the control group. In addition, increased physical activity preceded any decrease in energy intake by several days which mirrors the development of human AN in which increased physical activity may be the first apparent symptom prior to onset of dramatic weight loss [25].

When AN rats were compared to control animals, refeeding on a standard LF diet caused comparable increases in total body weight and subcutaneous fat accumulation. However, leptin concentrations were lower in the AN rats compared to controls and were also lower in AN rats than would be expected based on total body fat. This phenomenon of leptin concentration underestimating body fat stores is similar to that seen in rodent

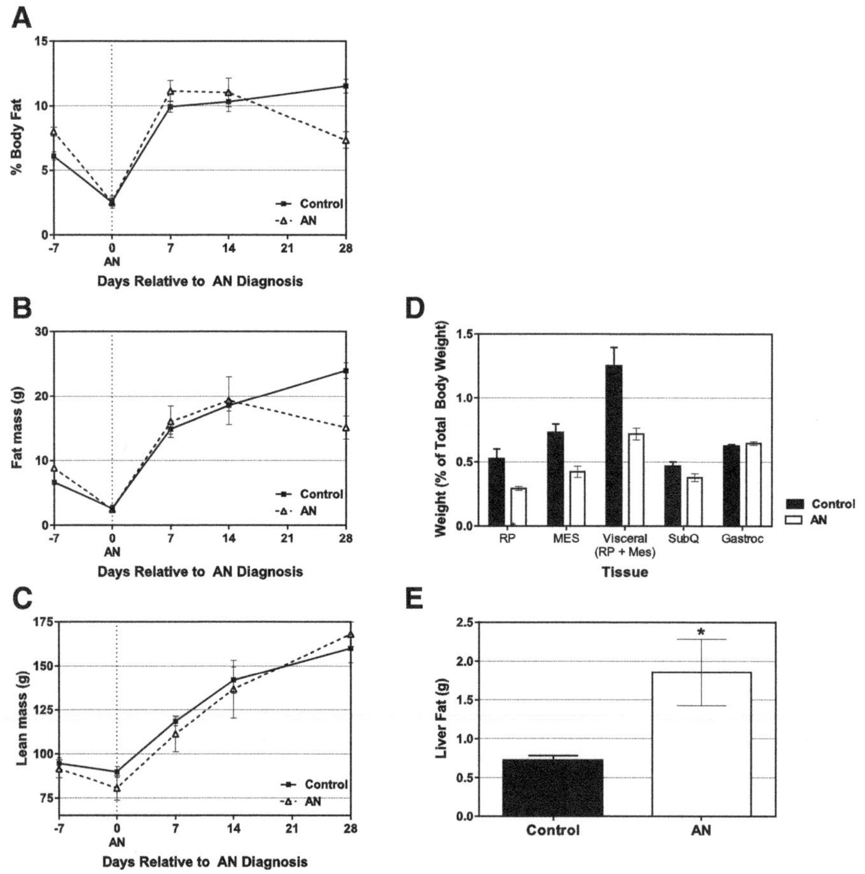

Fig. 4 Body composition and regional adiposity of AN and control rats. **a** Percent body fat, **b** Absolute fat mass (g), and **c** Absolute lean mass were measured by qMR for AN and control rats at weekly intervals throughout the study. At the end of the study, **d** Regional fat distribution was assessed by weighing each fat pad and expressing the weight as a % of totally body weight. **e** Fat (g) in the liver was measured by qMR at end of study. All data shows group mean ± SEM

models of obesity whereby formerly obese rats that lose weight do not have restored leptin concentrations after weight regain [23]. In our AN model, however, the effects are more dramatic than in the models of obesity. Although the underlying mechanism for this effect is unknown, the fact that the same amount of adipose tissue is secreting different amounts of leptin suggests that the adipo-insulin and adipo-leptin axes are perturbed in these animals.

Despite similar increases in total body fat, AN rats exhibited dramatically higher liver fat compared to controls. It is likely that the high accumulation of liver fat is due, at least in part, to increased de novo lipogenesis from excess carbohydrate intake during the refeeding period [26]. In addition, fat gain appeared to plateau in the AN rats during the second week of refeeding. In models of obesity-associated weight loss and weight regain, exercise appears to decrease the formation of new adipocytes via adipogenesis [27–29]. Thus, we would speculate that the exercise during the AN development phase, combined with the increase in caloric intake during the refeeding period, resulted in decreased formation of new adipocytes early in the regain period. If this is the case: 1) existing adipocytes likely reached their storage capacity during the first week of refeeding, and, after this time, excess nutrients were deposited in non-adipose storage sites, such as the liver, and 2) the lower number of total adipocytes may, in part, explain the lower leptin concentrations observed in AN rats. An alternative explanation is that the cessation of exercise could also contribute to hepatic de novo lipogenesis and the noticeable increase in lipid accumulation in the liver of AN rats, as cessation of daily exercise has been shown to promote hepatic steatosis in hyperphagic/obese rats [30]. Future studies could include use of tracers to directly address the etiology of lipid accumulation. Regardless of the underlying mechanism, this increase in fat accumulation in the liver is cause for concern, as

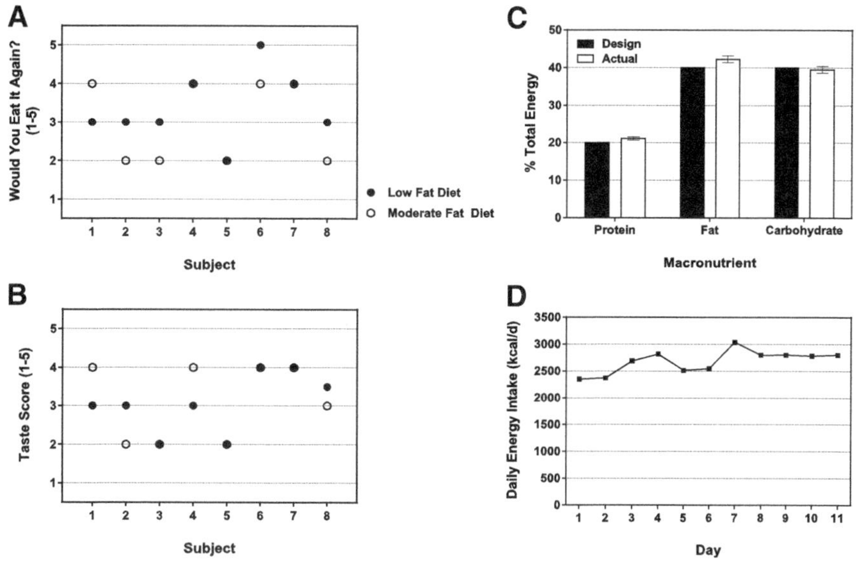

Fig. 5 Lower carbohydrate, higher fat diet acceptability and feasibility in female adolescent AN patients. Eight female inpatients diagnosed with AN rated the taste and acceptability of the standard LF diet, and a test diet high in protein with moderate fat (MF) using a validated five face scale. **a** Results of the face scale for willingness to consume the diet in the future and **b** taste after consuming both the LF and MF diets. The MF diet utilized only foods available from the hospital food service department. Daily menus from the complete option list for MF diet were analyzed for **c** macronutrient targets ((20 % protein, 40 % fat, 40 % carbohydrate) and **d** fidelity to daily caloric goals

liver fat is associated with insulin resistance [31] and the development of type 2 diabetes, independent of total adiposity [32].

It is not known if patients with AN develop increased liver fat during the refeeding process. Further research is needed to determine if human subjects undergoing weight restoration have similar findings. To counter the negative effects of a LF diet on fat accumulation in the liver, observed on the AN group, it may be optimal to adjust the composition of the diet during weight restoration in AN to a diet with lower carbohydrate and increased fat content. Although previous AN research has shown that the percentage of fat and protein is not lower in acute inpatient AN than in age and sex matched adolescents, the absolute amounts of fat and protein intake are low [16]. Thus, it is possible that increasing the fat and protein content of an AN refeeding diet may be beneficial. Indeed, during the timed food restriction, induction phase of ABA, a high fat diet can prevent AN in rats [33, 34]. This effect is due to both the preservation of caloric intake during the AN induction phase and decreased physical activity relative to standard rat chow which is a high carbohydrate food [34].

We would hypothesize that a diet higher in both fat and protein, and lower in carbohydrate, could ameliorate the fat accumulation observed in the liver in the current model and could also increase the rate of weight gain (by decreasing de novo lipogenesis with a concomitant decrease in TEE). This strategy would agree with the recommendation to limit AN refeeding diets to less than 40 % of calories from carbohydrate to reduce the risk of refeeding syndrome [35]. However, if both fat and protein are to be used to replace dietary carbohydrate, caution must be exercised as there are selected reports of hyperammonemia with high protein intake after substantial weight loss [36]. Although these data are from case reports and are rare in AN patients [37], it is important that refeeding diets with higher protein contents be tested in a pre-clinical model, such as that described herein, before being administered clinically.

Although it is possible that higher fat and protein refeeding diets may be beneficial, it is commonly believed that AN patients have an aversion to fat although the data supporting this assumption are equivocal [38]. To address this possible concern, we conducted a feasibility study in adolescent females with AN, which showed that a MF diet is both acceptable and palatable to patients with AN and that such a diet can be delivered successfully in an inpatient clinical setting. In the single patient with AN who consumed the MF diet for 10 consecutive days during weight restoration, all study parameters for macronutrient content were achieved in addition to following the program's standard of care guidelines for calorie changes over time, rate of weight gain, monitoring food avoidance behaviors and enhancing reward systems, and behavioral motivation, etc.

The measured average macronutrient content of the clinical refeeding diet utilized in the treatment program in this study matches that for a similar sample of subjects measured retrospectively at the time of medical hospitalization for malnutrition and bradycardia [16]. As part of treatment, parents work closely with dieticians to plan the patient's meals based on a specific number of protein, carbohydrate, and satiety (fat) foods to achieve the daily caloric goal for weight restoration so the macronutrient content of these inpatient diets may be somewhat limited by this process.

The onset of AN and maintenance of the illness is associated with decreased caloric intake over a sustained period of time, ranging from months to years. Further studies are needed to determine optimal macronutrient composition and rate of weight gain for the weight restoration phase of treatment of AN, and if sustained change in dietary composition improves outcomes. It is possible that the cognitive changes associated with AN (body image distortion, fear of fat, harm avoidance and cognitive rigidity) may also respond to changes in dietary composition during weight restoration.

Conclusion

We have made subtle changes to the standard rat ABA model such that the development of AN more closely mimics the human condition. In this model, refeeding a LF diet to restore body weight in AN rats caused depressed TEE and REE which facilitated rapid regain. However, this weight gain was metabolically unhealthy as it caused elevated lipid accumulation in the liver. Future studies should explore if this finding also occurs in human subjects with AN undergoing weight restoration. Further, it is necessary to investigate the use of other diets with different macronutrient ratios, such as lower carbohydrate, higher fat diets, in pre-clinical models to develop the optimal clinical refeeding diets for the weight restoration phase of AN treatment. Our preliminary data suggest that such diets are acceptable and feasible to deliver clinically in an inpatient hospital setting.

Ethics approval and consent to participate

Rodent studies were approved by the University of Colorado Anschutz Medical Campus Institutional Animal Care and Use Committee (IACUC). Human studies were conducted according to Declaration of Helsinki guidelines and all procedures were approved by the University of Colorado Anschutz Medical Campus Combined Institutional Review Board (COMIRB). All participants provided written assent with the written informed consent of a parent or guardian.

Consent for publication

Consent to publish has been obtained from all individuals or their parent or legal guardian.

Abbreviations

AN: anorexia nervosa; ABA: activity based anorexia; BMI: Body Mass Index; EDU: Children's Hospital Colorado Eating Disorders Unit; LAP: lean/activity-prone; LF: Low fat diet (12 % kcal fat); MF: Moderate fat diet (25 % kcal fat); MR: Metabolic rate; N: Urinary nitrogen; NDSR: Nutrition Data System for Research; NREE: non-resting energy expenditure; qMR: Quantitative Magnetic Resonance; TEE: total energy expenditure; vCO_2: carbon dioxide production; vO_2: oxygen consumption.

Competing interests

The authors declare that they have no competing interests.

Authors' contributions

EDG participated in the design and execution of the animal studies, and drafted the manuscript; JAH designed, executed, and coordinated both the rodent and human studies, conducted data analysis and interpretation, and drafted the manuscript; JOH designed and coordinated the human studies; PSM contributed to the design, execution, and data analysis/interpretation for the rodent study; ZP performed all statistical analyses. All authors read and approved the final manuscript.

Acknowledgements

This work was supported by the National Institutes of Health to PSM (R01 DK038088) and a Pilot Award from the Colorado Clinical Translational Research Institute to JAH (UL1 TR001082). We appreciate the support from the core facilities of the Colorado Nutrition Obesity Research Center (NORC, P30 DK48520).

Author details

[1]Center for Human Nutrition, University of Colorado Anschutz Medical Campus, Aurora, CO, USA. [2]Division of Endocrinology, Diabetes and Metabolism, School of Medicine, University of Colorado Anschutz Medical Campus, Aurora, CO, USA. [3]Department of Psychiatry, School of Medicine, University of Colorado Anschutz Medical Campus, Aurora, CO, USA. [4]Biostatistics Core, Children's Hospital Colorado Research Institute, Aurora, CO, USA. [5]Department of Pediatrics, School of Medicine, University of Colorado Anschutz Medical Campus, Aurora, CO, USA.

References

1. American Psychiatric Association. DSM-5 Task Force: Diagnostic and statistical manual of mental disorders: DSM-5. 5th ed. Arlington: American Psychiatric Association; 2013.
2. Sigel EJ. Eating Disorders. In: William Hay ML, Deterding R, Abzug M, editors. Current diagnosis and treatment pediatrics. 22nd ed. United States: McGraw-Hill; 2014.
3. Mehler PS, Brown C. Anorexia nervosa - medical complications. J Eat Disord. 2015;3:11.
4. Schwartz BI, Mansbach JM, Marion JG, Katzman DK, Forman SF. Variations in admission practices for adolescents with anorexia nervosa: a North American sample. J Adolesc Health. 2008;43:425–31.
5. Kahlhofer J, Lagerpusch M, Enderle J, Eggeling B, Braun W, Pape D, Muller MJ, Bosy-Westphal A. Carbohydrate intake and glycemic index affect substrate oxidation during a controlled weight cycle in healthy men. Eur J Clin Nutr. 2014;68:1060–6.
6. Lagerpusch M, Enderle J, Eggeling B, Braun W, Johannsen M, Pape D, Muller MJ, Bosy-Westphal A. Carbohydrate quality and quantity affect glucose and lipid metabolism during weight regain in healthy men. J Nutr. 2013;143:1593–601.
7. Kliewer KL, Ke JY, Lee HY, Stout MB, Cole RM, Samuel VT, Shulman GI, Belury MA. Short-term food restriction followed by controlled refeeding promotes gorging behavior, enhances fat deposition, and diminishes insulin sensitivity in mice. J Nutr Biochem. 2015;26:721–8.
8. Epling WF, Pierce WD. Activity-based anorexia in rats as a function of opportunity to run on an activity wheel. Nutr Behav. 1984;2:37–49.
9. Gutierrez E. A rat in the labyrinth of anorexia nervosa: contributions of the activity-based anorexia rodent model to the understanding of anorexia nervosa. Int J Eat Disord. 2013;46:289–301.

10. Casper RC, Sullivan EL, Tecott L. Relevance of animal models to human eating disorders and obesity. Psychopharmacology. 2008;199:313–29.
11. Klenotich SJ, Dulawa SC. The activity-based anorexia mouse model. Methods Mol Biol. 2012;829:377–93.
12. Dixon DP, Ackert AM, Eckel LA. Development of, and recovery from, activity-based anorexia in female rats. Physiol Behav. 2003;80:273–9.
13. Chowdhury TG, Rios MB, Chan TE, Cassataro DS, Barbarich-Marsteller NC, Aoki C. Activity-based anorexia during adolescence disrupts normal development of the CA1 pyramidal cells in the ventral hippocampus of female rats. Hippocampus. 2014;24:1421–9.
14. Chowdhury TG, Barbarich-Marsteller NC, Chan TE, Aoki C. Activity-based anorexia has differential effects on apical dendritic branching in dorsal and ventral hippocampal CA1. Brain Struct Funct. 2014;219:1935–45.
15. Wable GS, Barbarich-Marsteller NC, Chowdhury TG, Sabaliauskas NA, Farb CR, Aoki C. Excitatory synapses on dendritic shafts of the caudal basal amygdala exhibit elevated levels of GABAA receptor alpha4 subunits following the induction of activity-based anorexia. Synapse. 2014;68:1–15.
16. Higgins J, Hagman J, Pan Z, MacLean P. Increased physical activity not decreased energy intake is associated with inpatient medical treatment for anorexia nervosa in adolescent females. PLoS One. 2013;8:e61559.
17. De Andrade PB, Neff LA, Strosova MK, Arsenijevic D, Patthey-Vuadens O, Scapozza L, Montani JP, Ruegg UT, Dulloo AG, Dorchies OM. Caloric restriction induces energy-sparing alterations in skeletal muscle contraction, fiber composition and local thyroid hormone metabolism that persist during catch-up fat upon refeeding. Front Physiol. 2015;6:254.
18. De Toro-Martin J, Fernandez-Millan E, Lizarraga-Mollinedo E, Lopez-Oliva E, Serradas P, Escriva F, Alvarez C. Predominant role of GIP in the development of a metabolic syndrome-like phenotype in female Wistar rats submitted to forced catch-up growth. Endocrinology. 2014;155:3769–80.
19. Jackman MR, Steig A, Higgins JA, Johnson GC, Fleming-Elder BK, Bessesen DH, MacLean PS. Weight regain after sustained weight reduction is accompanied by suppressed oxidation of dietary fat and adipocyte hyperplasia. Am J Physiol Regul Integr Comp Physiol. 2008;294:R1117–29.
20. MacLean PS, Higgins JA, Johnson GC, Fleming-Elder BK, Peters JC, Hill JO. Metabolic adjustments with the development, treatment, and recurrence of obesity in obesity-prone rats. Am J Physiol Regul Integr Comp Physiol. 2004; 287:R288–97.
21. Giles ED, Jackman MR, Johnson GC, Schedin PJ, Houser JL, MacLean PS. Effect of the estrous cycle and surgical ovariectomy on energy balance, fuel utilization, and physical activity in lean and obese female rats. Am J Physiol Regul Integr Comp Physiol. 2010;299:R1634–42.
22. Weir JB. New methods for calculating metabolic rate with special reference to protein metabolism. J Physiol. 1949;109:1–9.
23. MacLean PS, Higgins JA, Jackman MR, Johnson GC, Fleming-Elder BK, Wyatt HR, Melanson EL, Hill JO. Peripheral metabolic responses to prolonged weight reduction that promote rapid, efficient regain in obesity-prone rats. Am J Physiol Regul Integr Comp Physiol. 2006;290:R1577–88.
24. Hames H, Seabrook JA, Matsui D, Rieder MJ, Joubert GI. A palatability study of a flavored dexamethasone preparation versus prednisolone liquid in children. Can J Clin Pharmacol. 2008;15:e95–8.
25. Davis C, Katzman DK, Kaptein S, Kirsh C, Brewer H, Kalmbach K, Olmsted MP, Woodside DB, Kaplan AS. The prevalence of high-level exercise in the eating disorders: etiological implications. Compr Psychiatry. 1997;38:321–6.
26. Schwarz JM, Linfoot P, Dare D, Aghajanian K. Hepatic de novo lipogenesis in normoinsulinemic and hyperinsulinemic subjects consuming high-fat, low-carbohydrate and low-fat, high-carbohydrate isoenergetic diets. Am J Clin Nutr. 2003;77:43–50.
27. Steig AJ, Jackman MR, Giles ED, Higgins JA, Johnson GC, Mahan C, Melanson EL, Wyatt HR, Eckel RH, Hill JO, MacLean PS. Exercise reduces appetite and traffics excess nutrients away from energetically efficient pathways of lipid deposition during the early stages of weight regain. Am J Physiol Regul Integr Comp Physiol. 2011;301:R656–67.
28. MacLean PS, Higgins JA, Giles ED, Sherk VD, Jackman MR. The role for adipose tissue in weight regain after weight loss. Obes Rev. 2015;16 Suppl 1:45–54.
29. MacLean PS, Higgins JA, Wyatt HR, Melanson EL, Johnson GC, Jackman MR, Giles ED, Brown IE, Hill JO. Regular exercise attenuates the metabolic drive to regain weight after long-term weight loss. Am J Physiol Regul Integr Comp Physiol. 2009;297:R793–802.
30. Rector RS, Thyfault JP, Laye MJ, Morris RT, Borengasser SJ, Uptergrove GM, Chakravarthy MV, Booth FW, Ibdah JA. Cessation of daily exercise dramatically alters precursors of hepatic steatosis in Otsuka Long-Evans Tokushima Fatty (OLETF) rats. J Physiol. 2008;586:4241–9.
31. Muller MJ, Lagerpusch M, Enderle J, Schautz B, Heller M, Bosy-Westphal A. Beyond the body mass index: tracking body composition in the pathogenesis of obesity and the metabolic syndrome. Obes Rev. 2012;13 Suppl 2:6–13.
32. Yki-Jarvinen H. Liver fat in the pathogenesis of insulin resistance and type 2 diabetes. Dig Dis. 2010;28:203–9.
33. Brown AJ, Avena NM, Hoebel BG. A high-fat diet prevents and reverses the development of activity-based anorexia in rats. Int J Eat Disord. 2008;41:383–9.
34. Barboriak JJ, Wilson AS. Effect of diet on self-starvation in the rat. J Nutr. 1972;102:1543–6.
35. Kohn MR, Madden S, Clarke SD. Refeeding in anorexia nervosa: increased safety and efficiency through understanding the pathophysiology of protein calorie malnutrition. Curr Opin Pediatr. 2011;23:390–4.
36. Bilsborough S, Mann N. A review of issues of dietary protein intake in humans. Int J Sport Nutr Exerc Metab. 2006;16:129–52.
37. Welsh E, Kucera J, Perloff MD. IAtrogenic hyperammonemia after anorexia. Arch Intern Med. 2010;170:486–8.
38. Segura-Garcia C, De Fazio P, Sinopoli F, De Masi R, Brambilla F. Food choice in disorders of eating behavior: Correlations with the psychopathological aspects of the diseases. Compr Psychiatry. 2014;55(5):1203–11.

Leptin receptor signaling is required for high-fat diet-induced atrophic gastritis in mice

Kyoko Inagaki-Ohara[1,2,3*], Shiki Okamoto[2], Kazuyo Takagi[2], Kumiko Saito[2], Seiya Arita[3], Lijun Tang[2], Tetsuji Hori[4], Hiroaki Kataoka[5], Satoshi Matsumoto[4] and Yasuhiko Minokoshi[2]

Abstract

Background: Obesity increases the risk for malignancies in various tissues including the stomach. Atrophic gastritis with precancerous lesions is an obesity-associated disease; however, the mechanisms that underlie the development of obesity-associated atrophic gastritis are unknown. Leptin is a hormone derived from stomach as well as adipose tissue and gastric leptin is involved in the development of gastric cancer. The aim of the current study is to investigate the involvement of leptin receptor signaling in the development of atrophic gastritis during diet-induced obesity.

Methods: Male C57BL/6, *ob/ob* and *db/db* mice were fed a high-fat diet (HFD) or a control diet (CD) from 1 week to 5 months. Pathological changes of the gastric mucosa and the expression of molecules associated with atrophic gastritis were evaluated in these mice.

Results: HFD feeding induced gastric mucosal hyperplasia with increased gastric leptin expression. Mucosal hyperplasia was accompanied by a higher frequency of Ki67-positive proliferating cells and atrophy of the gastric glands in the presence of inflammation, which increased following HFD feeding. Activation of ObR signaling-associated molecules such as ObR, STAT3, Akt, and ERK was detected in the gastric mucosa of mice fed the HFD for 1 week. The morphological alterations associated with gastric mucosal atrophy and the expression of Muc2 and Cdx2 resemble those associated with human intestinal metaplasia. In contrast to wild-type mice, leptin-deficient *ob/ob* mice and leptin receptor-mutated *db/db* mice did not show increased Cdx2 expression in response to HFD feeding.

Conclusion: Together, these results suggest that activation of the leptin signaling pathway in the stomach is required to develop obesity-associated atrophic gastritis.

Keywords: Leptin, Atrophic gastritis, High-fat diet, Obesity

Background

Gastric carcinoma (GC) typically arises on a background of atrophic gastritis, intestinal metaplasia, and dysplasia of gastric mucosa, and is the second leading cause of cancer-related deaths worldwide [1]. Obesity augments the risk of a higher prevalence of gastritis [2, 3], atrophic gastritis [4–6], and gastric cardia adenocarcinoma [7–9].

* Correspondence: k-inagaki@pu-hiroshima.ac.jp
[1]Research Institute, National Center for Global Health and Medicine (NCGM), 1-21-1, Toyama Shinjuku, Tokyo 162-0052, Japan
[2]Division of Endocrinology and Metabolism, Department of Developmental Physiology, National Institute for Physiological Sciences (NIPS), 38 Nishigonaka Myodaiji, Okazaki, Aichi 444-8585, Japan
Full list of author information is available at the end of the article

Infection with *Helicobacter pylori*, a bacterium that infects humans and colonizes the stomach, is the predominant cause of precancerous lesions in the mucosal lining of the stomach [10]. Although *H. pylori* infection is not confined to morbidly obese patients, obesity increases the prevalence of chronic gastritis and GC [2]. Furthermore, obesity is not only a risk factor for certain tumors but is also associated with an increased mortality rate [11]. Thus, obesity potentially affects the development of gastritis into gastric tumorigenesis. Therefore, it is imperative to identify signaling molecules associated with both obesity and precancerous lesions to aid in the management of high-risk individuals.

Leptin, a product of the obese (*ob*) gene, is primarily produced by adipocytes and acts on its receptor (ObR) in the hypothalamus to suppress food intake and increase energy expenditure [12]. ObR belongs to the class I cytokine receptor family, and its structure is highly homologous to that of gp130, the common signal-transducing receptor for the interleukin-6 (IL-6) family of cytokines [13]. Of the six alternate splice variants of ObR, only the long isoform, ObRb, transduces a signal cascade that activates downstream Janus kinase 2 and signal transducer and activator of transcription 3 (JAK2-STAT3), phosphoinositide 3-kinase (PI3K), and extracellular signal-regulated kinase 1/2 (ERK1/2) [14]. In addition to its role in energy homeostasis, leptin exerts pleiotropic effects on angiogenesis, hematopoiesis, and immunity as well [14]. Leptin and ObR are also expressed in various tissues including the gastrointestinal tract [15]. Additionally, the stomach can spontaneously express leptin and ObR, leading to the augmentation of leptin receptor signaling in the stomach during GC development [16–18]. We have previously demonstrated the significance of leptin signaling in the stomach and its role in the development of intestinal-type gastric tumor using a murine model [19]. Dysfunction of central sympathetic regulation of leptin signaling promotes leptin resistance. Despite high levels of circulating plasma leptin, obese individuals do not respond to its appetite-suppressing effects, indicating their leptin resistance [20]. Because leptin is crucial to the development of gastrointestinal malignancies and provides a link between obesity and tumorigenicity [17], a better understanding of the dysregulation of gastric leptin signaling and its role in obesity-induced gastric pathology is necessary.

Methods

Animals and diets

Male C57BL/6J (wild-type: WT), *ob/ob*, and *db/db* mice (CLEA Japan, Tokyo, Japan) were studied at 7 weeks of age. The animals were housed individually in plastic cages at 24 °C ± 1 °C with lights on from 0600 to 1800 h. The mice were provided with either a control-diet (CD, 10 % of calories from fat, D12450J) or a high-fat diet (HFD, 60 % of calories from fat, D12492) (Research Diets Inc., New Brunswick, NJ) and water *ad libitum*. The ethics committee for animal experiments of the National Institute for Physiological Sciences approved all animal experiments.

Histopathological analysis of the gastric mucosa

Paraffin-embedded gastric sections of 10 % formalin-fixed tissues were obtained from the HFD- and CD-fed mice and were stained with hematoxylin and eosin (H&E), and assessed for alterations in the gastric mucosa. The assessment of mucosal alterations in the stomach was based on a summation of scores for hyperplasia (0, non-substantial alteration; 1, low; 2, moderate; 3, high), cell infiltration (0, non-substantial alteration; 1, low; 2, moderate; 3, high), loss of gastric glandular cells (0, non-substantial alteration; 4, low; 5, moderate; 6, high), Alcian blue staining (0, non-substantial alteration; 4, focal; 5, diffuse; 6, very strong diffuse), and dysplasia (0, non-substantial alteration; 7, low). Each criterion was independently blind-scored by two individuals using criteria that were previously defined [19].

Intragastric pH measurements

Gastric pH was measured according to a published method [21]. In brief, mice were sacrificed after anesthetization by carbon dioxide inhalation. Following stomach removal, the gastric lumen was removed and washed with 0.5 ml saline (150 mM, pH 7.0), and the pH of the collected gastric fluid was measured using a pH meter (Mettler, Toledo, OH).

Immunohistochemical analysis

Paraffin-embedded sections of 10 % formalin-fixed tissues were stained either with H&E or with periodic-acid Schiff (PAS) and Alcian blue. For antigen retrieval, deparaffinized and rehydrated specimens were treated with 3 % hydrogen peroxide in methanol to block endogenous peroxidase activity and then were heated in a microwave using a Retrievagen A kit (BD Biosciences, San Jose, CA), followed by overnight incubation with primary antibodies (Abs) at 4 °C as listed in Additional file 1: Table S1. Subsequently, the slides were stained with a biotinylated anti-rabbit IgG or anti-goat IgG Ab and streptavidin-labeled peroxidase using a Histofine SAB-PO kit (Nichirei Biosciences Inc., Tokyo, Japan) and developed using 3, 3′-diaminobenzidine (DAB) solution (ImmPact™ DAB, Vector Laboratories, Burlingame, CA) according to the manufacturer's protocol, followed by hematoxylin counterstaining. For immunofluorescence staining, the slides were incubated with the primary Abs (Additional file 1: Table S1) and then reacted with Alexa 488-conjugated rabbit or mouse IgG Ab or Alexa 556-conjugated goat IgG Ab, as appropriate. The stained slides were mounted using ProLong Gold Antifade reagent with 4′,6-diamidino-2-phenylindole (DAPI) (Life Technologies, Carlsbad, CA) for detection using a fluorescence microscope (Olympus, Tokyo, Japan).

Western blot analysis

Gastric epithelial cells were isolated and prepared according to a modification of a previously published method [22]. Dissected small segments of the stomach were agitated at room temperature for 10 min in a Hank's balanced salt solution (HBSS) (Thermo Fisher Scientific Inc., Waltham, MA) medium containing 1 mM DTT. After removal of the supernatant, the tissues were stirred at 37 °C for 10 min in HBSS containing

10 mM EDTA. After removal of the supernatant, the tissue suspension was passed through a nylon mesh to remove debris and centrifuged through a 25/40 % discontinuous Percoll (Sigma-Aldrich, St. Louis, MO) gradient at 600 × *g* at 20 °C for 20 min. The cells collected from the interface of 25/40 % were the epithelial cells. Lysates were prepared from tissues and cells and analyzed by western blotting, according to a previously published method [23]. The Abs used in western blotting are summarized in Additional file 1: Table S1.

Laser-capture microdissection

The above-described paraffin-embedded gastric tissues were cut into 6-μm-thick sections and mounted onto membrane slides (MembraneSlide 1.0 PEN, Carl Zeiss Microscopy, LLC, Thornwood, NY). Paraffin was removed by rinsing the sections with xylene, after which the sections were immersed in a series of 100 % to 70 % ethanol baths and air-dried. Mucosal sections of gastric epithelia were cut and collected onto AdhesiveCaps (PALM, Microlaser Technologies, Bernried, Germany) by a laser-capture microdissection (LMD) system (PALM MB-III, Microlaser Technologies).

Quantitative reverse transcription-polymerase chain reaction (qRT-PCR)

Total RNA from the LMD samples and from murine gastric mucosa was extracted using AllPrep FFPE DNA/RNA and RNeasy Mini kits (Qiagen, Valencia, CA), respectively, according to the manufacturer's protocols. cDNA was synthesized from approximately 100–200 ng RNA from the LMD sections or 1–2 μg RNA from gastric mucosal cells using the ReverTra Ace® qPCR RT Kit (TOYOBO, Co., Ltd., Osaka, Japan) according to the manufacturer's protocol. qRT-PCR was carried out using the Power SYBR Green PCR Master Mix (Life Technologies, Carlsbad, CA) with specific primer sets (400 nM at the final concentration, Additional file 2: Table S2) according to the manufacturers' protocol. Relative changes in gene expression were calculated using the ΔΔCt method, and the 18S rRNA gene was used for normalization.

Quantitative analysis of immunohistochemical staining

For microscopic measurements, leptin-stained gastric mucosa samples were photographed using a microscope (Olympus), and quantitative analysis was performed using ImageJ software (http://rsb.info.nih.gov/ij/index.html). Mucosal height was measured between the base of the gastric glands and the neck zone.

Plasma assay

Serum was collected from blood obtained by cardiocentesis under anesthetization and stored at −80 °C. Insulin (Mouse Insulin ELISA kit, Shibayagi, Gunma, Japan), leptin (Leptin ELISA, Millipore, St. Charles, MO), glucose (Glucose CII-test, Wako, Osaka, Japan), and non-esterified fatty acid (NEFA) (NEFA C-test, Wako) levels in the sera were measured according to the manufacturers' protocols.

Statistical analysis

The Mann–Whitney *U* test and the Kruskal-Wallis test were used to determine significant differences. A *p*-value of less than 0.05 was considered significant. Statistical analyses were performed using Prism software version 6 (GraphPad, San Diego, CA, USA).

Results

HFD-fed mice develop atrophic gastritis

To determine how diet-induced obesity affects the pathogenesis of gastric mucosa, C57BL/6 mice were fed either HFD (60 % calories from fat) or CD (10 % calories from fat) and the histological changes of the gastric mucosa were examined in a time-dependent manner. Compared to the CD-fed mice, the HFD-fed mice exhibited rapid weight gain at a rate of > 2 g per week during the first 12 weeks. Thereafter, a moderate increase of 1 g per week was observed from 12 to 20 weeks (Fig. 1a). The cardial mucosa showed hyperplasia at 1 week, prior to any significant difference in body weight gain between the CD- and HFD-fed groups (1.5 ± 0.29 in CD *vs.* 1.8 ± 0.4 in HFD, $p > 0.05$) (Fig. 1a and 1b). At 3 weeks, a reduced parietal cell number and morphological alterations of the foveola in the stomach were observed, followed by glandular metaplasia and a complete loss of zymogenic and parietal cells at 12 weeks after the initiation of HFD feeding (Fig. 1b). Although the hyperplastic change of the gastric foveolar epithelium was seen at 1 week in the HFD-fed mice, few $CD45^+$ infiltrated cells were present in HFD-fed mice (Fig. 1b and 1d). However, after 3 weeks of feeding, a substantial amount of infiltrated cells were seen to have invaded the interglandular and basal spaces in accordance with the development of hyperplasia (Fig. 1b and 1d). In the antrum, slight mucosal hyperplasia was observed in HFD-fed mice at 1 week after diet initiation. Both the cardia and antrum displayed a replacement of normal glandular cells such as parietal and G cells with atypical and irregular cells after 3 weeks of HFD feeding (Fig. 1b). Furthermore, mildly dysplastic epithelia, with cells showing enlarged nuclei, nuclear pseudostratification, and distinct nucleoli, became apparent in the hyperplastic lesions of HFD-fed mice at 12 weeks after feeding (Fig. 1c). A high frequency of Ki67-positive proliferating cells was observed in the hyperplastic and dysplastic stomach lesions of the HFD-fed mice, whereas these cells presented a defined proliferating zone in the CD-fed mice (Fig. 1e). These alterations rapidly progressed by 8 weeks of feeding (Fig. 2c). At 20 weeks of feeding, the folds of the glossy gastric mucosa were flat with a pale appearance, and polyp-like

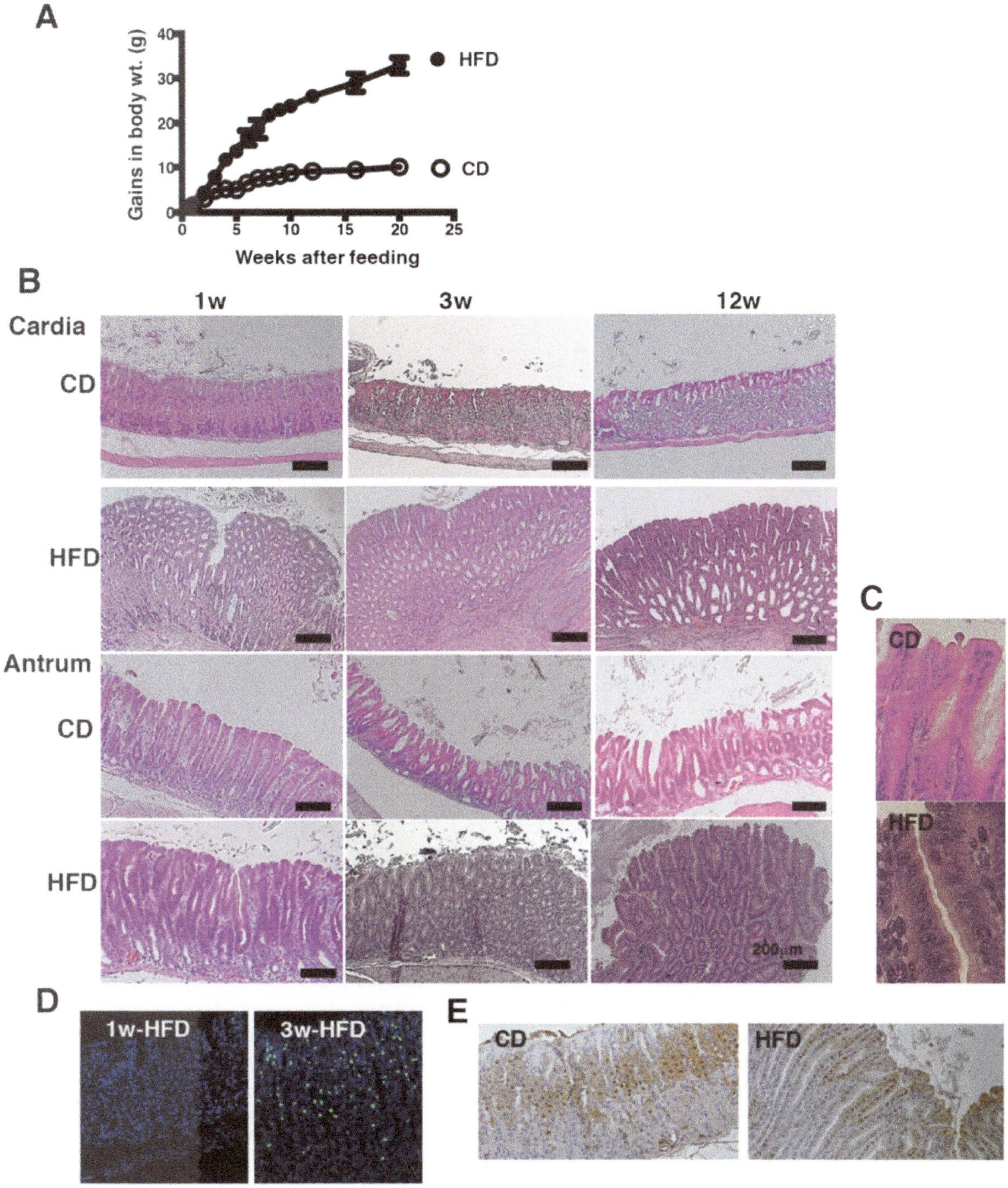

Fig. 1 Pathological changes of gastric mucosa owing to HFD-feeding. **a** Alteration of gains in body weights of C57BL/6 J mice fed CD ($n = 10$) or HFD ($n = 10$) during 20 weeks. **b** Representative H&E-sections of the gastric cardia and antrum from mice fed CD or HFD for 1, 3, and 12 weeks. **c** Magnified image of the gastric antrum in mice fed CD and HFD in Fig. 1b at 12 weeks after feeding (magnification, ×400). The cell nucleolus, nuclear hypertrophy, dyspolarity, and pseudostratification were observed. **d** CD45 staining of the gastric mucosa of 1 and 3 week HFD-fed mice. **e** Ki67-staining in the gastric mucosa of mice fed CD or HFD for 3 weeks. 5–10 mice were used in each analysis, and representative data are shown

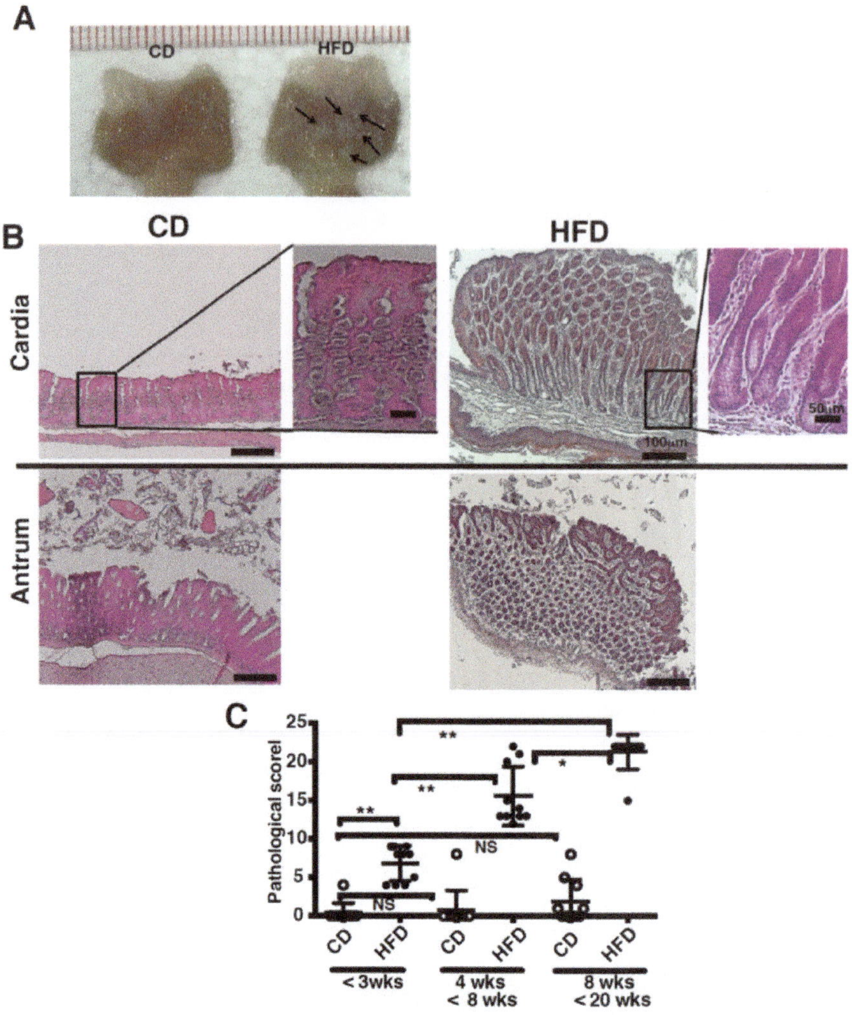

Fig. 2 Development of gastric mucosal atrophy in diet-induced obese mice. **a** The gastric lumen was opened along the outer curvature of mice fed CD or HFD for 20 weeks. Arrows indicate the polyp-like lesions in the stomach of HFD-fed mice. **b** Representative H&E-sections of the gastric cardia and antrum from mice fed CD or HFD for 20 weeks. **c** The histological scores from the stomachs of mice fed CD or HFD (<3 weeks, 4–8 weeks, 8–20 weeks of feeding; 10 mice per group) were graded according to the diagnostic criteria described in the Methods. Results were analyzed by the Kruskal-Wallis test, followed by a Dunn's multiple comparison test. * $p < 0.05$, ** $p < 0.01$, NS; not significant

lesions were observed in the cardia and fundic regions of HFD-fed mice (arrows in Fig. 2a). At this point, the cell infiltration was complete, and the normal gastric glands were replaced by intestinal crypt-like structures at the cardial basal mucosa of HFD-fed mice (Fig. 2b). These results indicate that HFD-feeding alters gastric epithelial integrity even at the early phase of feeding and suggest that the occurrence of mucosal hyperplasia in the stomach was initiated by inflammation-independent events.

Upregulation of intestinal markers in the gastric mucosa

We further examined whether the gastric mucosa in HFD-fed mice exhibited features of intestinal mucosa. We observed that the frequency of Alcian blue-stained goblet cells, which are intestinal mucus cells, increased as they spread across the gastric mucosa in HFD-fed mice (Fig. 3a). Muc2, an intestinal type of mucin, was ectopically expressed in the gastric mucosa only of HFD-fed mice (Fig. 3a), indicating that gastric mucin was converted to the intestinal type as has been observed in most human gastric carcinomas [24]. The results of gene expression analysis were consistent with the immunohistological findings. The mRNA expression of *Muc2* and *Tff3* (a peptide co-expressed with Muc2) increased, whereas that of the gastric-type mucins, *Muc1*, *Muc5ac*, and *Muc6*, remained unaltered or decreased in the

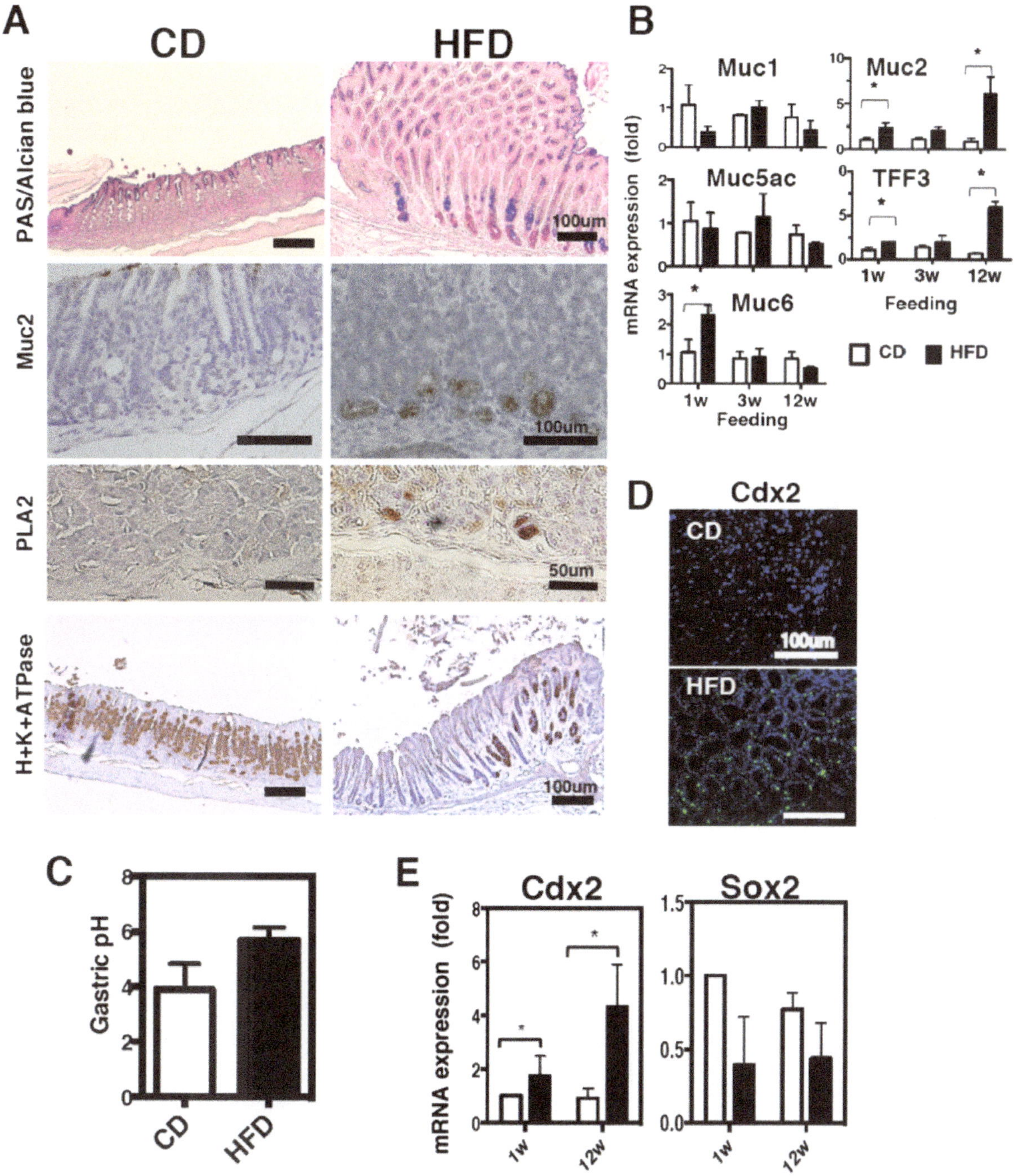

Fig. 3 Alteration of intestinal characteristics in the gastric mucosa of HFD-fed mice. Gastric sections stained for PAS-Alcian blue, Muc2, PLA2, and H^+K^+ ATPase (**a**), and Cdx2 (**d**) in mice fed CD or HFD for 20 weeks. Gene expression of mucins (**b**), and *Cdx2* and *Sox2* (**e**) in the gastric mucosa of mice fed CD or HFD at 1 to 12 weeks after feeding. We utilized 5–10 mice in each analysis, and representative data are shown. **c** The gastric pH in the gastric lumen was measured according to the description provided in the Methods. Values represent the means ± SD of 5 mice. The results were analyzed by the Kruskal-Wallis test. * $p < 0.05$

stomachs of HFD-fed mice (Fig. 3b). The cardia of HFD-fed mice also showed ectopic expression of phospholipase A2 (PLA2), an intestinal Paneth cell marker (Fig. 3a). In contrast, the expression of $H^{+}K^{+}$-ATPase, a marker of parietal cells that secrete gastric acid, decreased with a concurrent elevation of gastric pH in the HFD-fed mice (Fig. 3a and 3c). In addition, the deregulation of transcription factor expression transposes into a metaplastic phenotype. Accordingly, the mRNA expression of *Cdx2*, an intestinal master transcription factor that is a marker of intestinal metaplasia, was higher in HFD-fed mice at 1 week (Fig. 3e). Furthermore, *Cdx2* mRNA expression was increased in the gastric mucosa of HFD-fed mice at 12 weeks in contrast to that observed in CD-fed mice, in which it was constant (Fig. 3d and 3e). Consistent with the ectopic *Cdx2* mRNA expression, the mRNA of *Sox2*, a transcription factor for stomach organogenesis [25], tended to be downregulated, indicating the development of intestinal metaplasia in the gastric mucosa in HFD-fed mice (Fig. 3e). Taken together, these results imply that HFD-feeding accelerates intestinal metaplasia.

HFD feeding activates early leptin receptor signaling during gastric intestinal metaplasia

Because of the early morphological alterations observed in the gastric mucosa, we examined the gene expression of stomach-specific hormones, peptides, and enzymes 1 week after HFD feeding. Leptin mRNA expression in particular was significantly higher in the stomach of HFD-fed mice; in contrast, ghrelin expression was lower in HFD-fed mice (Fig. 4a). The expression of other genes such as *Atp4a*, *Atp4b*, *Pga*, and *Pgc*, which encode to $H^{+}K^{+}$-ATPase, pepsinogen A, and pepsinogen C, respectively, did not show significant differences between CD- and HFD-fed mice, although the expression of *Atp4a* and *Atp4b* tended to decrease (Fig. 4a). Normally, leptin is expressed in chief and parietal cells [26, 27]; however, HFD-fed mice exhibited strong leptin expression in the hyperplastic gastric epithelia (Fig. 4b and 4c). Even though the serum leptin concentration was similar between CD- and HFD-fed mice at 1 week after feeding (Fig. 4d), the leptin expression in the hyperplastic region of the stomach was consistent with the structural changes observed on H&E stained sections at 1 week (Fig. 1b). The leptin expression continued to increase to 12 weeks post HFD feeding, after which the expression approximately recovered to the level observed in CD-fed mice at 20 weeks (Fig. 4b and 4c). Concomitant with the high leptin expression at 1 week, phosphorylation of ObRb, STAT3, Akt, and ERK, which are molecules associated with leptin receptor signaling, was detected in the gastric mucosa of HFD-fed WT mice (Fig. 5a). These molecules remained activated at 4 weeks after feeding. In contrast, leptin-deficient *ob/ob* and ObR mutated *db/db* mice did not show phosphorylated ObRb, and only exhibited slightly activated STAT3, Akt, and ERK. In support of the validity of these findings, the isotype-control Ab did not react specifically and no expression of p-ObRb was detected in *db/db* mice (Fig. 5b and 5c).

Chronic inflammation can trigger atrophic gastritis. IL-6 and IL-11, which are predominantly expressed in the stomach, modulate inflammatory responses during neoplastic progression [28, 29]. In particular, IL-11 expression increases in atrophic gastritis and in intestinal metaplasia of the fundic mucosa [30]. To identify potential initiators of intestinal metaplasia, we examined the expression of leptin, IL-6, and IL-11 in the gastric mucosa. Whereas leptin was expressed at 1 week after feeding, *Il6* and *Il11* mRNA levels did not increase in the gastric cardia of HFD-fed mice until 3 weeks after diet initiation (Fig. 6a). At 12 weeks, IL-11 expression accompanied an increased number of $CD45^{+}$ infiltrated cells (Fig. 6a and 6b). These findings suggest that HFD-induced leptin expression and downstream activation precedes the induction of inflammatory cytokines during intestinal metaplasia.

Lack of leptin signaling suppresses gastric intestinal metaplasia

HFD feeding activated leptin signaling, leading to intestinal metaplasia in WT mice. Conversely, the absence of leptin signaling should therefore suppress HFD-induced gastric pathology. To investigate the role of leptin signaling in the development of intestinal metaplasia, we examined gastric mucosal changes in leptin-deficient *ob/ob* mice and leptin receptor-mutated *db/db* mice. The *ob/ob* and *db/db* mice showed a higher body weight than did WT mice; however, no significant difference in body weights was observed between CD- and HFD-fed mice at 1 week after feeding (Additional file 3: Figure S1a). The *ob/ob* and *db/db* mice fed the CD for 1 week exhibited hyperinsulinemia, whereas only HFD-fed *ob/ob* mice showed increased insulin levels. HFD-fed *db/db* mice showed insulin levels similar to those of CD-fed *db/db* mice, because of their insulin resistance (Additional file 3: Figure S1b). The *db/db* mice also exhibited hyperleptinemia and hypergluconemia. However, the non-esterified fatty acid (NEFA) concentration did not vary among WT, *ob/ob*, and *db/db* mice fed with either CD or HFD (Additional file 3: Figure S1b). Histopathological analysis revealed that compared to the WT mice, *ob/ob* and *db/db* mice that were obese and insulin- or leptin- resistant showed few morphological changes such as hyperplasia of the gastric cardial mucosa at 1 week after initiation of HFD feeding (Fig. 7a). Mucosal height analysis was consistent with the histological findings (Fig. 7c). Furthermore, immunohistochemical analysis revealed increased colocalization of Cdx2 and leptin in the gastric mucosa of WT mice fed the HFD for 1 week (Fig. 8a), whereas *db/db*

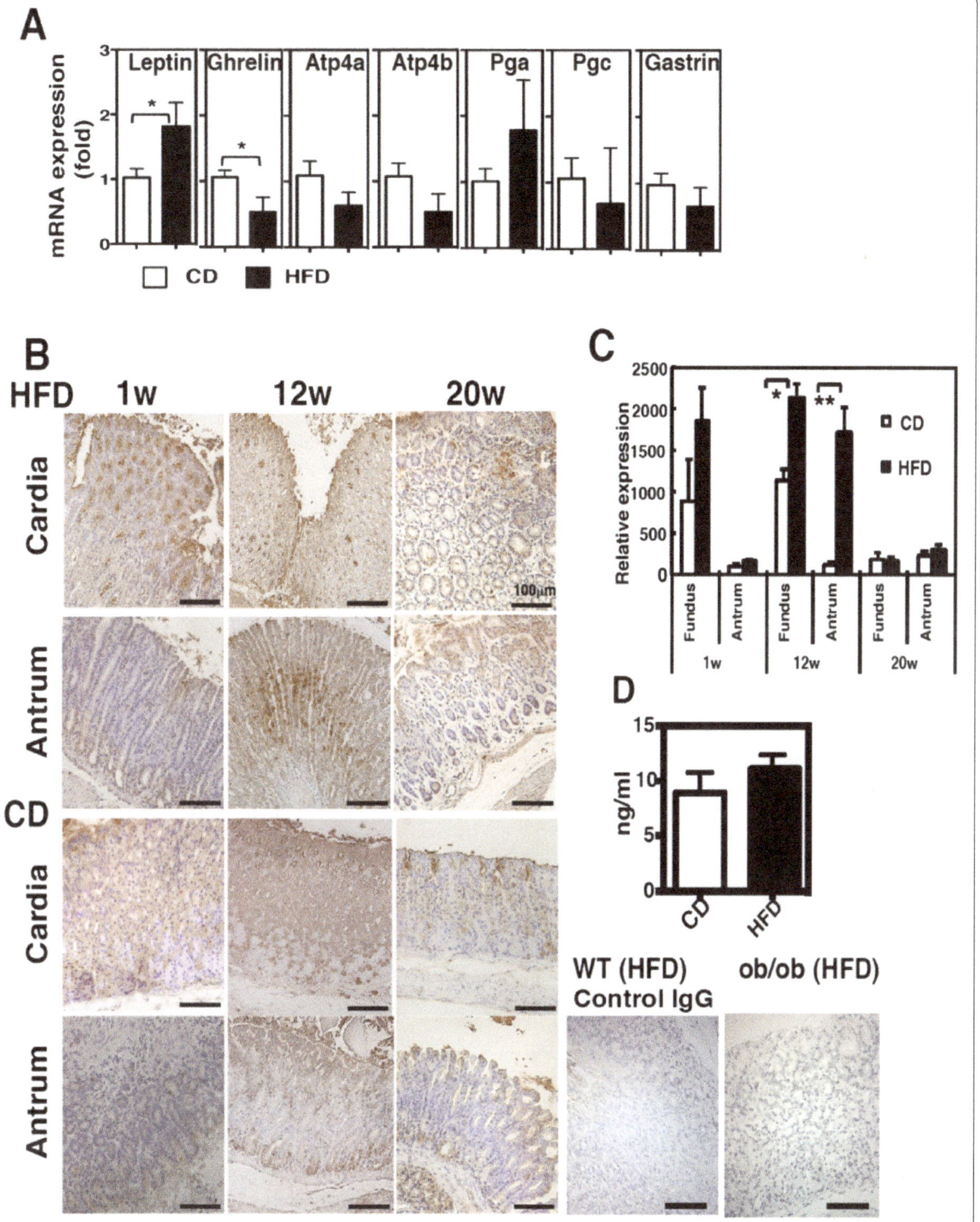

Fig. 4 (See legend on next page.)

(See figure on previous page.)
Fig. 4 Enhancement of gastric leptin expression in the early period of HFD feeding. **a** Gene expression of gastric-specific molecules at 1 week after CD and HFD feeding. **b** Gastric sections stained for leptin in mice fed CD or HFD for 1, 12, and 20 weeks. **c** Quantification of leptin expression in (**b**). The data are presented as the relative expression at each time-point to the expression level in the antrum of CD-fed mice after 1 week. **d** Serum leptin concentration in mice fed CD and HFD for 1 week. The values represent the means ± SD of 5 mice. The results were analyzed by the Mann–Whitney *U* test. * $p < 0.05$, ** $p < 0.01$

mice did not show Cdx2 expression in leptin-positive cells. In contrast, *ob/ob* mice showed little Cdx2 and no leptin expression. Similarly, co-localization of phosphorylated ObRb and Cdx2 was detected in HFD-fed WT mice, but not in HFD-fed *ob/ob* or *db/db* mice, which showed only some phosphorylation of ObRb or Cdx2, respectively. CD-fed ob/ob and db/db mice showed a drastic increase in body weight but only slight hyperplasia in the gastric mucosa compared to WT mice at 3 weeks (Fig. 7b and 7c). Despite having higher body weights, *ob/ob* and *db/db* mice fed the HFD for 3 weeks exhibited less hyperplasia than did WT mice fed the HFD for 20 weeks. After 20 weeks of HFD feeding, the WT mice presented an irregular and fused structure in the cardia (Fig. 7b). HFD feeding did not increase the expression of Cdx2 and Muc2 in the gastric mucosa of *ob/ob* and *db/db* mice (Fig. 8b). These results suggest that leptin signaling in the stomach is an important factor that leads to metaplastic pathology in obesity-related gastritis.

Discussion

This study presents the first evidence supporting the theory that HFD-induced enhanced leptin receptor signaling in the gastric mucosa causes atrophic gastritis in a murine model. We found that HFD feeding triggers leptin production and the activation of leptin-ObR signaling in the gastric mucosa, promoting atrophic gastritis and intestinal metaplasia. Given the higher frequency of gastritis in obese patients [31, 32], our results substantiate the role of leptin receptor signaling in obesity-induced atrophic gastritis. *H. pylori* infection is considered a major cause of chronic gastritis and GC [33, 34]; however, very few *H. pylori*-infected patients develop GC [35]. Furthermore, the frequency of gastritis is significantly higher in morbidly obese patients, whereas the prevalence of *H. pylori* infection is similar in obese and non-obese individuals [2]. Thus, obesity is an important factor accounting for the prevalence of histologic gastritis and the transformation of gastric mucosal cells in addition to *H. pylori* infection.

In addition to adipose tissue, the placenta [36] and mammary glands [37, 38] also produce leptin, which supports trophoblast cell proliferation to regulate fetal growth and development [39, 40] and the development of the mammary gland, respectively. In those tissues, leptin is produced in both normal and malignant cells, and its overexpression has been demonstrated in neoplastic cells [36, 41]. Elevated expression of leptin and ObRb is associated with faster tumor recurrence and mortality in human grade-III invasive breast tumors [42, 43]. Tumor cells derived from MMTV-Wnt1 mice, a widely used model of mammary tumors, show decreased growth in *ob/ob* mice compared with cells from diet-induced obese mice that have functional leptin signaling [44]. Our data show that *ob/ob* and *db/db* mice show no activation of the ObR, a marked decrease in the activation of STAT3, Akt, and ERK (Fig. 5a), and exhibit less progression of gastric hyperplasia even though these mice are more obese than HFD-fed WT mice (Fig. 7). Furthermore, *ob/ob* and *db/db* mice do not spontaneously develop gastric tumors although these mice exhibit extraordinary obesity. Thus, the results of our study together with those of the previous reports imply that leptin signaling is critically involved in the control of epithelium development in a variety of tissues. Although the significance of leptin expression and its signaling in the stomach remains uncertain, considering the constitutive expression of leptin and ObRb in the stomach [45, 46], leptin might be necessary for the maintenance of gastric mucosal homeostasis.

Leptin is considered to represent a key player in obesity-associated gastrointestinal malignancies because of its roles in angiogenesis, apoptosis, cell proliferation, and cell migration, which support the milieu of tumor development and progression [17]. Recently, leptin was shown to contribute to mucin production and the formation of gastrointestinal neoplasms by modulating mTOR-, STAT3-, and ERK-dependent pathways [47] in addition to PKC-, PI3K-, and MAPK-dependent pathways [48, 49]. The mechanisms underlying the induction of gastric atrophy are not defined; however, transcription factors responsible for cell differentiation have been reported to be potently involved in gastric tumorigenesis. Transcription factors such as Cdx2 and Sox2 are critical for cell self-renewal and the maintenance of cells in appropriate proportions [50]. Sox2 is a primary regulator of gastric differentiation that maintains gastric mucosal features and regulates the expression of gastric mucus genes, such as *Muc5ac* [51], and it is downregulated during the development of gastric adenocarcinoma [52, 53]. In contrast, Cdx2 is essential for intestinal epithelium differentiation to regulate the expression of Muc2 [54, 55] and Tff3 [56], and it is upregulated during the progression of gastric tumors [57]. Recently, the binding of phosphorylated STAT3 to the Cdx2 promoter region was shown to

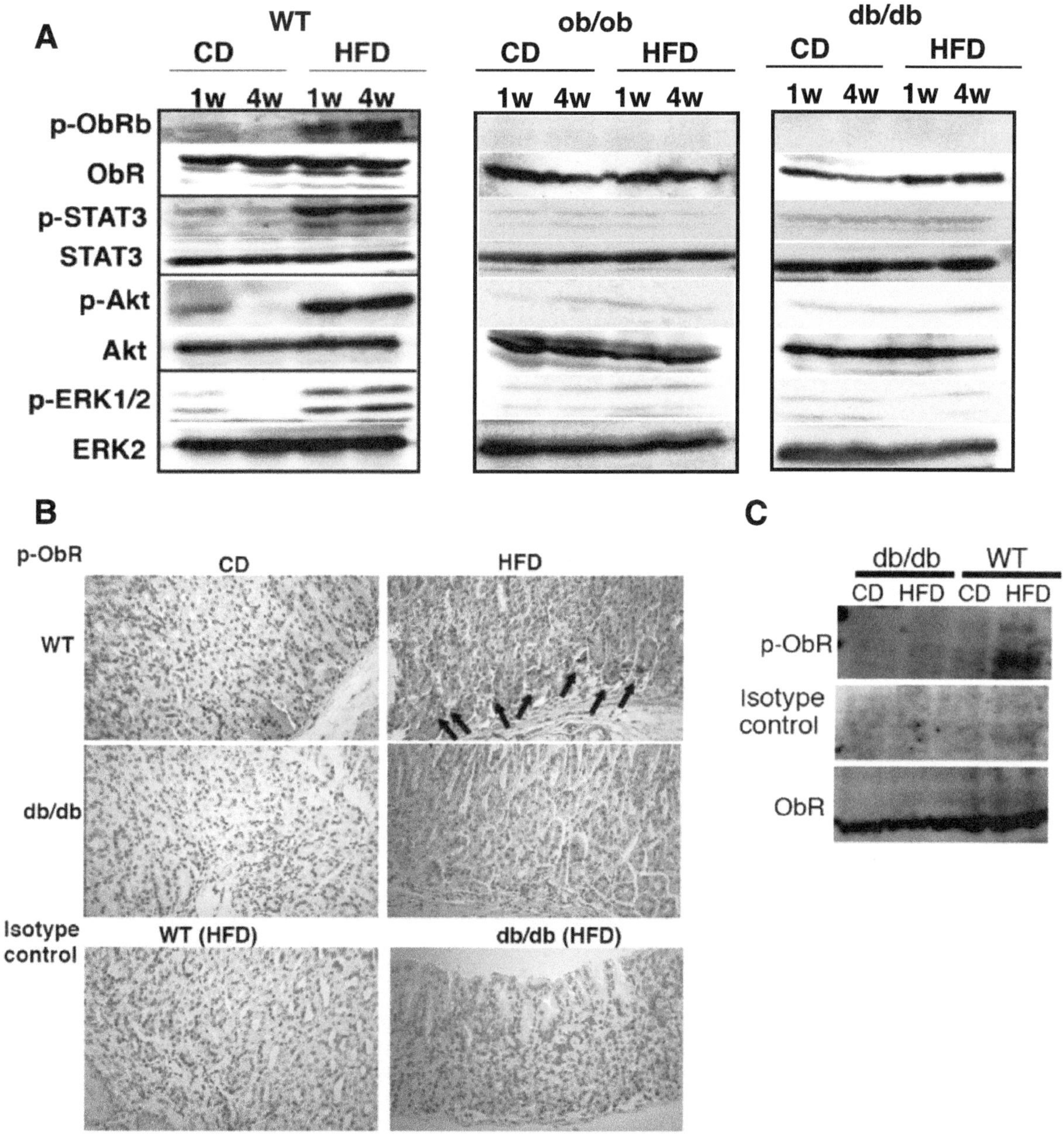

Fig. 5 Upregulation of leptin receptor signaling in the gastric mucosa of HFD-fed WT mice. **a** Western blot analysis of the phosphorylation of ObRb, STAT3, Akt and ERK1/2 in the gastric mucosa of WT, *ob/ob* and *db/db* mice fed CD and HFD for 1 and 4 weeks. A total of 3 mice were used in each diet group per one experiment. Each experiment was repeated twice and representative data are shown. **b** Immunohistochemistry and (**c**) western blot analysis of phosphorylation of ObR in the gastric mucosa of *db/db* mice and WT mice fed CD or HFD for 3 weeks. We utilized 3 mice in each analysis, and representative data are shown. Arrows indicate phosphorylated ObR-positive cells

upregulate Cdx2 but downregulate Sox2 in two gastric cell lines, MKN45 and NUGC4 [58]. In this study, we showed that HFD feeding induces Cdx2 and Muc2 expression associated with increased leptin levels (Figs. 3 and 8), suggesting the possibility that leptin acts to suppress cellular protection against gastric mucosal malignancies in the early stage of atrophic gastritis.

Atrophic gastritis is characterized by an alteration of the differentiation of gastric mucosal cells such as the loss of parietal and chief cells and replacement of the

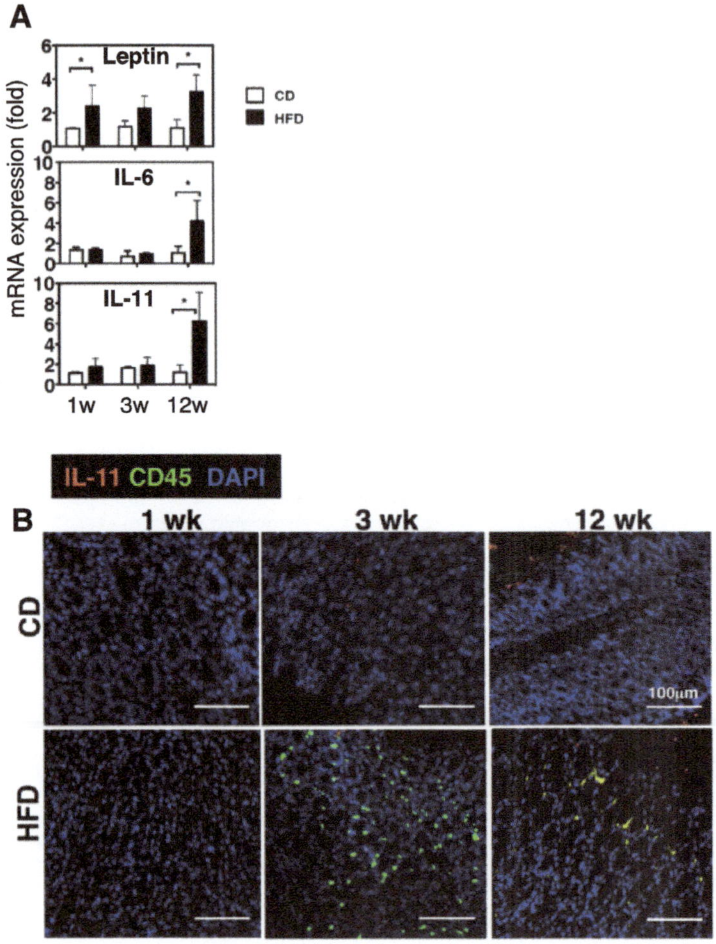

Fig. 6 Delayed induction of proinflammatory cytokines in the gastric mucosa after HFD-feeding. **a** Gene expression of leptin, *Il6*, and *Il11* in the gastric mucosa of CD- and HFD-fed mice after 1, 3, and 12 weeks. The values represent the means ± SD of 4 mice. The results were analyzed by the Kruskal-Wallis test. * $p < 0.05$, $p < 0.01$. **b** Immunohistological staining of the stomach sections of the CD and HFD-fed mice with Abs against IL-11 and CD45

destroyed glandular structure with a diffuse intestinal mucous metaplasia [59]. Variations in the pathology of atrophic gastritis have been reported to some degree in genetically engineered mice such as Atp4a$^{-/-}$ and gastrin$^{-/-}$ mice, which are used as models of parietal and glandular cell loss. However, Atp4a$^{-/-}$ mice exhibit the same expression levels of Muc2 and Tff3 in the gastric mucosa as control Atp4a$^{+/+}$ mice, indicating incomplete intestinalization of the gastric mucosa in these mice [60]. Gastrin is secreted from G-cells to stimulate acid secretion and cell proliferation of the fundic mucosa [61]. Gastrin$^{-/-}$ mice develop antral gastric neoplasia with increased levels of Muc2 and villin (an intestinal-specific actin bundling protein) in the gastric mucosa in the presence of gastric inflammation but not in the fundus [62, 63]. As proinflammatory cytokines involved in atrophic gastritis, IL-6 and IL-11 cause an inflammatory response in the stomach and play important roles in angiogenesis and cell proliferation during the progression of neoplasia [28, 29]; thus, they are used as biomarkers of aggressive tumors [64]. In particular, IL-11, which is mainly expressed in the fundic mucosa, might play a pivotal role in atrophic gastritis and the progression of GC [30, 65]. Chronic treatment of WT mice with recombinant IL-11 induces atrophy in the gastric fundus, including the cardia, with reduced parietal cells and highly phosphorylated STAT3, but no features of intestinalization of the gastric mucosa such as the appearance of goblet cells, Muc2, and Cdx2. These reports raise the question of which molecules are directly involved in the atrophy of the gastric mucosa associated with metaplasia. In our study, the increase of gastric leptin expression is observed during the early period after the initiation of HFD feeding and its

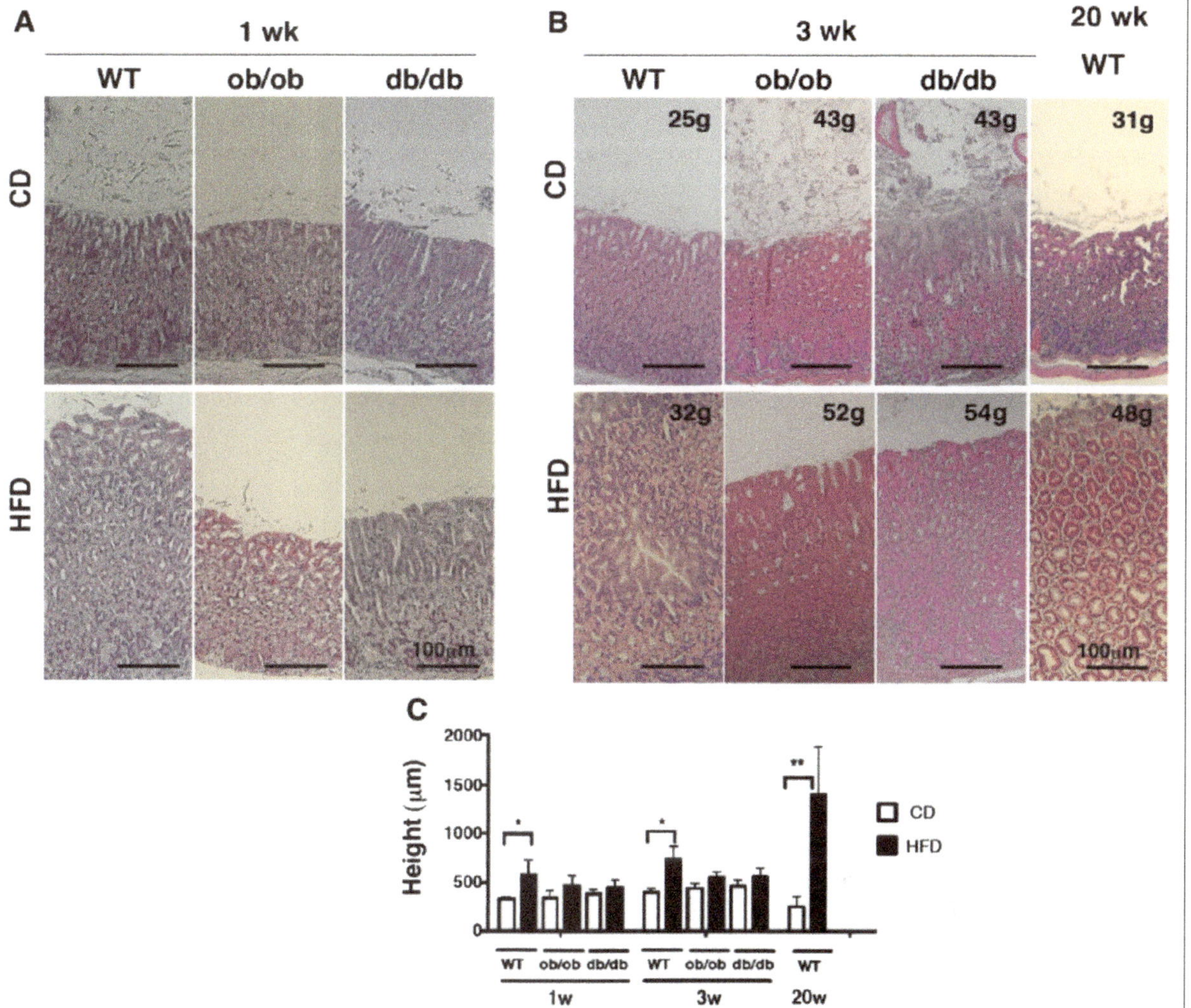

Fig. 7 Suppressed alteration of gastric morphology in HFD-fed mice devoid of leptin signaling. Representative H&E-sections of the gastric mucosa from WT, *ob/ob* and *db/db* mice fed CD or HFD for 1 (**a**) and 3 weeks (**b**). Each value in the images indicates the body weight of the mouse from which the gastric mucosa was obtained and stained with H&E-stain. **c** Measurement of mucosal height in the gastric fundus of WT, *ob/ob* and *db/db* mice at 1 and 3 weeks and of WT mice at 20 weeks after feeding. The values represent the means ± SD of 4 mice. The results were analyzed by the Kruskal-Wallis test. * $p < 0.05$, ** $p < 0.01$

subsequent reduction is consistent with the loss of normal parietal and chief cells, which constitutively produce leptin and ObR [26, 27], in the gastric mucosa of HFD-fed mice in accordance with the development of intestinal metaplasia after 20 weeks of HFD feeding (Figs. 1, 2 and 3). Our results might therefore directly indicate the involvement of leptin receptor signaling in the initiation of obese-associated gastric atrophy.

The involvement of gastric leptin in diet-induced obesity-associated gastric atrophy has not previously been investigated, although the elevation of serum leptin contributes to tumorigenesis in the stomach of obese mice infected with *H. felis* [66]. In the current study, we showed rapid (1 week) mucosal morphological changes in the gastric cardia (Fig. 1b) in accordance with high expression of gastric leptin at this time (Fig. 4d). Furthermore, prior to the production of IL-11, leptin expression in the cardial gastric mucosa increases, concurrent with the hyperplastic lesions observed in the early period after HFD feeding (Fig. 4b and 6). The localization of leptin-producing cells within cardial mucosal lesions occurs during the early stage of atrophy in HFD-fed mice. Furthermore, the increased leptin levels and activation of ObRb resulted in increased levels of phosphorylated STAT3 in the HFD-fed mice (Fig. 5a). Notably, because *ob/ob* and *db/db* mice do not transduce leptin receptor signaling and do not show

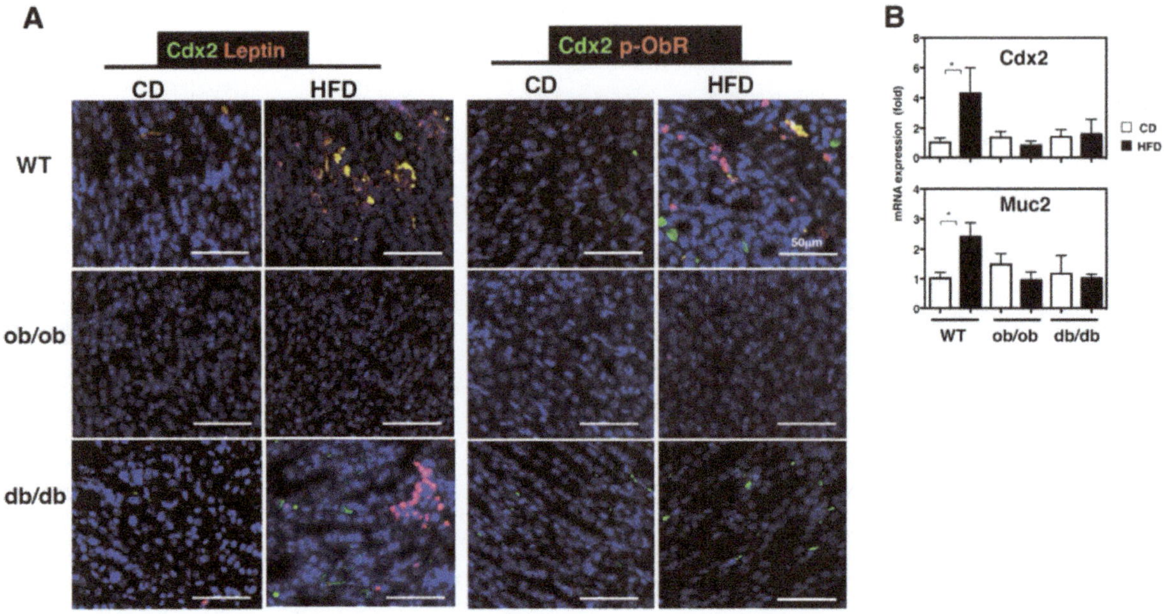

Fig. 8 Downregulation of intestinal epithelial markers in mice devoid of leptin signaling. **a** Immunohistological staining of the stomach sections of the CD and HFD-fed mice with Abs against leptin, Cdx2, and p-ObRb. **b** Gene expression of *Cdx2* and *Muc2* in the gastric mucosa of mice fed CD or HFD for 1 week. The values represent the means ± SD of 4 mice. The results were analyzed by the Kruskal-Wallis test. $*p < 0.01$

morphological alterations such as loss of glandular structure (Fig. 5a and 7), the elevation of gastric leptin by HFD feeding might initiate a reduction of glandular structure by diffuse metaplasia, i.e., a loss of parietal and chief cells. Since most parietal and chief cells residing in the fundic mucosa of the stomach express leptin and ObRb [26, 45, 46], it would be interesting to investigate how these cells respond to food-based stimulants such as fatty acids in the HFD.

In summary, we demonstrated the development of atrophic gastritis using a murine model of diet-induced obesity with an enhanced leptin-ObRb signaling pathway. The expression and unique localization of the leptin-ObR signaling pathway predominantly indicates a role in the early phase of human GC. The significance of this study lies in the potential and invaluable use of leptin and ObR as biomarkers or as new therapeutic targets for the diagnosis and treatment of atrophic gastritis.

Conclusion

In this study, we show that diet-induced obese WT mice exhibit overexpression of leptin and activation of leptin receptor signaling in the gastric mucosa, leading to atrophic gastritis with intestinal metaplasia of the gastric mucosa. These pathological features are less severe in *ob/ob* and *db/db* mice, which lack leptin receptor signaling, than in the WT mice. Therefore, leptin receptor signaling in the stomach is a critical checkpoint for the onset of gastric neoplasia, and preventive therapeutics targeting gastric leptin receptor signaling might be developed against GC.

Additional files

Additional file 1: Table S1. Antibody list: Antibodies used for western blotting and immunohistochemistry. (DOCX 127 kb)

Additional file 2: Table S2. Primers used for quantitative PCR. (DOCX 100 kb)

Additional file 3: Figure S1. Alteration of index associated with obesity. Body weight (A), insulin, leptin, glucose and NEFA in sera (B) in CD- and HFD-fed WT, ob/ob and db/db mice were measured 1 week after feeding. Results were analyzed by the Kruskal Wallis test. $*p < 0.01$. (EPS 1473 kb)

Abbreviations

CD: Control diet; DTT: Dithiothreitol; EDTA: Ethylenediaminetetraacetic acid; ELISA: Enzyme-linked immunosorbent assay; GC: Gastric carcinoma; HFD: High fat diet; LMD: Laser-capture microdissection; NEFA: Non-esterified fatty acid; WT: Wild-type.

Competing interests

The authors declare they have no competing interests.

Authors' contributions

K I-O conceived and designed the project and executed the experiments and wrote the manuscript. KT, LT, KS, and SA assisted with the animal care and plasma assay experiments, TH and SM set up LMD. SO and YM analyzed the data and provided constructive discussion. All authors read and approved the final manuscript.

Acknowledgments
This work was supported by Grants-in-Aid for Scientific Research (C) from the Ministry of Education, Culture, Sports, Science and Technology of Japan (23590272 and 26461391) and a PUH Research Grant Program (A)(Prefectural University of Hiroshima) awarded to K. I-O. We would like to thank Professor Takao Shimizu, Professor Masashi Mizokami (NCGM), Dr. Masanobu Nanno (Yakult Honsha Co. Ltd), and Professor Masao Mitsuyama (Kyoto University) for their continuous encouragement and support.

Author details
[1]Research Institute, National Center for Global Health and Medicine (NCGM), 1-21-1, Toyama Shinjuku, Tokyo 162-0052, Japan. [2]Division of Endocrinology and Metabolism, Department of Developmental Physiology, National Institute for Physiological Sciences (NIPS), 38 Nishigonaka Myodaiji, Okazaki, Aichi 444-8585, Japan. [3]Division of Host Defense, Department of Life Sciences, Faculty of Life and Environmental Sciences, Prefectural University of Hiroshima, 562 Nanatsuka, Shobara, Hiroshima 727-0023, Japan. [4]Yakult Central Institute for Microbiological Research, 5-11 Izumi, Kunitachi, Tokyo 186-8650, Japan. [5]Section of Oncopathology and Regenerative Biology, Department of Pathology, Faculty of Medicine, University of Miyazaki, 5200 Kihara, Kiyotake, Miyazaki 889-1692, Japan.

References

1. Vannella L, Lahner E, Annibale B. Risk for gastric neoplasias in patients with chronic atrophic gastritis: a critical reappraisal. World J Gastroenterol. 2012;18:1279–85.
2. Dutta SK, Arora M, Kireet A, Bashandy H, Gandsas A. Upper gastrointestinal symptoms and associated disorders in morbidly obese patients: a prospective study. Dig Dis Sci. 2009;54:1243–6.
3. Renshaw AA, Rabaza JR, Gonzalez AM, Verdeja JC. Helicobacter pylori infection in patients undergoing gastric bypass surgery for morbid obesity. Obes Surg. 2001;11:281–3.
4. Tanaka M, Fukui M, Kuroda M, Yamazaki M, Hasegawa G, Oda Y, et al. Pepsinogen I/II ratio is related to glucose, triacylglycerol, and uric acid levels. Nutrition. 2012;28:418–21.
5. Torisu T, Matsumoto T, Takata Y, Ansai T, Soh I, Awano S, et al. Atrophic gastritis, but not antibody to Helicobacter pylori, is associated with body mass index in a Japanese population. J Gastroenterol. 2008;43:762–6.
6. Watabe H, Mitsushima T, Derakhshan MH, Yamaji Y, Okamoto M, Kawabe T, et al. Study of association between atrophic gastritis and body mass index: a cross-sectional study in 10,197 Japanese subjects. Dig Dis Sci. 2009;54:988–95.
7. O'Doherty MG, Freedman ND, Hollenbeck AR, Schatzkin A, Abnet CC. A prospective cohort study of obesity and risk of oesophageal and gastric adenocarcinoma in the NIH-AARP Diet and Health Study. Gut. 2012;61:1261–8.
8. Cho Y, Lee DH, Oh HS, Seo JY, Lee DH, Kim N, et al. Higher prevalence of obesity in gastric cardia adenocarcinoma compared to gastric non-cardia adenocarcinoma. Dig Dis Sci. 2012;57:2687–92.
9. Lagergren J, Bergstrom R, Nyren O. Association between body mass and adenocarcinoma of the esophagus and gastric cardia. Ann Intern Med. 1999;130:883–90.
10. Bhandari A, Crowe SE. Helicobacter pylori in gastric malignancies. Curr Gastroenterol Rep. 2012;14:489–96.
11. Chung WK, Leibel RL. The links between obesity, leptin, and prostate cancer. Cancer J. 2006;12:178–81.
12. Friedman JM, Halaas JL. Leptin and the regulation of body weight in mammals. Nature. 1998;395:763–70.
13. Tartaglia LA, Dembski M, Weng X, Deng N, Culpepper J, Devos R, et al. Identification and expression cloning of a leptin receptor. OB-R Cell. 1995;83:1263–71.
14. La Cava A, Matarese G. The weight of leptin in immunity. Nat Rev Immunol. 2004;4:371–9.
15. Guilmeau S, Buyse M, Bado A. Gastric leptin: a new manager of gastrointestinal function. Curr Opin Pharmacol. 2004;4:561–6.
16. Ishikawa M, Kitayama J, Nagawa H. Expression pattern of leptin and leptin receptor (OB-R) in human gastric cancer. World J Gastroenterol. 2006;12:5517–22.
17. Howard JM, Pidgeon GP, Reynolds JV. Leptin and gastro-intestinal malignancies. Obes Rev. 2010;11:863–74.
18. Zhao L, Shen ZX, Luo HS, Shen L. Possible involvement of leptin and leptin receptor in developing gastric adenocarcinoma. World J Gastroenterol. 2005;11:7666–70.
19. Inagaki-Ohara K, Mayuzumi H, Kato S, Minokoshi Y, Otsubo T, Kawamura YI, et al. Enhancement of leptin receptor signaling by SOCS3 deficiency induces development of gastric tumors in mice. Oncogene. 2014;33:74–84.
20. Myers MG, Cowley MA, Munzberg H. Mechanisms of leptin action and leptin resistance. Annu Rev Physiol. 2008;70:537–56.
21. Martinez V, Curi AP, Torkian B, Schaeffer JM, Wilkinson HA, Walsh JH, et al. High basal gastric acid secretion in somatostatin receptor subtype 2 knockout mice. Gastroenterology. 1998;114:1125–32.
22. Inagaki-Ohara K, Chinen T, Matsuzaki G, Sasaki A, Sakamoto Y, Hiromatsu K, et al. Mucosal T cells bearing TCRgammadelta play a protective role in intestinal inflammation. J Immunol. 2004;173:1390–8.
23. Inagaki-Ohara K, Sasaki A, Matsuzaki G, Ikeda T, Hotokezaka M, Chijiiwa K, et al. Suppressor of cytokine signalling 1 in lymphocytes regulates the development of intestinal inflammation in mice. Gut. 2006;55:212–9.
24. Lauren P. The Two Histological Main Types of Gastric Carcinoma: Diffuse and So-Called Intestinal-Type Carcinoma. An Attempt at a Histo-Clinical Classification. Acta Pathol Microbiol Scand. 1965;64:31–49.
25. Chalmers AD, Slack JM, Beck CW. Regional gene expression in the epithelia of the Xenopus tadpole gut. Mech Dev. 2000;96:125–8.
26. Cinti S, Matteis RD, Pico C, Ceresi E, Obrador A, Maffeis C, et al. Secretory granules of endocrine and chief cells of human stomach mucosa contain leptin. Int J Obes Relat Metab Disord. 2000;24:789–93.
27. Mix H, Widjaja A, Jandl O, Cornberg M, Kaul A, Goke M, et al. Expression of leptin and leptin receptor isoforms in the human stomach. Gut. 2000;47:481–6.
28. Howlett M, Menheniott TR, Judd LM, Giraud AS. Cytokine signalling via gp130 in gastric cancer. Biochim Biophys Acta. 2009;1793:1623–33.
29. Matsuo K, Oka M, Murase K, Soda H, Isomoto H, Takeshima F, et al. Expression of interleukin 6 and its receptor in human gastric and colorectal cancers. J Int Med Res. 2003;31:69–75.
30. Howlett M, Chalinor HV, Buzzelli JN, Nguyen N, van Driel IR, Bell KM, et al. IL-11 is a parietal cell cytokine that induces atrophic gastritis. Gut. 2012;61:1398–409.
31. Yamamoto S, Watabe K, Takehara T. Is obesity a new risk factor for gastritis? Digestion. 2012;85:108–10.
32. Delgado-Aros S, Locke 3rd GR, Camilleri M, Talley NJ, Fett S, Zinsmeister AR, et al. Obesity is associated with increased risk of gastrointestinal symptoms: a population-based study. Am J Gastroenterol. 2004;99:1801–6.
33. Coussens LM, Zitvogel L, Palucka AK. Neutralizing tumor-promoting chronic inflammation: a magic bullet? Science. 2013;339:286–91.
34. Ahmed N, Sechi LA. Helicobacter pylori and gastroduodenal pathology: new threats of the old friend. Ann Clin Microbiol Antimicrob. 2005;4:1.
35. Fox JG, Wang TC. Inflammation, atrophy, and gastric cancer. J Clin Invest. 2007;117:60–9.
36. Masuzaki H, Ogawa Y, Sagawa N, Hosoda K, Matsumoto T, Mise H, et al. Nonadipose tissue production of leptin: leptin as a novel placenta-derived hormone in humans. Nat Med. 1997;3:1029–33.
37. Smith-Kirwin SM, O'Connor DM, De Johnston J, Lancey ED, Hassink SG, Funanage VL. Leptin expression in human mammary epithelial cells and breast milk. J Clin Endocrinol Metab. 1998;83:1810–3.
38. Aoki N, Kawamura M, Matsuda T. Lactation-dependent down regulation of leptin production in mouse mammary gland. Biochim Biophys Acta. 1999;1427:298–306.
39. Cameo P, Bischof P, Calvo JC. Effect of leptin on progesterone, human chorionic gonadotropin, and interleukin-6 secretion by human term trophoblast cells in culture. Biol Reprod. 2003;68:472–7.
40. Henson MC, Castracane VD. Leptin in pregnancy: an update. Biol Reprod. 2006;74:218–29.
41. Hu X, Juneja SC, Maihle NJ, Cleary MP. Leptin–a growth factor in normal and malignant breast cells and for normal mammary gland development. J Natl Cancer Inst. 2002;94:1704–11.
42. Garofalo C, Koda M, Cascio S, Sulkowska M, Kanczuga-Koda L, Golaszewska J, et al. Increased expression of leptin and as a marker of breast cancer progression: possible role of obesity-related stimuli. Clin Cancer Res. 2006;12:1447–53.
43. Maccio A, Madeddu C, Gramignano G, Mulas C, Floris C, Massa D, et al. Correlation of body mass index and leptin with tumor size and stage of disease in hormone-dependent postmenopausal breast cancer: preliminary results and therapeutic implications. J Mol Med (Berl). 2010;88:677–86.
44. Zheng Q, Dunlap SM, Zhu J, Downs-Kelly E, Rich J, Hursting SD, et al. Leptin deficiency suppresses MMTV-Wnt-1 mammary tumor growth in obese mice and abrogates tumor initiating cell survival. Endocr Relat Cancer. 2011;18:491–503.

45. Bado A, Levasseur S, Attoub S, Kermorgant S, Laigneau JP, Bortoluzzi MN, et al. The stomach is a source of leptin. Nature. 1998;394:790–3.
46. Sobhani I, Bado A, Vissuzaine C, Buyse M, Kermorgant S, Laigneau JP, et al. Leptin secretion and leptin receptor in the human stomach. Gut. 2000;47:178–83.
47. Chang MS, Byeon SJ, Yoon SO, Kim BH, Lee HS, Kang GH, et al. Leptin, MUC2 and mTOR in appendiceal mucinous neoplasms. Pathobiology. 2012;79:45–53.
48. Plaisancie P, Ducroc R, El Homsi M, Tsocas A, Guilmeau S, Zoghbi S, et al. Luminal leptin activates mucin-secreting goblet cells in the large bowel. Am J Physiol Gastrointest Liver Physiol. 2006;290:G805–12.
49. El Homsi M, Ducroc R, Claustre J, Jourdan G, Gertler A, Estienne M, et al. Leptin modulates the expression of secreted and membrane-associated mucins in colonic epithelial cells by targeting PKC, PI3K, and MAPK pathways. Am J Physiol Gastrointest Liver Physiol. 2007;293:G365–73.
50. Al-Marzoqee FY, Khoder G, Al-Awadhi H, John R, Beg A, Vincze A, et al. Upregulation and inhibition of the nuclear translocation of Oct4 during multistep gastric carcinogenesis. Int J Oncol. 2012;41:1733–43.
51. Park ET, Gum JR, Kakar S, Kwon SW, Deng G, Kim YS. Aberrant expression of SOX2 upregulates MUC5AC gastric foveolar mucin in mucinous cancers of the colorectum and related lesions. Int J Cancer. 2008;122:1253–60.
52. Tsukamoto T, Inada K, Tanaka H, Mizoshita T, Mihara M, Ushijima T, et al. Down-regulation of a gastric transcription factor, Sox2, and ectopic expression of intestinal homeobox genes, Cdx1 and Cdx2: inverse correlation during progression from gastric/intestinal-mixed to complete intestinal metaplasia. J Cancer Res Clin Oncol. 2004;130:135–45.
53. Tsukamoto T, Mizoshita T, Mihara M, Tanaka H, Takenaka Y, Yamamura Y, et al. Sox2 expression in human stomach adenocarcinomas with gastric and gastric-and-intestinal-mixed phenotypes. Histopathology. 2005;46:649–58.
54. Mesquita P, Jonckheere N, Almeida R, Ducourouble MP, Serpa J, Silva E, et al. Human MUC2 mucin gene is transcriptionally regulated by Cdx homeodomain proteins in gastrointestinal carcinoma cell lines. J Biol Chem. 2003;278:51549–56.
55. Yamamoto H, Bai YQ, Yuasa Y. Homeodomain protein CDX2 regulates goblet-specific MUC2 gene expression. Biochem Biophys Res Commun. 2003;300:813–8.
56. Shimada T, Koike T, Yamagata M, Yoneda M, Hiraishi H. Regulation of TFF3 expression by homeodomain protein CDX2. Regul Pept. 2007;140:81–7.
57. Mutoh H, Sakurai S, Satoh K, Tamada K, Kita H, Osawa H, et al. Development of gastric carcinoma from intestinal metaplasia in Cdx2-transgenic mice. Cancer Res. 2004;64:7740–7.
58. Cobler L, Pera M, Garrido M, Iglesias M, de Bolos C. CDX2 can be regulated through the signalling pathways activated by IL-6 in gastric cells. Biochim Biophys Acta. 1839;2014:785–92.
59. Rugge M, Correa P, Dixon MF, Fiocca R, Hattori T, Lechago J, et al. Gastric mucosal atrophy: interobserver consistency using new criteria for classification and grading. Aliment Pharmacol Ther. 2002;16:1249–59.
60. Judd LM, Andringa A, Rubio CA, Spicer Z, Shull GE, Miller ML. Gastric achlorhydria in H/K-ATPase-deficient (Atp4a(−/−)) mice causes severe hyperplasia, mucocystic metaplasia and upregulation of growth factors. J Gastroenterol Hepatol. 2005;20:1266–78.
61. Wang TC, Koh TJ, Varro A, Cahill RJ, Dangler CA, Fox JG, et al. Processing and proliferative effects of human progastrin in transgenic mice. J Clin Invest. 1996;98:1918–29.
62. Friis-Hansen L, Sundler F, Li Y, Gillespie PJ, Saunders TL, Greenson JK, et al. Impaired gastric acid secretion in gastrin-deficient mice. Am J Physiol. 1998;274:G561–8.
63. Zavros Y, Eaton KA, Kang W, Rathinavelu S, Katukuri V, Kao JY, et al. Chronic gastritis in the hypochlorhydric gastrin-deficient mouse progresses to adenocarcinoma. Oncogene. 2005;24:2354–66.
64. Necula LG, Chivu-Economescu M, Stanciulescu EL, Bleotu C, Dima SO, Alexiu I, et al. IL-6 and IL-11 as markers for tumor aggressiveness and prognosis in gastric adenocarcinoma patients without mutations in Gp130 subunits. J Gastrointestin Liver Dis. 2012;21:23–9.
65. Ernst M, Thiem S, Nguyen PM, Eissmann M, Putoczki TL. Epithelial gp130/Stat3 functions: an intestinal signaling node in health and disease. Semin Immunol. 2014;26:29–37.
66. Ericksen RE, Rose S, Westphalen CB, Shibata W, Muthupalani S, Tailor Y, et al. Obesity accelerates Helicobacter felis-induced gastric carcinogenesis by enhancing immature myeloid cell trafficking and TH17 response. Gut. 2014;63:385–94.

Human serum preβ1-high density lipoprotein levels are independently and negatively associated with coronary artery diseases

Yunqin Chen[1,2†], Jibin Dong[3†], Xueying Chen[1†], Hui Jiang[1], Ahmed Bakillah[2], Xiaojin Zhang[4], Zhiqiang Li[1], Jia Yin[5], Donghui Liang[5], Yunzeng Zou[1], Mahmood Hussain[2], Marina Cuchel[6], Daniel Rader[5], Haozhu Chen[1], Junbo Ge[1*] and Xian-Cheng Jiang[2*]

Abstract

Background: Serum preβ1-high density lipoprotein (preβ1-HDL) was defined by two-dimensional non-denaturing linear gel electrophoresis and apolipoprotein A-I immuno-blotting. Serum preβ1-HDL seems to play an important role in reverse cholesterol transport, a well-known anti-atherosclerosis process. However, there are still debatable questions for its quantification and coronary artery disease (CAD) relevance.

Methods: We isolated the preβ1-HDL using a new native polyacrylamide gel electrophoresis (PAGE) system and lipid pre-staining serum. We established a two-demensional gel electrophoresis system.

Results: We measured the preβ1-HDL in Tangier disease patients and subjects with cholesterol ester transfer protein (CETP) mutation. The preβ1-HDL is clearly separated from lipid-free apoA-I monomer and cannot be converted into other HDL particles under lecithin-cholesterol acyltransferase (LCAT) inhibition. This preβ1-HDL is a spheroidal particle with the highest apoA-1/cholesterol ratio and highest density (≥1.21 g/ml), as compared with all other HDLs. Importantly, we found that serum from subjects with Tangier disease or with cholesterol ester transfer protein (CETP) mutation have no detectible preβ1-HDL particles. We recruited a total of 102 subjects underwent diagnostic coronary angiography and measured their preβ1-HDL levels. Among them, 56 had no stenosis of coronary artery and 46 were diagnosed as CAD, which was predefined as the presence of a luminal diameter stenosis ≥50 % in at least 1 major coronary artery territory. We found that preβ1-HDL is independently and negatively associated with the severity of the coronary artery stenosis (Gensini score).

Conclusion: We established a novel and simple method for human serum preβ1-HDL quantification. We found that human lower preβ1-HDL is an independent predictor for severer coronary artery stenosis.

Keywords: preβ1-high density lipoprotein, Native PAGE system, Coronary artery diseases

* Correspondence: ge.junbo@zs-hospital.sh.cn; xjiang@downstate.edu
†Equal contributors
[1]Shanghai Institute of Cardiovascular Diseases, Zhongshan Hospital, Fudan University, Shanghai, China
[2]Department of Cell Biology, SUNY Downstate Medical Center, 450 Clarkson Ave, Box 5, Brooklyn, NY 11203, USA
Full list of author information is available at the end of the article

Background

HDL cholesterol concentration in the blood is inversely proportional to coronary artery disease (CAD) risk [1]. This relationship is thought to be mediated by the ability of HDL to transport excess cholesterol from peripheral tissues back to the liver for excretion, a process known as reverse cholesterol transport [2]. An understanding of the molecular events in HDL formation is thus prerequisite for the development of therapeutic strategies to raise HDL cholesterol levels and protect against atherosclerosis. However, recent research has indicated that HDL particles are very heterogeneous, and indeed increasing total HDL cholesterol does not reduce CAD risk [3–8]. Thus, it is important to characterize each HDL particle subclass in terms of its pro- or anti-atherogenicity.

There are many subclasses of HDL depending on the analytical technique used for separation. HDL can be separated from non-HDL by chemical precipitation methods [9–11]. Likewise, HDL can be separated into HDL_2 and HDL_3 by ultracentrifugation [12, 13]. HDL particle size distribution can also be assessed by native PAGE [14, 15]. Two-dimensional nondenaturing linear gel electrophoresis, immunoblotting, and image analysis were first utilized by Castro and Fielding in 1988 to describe preβ1-HDL, preβ2-HDL, and αHDL [16]. Although free apoA-I was not seen on the two-dimensional gel in that first paper [16], Francone et al. from the same lab clearly showed that lipid-free apoA-I could be separated from preβ1-HDL [17]. In 1993, Asztalos et al. used a modified two-dimensional gel system to define 12 subfractions of HDL, including preβ1-HDL and preβ2-HDL, but they did not indicate whether the preβ1-HDL they identified contained lipid-free apoA-I or not [18]. Since then, the same method has been utilized in many clinical studies, including those concerning CAD patients, and the results suggest that an elevated level of preβ1-HDL is a risk factor for CAD [19–21]. The same method was used to show that subjects with Tangier disease still have preβ1-HDL but that HDL maturation is impaired [22]. Miyazaki et al. very recently showed that in their hand the so-called "preβ1-HDL" is, in fact, lipid-free monomolecular apoA-I [23]. Thus, it is necessary to re-valuate how preβ1-HDL is defined and measured. In this study, we established a direct measurement for preβ1-HDL in human serum. Moreover, we found no detectible preβ1-HDL in Tangier patients and in the subjects with cholesterol ester transfer protein (CETP) mutation. Importantly, preβ1-HDL is reduced in CAD patients.

Methods

A new native polyacrylamide gel electrophoresis (PAGE) system

We used the following six solutions (also see Fig. 1a). 1) Solution A: Acrylamide (9.60 g; Fluca) and 0.25 g N,N'-methylenebisacrylamide (Fluca) in deionized water to 100 ml final volume. 2) Solution B: Tris (18.30 g) to 24 ml of 1 N HCl and diluted to 100 ml final volume with deionized water. 3) Solution C: Acrylamide (19.60 g) and 0.40 g N,N'-methylenebisacrylamide in deionized water to 100 ml final volume. 4) Solution D: Tris (6.06 g) and 1.17 g EDTA-Na_2 in deionized water to 100 ml final volume. 5) Staining solution: Sudan Black-B (0.125 g; Sigma) to 25 ml isopropanol:ethylene glycol (4:1, V/V), mixed well, and incubated in a water bath at 37 °C overnight. 6) Running buffer: Tris (6.0 g) and 28.8 g glycine in deionized water to 1000 ml final volume, and then diluted 10-fold with deionized water before use.

The gradient gels in 6 × 100 mm glass tubes were prepared as indicated in Fig. 1a. Each tube gel comprised three layers differing in polyacrylamide concentration (7.0, 3.6, and 3.0 %) and height (45 mm, 40 mm, and 7 mm, respectively). Each gel tube was inserted vertically into an electrophoretic cell (DYY-III 27B Model, Liuyi Inc., Beijing). The upper and lower chambers of the electrophoretic cell contained ~400 ml and ~600 ml running buffer, respectively. Serum (100 μl) was mixed with 10 μl of staining solution, and 50 μl was loaded on the top of the tube gel; electrophoresis was carried out for 2.5 h at 100 V. After electrophoresis, each tube was subjected to densitometry (604 nm; Model CS-9301, Shimadzu, Inc. Japan). The sum of the peak areas was taken as the total amount of blood lipids, and the percentage of each lipoprotein fraction was calculated automatically by the densitometer.

A new two- dimensional gel electrophoresis system

Serum (4 μl) was applied to a 0.75 % agarose gel (2 mm thick) and subjected to electrophoresis with a Sub-Cell® GT Cell apparatus (Bio-Rad) in a buffer containing 25 mM Tris (pH 8.6) at 100 V for 1.5 h. Gel strips were then excised and placed on top of nonlinear gradient slab gels. Slab gels were prepared as shown in Fig. 2a and had the same gradient setting as tube gels (Fig. 1a). The second-dimension electrophoresis was carried out in an XCell SureLock™ Mini-Cell apparatus (Life Technologies) in a buffer containing 5 mM Tris and 38.4 mM glycine (pH 8.4) at 100 V for 3 h. The separated proteins were transferred to a nitrocellulose membrane. Immunoblotting for apoA-I was performed using polyclonal anti-human apoA-I (Abcam). Horseradish peroxidase–conjugated rabbit polyclonal anti-goat lgG (Novus Biologicals) was used as a secondary antibody. The SuperSignal Westen detection Kit (Pierce) was used for detection.

Ultracentrifugation

Human serum (6 ml) was adjusted to 1.30 g/ml by adding 2.93 g of KBr. The sample was then added into a

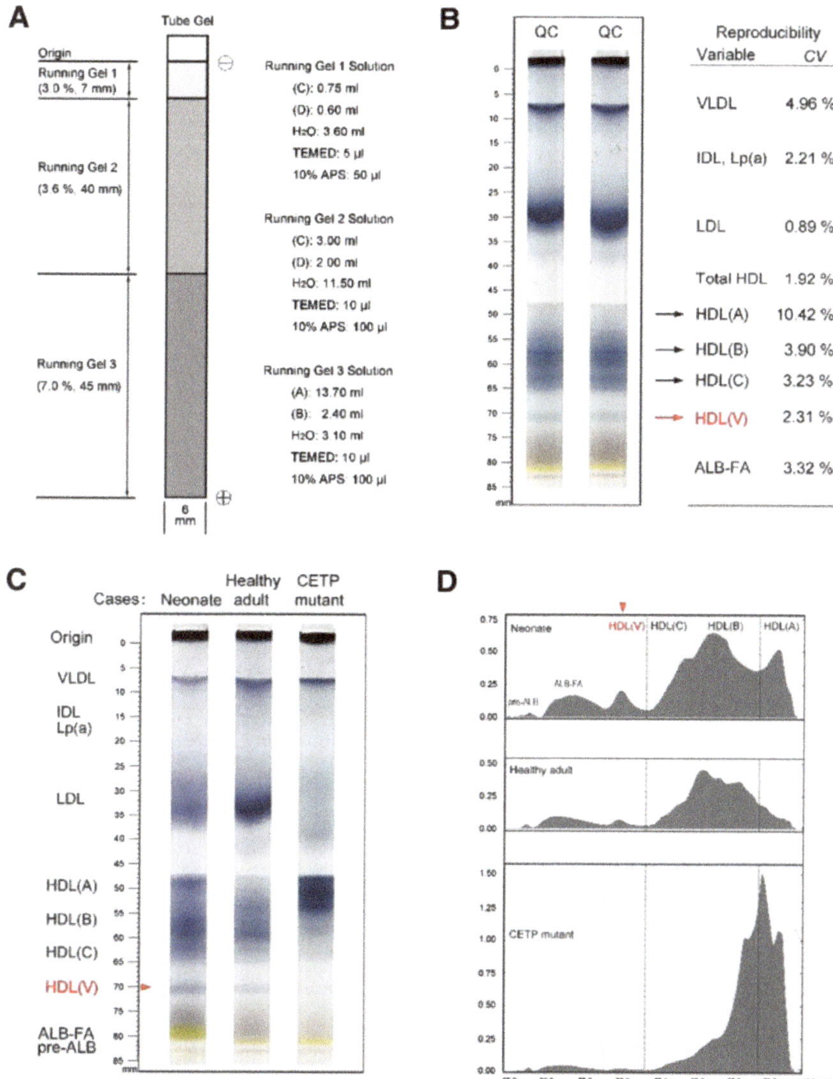

Fig. 1 Native PAGE system to separate HDL subclasses. **a** Diagram depicting gel preparation in our new system. Electrophoresis proceeded in the downward direction. Solutions A–D are described in Methods. TEMED, N,N,N′,N′-tetramethylethylenediamine; APS, ammonium persulfate. **b** Tube-gel PAGE of human serum. HDL (V) was indicated in red. CV, interassay coefficient of variation; QC, quality control. **c** Samples were from: a normal neonate, a normal adult, a patient with acute myocardial infarction (AMI), and an adult carrying a *CETP* mutation. HDL (V) was indicated in red. **d** Representative densitometric scans

28 ml ultracentrifuge (polyallomer) tube and overlaid with KBr solution (1.063 g/ml) till full. Ultracentrifugation was performed (Rotor: 50.2Ti) with a Beckman L8-M at 40,000 rpm at 10 °C for 10 h. Fractions (1 ml of each) were collected with a long needle from the bottom to top. The density of each fraction was weighed (800 μl was weighed on a scale, Explorer, OHAUS). Each fraction was desalted and concentrated through centricon filters (Millipore) to a final volume of 0.5 ml. These samples were then used for tube gel and two-dimensional gel electrophoresis.

Electron microscopy

The HDL subclasses were eluted from gels, dialyzed against a solution of 0.4 % NH_4HCO_3, and then processed as described [24]. An aliquot of lipoprotein solution was mixed with an equal volume of 2 % sodium phosphotungstate (pH 7.4). A small droplet was applied to a Formvar-grid, where it remained for 30 s. The size and morphology of lipoprotein particles were immediately observed under a transmission electron microscope (JEM-1200EX, Japan) operating at 80 KV. Micrographs were recorded at instrument magnifications of 100 K.

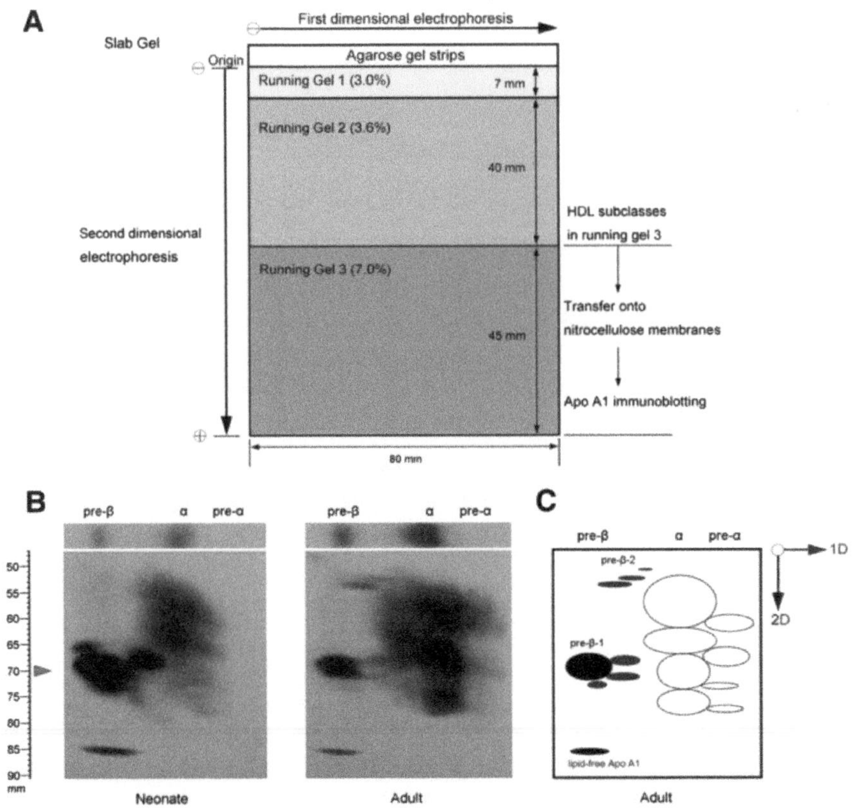

Fig. 2 Distribution of apoA-I in human serum determined by nondenaturing two-dimensional nonlinear gradient gel electrophoresis. **a** Schematic diagram of the gel system. **b** Human serum (4 μl) from each of a neonate and adult was subjected to electrophoresis on a 0.75 % agarose gel (first dimension) for 1 h. The lane was then excised and placed on a nonlinear gradient polyacrylamide slab gel (second dimension) and subjected to electrophoresis for 3 h. Serum proteins were transferred to a nitrocellulose membrane, and human apoA-I was visualized with goat anti-human apoA-I. The red arrowhead indicates the distance of particle migration in the electrophoresis. **c** Diagram showing HDL subspecies (in adults) isolated by two-dimensional gel electrophoresis

The diameter of 100 scattered particles in each lipoprotein fraction was measured using the software of Image-Pro Plus 6.0 (Media Cybernetics, Inc. USA).

Human study population

The study complied with the Declaration of Helsinki, and was approved by the hospital ethical review board (Zhongshan Hospital, Fudan University, Shanghai, China). A total of 102 subjects underwent diagnostic coronary angiography in Zhongshan Hospital, Fudan University were included in this study, among which, 56 had no stenosis of coronary artery and 46 were diagnosed as CAD, which was predefined as the presence of a luminal diameter stenosis ≥50 % in at least 1 major coronary artery territory (left anterior descending, left circumflex or right coronary artery or their major branches). The severity of the coronary artery stenosis was evaluated by Gensini score [25], which is computed by assigning a severity score to each coronary stenosis according to the degree of luminal narrowing and its geographic importance. Reductions in the lumen diameter of 25 %, 50 %, 75 %, 90 %, 99 % and complete occlusion were given score of 1, 2, 4, 8, 16 and 32, respectively. Each principal vascular segment was assigned a multiplier in accordance with the functional significance of the myocardial area supplied by that segment, that is, the LM was assigned the significant multiplier × 5; the proximal segment of the LAD × 2.5; the proximal segment of the LCX × 2.5; the mid segment of the LAD × 1.5; the RCA, the distal segment of the LAD, the posterolateral artery, and the obtuse marginal artery × 1; and others × 0.5. Diabetes mellitus (DM) was diagnosed by clinical history, use of hypoglycemic medications or a fasting blood sugar level >7.0 mmol/L (125 mg/dL); hypertension was defined in patients receiving antihypertensive treatment or with known diagnosis of hypertension (blood pressure ≥140/90 mmHg).

Statistical analysis

Continuous variables were reported as means ± standard deviation (SD). Comparisons among more than two groups were performed by analysis of variance (ANOVA), followed by least significant difference (LSD) test for multiple comparisons. The Pearson's $\chi 2$ test was used to assess statistical differences in dichotomous and categorical variables. Univariate linear regression analysis was used to determine correlation between Gensini score and HDL-(V) (preβ1-HDL) levels. Attempts were also made to predict CAD by multivariate logistic regression analysis, using CAD as the dependent variable, and age, gender, BMI, smoking history, hypertension, DM, HDL-(V) (preβ1-HDL), HDL-(A), HDL-(B), and HDL-(C) levels as independent variables. To further investigate the relationships between Gensini score and clinical characteristics or laboratory parameters, multivariate linear regression analysis was performed by using Gensini score as the dependent variable, and age, gender, BMI, smoking history, hypertension, DM, HDL-(A), HDL-(B), HDL-(C), and HDL-(V) (preβ1-HDL) levels as independent variables. P values < 0.05 were considered statistically significant. All analyses were done using SPSS version 16 analytical software (SPSS Inc., Chicago, IL).

Biochemical detection

Blood lipids were determined according to standard procedures [26] in the clinical laboratory of Zhongshan Hospital. Lipid concentrations were measured on a Hitachi 911 automatic analyzer, using reagents from Roche Diagnostics. Cholesterol and triglyceride concentrations were determined enzymatically using CHOD-PAP and lipase/GPO/PAP methods, respectively. HDL-cholesterol (HDL-C) concentration was measured with the phosphotungstic acid and $MgCl_2$ precipitation approach. LDL-cholesterol (LDL-C) was measured by a direct method, not calculated. The levels of apoAI, apoB, apoE, and Lipoprotein (a) [Lp (a)] were determined by immunoturbidimetric assays.

Other human samples

Three *CETP* mutant (with G → A in the splice donor site of intron 14 [27]) serums were a gift from Dr. Akihiro Inazu, Department of Clinical Laboratory Science, Kanazawa.

Six Tangier disease serums were from Division of Translational Medicine and Human Genetics, Perelman School of Medicine, University of Pennsylvania.

Results

The makeup of the native polyacrylamide gels that we developed is shown in Fig. 1a. Non-gradient polyacrylamide gels of 3.0, 3.6, and 7.0 % acrylamide were used for VLDL, LDL, and HDL separation, respectively. Moreover, this system could separate HDL (HDL total) into four fractions denoted here as HDL-(A), (B), (C), and (V) (Fig. 1b). The precision of the assays was established by carrying out ten assays for each of the HDL subclasses in a pooled human adult serum sample. The interassay coefficient of variation for each HDL subclass is shown in Fig. 1b.

We next sought to determine the distribution of these HDL subclasses in different human serum samples. We found that neonates had significantly higher HDL (A) than healthy adults and HDL (B) was the predominant HDL particle in healthy adults. Subjects carrying a *CETP* mutation had much higher HDL (A) levels than all the tested samples (Fig. 1c, d). Importantly, we found that our system could quantitatively separate HDL-(V) from the other subclasses. The order of its abundance was as follows: neonates > healthy adults > persons with a *CETP* mutation.

To characterize these HDL subclasses, we created a new system for two-dimensional gel electrophoresis. All serum lipoproteins were first separated by agarose gel electrophoresis (Fig. 2a). The gel strips were then excised and placed on top of a nonlinear gradient slab gel. As shown in Fig. 2b, this new system yielded patterns comparable with those reported by Francone et al. [17]. We also noticed that human adults had much higher α-HDL and preβ2-HDL compared with neonates, whereas neonates had not only higher preβ1-HDL but also more preβ1-HDL subspecies (Fig. 2b, c).

To further characterize HDL particles, we isolated them by ultracentrifugation (Fig. 3a) and then subjected the Sudan Black pre-stained particles (with different densities) to electrophoresis on our native PAGE gel. We found that HDL-(V), which was well separated from the other HDLs, had the highest density (Fig. 3b). Two-dimensional gel electrophoresis showed that HDL-(V) is, in fact, preβ1-HDL [17], which had a density about 1.21 g/ml (Fig. 3c).

To further evaluate that HDL-(V) is preβ1-HDL, we treated human serum with DTNB (1 mM) to inhibit LCAT [28] and then ran the pre-stained serum on the native PAGE gel. We found that without DTNB treatment, HDL-(V) gradually disappeared during the 6-h incubation, indicating a LCAT-mediated process for HDL maturation, from preβ1-HDL (nascent HDL) to matured HDL. However, DTNB treatment could prevent this process (Fig. 4).

We next determined the particle size of the isolated HDL subclasses using electron microscopy with a negative-staining approach. A scattered pattern of isolated HDL particles was observed at 100,000× magnification (Fig. 5a). All particles were spheroidal. The preβ1-HDLs were visualized as small dot-like particles rather than disc-

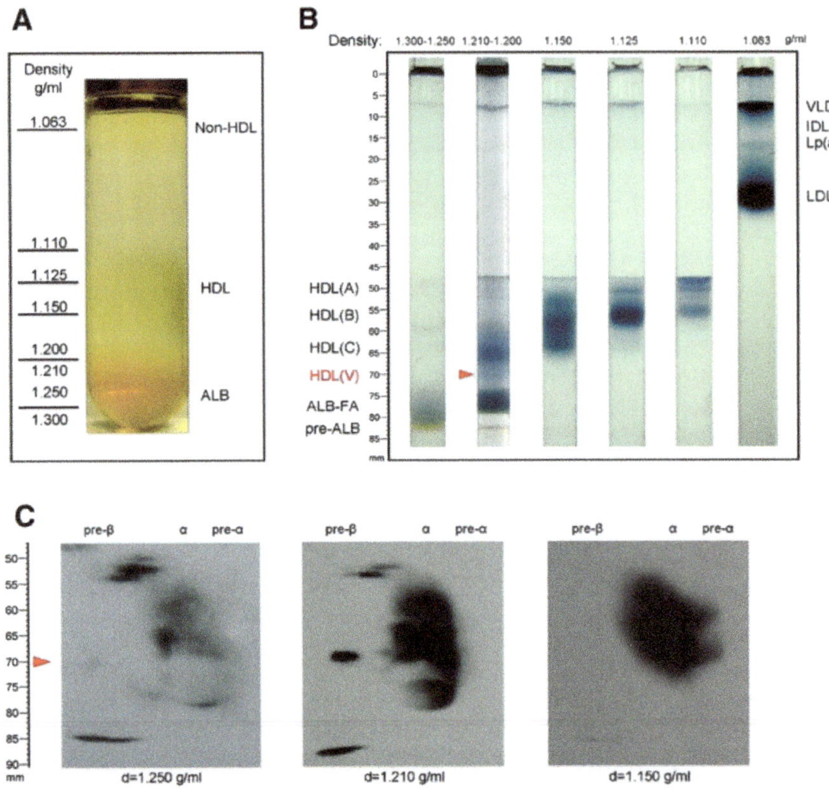

Fig. 3 HDL (V) is preβ1-HDL. To prove that HDL-(V) is preβ1-HDL, we isolated different HDL fractions by ultracentrifugation. **a** Isolation of non-HDL and HDL particles using ultracentrifugation. **b** Each fraction was subjected to our new PAGE system. The red arrowhead indicates HDL (V). **c** Each fraction was subjected to our new two-dimensional gel electrophoresis and then immunoblotted with anti-apoA-I. HDL-(V) exhibited an electrophoretic pattern identical to that preβ1-HDL

like ones in which they exhibited a weak contrast. The mean diameter of the HDL particles was as follows: (A) = 11 nm, (B) = 9 nm, (C) = 7 nm, and preβ1-HDL = 5 nm. We also measured apoA-I and cholesterol levels in each fraction and found that preβ1-HDL had the highest apoA-I/cholesterol ratio, indicating that although it is lipid poor it is not lipid free (Fig. 5b). This was consistent with the results obtained from our native PAGE because the lipids in each HDL were pre-stained with Sudan Black (Fig. 1b, c).

We analyzed Tangier patient pre-stained serum (pooled from 5 samples) on our native PAGE gel and found that there was no preβ1-HDL (Fig. 6a). However, when we ran the same sample on our two-dimensional gel, we found there was a preβ1-HDL-like spot (Fig. 6b), suggesting that the two-dimensional gel cannot distinguish real preβ1-HDL particles and preβ1-HDL-like apoA-I aggregates. To see the lipid-free apoA-I aggregate does exist, we ran purified apoA-I (Sigma) on the two-dimensional gel and found the apoA-I sample contains preβ1-HDL-like/lipid-free apoA-I aggregates (Fig. 6c). Thus, the two-dimensional gel system cannot precisely quantify preβ1-HDL in human serum.

Further, we utilized our one-dimensional method to measure preβ1-HDL levels in 102 human subjects. Concerning that Gensini sore > 60 was related to severe coronary artery stenosis and poor prognosis [25], all these 102 subjects were divided into three groups according to Gensini score (group 1, Gensini score = 0, $n = 56$; group 2, Gensini score 0 ~ 60, $n = 22$; group 3, Gensini score > 60, $n = 24$). Clinical characteristics and parameters of the three groups and significant differences are shown in Table 1. Smoking history, levels of HDL-C, preβ1-HDL, HDL-(A), HDL-(B), and IDL were significantly different in the three groups. Further multiple comparisons by LSD test showed significant difference between every two groups in smoking history, levels of preβ1-HDL, and IDL (Table 1, Fig. 7a).

By multivariate logistic regression analysis (Table 2), both smoking history and preβ1-HDL (aOR = 0.13, $p = 0.05$) levels in CAD patients were found to be independently associated with CAD.

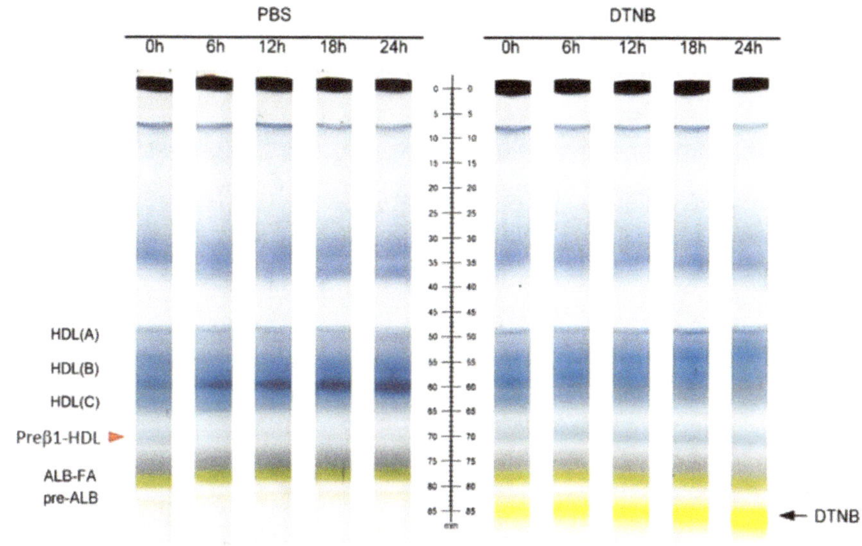

Fig. 4 LCAT inhibition blocks preβ1-HDL conversion. Human serum was treated with or without DTNB (1.8 mM) and then pre-stained with Sudan Black. The sample was run on the gel

To study the relationship between the severity of coronary artery stenosis and preβ1-HDL levels, univariate linear regression analysis was performed to show a negative correlation between Gensini score and preβ1-HDL levels ($r = -0.394$, $p < 0.0001$, Fig. 7b). Further, using multivariate linear regression analysis, DM (B = 43.57, $p = 0.01$) and preβ1-HDL levels (B = −37.33, $p = 0.01$) were independently associated with Gensini score after adjusted for age, gender, BMI, hypertension, HDL-(A), HDL-(B), and HDL-(C) levels (Table 3). Thus, preβ1-HDL levels are independent predictors of higher Gensini score.

Discussion

In this study, we 1) developed a new native PAGE system which quantitatively separates a smaller HDL particles from other HDL particles; 2) demonstrated that this HDL fraction is preβ1-HDL, which can be converted to other HDLs by LCAT; 3) found that preβ1-HDL particles thus isolated are spheroidal with the highest apoA-I/cholesterol ratio and highest density (≥1.21 g/ml), compared with all other HDL particles; 4) found that neonates have significantly higher and more complex preβ-HDLs than adults; 5) found that Tangier patients and *CETP* mutation have no detectable preβ-HDLs; 6) found

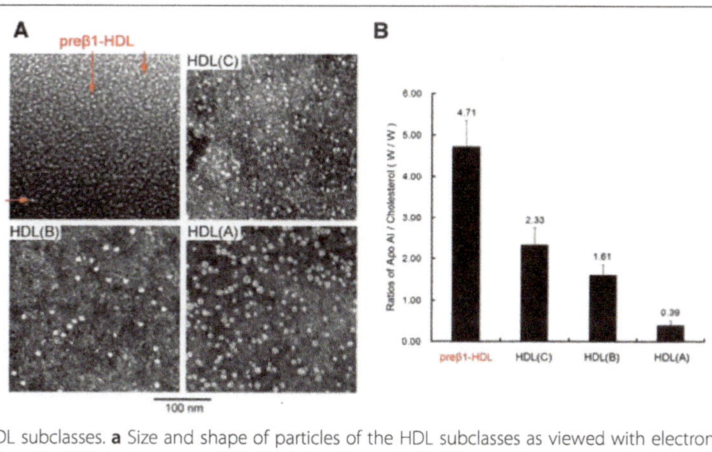

Fig. 5 Characterization of HDL subclasses. **a** Size and shape of particles of the HDL subclasses as viewed with electron microscopy. The mean diameter of the particles of preβ1-HDL (red arrows), HDL-(C), HDL-(B), and HDL-(A) was 5 nm, 7 nm, 9 nm, and 11 nm, respectively. The bar indicates 100 nm. **b** ApoA-I/cholesterol ratios in 9 separated samples

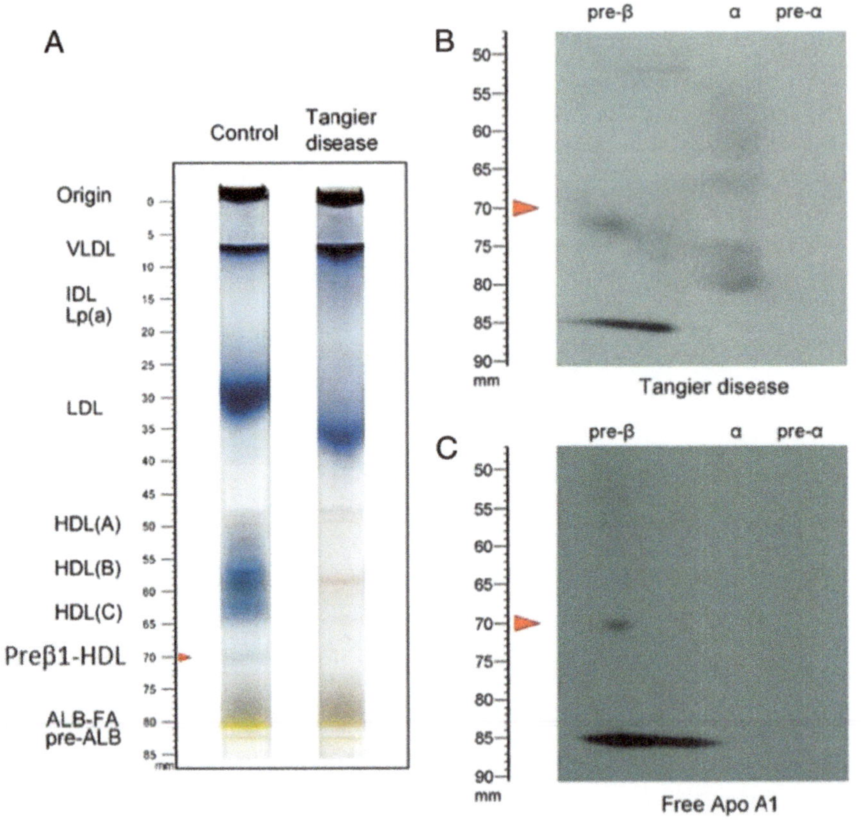

Fig. 6 A two-dimensional gel system cannot precisely quantify preβ1-HDL. **a** Tangier patient (pooled from 5 subjects) and control serum running on the native PAGE system as shown in Fig. 1. **b** Tangier sample running on the two-dimensional gel system. **c** purified apoA-I (200 ng) running on the two-dimensional gel system

that the existing two-dimensional gel system cannot precisely quantify preβ1-HDL in human serum; and 7) found that preβ1-HDL is significantly related to the severity of coronary artery stenosis in a negative manner.

One of the key accomplishments of this study is that we established a simple and fast method for preβ1-HDL quantification. It has been reported that HDL subclasses can be defined by either of two gradient PAGE systems [14, 15], but the resolution of neither system is ideal. The novelty of our system is that we assemble three different polyacrylamide gels (3.0, 3.6, and 7.0 % acrylamide) to separate VLDL, LDL, and HDL and also to separate HDL subclasses in a single-step electrophoresis. The biggest difference between our native PAGE system and previous systems is that we can clearly resolve HDL (V), i.e. preβ1-HDL (Fig. 1b), whereas other systems cannot detect this fraction [14, 15]. Moreover, our system has a small inter-assay coefficient of variation (Fig. 1b).

The second key accomplishment of this study is that we established a new system for HDL two-dimensional gel electrophoresis. It has been reported that HDL subclasses can be defined on two-dimensional systems (agarose/linear gradient polyacrylamide gel) [17, 20]. Based on these reported systems, we established our own agarose/nonlinear gradient PAGE system applicable to any typical research or clinical laboratory (Fig. 2).

Preβ1-HDL has unique characteristics. We found that preβ1-HDL particles isolated with our PAGE system have higher density (≥1.21 g/ml; Fig. 3a, b) than other HDLs, and this was confirmed by two-dimensional gels (Fig. 3c). With respect to particle structure, many studies have postulated that preβ1-HDL is discoidal [29–32], but no report has shown this directly. Discoidal HDL, having an electrophoretic mobility like that of preβ1-HDL, can be synthesized in vitro to serve as a model for plasma preβ-HDL [31, 33]. Our electron microscopy analysis revealed no discoidal particles but rather only spheroidal particles (Fig. 5a), similar to a previous report [23]. Moreover, we also found that preβ1-HDL contains lipids (Figs. 1b, c and 5b), which is different from the previous report [23].

Plasma preβ1-HDL plays an important role in cholesterol efflux, but it remains controversial whether preβ1-HDL is the

Table 1 Group comparisons for different variables in different Gensini score groups: Continuous variables are given as means ± SD and evaluated using analysis of variance (ANOVA), followed by least significant difference (LSD) test for multiple comparisons. Dichotomous and categorical variables are given as percentages and and compared using Pearson's χ^2 test

Variable	Group 1 (Gensini score = 0, *n* = 56)	Group 2 (Gensini score = 0 ~ 60, *n* = 22)	Group 3 (Gensini score >60, *n* = 24)	*p* value
Male (N%)	43 (76.8 %)	18 (81.8 %)	18 (75.0 %)	0.845
Age (years)	59.75 ± 12.67	57.82 ± 13.83	65.83 ± 9.70	0.062
BMI (kg/m^2)	23.85 ± 4.21	25.58 ± 3.18	23.39 ± 3.30	0.122
Smoking (N%)	3 (18.8 %)	15 (68.2 %)	13 (54.2 %)	0.009
				0.003 (Group 1 vs. 2)
				0.025 (Group 1 vs. 3)
				0.331 (Group 2 vs. 3)
Hypertension (N%)	9 (56.2 %)	12 (54.5 %)	14 (58.3 %)	0.967
DM (N%)	2 (12.5 %)	4 (18.2 %)	6 (25.0 %)	0.609
TC (mmol/L)	4.35 ± 0.74	4.20 ± 1.14	4.52 ± 1.10	0.507
TG (mmol/L)	1.29 ± 0.56	1.62 ± 0.93	1.71 ± 1.27	0.077
HDL-C (mmol/L)	1.39 ± 0.31	1.09 ± 0.19	1.14 ± 0.29	<0.0001
				<0.0001 (Group 1 vs. 2)
				<0.0001 (Group 1 vs. 3)
				0.507 (Group 2 vs. 3)
LDL-C (mmol/L)	2.39 ± 0.58	2.38 ± 0.90	2.62 ± 0.84	0.381
ApoAI (mg/mL)	0.97 ± 0.13	0.98 ± 0.15	1.08 ± 0.23	0.078
ApoB (mg/mL)	0.70 ± 0.19	0.82 ± 0.29	0.88 ± 0.30	0.143
ApoE (mg/L)	43.52 ± 12.78	46.05 ± 17.38	51.87 ± 20.65	0.309
Lp (a) (mg/L)	187.40 ± 182.46	191.16 ± 179.62	188.22 ± 191.16	0.998
HDL-(A) (%)	1.94 ± 0.77	1.48 ± 0.64	1.81 ± 0.71	0.048
				0.014 (Group 1 vs. 2)
				0.451 (Group 1 vs. 3)
				0.135 (Group 2 vs. 3)
HDL-(B) (%)	19.11 ± 6.73	13.70 ± 4.77	15.46 ± 6.24	0.001
				0.011 (Group 1 vs. 2)
				0.018 (Group 1 vs. 3)
				0.343 (Group 2 vs. 3)
HDL-(C) (%)	10.45 ± 2.36	11.15 ± 2.97	9.69 ± 2.89	0.171
Preβ1-HDL (%)	1.69 ± 0.34	1.48 ± 0.47	1.24 ± 0.42	<0.0001
				0.032 (Group 1 vs. 2)
				<0.0001 (Group 1 vs. 3)
				0.047 (Group 2 vs. 3)
LDL (%)	41.90 ± 5.88	42.81 ± 7.02	44.34 ± 5.92	0.268
IDL (%)	3.58 ± 1.06	5.14 ± 1.71	6.02 ± 2.28	<0.0001
				<0.0001 (Group 1 vs. 2)
				<0.0001 (Group 1 vs. 3)
				0.006 (Group 2 vs. 3)
VLDL (%)	16.37 ± 6.10	20.12 ± 8.38	17.95 ± 8.24	0.116

BMI body mass index, *DM* diabetes mellitus, *TC* total cholesterol, *TG* triglyceride, *HDL-C* high density lipoprotein cholesterol, *LDL-C* low density lipoprotein cholesterol, *ApoAI* apolipoprotein A, *ApoB* apolipoprotein B, *ApoE* apolipoprotein E, *Lp (a)* Lipoprotein (a). The sum of the peak areas (after scanning see Fig. 1) was taken as the total amount of plasma lipoproteins, and the percentage (%) of each lipoprotein fraction was calculated automatically by the densitometer

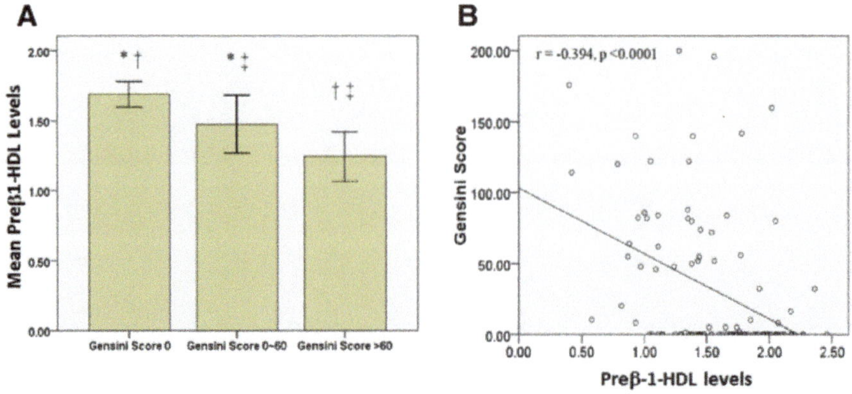

Fig. 7 Comparisons of preβ1-HDL levels in patients having different Gensini score. **a** There were 56, 22 and 24 individuals having Gensini score 0, 0 ~ 60 and >60, respectively. Mean preβ1-HDL levels among the 3 groups were significant different by ANOVA test ($p < 0.0001$). By LSD test, there were significant different preβ1-HDL levels between Gensini score 0 and 0 ~ 60 (* $p = 0.0032$), 0 and >60 († $p < 0.0001$), and 0 ~ 60 and >60 (‡ $p = 0.047$). **b** Univariate linear regression analysis showed a negative correlation between Gensini score and preβ1-HDL levels ($r = -0.394$, $p < 0.0001$)

substrate or the first product of ABCA1-mediated cholesterol efflux [34, 35]. It has been reported that "preβ1-HDL-like" lipid-poor apoA-1 or nascent HDL is formed when lipid-free apoA-1 retrieves phospholipids and cholesterol from cells mediated by ABCA1 in experiments using various culture cells [36, 37]. Thus, the levels of preβ1-HDL should be an indicator of the capacity for HDL production and reverse cholesterol transport, and preβ1-HDL should be expected to have an anti-atherogenic function. However, the results from literatures suggest that an elevated level of preβ1-HDL is a risk factor for CAD [19–21]. This could be due the two-dimensional electrophoresis cannot separate preβ1-HDL from the lipid-free apoA-I. Our new two-dimensional gel system not only separated preβ1-HDL from the lipid-free apoA-I, but also demonstrated a complex pattern of preβ1-HDL, which was not reported before (Fig. 2b, c).

Two-dimensional electrophoresis system is not suitable for preβ1-HDL measurement. It has been reported that patients with Tangier disease have preβ1-HDLs, but not mature HDL [22]. However, when we carefully re-checked the two-dimensional electrophoresis gel presented in current study, the homozygous patient might only have lipid-free apoA-I (as recently suggested by Miyazaki et al. [23]). Importantly, we found that samples from subjects with Tangier disease do not contain preβ1-HDLs when using our one-dimensional native PAGE gel (Fig. 6a), however, when we examined the sample on our two-dimensional gel system, we did find a preβ1-HDL-like spot (Fig. 6b), probably consisting in preβ1-HDL-like/lipid-free apoA-I aggregates (Fig. 6c). Thus, the two-dimensional gel system cannot precisely quantify preβ1-HDL in human serum. It is reasonable to

Table 2 Logistic regression predictors of CAD: Logistic regression analysis was performed by using CAD as the dependent variable, and age, gender, BMI, smoking history, hypertension, DM, preβ1-HDL, HDL-(A), HDL-(B), and HDL-(C) as independent variables

Variables	*p* value	aOR	95.0 % C.I. for aOR
Age (years)	0.31	1.04	(0.96-1.14)
Male gender	0.43	1.93	(0.37-9.99)
BMI (kg/m^2)	0.27	1.14	(0.90-1.45)
Smoking	0.03	9.77	(1.28-74.64)
Hypertension	0.97	1.03	(0.17-6.22)
DM	0.95	1.08	(0.10-11.67)
HDL-(A)	0.10	4.75	(0.73-30.86)
HDL-(B)	0.11	0.84	(0.68-1.04)
HDL-(C)	0.52	0.91	(0.68-1.22)
Preβ1-HDL	0.05	0.13	(0.02-1.02)

Table 3 Predictors of Gensini score by multivariate linear regression: Multivariate linear regression analysis was performed by using Gensini score as the dependent variable, and age, gender, BMI, smoking history, hypertension, DM, HDL-(A), HDL-(B), HDL-(C), and preβ1-HDL levels as independent variables

Variables	*p* value	B	95 % confidence interval for B
Age (years)	0.10	1.10	(−0.23-2.43)
Male gender	0.62	8.22	(−24.80-41.24)
BMI (kg/m^2)	0.25	−2.39	(−6.46-1.69)
Smoking	0.44	11.74	(−18.77-42.25)
Hypertension	0.58	8.60	(−22.75-39.95)
DM	0.01	43.57	(10.06-77.07)
HDL-(A)	0.31	13.06	(−12.65-38.76)
HDL-(B)	0.32	−1.73	(−5.20-1.74)
HDL-(C)	0.50	−1.86	(−7.09-3.38)
Preβ1-HDL	0.01	−37.33	(−66.61- -8.05)

infer that Tangier patients have only lipid-free apoA-I (which could be monomer and polymer or aggregate) but have no preβ1-HDL, since they have no ABCA1-mediated cholesterol efflux and preβ1-HDL cannot be formed, thus, no apoA-I-containing mature HDL can be produced.

Using our new one-dimensional PAGE system, we can precisely separate preβ1-HDL from the rest of HDL. This relatively simple method helped us to re-evaluate the relationship between preβ1-HDL and CAD. We found that preβ1-HDL levels are independently and negatively associated with the severity of the coronary artery stenosis (Table 3, Fig. 7a, b).

Interestingly, we also found that subjects carrying a *CETP* mutation have not only larger HDLs but also no detectible preβ1-HDL with our system (Fig. 1c). This preβ1-HDL deficiency may be one of the reasons why CETP inhibitors, to date, do not work in the expected direction, i.e., to reduce the incidence of cardiovascular diseases.

Another interesting observation from this study is that neonates have much higher and more complex preβ1-HDLs than adults, indicating that there are age-related changes in the characteristics of circulating preβ1-HDLs. If we can slow down such changes, we may find a new way to slow down the development of atherosclerosis.

We also observed some interesting phenomena, few of which have been reported before (Table 1). We found that 1) in healthy adults, HDL-(B) is the major HDL particle, and 2) neonates have a dramatically different pattern of HDL subclasses compared with healthy adults. Although we do not know the physiological relevance of these differences, we now have, at least, a way to view them.

There are some limitations of our system. The preparation of tube gels is time consuming; however, this process can be standardized. Further optimization is needed to improve the resolution of HDL-(A), −(B), and -(C). Regardless, the simple method for preβ1-HDL quantification we developed is suitable for clinical applications and may also be appropriate for screening potential drugs that may increase the level of circulating preβ1-HDLs.

Conclusion

We established a novel and simple method for human serum preβ1-HDL quantification. We found that human lower preβ1-HDL is an independent predictor for severer coronary artery stenosis.

Abbreviations

CETP: cholesteryl ester transfer protein; HDL: high density lipoprotein; LCAT: lecithin-cholesterol acyltransferase; PAGE: polyacrylamide gel electrophoresis.

Competing interests

The authors declare that they have no competing interests.

Authors' contributions

YC, JD, JG, XCJ conceived and designed the experiments. YC, JD, HJ, AB, XZ, ZL, JY, DL conducted the experiments. XC conducted statistical analysis. MC and DR provided human samples, read and edited the manuscript. MMH, YZ, and HC involved in critical editing of manuscript. XCJ wrote the paper. All authors read and approved the final manuscript.

Acknowledgments

This work was supported by grants from National Natural Science Foundation of China (No. 31100851, No. 30500205, No. 30873351 and No. 81373869) and from Shanghai Municipal Commission of Health and Family Planning (No. 20134127). This work also partially supported by a NIH grant (R56HL121409).

We thank Chunjie Yang (Shanghai Institute of Cardiovascular Diseases) and Jong Wu and Weiyun Wu (Department of Clinical Laboratory of Zhongshan Hospital) for their technical support. We thank Dr. Akihiro Inazu, Department of Clinical Laboratory Science, Kanazawa University for providing *CETP* mutant serums.

Author details

[1]Shanghai Institute of Cardiovascular Diseases, Zhongshan Hospital, Fudan University, Shanghai, China. [2]Department of Cell Biology, SUNY Downstate Medical Center, 450 Clarkson Ave, Box 5, Brooklyn, NY 11203, USA. [3]School of Pharmacy, Fudan University, Shanghai, China. [4]Obstetrics & Gynecology Hospital, Fudan University, Shanghai, China. [5]Southern Medical University, Guangzhou, China. [6]Division of Translational Medicine and Human Genetics, Perelman School of Medicine, University of Pennsylvania, Philadelphia, USA.

References

1. Assmann G, Gotto Jr AM. HDL cholesterol and protective factors in atherosclerosis. Circulation. 2004;109:III8–14.
2. Glomset JA. The plasma lecithins:cholesterol acyltransferase reaction. J Lipid Res. 1968;9:155–67.
3. Lincoff AM, Wolski K, Nicholls SJ, Nissen SE. Pioglitazone and risk of cardiovascular events in patients with type 2 diabetes mellitus: a meta-analysis of randomized trials. JAMA. 2007;298:1180–8.
4. Kastelein JJ, van Leuven SI, Burgess L, Evans GW, Kuivenhoven JA, Barter PJ, Revkin JH, Grobbee DE, Riley WA, Shear CL et al. Effect of torcetrapib on carotid atherosclerosis in familial hypercholesterolemia. N Engl J Med. 2007;356:1620–30.
5. Bots ML, Visseren FL, Evans GW, Riley WA, Revkin JH, Tegeler CH, Shear CL, Duggan WT, Vicari RM, Grobbee DE, Kastelein JJ. Torcetrapib and carotid intima-media thickness in mixed dyslipidaemia (RADIANCE 2 study): a randomised, double-blind trial. Lancet. 2007;370:153–60.
6. Fayad ZA, Mani V, Woodward M, Kallend D, Abt M, Burgess T, Fuster V, Ballantyne CM, Stein EA, Tardif JC et al. Safety and efficacy of dalcetrapib on atherosclerotic disease using novel non-invasive multimodality imaging (dal-PLAQUE): a randomised clinical trial. Lancet. 2011;378:1547–59.
7. Barter PJ, Rye KA. Cholesteryl ester transfer protein inhibition as a strategy to reduce cardiovascular risk. J Lipid Res. 2012;53:1755–66.
8. Voight BF, Peloso GM, Orho-Melander M, Frikke-Schmidt R, Barbalic M, Jensen MK, Hindy G, Holm H, Ding EL, Johnson T et al. Plasma HDL cholesterol and risk of myocardial infarction: a mendelian randomisation study. Lancet. 2012;380:572–80.
9. Burstein M, Scholnick HR. Lipoprotein-polyanion-metal interactions. Adv Lipid Res. 1973;11:67–108.
10. Warnick GR, Benderson J, Albers JJ. Dextran sulfate-Mg2+ precipitation procedure for quantitation of high-density-lipoprotein cholesterol. Clin Chem. 1982;28:1379–88.
11. Briggs CJ, Anderson D, Johnson P, Deegan T. Evaluation of the polyethylene glycol precipitation method for the estimation of high-density lipoprotein cholesterol. Ann Clin Biochem. 1981;18:177–81.
12. Delalla OF, Elliott HA, Gofman JW. Ultracentrifugal studies of high density serum lipoproteins in clinically healthy adults. Am J Physiol. 1954;179:333–7.
13. Havel RJ, Eder HA, Bragdon JH. The distribution and chemical composition of ultracentrifugally separated lipoproteins in human serum. J Clin Invest. 1955;34:1345–53.

14. Alabakovska SB, Todorova BB, Labudovic DD, Tosheska KN. LDL and HDL subclass distribution in patients with end-stage renal diseases. Clin Biochem. 2002;35:211–6.
15. Oravec S, Dostal E, Dukat A, Gavornik P, Kucera M, Gruber K. HDL subfractions analysis: a new laboratory diagnostic assay for patients with cardiovascular diseases and dyslipoproteinemia. Neuro Endocrinol Lett. 2011;32:502–9.
16. Castro GR, Fielding CJ. Early incorporation of cell-derived cholesterol into pre-beta-migrating high-density lipoprotein. Biochemistry. 1988;27:25–9.
17. Francone OL, Gurakar A, Fielding C. Distribution and functions of lecithin:cholesterol acyltransferase and cholesteryl ester transfer protein in plasma lipoproteins. Evidence for a functional unit containing these activities together with apolipoproteins A-I and D that catalyzes the esterification and transfer of cell-derived cholesterol. J Biol Chem. 1989; 264:7066–72.
18. Asztalos BF, Sloop CH, Wong L, Roheim PS. Two-dimensional electrophoresis of plasma lipoproteins: recognition of new apo A-I-containing subpopulations. Biochim Biophys Acta. 1993;1169:291–300.
19. Lamon-Fava S, Herrington DM, Reboussin DM, Sherman M, Horvath KV, Cupples LA, White C, Demissie S, Schaefer EJ, Asztalos BF. Plasma levels of HDL subpopulations and remnant lipoproteins predict the extent of angiographically-defined coronary artery disease in postmenopausal women. Arterioscler Thromb Vasc Biol. 2008;28:575–9.
20. Asztalos BF, Cupples LA, Demissie S, Horvath KV, Cox CE, Batista MC, Schaefer EJ. High-density lipoprotein subpopulation profile and coronary heart disease prevalence in male participants of the Framingham Offspring Study. Arterioscler Thromb Vasc Biol. 2004;24:2181–7.
21. Asztalos BF, Collins D, Cupples LA, Demissie S, Horvath KV, Bloomfield HE, Robins SJ, Schaefer EJ. Value of high-density lipoprotein (HDL) subpopulations in predicting recurrent cardiovascular events in the Veterans Affairs HDL Intervention Trial. Arterioscler Thromb Vasc Biol. 2005;25:2185–91.
22. Asztalos BF, Brousseau ME, Mcnamara JR, Horvath KV, Roheim PS, Schaefer EJ. Subpopulations of high density lipoproteins in homozygous and heterozygous Tangier disease. Atherosclerosis. 2001;156:217–25.
23. Miyazaki O, Ogihara J, Fukamachi I, Kasumi T. Evidence for the presence of lipid-free monomolecular apolipoprotein A-1 in plasma. J Lipid Res. 2014;55: 214–25.
24. Forte TM, Nordhausen RW. Electron microscopy of negatively stained lipoproteins. Methods Enzymol. 1986;128:442–57.
25. Gensini GG. A more meaningful scoring system for determining the severity of coronary heart disease. Am J Cardiol. 1983;51:606.
26. Stein EA, Myers GL. National Cholesterol Education Program recommendations for triglyceride measurement: executive summary. The National Cholesterol Education Program Working Group on lipoprotein measurement. Clin Chem. 1995;41:1421–6.
27. Brown ML, Inazu A, Hesler CB, Agellon LB, Mann C, Whitlock ME, Marcel YL, Milne RW, Koizumi J, Mabuchi H et al. Molecular basis of lipid transfer protein deficiency in a family with increased high-density lipoproteins. Nature. 1989;342:448–51.
28. Bisgaier CL, Sachdev OP, Lee ES, Williams KJ, Blum CB, Glickman RM. Effect of lecithin:cholesterol acyltransferase on distribution of apolipoprotein A-IV among lipoproteins of human plasma. J Lipid Res. 1987;28:693–703.
29. Sviridov D, Miyazaki O, Theodore K, Hoang A, Fukamachi I, Nestel P. Delineation of the role of pre-beta 1-HDL in cholesterol efflux using isolated pre-beta 1-HDL. Arterioscler Thromb Vasc Biol. 2002;22:1482–8.
30. von Eckardstein A, Nofer JR, Assmann G, High density lipoproteins and arteriosclerosis. Role of cholesterol efflux and reverse cholesterol transport. Arterioscler Thromb Vasc Biol. 2001;21:13–27.
31. Favari E, Calabresi L, Adorni MP, Jessup W, Simonelli S, Franceschini G, Bernini F. Small discoidal pre-beta1 HDL particles are efficient acceptors of cell cholesterol via ABCA1 and ABCG1. Biochemistry. 2009;48:11067–74.
32. Asztalos BF, Schaefer EJ, Horvath KV, Yamashita S, Miller M, Franceschini G, Calabresi L. Role of LCAT in HDL remodeling: investigation of LCAT deficiency states. J Lipid Res. 2007;48:592–9.
33. Davidson WS, Thompson TB. The structure of apolipoprotein A-I in high density lipoproteins. J Biol Chem. 2007;282:22249–53.
34. Rye KA, Barter PJ. Formation and metabolism of prebeta-migrating, lipid-poor apolipoprotein A-I. Arterioscler Thromb Vasc Biol. 2004;24:421–8.
35. Wroblewska M. The origin and metabolism of a nascent pre-beta high density lipoprotein involved in cellular cholesterol efflux. Acta Biochim Pol. 2011;58:275–85.
36. Ji A, Wroblewski JM, Cai L, de Beer MC, Webb NR, van der Westhuyzen DR. Nascent HDL formation in hepatocytes and role of ABCA1, ABCG1, and SR-BI. J Lipid Res. 2012;53:446–55.
37. Duong PT, Weibel GL, Lund-Katz S, Rothblat GH, Phillips MC. Characterization and properties of pre beta-HDL particles formed by ABCA1-mediated cellular lipid efflux to apoA-I. J Lipid Res. 2008;49:1006–14.

Alterations in protein and amino acid metabolism in rats fed a branched-chain amino acid- or leucine-enriched diet during postprandial and postabsorptive states

Milan Holecek[1*], Pavel Siman[2], Melita Vodenicarovova[1] and Roman Kandar[3]

Abstract

Background: Many people believe in favourable effects of branched-chain amino acids (BCAAs; valine, leucine, and isoleucine), especially leucine, on muscle protein balance and consume BCAAs for many years. We determined the effects of the chronic intake of a BCAA- or leucine-enriched diet on protein and amino acid metabolism in fed and postabsorptive states.

Methods: Rats were fed a standard diet, a diet with a high content of valine, leucine, and isoleucine (HVLID), or a high content of leucine (HLD) for 2 months. Half of the animals in each group were sacrificed in the fed state on the last day, and the other half were sacrificed after overnight fast. Protein synthesis was assessed using the flooding dose method (L-[3,4,5-^{3}H]phenylalanine), proteolysis on the basis of chymotrypsin-like activity (CHTLA) of proteasome and cathepsin B and L activities.

Results: Chronic intake of HVLID or HLD enhanced plasma levels of urea, alanine and glutamine. HVLID also increased levels of all three BCAA and branched-chain keto acids (BCKA), HLD increased leucine, ketoisocaproate and alanine aminotransferase and decreased valine, ketovaline, isoleucine, ketoisoleucine, and LDL cholesterol. Tissue weight and protein content were lower in extensor digitorum longus muscles in the HLD group and higher in kidneys in the HVLID and HLD groups. Muscle protein synthesis in postprandial state was higher in the HVLID group, and CHTLA was lower in muscles of the HVLID and HLD groups compared to controls. Overnight starvation enhanced alanine aminotransferase activity in muscles, and decreased protein synthesis in gastrocnemius (in HVLID group) and extensor digitorum longus (in HLD group) muscles more than in controls. Effect of HVLID and HLD on CHTLA in muscles in postabsorptive state was insignificant.

Conclusions: The results failed to demonstrate positive effects of the chronic consumption of a BCAA-enriched diet on protein balance in skeletal muscle and indicate rather negative effects from a leucine-enriched diet. The primary effects of both diets are an activated catabolism of BCAAs, which leads to an enhanced production of BCKA, alanine and glutamine and their utilization in visceral tissues and an impaired protein synthesis in postabsorptive state, particularly in fast-twitch (white) muscles.

Keywords: Nutritional supplements, Glutamine, Protein synthesis, Proteolysis, Muscle, Starvation

* Correspondence: holecek@lfhk.cuni.cz
[1]Department of Physiology, Faculty of Medicine in Hradec Kralove, Charles University in Prague, Simkova 870, Hradec Kralove 500 38, Czech Republic
Full list of author information is available at the end of the article

Background

The branched-chain amino acids (BCAAs) valine, leucine and isoleucine are essential substrates and important regulators in the synthesis of body proteins, substrates for energy production and precursors for the formation of other amino acids. The stimulatory effect of BCAAs on protein synthesis and the inhibitory effect on proteolysis have been known for many years [1–3]. Particularly, leucine was implicated in the stimulation of protein synthesis in skeletal muscle. Leucine enhances insulin release from β-cells of the pancreas and directly stimulates protein synthesis through the mammalian target of rapamycin (mTOR) signalling pathway and the phosphorylation of translation initiation factors and ribosomal proteins [4, 5]. The inhibitory effect of BCAAs on proteolysis is likely mediated by several metabolites of BCAAs, particularly branched-chain keto acids and beta-hydroxy-beta-methylbutyrate [6, 7].

The initial site for most BCAA catabolism is skeletal muscle because of the high activity of BCAA aminotransferase, which enables the transfer of the amino group of BCAAs to α-ketoglutarate to form glutamate and branched-chain keto acids (BCKA), i.e., α-ketoisocaproate (KIC, ketoleucine), α-keto-β-methylvalerate (KMV, ketoisoleucine) and α-ketoisovalerate (KIV, ketovaline). The enhanced availability of glutamic acid increases the flux through glutamine synthetase and alanine aminotransferase leading to enhanced synthesis of glutamine and alanine. These amino acids are released together with most of the BCKA from skeletal muscle to the blood [8–10]. Overall, an enhanced intake of BCAAs should lead to enhanced BCAA catabolism and the release of glutamine, alanine and BCKA from muscles to the blood stream (Fig. 1).

The unique effects of BCAAs on protein metabolism led to the use of BCAAs in patients with cachectic disorders and as popular dietary supplements, especially in athletes. However, chronic and excessive intake of the BCAAs raises concerns of their adverse side effects. The chronic intake of high amounts of BCAAs may induce an imbalance in amino acid concentrations in body fluids, alter various biochemical pathways and cellular functions, and the response of the body to different physiological and pathological conditions, such as starvation, exercise, trauma, infection, and cancer development. Unfortunately, few studies have investigated the long-term effects of BCAA supplementation, and there is a lack of information on the side effects and consequences of the long-term intake of these supplements.

We determined how the chronic intake of a BCAA- or leucine-enriched diet affected protein and amino acid homeostasis, particularly the effect on protein balance in skeletal muscle and on the concentrations of free amino acids in extracellular and intracellular spaces, especially BCAA, alanine, and glutamine levels. Various types of hindlimb muscles were examined, including m. soleus (SOL, slow-twitch, red muscles), m. extensor digitorum longus (EDL, fast-twitch, white muscle), and m. gastrocnemius (GM, both fibre types), because of reported differences in protein, BCAA and glutamine metabolism in slow-twitch and fast-twitch muscles [11–13].

The effects of BCAA- or leucine-enriched diet have been examined in two nutritionally different conditions—in fed and overnight fasted animals. In fed (postprandial) state are concentrations of nutrients in body fluids closely related to composition of the food and anabolic response of the body mediated by enhanced secretion of insulin. After overnight fast (in postabsorptive state) is the effect of food composition on concentration of nutrients in extracellular fluid smaller and the main role play gradual decrease in insulin/glucagon ratio and enhanced catabolism of glycogen, lipids, and proteins.

Methods

Animals and material

Male Wistar rats (BioTest, Konarovice, CR) were housed in standardised cages in quarters with controlled temperature and a 12-h light–dark cycle. All rats received the standard laboratory diet (SLD) ST-1 (Velas, CR) and drinking water *ad libitum*. All procedures

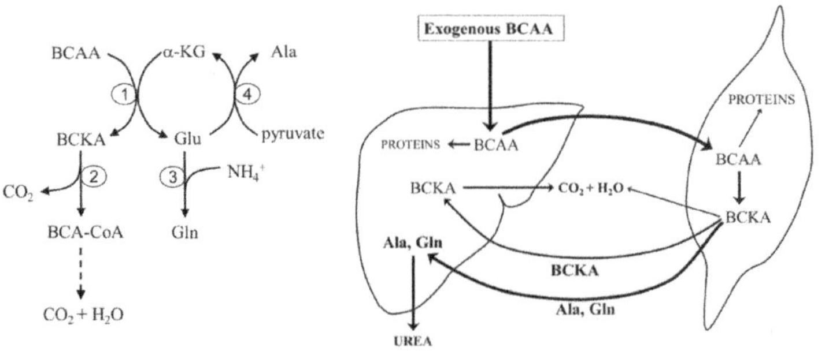

Fig. 1 The primary pathways of BCAA catabolism in skeletal muscle and the supposed response of skeletal muscle and liver to surplus exogenous BCAAs. 1, BCAA aminotransferase; 2, BCKA dehydrogenase; 3, glutamine synthetase; 4, alanine aminotransferase (ALT)

involving animals were performed according to the guidelines set by the Institutional Animal Care and Use Committee of Charles University. Animal Care and Use Committee of Charles University in Prague, Faculty of Medicine in Hradec Kralove specifically approved this study. L-[3,4,5-^{3}H]phenylalanine was purchased from American Radiolabeled Chemical, Inc. (St. Louis, MO, USA). Chemicals were obtained from Sigma Chemical (St. Louis, MO, USA), Lachema (Brno, CR), Waters (Milford, MA, ISA), Biomol (Hamburg, Germany), and Merck (Darmstadt, Germany).

Experimental design

A total of 120 male Wistar rats weighing approximately 200 g each were randomly divided into three groups fed an SLD or a diet in which 10 % of the basal diet was replaced by a mixture of valine, leucine, and isoleucine in ratios of 1 : 1 : 1 (HVLID, high valine, leucine, and isoleucine diet) or leucine (HLD, high leucine diet). The mixtures were used to prepare pellets with the same physical properties and consistency. Estimated contents of L-valine, L-leucine, and L-isoleucine (g/kg diet) are shown in Table 1. These contents resemble a high-dose supplementation in which adverse outcomes for the monitored variables were not reported [14–16].

The animals consumed tested diets for 2 months and were sacrificed between 7 and 8 a.m. on the last day of the study protocol. Half of the animals in each group were sacrificed in the fed state, and the other half were sacrificed after an overnight fast. Two separate studies were performed. Tissue protein synthesis rates were measured using the flooding dose method (L-[3,4,5-^{3}H]phenylalanine) in the first study. Alterations in amino acid concentrations in body fluids and various parameters of protein and amino acid metabolism were estimated in the second study.

Protein synthesis

The rats were injected intravenously with a flooding dose of L-[3,4,5-^{3}H]phenylalanine (50 μCi/100 g b.w.) combined with unlabelled L-phenylalanine (150 μmol/100 g b.w.) 10 min before the sacrifice by exsanguination via the abdominal aorta [17]. Small pieces (approximately 0.1 g) of soleus (SOL), gastrocnemius (GM), and extensor digitorum longus (EDL) muscles, liver, kidneys,

Table 1 Estimated contents of L-valine, L-leucine, and L-isoleucine in experimental diets (g/kg diet)

Diet	Valine (g/kg)	Leucine (g/kg)	Isoleucine (g/kg)
SLD	14	21	12
HVLID	46	50	44
HLD	13	120	11

SLD standard laboratory diet; *HVLID* diet with high content of valine, leucine, and isoleucine; *HLD* high leucine diet

and jejunum were quickly removed and frozen in liquid nitrogen. Tissue samples were homogenized in 6 % (v/v) perchloric acid, and the precipitated proteins were collected via centrifugation for 5 min at 12,000 g. The supernatant was used for the measurement of L-[3,4,5-^{3}H]phenylalanine specific activity. The pellet was washed three times and hydrolysed in 2 N NaOH. Aliquots were taken for protein content [18] and radioactivity measurements. The fractional rate of protein synthesis (FRPS) was calculated according the formula derived by McNurlan et al. [19]:

$$FRPS\ (\%\ per\ day) = (S_b \cdot 100)/(t \cdot S_a)$$

where S_b and S_a are the specific activities (dpm/nanomole) of protein-bound phenylalanine and tissue-free phenylalanine in the acid-soluble fraction of tissue homogenates, respectively, and t is the time (days) between isotope injection and tissue immersion into liquid nitrogen. The value of 274 μmol phenylalanine/g protein was used for the calculation of protein-bound phenylalanine specific activity [20]. Sample radioactivity was measured using a liquid scintillation radioactivity counter LS 6000 (Beckman Instruments, Fullerton, CA, USA).

Amino acid concentrations in blood plasma and tissues

Amino acid concentrations were determined in the supernatants of deproteinised blood plasma and tissue samples using high-performance liquid chromatography (Aliance 2695, Waters, Milford, MA, USA) after derivatisation with 6-aminoquinolyl-N-hydroxysuccinimidyl carbamate. The intracellular concentration of each amino acid was calculated by subtracting the free extracellular portion from the total amount, assuming the plasma concentration to be equal to the concentration in the interstitial fluid as described by Bergstrőm et al. [21]. Total tissue water was measured from the tissue weight obtained after drying for 24 h at 90 °C. The determination of extra- and intracellular water was based on the chloride method according to Graham et al. [22]. BCKA concentrations in blood plasma were measured using liquid chromatograph (Shimadzu, Kyoto, Japan) after precolumn derivatisation with o-phenylenediamine [23].

Chymotrypsin-like activity (CHTLA)

The chymotrypsin-like activity of proteasomes was determined using the fluorogenic substrate Suc-LLVY-MCA [24] as follows. The muscles were homogenised in 0.4 ml of ice-cold 20 mM Tris buffer, pH 7.5, containing 2 mM ATP, 5 mM $MgCl_2$ and 1 mM dithiothreitol. The homogenates were centrifuged for 10 min at 18,000 g at 4 °C. Cellular supernatants (0.1 ml) were incubated with 0.1 ml of substrate Suc-LLVY-MCA (0.1 mM) with or without inhibitor MG132 (0.02 mM) for 1 h on ice. A volume of 0.4 ml of 100 mM sodium acetate buffer (pH 4.3) was added to stop the reaction. Sample fluorescence was immediately determined at an excitation wavelength of 340 nm and emission wavelength of 440 nm (Tecan Infinite^{TM} 200). The standard curve was established for 7-amino-4-methylcoumarin (AMC), which permitted the expression of CHTLA as nmol of AMC/g protein/hour. The activity was adjusted for the protein concentration of the supernatant. Differences after the subtraction of inhibited from non-inhibited activities were used for calculations.

Cathepsin B and L activities

The activities of cathepsin B and L were determined using the fluorogenic substrate Z-FA-MCA [25, 26] as follows. Tissue samples (approximately 20 mg) were homogenised in 0.6 ml of ice-cold 300 mM sodium acetate buffer, pH 5.0, containing 4 mM EDTA, 8 mM dithiothreitol and 0.2 % Triton X-100 (v/v). The homogenates were allowed to stand for 30 min on ice and centrifuged for 30 min at 18,000 g at 4 °C. Cellular supernatant (0.01 ml) were incubated with 0.19 ml of substrate Z-FA-MCA (0.1 mM) with or without the inhibitor Z-FF-FMK (0.04 mM) for 30 min at 37 °C. The reaction was stopped by the addition of 1 ml of 100 mM sodium acetate buffer, pH 4.3, and the activities of cathepsin B and L were determined as described above for CHTLA.

Other techniques

Glutamine synthetase activity was determined using a colorimetric assay based on the formation of γ-glutamyl-hydroxamate [27]. The catalytic concentration of alanine aminotransferase was determined from the rate of decrease of NADH, measured at 340 nm, by lactate dehydrogenase [28]. Enzyme activities are reported per milligram of protein of reaction mixture. Plasma levels of urea, creatinine, ALT, AST, glucose, triglycerides, and cholesterol were measured using commercial tests (Boehringer, Mannheim, Germany; Elitech, Sées, France and Lachema, Brno, CR).

Statistics

Results are expressed as means ± SE. Analysis of variance (ANOVA) followed by Bonferroni multiple comparison post hoc analysis was used to detect differences between multiple independent groups. NCSS 2001 statistical software (Kaysville, UT, USA) was used for analyses. Differences were considered significant at $P < 0.05$.

Results

Effects of HVLID and HLD on food intake, body weight and blood biochemistry

The intake of HVLID was lower than the intake of SLD and HLD in the initial phase of the study. Differences in daily food intake were not significant beginning the second week. There were no differences in body weight gain between animals receiving the various diets (Fig. 2). Higher blood plasma concentrations of urea were observed in animals that chronically consumed HVLID or HLD. In HLD fed animals we observed higher ALT activity and lower concentration of LDL cholesterol and atherogenicity index than in controls (Table 2).

Effects of HVLID and HLD on amino acid and BCKA concentrations in blood plasma

Plasma concentrations of BCAA, BCKA, alanine, and glutamine increased significantly in animals fed HVLID. Enhanced concentrations of leucine, KIC, glutamine and alanine were also found in animals fed HLD, but concentrations of valine, isoleucine, KIV and KMV were significantly lower than controls. Overnight starvation decreased the plasma concentration of most amino acids in controls and normalised alterations induced by the intake of HVLID or HLD (Table 3 and Fig. 3).

Effects of HVLID and HLD on amino acid concentrations in tissues

HVLID increased levels of valine, leucine, and isoleucine and HLD increased leucine and decreased valine and isoleucine concentrations in all muscle types (Table 4). In other tissues the effects of HVLID and HLD were less significant (Table 5). Alanine concentrations were higher in all muscle types of animals that consumed HVLID or HLD and in the jejunum and kidneys of animals that consumed HLD. Glutamine concentrations increased significantly only in muscles of the HLD group. Most of the alterations in intracellular amino acid concentrations that were induced by the chronic intake of HVLID or HLD in the postprandial state disappeared after an overnight fast.

Effects of HVLID and HLD on glutamine synthetase and alanine aminotransferase activities

The effect of chronic HVLID or HLD consumption on glutamine synthetase and alanine aminotransferase in muscles was not significant. Overnight starvation had no effect on glutamine synthetase, but a significant increase in alanine aminotransferase activity in muscles was found in the SOL and MG of animals fed various diets and the EDL of animals fed SLD before an overnight fast (Figs. 4 and 5).

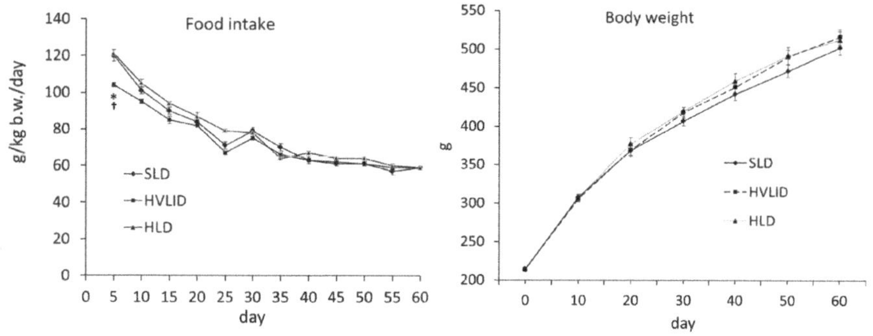

Fig. 2 Food intake and body weight changes in rats fed an SLD, HVLID and HLD. Means ± SE, $p < 0.05$. *compared to the SLD group; † HLD group vs. HVLID group

Effects of HVLID and HLD on protein synthesis

The fractional rate of protein synthesis (Fig. 6) was higher in the postprandial state in MG and SOL of animals fed an HVLID and in the jejunum of animals fed an HLD. A decrease in protein synthesis was found in muscles after an overnight fast. The decrease was more pronounced in gastrocnemius muscles of animals that consumed HVLID and in EDL muscles of animals that consumed HLD. Higher values of protein synthesis were observed in the postabsorptive state in the kidneys of HVLID and HLD groups compared to controls.

Effects of HVLID and HLD on protein breakdown

Consumption of HVLID decreased CHTLA activities in the muscles; HLD decreased CHTLA activities in the muscles, liver, jejunum, and kidneys (Fig. 7). Cathepsin B and L activities (Table 6) increased in the jejunum of the HVLID group. Lower activities were found in the SOL and jejunum of animals that consumed HLD compared to animals fed by HVLID. Effect of HVLID and HLD on CHTLA in muscles in postabsorptive state was insignificant. Cathepsin B and L activities in the jejunum and EDL of HVLID and HLD groups were lower than controls fed SLD before an overnight fast.

Effects of HVLID and HLD on weight and protein content of tissues

The effect of HVLID on muscle weight and protein content was not significant, but lower weight and protein content was found in EDL of animals that consumed HLD. Chronic intake of HVLID and HLD significantly increased the weight and protein content of the kidneys.

Table 2 Changes in blood plasma

	Fed animals			Overnight starved animals		
	SLD ($n = 10$)	HVLID ($n = 10$)	HLD ($n = 9$)	SLD + S ($n = 10$)	HVLID + S ($n = 10$)	HLD + S ($n = 10$)
Glucose (mmol/l)	9.67 ± 0.21	chylosity	8.58 ± 0.29 [a]	7.17 ± 0.18 [b]	8.84 ± 0.28 [a]	7.96 ± 0.24
Urea (mmol/l)	7.32 ± 0.21	9.60 ± 0.14 [a]	8.86 ± 0.32 [a]	6.31 ± 0.25 [b]	8.23 ± 0.24 [a,b]	9.00 ± 0.36 [a]
Creatinine (μmol/l)	27.9 ± 1.0	29.4 ± 1.1	27.6 ± 0.6	30.2 ± 1.3	30.9 ± 1.7	29.9 ± 0.85
ALT (μkat/l)	0.88 ± 0.05	0.97 ± 0.06	1.22 ± 0.03 [a,c]	0.68 ± 0.04 [b]	0.59 ± 0.05 [a]	0.86 ± 0.06 [a,b,c]
AST (μkat/l	1.35 ± 0.15	1.33 ± 0.05	1.16 ± 0.06	1.26 ± 0.05	1.29 ± 0.06	1.15 ± 0.05
Cholesterol (mmol/l)	1.64 ± 0.11	1.49 ± 0.08	1.54 ± 0.12	1.42 ± 0.10	1.47 ± 0.06	1.30 ± 0.07
HDL cholesterol (mmol/l)	1.08 ± 0.12	0.99 ± 0.04	1.31 ± 0.10 [c]	1.24 ± 0.09	1.02 ± 0.04	1.16 ± 0.07
LDL cholesterol (mmol/l)	0.29 ± 0.03	chylosity	0.17 ± 0.03 [a]	0.20 ± 0.03 [b]	0.28 ± 0.02	0.12 ± 0.01 [c]
Atherogenicity index	0.39 ± 0.03	0.51 ± 0.05 [a]	0.19 ± 0.02 [a,c]	0.14 ± 0.02 [b]	0.47 ± 0.03 [a]	0.12 ± 0.02 [c]
Triglycerides (mmol/l)	1.25 ± 0.07	0.72 ± 0.08 [a]	0.95 ± 0.06	0.79 ± 0.10 [b]	0.60 ± 0.07	0.86 ± 0.11
Total protein (g/l)	63.1 ± 0.7	63.0 ± 0.7	64.6 ± 1.2	58.0 ± 0.6 [b]	61.4 ± 0.8 [a]	60.3 ± 0.7 [b]
Albumins (mmol/l)	35.3 ± 1.4	34.7 ± 1.1	35.7 ± 1.8	33.1 ± 0.8	34.8 ± 1.6	33.7 ± 1.2

Means ± SE, $p < 0.05$

SLD standard laboratory diet; *SLD + S* rats fed SLD starved overnight before sacrifice; *HVLID* diet with high content of valine, leucine, and isoleucine; *HVLID + S* rats fed HVLID starved overnight before sacrifice; *HLD* high leucine diet; *HLD + S* rats fed HLD starved overnight before sacrifice

[a] compared to the corresponding control (SLD or SLD + S)

[b] compared to the corresponding fed group

[c] HLD (HLD + S) vs. HVLID (HVLID + S). Atherogenicity index was calculated as: (cholesterol-HDL cholesterol)/HDL cholesterol

Table 3 Amino acid concentrations (μmol/l) in blood plasma

	Fed animals			Overnight starved animals		
	SLD ($n = 10$)	HVLID ($n = 10$)	HLD ($n = 9$)	SLD + S (n =10)	HVLID + S ($n = 10$)	HLD + S ($n = 10$)
Asp	17 ± 1	34 ± 3 [a]	25 ± 3	11 ± 1	26 ± 3 [a]	24 ± 6 [a]
Glu	129 ± 8	111 ± 6	108 ± 4	101 ± 6	129 ± 11	128 ± 10
Ser	254 ± 12	239 ± 4	217 ± 6 [a]	241 ± 8	232 ± 7	236 ± 7
Asn	70 ± 4	78 ± 2	64 ± 2 [c]	59 ± 2 [b]	67 ± 2 [b]	64 ± 2
Gly	306 ± 23	219 ± 6 [a]	191 ± 10 [a]	392 ± 15 [b]	319 ± 12 [a,b]	281 ± 10 [a,b]
Gln	713 ± 25	825 ± 12 [a]	808 ± 19 [a]	623 ± 10 [b]	678 ± 16 [b]	690 ± 14 [a,b]
His	66 ± 3	65 ± 2	57 ± 1 [a,c]	54 ± 2 [b]	56 ± 1 [b]	54 ± 2
Tau	324 ± 16	467 ± 50	437 ± 52	227 ± 17	528 ± 57 [a]	520 ± 31 [a]
Thr	284 ± 17	206 ± 6 [a]	206 ± 5 [a]	232 ± 14 [b]	230 ± 7	226 ± 6
Ctr	82 ± 4	87 ± 3	79 ± 3	60 ± 2 [b]	74 ± 2 [a,b]	69 ± 2
Ala	527 ± 27	667 ± 25 [a]	627 ± 13 [a]	364 ± 16 [b]	379 ± 12 [b]	412 ± 14 [b]
Arg	188 ± 9	175 ± 5	165 ± 6 [a]	150 ± 3 [b]	165 ± 5	157 ± 4
Pro	262 ± 16	251 ± 7	244 ± 6	131 ± 5 [b]	147 ± 3 [b]	140 ± 3 [b]
Tyr	94 ± 15	77 ± 3 [a]	71 ± 2 [a]	89 ± 3	85 ± 3	83 ± 3 [b]
Cys	123 ± 5	122 ± 2	106 ± 3	123 ± 3	138 ± 5	126 ± 5 [b]
Val	262 ± 8	444 ± 30 [a]	158 ± 6 [a,c]	213 ± 7	213 ± 4 [b]	206 ± 6
Met	63 ± 3	63 ± 1	56 ± 1 [a]	55 ± 1 [b]	52 ± 1 [b]	52 ± 1
Orn	67 ± 3	68 ± 5	69 ± 3	44 ± 2 [b]	52 ± 2 [b]	48 ± 2 [b]
Lys	339 ± 5	332 ± 9	324 ± 13	334 ± 9	417 ± 13 [b]	440 ± 11 [b]
Ile	135 ± 19	227 ± 21 [a]	91 ± 9 [a,c]	122 ± 6	122 ± 2 [b]	134 ± 9 [b]
Leu	228 ± 18	317 ± 21 [a]	543 ± 35 [a,c]	177 ± 7	195 ± 4 [b]	189 ± 6 [b]
Phe	72 ± 3	71 ± 1	73 ± 1	69 ± 2	72 ± 2	70 ± 2
BCAA	625 ± 37	988 ± 71 [a]	793 ± 40 [a,c]	513 ± 20	530 ± 9 [b]	529 ± 20 [b]
Σ - BCAA	3975 ± 151	4157 ± 87	3928 ± 94	3361 ± 86 [b]	3846 ± 75 [a]	3819 ± 74 [a]

Means ± SE, $p < 0.05$
[a] compared to the corresponding control (SLD or SLD + S)
[b] compared to the corresponding fed group
[c] HLD (HLD + S) vs. HVLID (HVLID + S). Abbreviations as indicated in Table 1

We also observed higher liver weights in HLD fed animals (Table 7).

Discussion

Only moderate changes in food intake and body weight gain were observed between animals that consumed various diets in the initial phase of our study. Therefore, alterations in food intake did not affect our findings, but food composition, i.e., the replacement of 10 % of the basal diet with BCAAs or leucine alone exerted significant effects.

Effects on amino acid concentration and metabolism

It is well established that the rate of BCAA degradation in skeletal muscle is highly responsive to changes in dietary intake. The K_m of BCAA aminotransferases for BCAAs is two- to four-fold higher than tissue BCAA concentrations [29]. Therefore, the rate of transamination leading to the production of glutamate and BCKA responds rapidly to changes in BCAA level. BCKA dehydrogenase activity in skeletal muscle is low, and most BCKA that is produced in muscle is released to the circulation and utilised in other tissues, especially the liver. The rise in plasma levels of all three BCKAs and ketoisocaproate in animals fed HVLID and HLD, respectively, indicates an enhanced load of these keto-acids in visceral tissues with unknown consequences. Enhanced KIC production from leucine may activate alternative pathways of KIC (ketoleucine) catabolism by the cytosolic enzyme KIC-dioxygenase in the liver. The result is an enhanced synthesis of ß-hydroxy-ß-methylbutyrate, which may be involved in the observed decrease in LDL cholesterol and muscle protein breakdown in animals fed HLD [30, 31].

To determine whether adaptive changes in enzyme activities in muscle tissue were involved in the rise in alanine and glutamine in blood plasma, alanine aminotransferase and glutamine synthetase activities

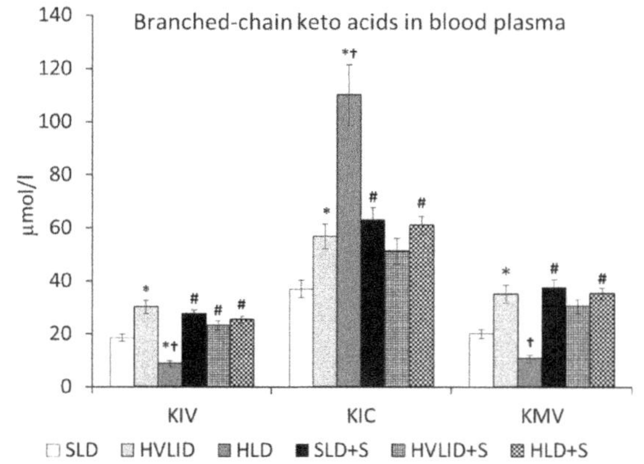

Fig. 3 Branched-chain keto acids in blood plasma. Means ± SE, $p < 0.05$. *compared to the corresponding control (SLD or SLD + S); # compared to the corresponding fed group; † HLD (HLD + S) group vs. HVLID (HVLID + S) group. KIC: α-ketoisocaproate (ketoleucine), KMV: α-keto-β-methylvalerate (ketoisoleucine), KIV: α-ketoisovalerate (ketovaline)

were measured in muscles. Although marked alterations have been reported in various conditions, such dexamethasone treatment [27], chronic consumption of HVLID and HLD was without notable adaptive changes in these enzymes. Therefore, the main mechanism leading to enhanced alanine and glutamine production in skeletal muscle should be an increased flux of glutamate through glutamine synthetase and alanine aminotransferase resulting from enhanced glutamate production by BCAA aminotransferase.

A chronically enhanced release of BCKA, alanine, and glutamine from muscle may be related to the observed hypertrophy of the kidneys. Enhanced glutamine load may activate ammonia production in various tissues, especially gut and kidneys, and in the case of impaired ammonia detoxification to urea in liver disease induce symptoms of hepatic encephalopathy [32]. Enhanced ammonia concentrations in blood after BCAA supplementation were found during exercise and following a leucine intake >500 $mg \cdot kg^{-1} \cdot d^{-1}$ [33, 34]. Nevertheless, alterations in aminoacidemia induced by BCAA intake may also have favourable effects. The example might be positive influence of glutamine on the immune system, protein balance, and gut integrity.

The drop in concentrations of valine and isoleucine in blood plasma and muscles in animals fed high amounts of leucine is likely due to the well-known phenomenon that is referred to as BCAA antagonism [35]. Leucine stimulates the BCKA dehydrogenase complex that controls the rate limiting step in BCAA catabolism leading to enhanced catabolism of all three BCAAs. Depletion of

Table 4 Amino acid concentrations in muscles (μmol/l of intracellular water)

	Fed animals			Overnight starved animals		
	SLD (n = 10)	HVLID (n = 10)	HLD (n = 9)	SLD + S (n =10)	HVLID + S (n = 10)	HLD + S (n = 10)
M. gastrocnemius						
Valine	269 ± 15	547 ± 28 [a]	166 ± 8 [a,c]	317 ± 9	352 ± 10 [b]	336 ± 19 [b]
Isoleucine	129 ± 10	227 ± 12 [a]	72 ± 5 [a,c]	182 ± 5 [b]	199 ± 5	181 ± 8 [b]
Leucine	193 ± 13	328 ± 19 [a]	533 ± 30 [a,c]	264 ± 7 [b]	302 ± 10	304 ± 18 [b]
Glutamine	5773 ± 244	5731 ± 212	6665 ± 236 [a,c]	3870 ± 141 [b]	3892 ± 148 [b]	4714 ± 103 [a,b,c]
Alanine	3188 ± 165	4838 ± 644[a]	4879 ± 183 [a]	3227 ± 103	3025 ± 61 [b]	3467 ± 115 [b]
M. soleus						
Valine	190 ± 8	452 ± 26 [a]	128 ± 9 [a,c]	229 ± 9	226 ± 6 [b]	215 ± 11 [b]
Isoleucine	92 ± 6	184 ± 12 [a]	49 ± 6 [a,c]	126 ± 5 [b]	116 ± 3 [b]	109 ± 6 [b]
Leucine	159 ± 10	287 ± 15	595 ± 93 [a,c]	231 ± 19	196 ± 4	216 ± 12 [b]
Glutamine	12,374 ± 279	13,849 ± 451	15,137 ± 835 [a]	11,887 ± 357	11,962 ± 529 [b]	13,656 ± 334
Alanine	3293 ± 99	3920 ± 151 [a]	3972 ± 204 [a]	3633 ± 131	3558 ± 132	3854 ± 112
M. ext.digitorum longus						
Valine	268 ± 9	552 ± 28 [a]	177 ± 7 [a]	336 ± 23 [b]	339 ± 8 [b]	330 ± 13 [b]
Isoleucine	124 ± 4	235 ± 12 [a]	82 ± 7 [a,c]	199 ± 12 [b]	194 ± 10 [b]	182 ± 13 [b]
Leucine	201 ± 8	354 ± 23 [a]	558 ± 27 [a,c]	297 ± 18 [b]	325 ± 38 [b]	297 ± 10 [b]
Glutamine	8413 ± 322	9216 ± 293	9935 ± 480 [a]	5880 ± 175 [b]	6137 ± 193 [b]	6838 ± 140 [b]
Alanine	3499 ± 136	4642 ± 111 [a]	5272 ± 235 [a,c]	3635 ± 143	3762 ± 115 [b]	3818 ± 110 [b]

Means ± SE, $p < 0.05$
[a] compared to the corresponding control (SLD or SLD + S)
[b] compared to the corresponding fed group
[c] HLD (HLD + S) vs. HVLID (HVLID + S). Abbreviations as indicated in Table 1

Table 5 Amino acid concentrations in liver, jejunum, and kidneys (μmol/l of intracellular water)

	Fed animals			Overnight starved animals		
	SLD (*n* = 10)	HVLID (*n* = 10)	HLD (*n* = 9)	SLD + S (*n* =10)	HVLID + S (*n* = 10)	HLD + S (*n* = 10)
Live						
Valine	430 ± 26	946 ± 51 [a]	438 ± 26 [c]	449 ± 31	469 ± 32 [b]	514 ± 25
Isoleucine	692 ± 65	555 ± 33 [a]	321 ± 13 [a,c]	308 ± 27 [b]	280 ± 19 [b]	307 ± 18
Leucine	603 ± 57	861 ± 50	1663 ± 158 [a]	545 ± 35	534 ± 38 [b,c]	580 ± 32 [b]
Glutamine	15,588 ± 308	15,253 ± 646	14,247 ± 749	15,644 ± 1006	16,574 ± 1052	18,694 ± 639 [a,b]
Alanine	6927 ± 340	6778 ± 321	6618 ± 335	3096 ± 378 [b]	3371 ± 362 [b]	4973 ± 224 [a,b,c]
Jejunum						
Valine	725 ± 75	1528 ± 195 [a]	918 ± 53 [c]	632 ± 94	569 ± 48	562 ± 42
Isoleucine	477 ± 51	990 ± 146 [a]	634 ± 47 [c]	406 ± 61	357 ± 34	357 ± 30
Leucine	790 ± 73	1589 ± 215	3367 ± 644 [a,c]	787 ± 109	623 ± 57	718 ± 48
Glutamine	1900 ± 202	1721 ± 148	1871 ± 149	1042 ± 79 [b]	1358 ± 102	1456 ± 105
Alanine	6032 ± 431	6036 ± 233	7338 ± 249 [a,c]	4107 ± 308	4495 ± 182	4,5003 ± 202
Kidney						
Valine	402 ± 33	675 ± 51 [a]	410 ± 34 [c]	404 ± 21	444 ± 26	444 ± 21
Isoleucine	308 ± 35	344 ± 27	295 ± 51	222 ± 11	239 ± 15	241 ± 17
Leucine	481 ± 33	503 ± 37	911 ± 73 [a,c]	481 ± 20	241 ± 80 [b]	483 ± 28 [b]
Glutamine	4335 ± 193	4051 ± 123	4110 ± 312	3233 ± 216 [b]	3249 ± 197	3324 ± 133 [b]
Alanine	2156 ± 84	2331 ± 132	2801 ± 113 [a,c]	1719 ± 81 [b]	1857 ± 63 [b]	2109 ± 64 [b]

Means ± SE, $p < 0.05$
[a] compared to the corresponding control (SLD or SLD + S)
[b] compared to the corresponding fed group
[c] HLD (HLD + S) vs. HVLID (HVLID + S). Abbreviations as indicated in Table 1

valine and isoleucine pools may also be due to their competition with leucine for transport via the L-carrier system.

Effects on protein metabolism in skeletal muscle

Higher protein synthesis rates and decreased CHTLA in the postprandial state in the muscles of animals fed an HVLID are consistent with most in vitro studies and/or studies that assessed the immediate response to BCAA administration [2, 36–38]. Therefore, our results confirm the regulatory effects of BCAAs on protein turnover, which may exert a positive influence on muscle protein balance. The marked decrease in CHTLA in muscles of animals fed an HLD is consistent with studies that

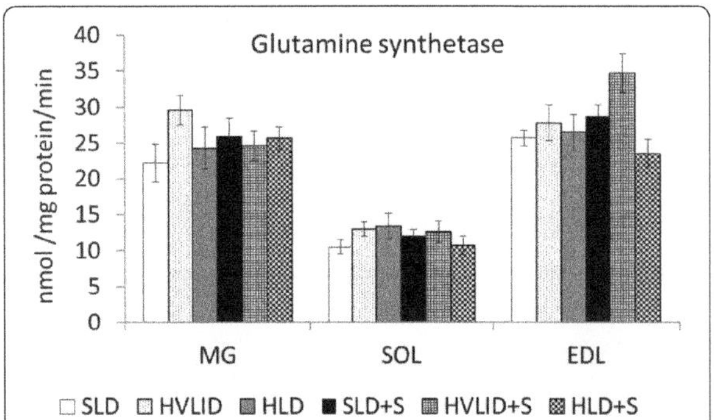

Fig. 4 Glutamine synthetase. Means ± SE, $p < 0.05$. *compared to the corresponding control (SLD or SLD + S); # compared to the corresponding fed group; † HLD (HLD + S) group vs. HVLID (HVLID + S) group

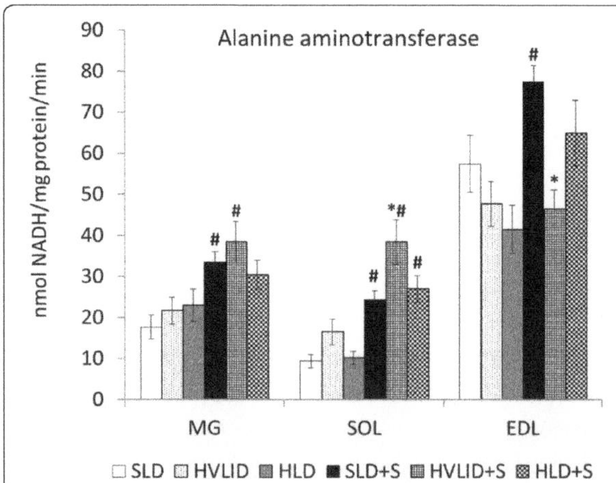

Fig. 5 Alanine aminotransferase. Means ± SE, $p < 0.05$. *compared to the corresponding control (SLD or SLD + S); # compared to the corresponding fed group; † HLD (HLD + S) group vs. HVLID (HVLID + S) group

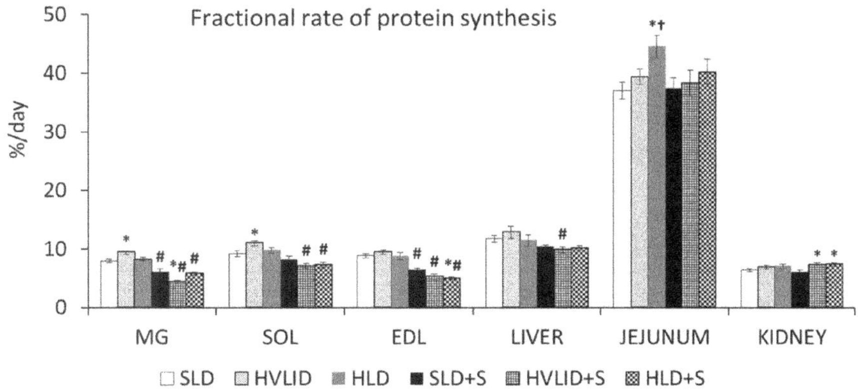

Fig. 6 Fractional rate of protein synthesis. Means ± SE, $p < 0.05$. *compared to the corresponding control (SLD or SLD + S); # compared to the corresponding fed group; † HLD (HLD + S) group vs. HVLID (HVLID + S) group

concluded that leucine administration may specifically induce a reduction in protein breakdown without increasing protein synthesis [39–41]. However, we failed to demonstrate a positive effect of BCAA on muscle protein balance and a negative effect in EDL muscles exerted chronic consumption of excessive amounts of leucine. This was indicated by insignificant changes in weight and protein content in muscles of animals consuming HVLID and the decrease in EDL muscles in the HLD group.

We suppose that the discrepancy between the positive effects of HVLID on protein synthesis and proteolysis and HLD on proteolysis and the insignificant changes in muscle protein content may be explained by metabolic alterations in the postabsorptive state that were induced in our study by an overnight fast. Decreased rates of protein synthesis and CHTLA activities in overnight-fasted animals fed a normal diet represent metabolic adaptation that spares muscle protein in starvation. The more pronounced decrease in protein synthesis gastrocnemius muscles in HVLID group and in EDL muscles in HLD group of overnight-starved animals indicate an impaired metabolic response that is clearly not beneficial for muscle protein balance.

The adverse effect of a leucine-enriched diet is likely related to decreased intracellular pools of valine and isoleucine and preferential leucine oxidation. Both valine and isoleucine catabolites may be utilised in the citric cycle and promote consumption of pyruvate from glycolysis while the end product of leucine is acetyl Co-A, which blocks the entry of pyruvate into the citric cycle. Therefore, preferential leucine oxidation may exert negative effect on glycolysis, ATP production, and muscle performance, and lead to elevations in alanine aminotransferase activities in blood plasma. Enhanced plasma alanine aminotransferase activity without alterations in other markers of hepatocellular damage was reported after dietary leucine excess in muscle disease patients and apparently healthy individuals [42–44].

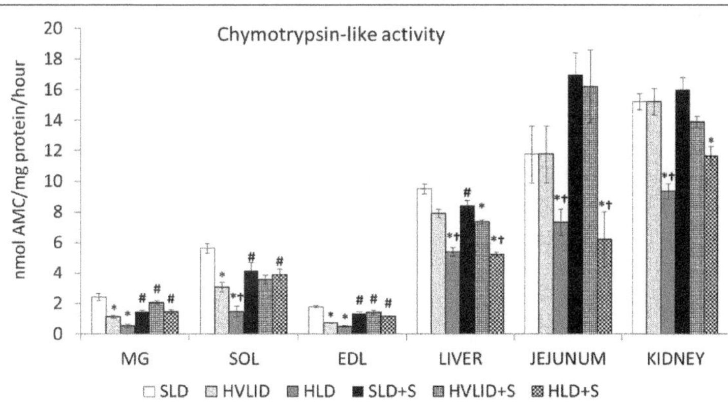

Fig. 7 Chymotrypsin-like activity. Means ± SE, $p < 0.05$. *compared to the corresponding control (SLD or SLD + S); #compared to the corresponding fed group; † HLD (HLD + S) group vs. HVLID (HVLID + S) group

Table 6 Cathepsin B and L activities (nmol AMC/mg protein/hour)

	Fed animals			Overnight starved animals		
	SLD ($n = 10$)	HVLID ($n = 10$)	HLD ($n = 9$)	SLD + S ($n = 10$)	HVLID + S ($n = 10$)	HLD ($n = 10$)
M. gastrocnemius	5.4 ± 1.1	4.3 ± 1.6	5.7 ± 1.2	6.5 ± 1.4	6.0 ± 0.9	5.9 ± 1.1
M. soleus	44.3 ± 2.6	51.4 ± 3.2	39.0 ± 2.1 [c]	55.4 ± 3.8 [b]	45.4 ± 1.6	27.4 ± 2.1 [a,b,c]
M. ext. digitorum longus	12.6 ± 1.4	11.5 ± 1.4	8.0 ± 1.4	10.1 ± 4.7	4.7 ± 1.6 [a,b]	1.6 ± 1.0 [a,b]
Liver	213 ± 10	233 ± 11	192 ± 12	346 ± 21 [b]	394 ± 14 [b]	372 ± 16 [b]
Jejunum	164 ± 7	214 ± 17 [a]	98 ± 24 [c]	270 ± 20	104 ± 16 [a,b]	99 ± 23 [a]
Kidney	1420 ± 47	1337 ± 96	831 ± 56	1566 ± 50	1126 ± 56	1021 ± 57

Means ± SE, $p < 0.05$
[a] compared to the corresponding control (SLD or SLD + S)
[b] compared to the corresponding fed group
[c] HLD (HLD + S) vs. HVLID (HVLID + S). Abbreviations as indicated in Table 1

The finding of more significant alterations in EDL muscles compared to SOL or gastrocnemius muscles presents additional evidence that muscles composed mostly of white, fast-twitch fibres are more sensitive to various physiological or pathological signals than muscles composed mostly of red, slow-twitch fibres [45, 46].

A number of variables can modify the response to starvation, e.g., duration of starvation, muscle type, and ageing. Combaret et al. [47] reported that the rates of proteasome-dependent proteolysis were 1.5–2 fold higher in muscles in postabsorptive state and that with aging tended to decrease in the postabsorptive state and

Table 7 Tissue weights, protein concentration, and protein content.

	Fed animals			Overnight starved animals		
	SLD ($n = 10$)	HVLID ($n = 10$)	HLD ($n = 9$)	SLD + S ($n = 10$)	HVLID + S ($n = 10$)	HLD + S ($n = 10$)
M. gastrocnemius						
- Weight (g/kg b.w.)	4.16 ± 0.20	4.45 ± 0.21	4.09 ± 0.23	4.67 ± 0.67	4.69 ± 0.12	4.29 ± 0.14
- Protein (mg/g)	240 ± 8	234 ± 8	231 ± 5	233 ± 6	245 ± 7	238 ± 6
- Protein (mg/kg b.w.)	996 ± 58	1047 ± 72	946 ± 56	1088 ± 56	1144 ± 30	1027 ± 57
M. soleus						
- Weight (g/kg b.w.)	0.43 ± 0.01	0.48 ± 0.02	0.40 ± 0.01 [c]	0.49 ± 0.01 [b]	0.51 ± 0.01	0.42 ± 0.01 [a,c]
- Protein (mg/g)	223 ± 14	218 ± 7	228 ± 11	225 ± 4	241 ± 5	243 ± 10
- Protein (mg/kg b.w.)	97 ± 3	104 ± 4	91 ± 6	110 ± 3	122 ± 5 [b]	102 ± 6 [c]
M. ext. digitorum longus						
- Weight (g/kg b.w.)	0.42 ± 0.01	0.43 ± 0.01	0.39 ± 0.00 [a,c]	0.45 ± 0.01	0.45 ± 0.01	0.41 ± 0.01 [a,c]
- Protein (mg/g)	271 ± 7	251 ± 6	272 ± 7	279 ± 8	262 ± 11	266 ± 8
- Protein (mg/kg b.w.)	114 ± 5	109 ± 4	97 ± 3 [a]	127 ± 4	118 ± 5	109 ± 3 [a]
Liver						
- Weight (g/kg b.w.)	35.87 ± 1.05	37.35 ± 0.68	39.35 ± 0.80 [a]	27.36 ± 0.49 [b]	26.96 ± 0.64 [b]	30.07 ± 0.7 [b,c]
- Protein (mg/g)	244 ± 8	242 ± 6	240 ± 8	320 ± 9 [b]	270 ± 6 [a,b]	278 ± 8 [a,b]
- Protein (mg/kg b.w.)	8780 ± 462	9010 ± 235	9434 ± 386	8718 ± 190	7272 ± 184 [b,c]	8350 ± 293
Jejunum						
- Protein (mg/g)	197 ± 7	181 ± 8	176 ± 5	199 ± 9	179 ± 12	166 ± 6
Kidney						
- Weight (g/kg b.w.)	3.21 ± 0.13	3.56 ± 0.07 [a]	3.61 ± 0.10 [a]	3.18 ± 0.07	3.53 ± 0.09 [a]	3.44 ± 0.07 [a]
- Protein (mg/g)	222 ± 8	229 ± 9	222 ± 4	213 ± 7	221 ± 5	222 ± 6
- Protein (mg/kg b.w.)	709 ± 28	815 ± 32 [a]	798 ± 19 [a]	674 ± 24	774 ± 9 [a]	761 ± 18 [a]

Means ± SE, $p < 0.05$
[a] compared to the corresponding control (SLD or SLD + S)
[b] compared to the corresponding fed group
[c] HLD (HLD + S) vs. HVLID (HVLID + S). Abbreviations as indicated in Table 1

increase in the postprandial state. A role may play alterations in insulin sensitivity, the BCKA dehydrogenase activity, and amino acid concentrations [35, 48]. It should be noted that only protein synthesis rates can be measured directly under in vivo conditions. Proteolysis can be estimated indirectly, e.g. by changes MuRF1 and MAFbx expression, rates of ubiquitination, and activities of enzymes of ubiquitin-proteasome system [49]. Therefore, the results of the present study cannot exclude significant effects of chronic consumption of HVLID or HLD on proteolysis in postabsorptive state in other experimental conditions.

Conclusions

To the best of our knowledge, this report is the first study to assess the metabolic response to BCAA and leucine supplementation in postprandial and postabsorptive states. We conclude that the chronic intake of a BCAA- or leucine-enriched diet significantly affects whole body metabolism as demonstrated by alterations in urea, alanine aminotransferase, and LDL cholesterol in blood, protein synthesis and proteolysis in various tissues, amino acid concentrations in blood and tissues, and liver and kidney weights. However, the results failed to demonstrate positive effects of the chronic consumption of BCAA or leucine-enriched diets on protein balance in skeletal muscle.

The non-significant effect of HVLID and rather negative effect of HLD on protein balance may be explained by depletion of valine and isoleucine pools in animals fed by an HLD and an impaired response to short-term starvation, which was characterised by impaired synthesis of muscle proteins, particularly in muscles with high content of white, fast-twitch fibres. These findings explain the discrepancy between the protein anabolic effects of BCAA or leucine on muscles that were reported under in vitro conditions and/or shortly after BCAA intake [2, 36–38] and their reduced or lack of effects following chronic administration [15, 50–52].

It should be noted that the present study was performed in healthy individuals without the adverse effects of signals that occur in several disorders, which lead to muscle wasting, and without the stimulatory effect of exercise on signalling pathways that activate protein synthesis. Further research is needed into the effects of chronic BCAA and leucine consumption in muscle-wasting disorders, the elderly, and during endurance exercise.

Abbreviations

AMC: 7-Amino-4-methylcoumarin; BCAA: Branched-chain amino acids (valine, leucine, and isoleucine); BCKA: Branched-chain keto acids; CHTLA: Chymotrypsin-like activity; FRPS: Fractional rate of protein synthesis; HLD: High leucine diet; HLD + S: Rats fed HLD starved overnight before sacrifice; HVLID: Diet with high content of valine, leucine, and isoleucine; HVLID + S: Rats fed HVLID starved overnight before sacrifice; KIC: α-Ketoisocaproate (ketoleucine); KMV: α-Keto-β-methylvalerate (ketoisoleucine); KIV: α-Ketoisovalerate (ketovaline); SLD: Standard laboratory diet; SLD + S: Rats fed SLD starved overnight before sacrifice.

Competing interest

The authors declare that they have no competing interests.

Authors' contributions

MH outlined the experiments, performed statistical analysis, and prepared the draft of the manuscript. MV, PS and RK were involved in data acquisition and their interpretation. All authors read and approved the final manuscript.

Acknowledgements

The authors wish to thank to R. Fingrova, L. Kriesfalusyova, and D. Jezkova for their technical assistance.

Funding

This project was supported by the program PRVOUK P37/02.

Author details

[1]Department of Physiology, Faculty of Medicine in Hradec Kralove, Charles University in Prague, Simkova 870, Hradec Kralove 500 38, Czech Republic. [2]Department of Biochemistry, Faculty of Medicine in Hradec Kralove, Charles University Prague, Hradec Kralove, Czech Republic. [3]Department of Biological and Biochemical Sciences, Faculty of Chemical Technology, University of Pardubice, Pardubice, Czech Republic.

References

1. Fulks RM, Li JB, Goldberg AL. Effects of insulin, glucose, and amino acids on protein turnover in rat diaphragm. J Biol Chem. 1975;250:290–8.
2. Buse MG, Reid SS. Leucine. A possible regulator of protein turnover in muscle. J Clin Invest. 1975;56:1250–61.
3. Li JB, Jefferson LS. Influence of amino acid availability on protein turnover in perfused skeletal muscle. Biochim Biophys Acta. 1978;544:351–9.
4. Garlick PJ. The role of leucine in the regulation of protein metabolism. J Nutr. 2005;135:1553S–6S.
5. Nair KS, Short KR. Hormonal and signaling role of branched-chain amino acids. J Nutr. 2005;135:1547S–52S.
6. Tischler ME, Desautels M, Goldberg AL. Does leucine, leucyl-tRNA, or some metabolite of leucine regulate protein synthesis and degradation in skeletal and cardiac muscle? J Biol Chem. 1982;257:1613–21.
7. Holecek M, Muthny T, Kovarik M, Sispera L. Effect of beta-hydroxy-beta-methylbutyrate (HMB) on protein metabolism in whole body and in selected tissues. Food Chem Toxicol. 2009;47:255–9.
8. Ruderman NB, Berger M. The formation of glutamine and alanine in skeletal muscle. J Biol Chem. 1974;249:5500–6.
9. Odessey R, Goldberg AL. Oxidation of leucine by rat skeletal muscle. Am J Physiol. 1972;223:1376–83.
10. Durschlag RP, Smith RJ. Regulation of glutamine production by skeletal muscle cells in culture. Am J Physiol. 1985;248:C442–8.
11. Yang Q, Birkhahn RH. Branched-chain transaminase and keto acid dehydrogenase activities in burned rats: evidence for a differential adaptation according to sex. Nutrition. 1997;13:640–5.
12. Hickson RC, Wegrzyn LE, Osborne DF, Karl IE. Glutamine interferes with glucocorticoid-induced expression of glutamine synthetase in skeletal muscle. Am J Physiol. 1996;270:E912–7.
13. Holecek M, Sispera L. Glutamine deficiency in extracellular fluid exerts adverse effects on protein and amino acid metabolism in skeletal muscle of healthy, laparotomized, and septic rats. Amino Acids. 2014;46:1377–84.
14. Elango R, Chapman K, Rafii M, Ball RO, Pencharz PB. Determination of the tolerable upper intake level of leucine in acute dietary studies in young men. Am J Clin Nutr. 2012;96:759–67.
15. Tsubuku S, Hatayama K, Katsumata T, Nishimura N, Mawatari K, Smriga M, et al. Thirteen-week oral toxicity study of branched-chain amino acids in rats. Int J Toxicol. 2004;23:119–26.
16. Mawatari K, Katsumata T, Uematsu M, Katsumata T, Yoshida J, Smriga M, et al. Prolonged oral treatment with an essential amino acid L-leucine does not affect female reproductive function and embryo-fetal development in rats. Food Chem Toxicol. 2004;42:1505–11.

17. Garlick PJ, McNurlan MA, Preedy VR. A rapid and convenient technique for measuring the rate of protein synthesis in tissue by injection of [^{3}H]phenylalanine. Biochem J. 1980;192:719–23.
18. Lowry OH, Rosebrough NJ, Farr AL, Randall RJ. Protein measurement with the Folin phenol reagent. J Biol Chem. 1951;193:265–75.
19. McNurlan MA, Tomkins AM, Garlick PJ. The effect of starvation on the rate of protein synthesis in rat liver and small intestine. Biochem J. 1979;178: 373–9.
20. Welle S. Methods for studying protein metabolism in humans. In: Human protein metabolism. New-York: Springer; 1999. p. 29–71.
21. Bergström J, Fürst P, Norée LO, Vinnars E. Intracellular free amino acid concentration in human muscle tissue. J Appl Physiol. 1974;36:693–7.
22. Graham JA, Lamb JF, Linton AL. Measurement of body water and intracellular electrolytes by means of muscle biopsy. Lancet. 1976;2(7527): 1172–6.
23. Kandar R, Zakova P, Jirosova J, Sladka M. Determination of branched chain amino acids, methionine, phenylalanine, tyrosine and α-keto acids in plasma and dried blood samples using HPLC with fluorescence detection. Clin Chem Lab Med. 2009;47:565–72.
24. Gomes-Marcondes MCC, Tisdale MJ. Induction of protein catabolism and the ubiquitin-proteasome pathway by mild oxidative stress. Cancer Lett. 2002;180:69–74.
25. Koohmaraie M, Kretchmar DH. Comparisons of four methods for quantification of lysosomal cysteine proteinase activities. J Anim Sci. 1990; 68:2362–70.
26. Tardy C, Autefage H, García V, Levade T, Andrieu-Abadie N. Mannose 6-phosphorylated proteins are required for tumor necrosis factor-induced apoptosis: defective response in I-cell disease fibroblasts. J Biol Chem. 2004; 279:52914–23.
27. Minet R, Villie F, Marcollet M, Meynial-Denis D, Cynober L. Measurement of glutamine synthetase activity in rat muscle by a colorimetric assay. Clin Chim Acta. 1997;268:121–32.
28. Gella FJ, Olivella T, Cruz Pastor M, Arenas J, Moreno R, Durban R, et al. A simple procedure for the routine determination of aspartate aminotransferase and alanine aminotransferase with pyridoxal phosphate. Clin Chim Acta. 1985;153:241–7.
29. Krebs HA. Some aspects of the regulation of fuel supply in omnivorous animals. Adv Enzyme Regul. 1972;10:397–420.
30. Nissen S, Sharp RL, Panton L, Vukovich M, Trappe S, Fuller JC. Beta-hydroxy-beta-methylbutyrate (HMB) supplementation in humans is safe and may decrease cardiovascular risk factors. J Nutr. 2000;130:1937–45.
31. Kovarik M, Muthny T, Sispera L, Holecek M. Effects of β-hydroxy-β-methylbutyrate treatment in different types of skeletal muscle of intact and septic rats. J Physiol Biochem. 2010;66:311–9.
32. Holecek M. Branched-chain amino acids and ammonia metabolism in liver disease: therapeutic implications. Nutrition. 2013;29:1186–91.
33. MacLean DA, Graham TE. Branched-chain amino acid supplementation augments plasma ammonia responses during exercise in humans. J Appl Physiol. 1993;74:2711–7.
34. Pencharz PB, Elango R, Ball RO. Determination of the tolerable upper intake level of leucine in adult men. J Nutr. 2012;142:2220S–4S.
35. Harper AE, Miller RH, Block KP. Branched-chain amino acid metabolism. Annu Rev Nutr. 1984;4:409–54.
36. Mitch WE, Clark AS. Specificity of the effects of leucine and its metabolites on protein degradation in skeletal muscle. Biochem J. 1984;222:579–86.
37. Lynch CJ, Hutson SM, Patson BJ, Vaval A, Vary TC. Tissue-specific effects of chronic dietary leucine and norleucine supplementation on protein synthesis in rats. Am J Physiol. 2002;283:E824–35.
38. Kobayashi H, Kato H, Hirabayashi Y, Murakami H, Suzuki H. Modulations of muscle protein metabolism by branched-chain amino acids in normal and muscle-atrophying rats. J Nutr. 2006;136:234S–6S.
39. Matthews DE. Observations of branched-chain amino acid administration in humans. J Nutr. 2005;135:1580S–4S.
40. Louard RJ, Barrett EJ, Gelfand RA. Overnight branched-chain amino acid infusion causes sustained suppression of muscle proteolysis. Metabolism. 1995;44:424–9.
41. Nair KS, Schwartz RG, Welle S. Leucine as a regulator of whole body and skeletal muscle protein metabolism in humans. Am J Physiol. 1992;263: E928–34.
42. Matsuzaki K, Kato H, Sakai R, Toue S, Amao M, Kimura T. Transcriptomics and metabolomics of dietary leucine excess. J Nutr. 2005;135:1571S–5S.
43. Lott JA, Landesman PW. The enzymology of skeletal muscle disorders. Crit Rev Clin Lab Sci. 1984;20:153–90.
44. Pertusi R, Dickerman RD, McConathy WJ. Evaluation of aminotransferase elevations in a bodybuilder using anabolic steroids: hepatitis or rhabdomyolysis? J Am Osteopath Assoc. 2001;101:391–4.
45. Kadlcikova J, Holecek M, Safranek R, Tilser I, Kessler BM. Effects of proteasome inhibitors MG132, ZL3VS and AdaAhx3L3VS on protein metabolism in septic rats. Int J Exp Pathol. 2004;85:365–71.
46. Muthny T, Kovarik M, Sispera L, Tilser I, Holecek M. Protein metabolism in slow- and fast-twitch skeletal muscle during turpentine-induced inflammation. Int J Exp Pathol. 2008;89:64–71.
47. Combaret L, Dardevet D, Rieu I, Pouch MN, Béchet D, Taillandier D, et al. A leucine-supplemented diet restores the defective postprandial inhibition of proteasome-dependent proteolysis in aged rat skeletal muscle. J Physiol. 2005;569:489–99.
48. Khatra BS, Chawla RK, Wadsworth AD, Rudman D. Effect of dietary branched-chain alpha-keto acids on hepatic branched-chain alpha-keto acid dehydrogenase in the rat. J Nutr. 1977;107:1528–36.
49. Attaix D, Ventadour S, Codran A, Béchet D, Taillandier D, Combaret L. The ubiquitin proteasome system and skeletal muscle wasting. Essays Biochem. 2005;41:173–86.
50. Mourier A, Bigard AX, de Kerviler E, Roger B, Legrand H, Guezennec CY. Combined effects of caloric restriction and branched-chain amino acid supplementation on body composition and exercise performance in elite wrestlers. Int J Sports Med. 1997;18:47–55.
51. Spillane M, Emerson C, Willoughby DS. The effects of 8 weeks of heavy resistance training and branched-chain amino acid supplementation on body composition and muscle performance. Nutr Health. 2012;21:263–73.
52. Nelson AR, Phillips SM, Stellingwerff T, Rezzi S, Bruce SJ, Breton I, et al. A protein-leucine supplement increases branched-chain amino acid and nitrogen turnover but not performance. Med Sci Sports Exerc. 2012;44:57–68.

PERMISSIONS

All chapters in this book were first published in Nutrition & Metabolism, by BioMed Central; hereby published with permission under the Creative Commons Attribution License or equivalent. Every chapter published in this book has been scrutinized by our experts. Their significance has been extensively debated. The topics covered herein carry significant findings which will fuel the growth of the discipline. They may even be implemented as practical applications or may be referred to as a beginning point for another development.

The contributors of this book come from diverse backgrounds, making this book a truly international effort. This book will bring forth new frontiers with its revolutionizing research information and detailed analysis of the nascent developments around the world.

We would like to thank all the contributing authors for lending their expertise to make the book truly unique. They have played a crucial role in the development of this book. Without their invaluable contributions this book wouldn't have been possible. They have made vital efforts to compile up to date information on the varied aspects of this subject to make this book a valuable addition to the collection of many professionals and students.

This book was conceptualized with the vision of imparting up-to-date information and advanced data in this field. To ensure the same, a matchless editorial board was set up. Every individual on the board went through rigorous rounds of assessment to prove their worth. After which they invested a large part of their time researching and compiling the most relevant data for our readers.

The editorial board has been involved in producing this book since its inception. They have spent rigorous hours researching and exploring the diverse topics which have resulted in the successful publishing of this book. They have passed on their knowledge of decades through this book. To expedite this challenging task, the publisher supported the team at every step. A small team of assistant editors was also appointed to further simplify the editing procedure and attain best results for the readers.

Apart from the editorial board, the designing team has also invested a significant amount of their time in understanding the subject and creating the most relevant covers. They scrutinized every image to scout for the most suitable representation of the subject and create an appropriate cover for the book.

The publishing team has been an ardent support to the editorial, designing and production team. Their endless efforts to recruit the best for this project, has resulted in the accomplishment of this book. They are a veteran in the field of academics and their pool of knowledge is as vast as their experience in printing. Their expertise and guidance has proved useful at every step. Their uncompromising quality standards have made this book an exceptional effort. Their encouragement from time to time has been an inspiration for everyone.

The publisher and the editorial board hope that this book will prove to be a valuable piece of knowledge for researchers, students, practitioners and scholars across the globe.

LIST OF CONTRIBUTORS

Chisa Takashina, Ichizo Tsujino, Taku Watanabe, aisuke Ikeda, Asuka Yamada and Takahiro Sato
First Department of Medicine, Hokkaido University Hospital, North 14, West 5, Kita-ku, Sapporo 060-8648, Japan

Shinji Sakaue, D Hiroshi Ohira and Masaharu Nishimura
First Department of Medicine, Hokkaido University Graduate School of Medicine, Sapporo, Japan

Yoshinori Otsuka
Department of Human Developmental Science, Faculty of Education, Hokkaido University, Sapporo, Japan

Noriko Oyama-Manabe
Department of Diagnostic and Interventional Radiology, Hokkaido University Hospital, Sapporo, Japan

Yoichi M. Ito
Department of Biostatistics, Hokkaido University Graduate School of Medicine, Sapporo, Japan

Rolando A. Garcia, James N. Roemmich and Kate J. Claycombe
USDA-ARS, Grand Forks Human Nutrition Research Center, 2420 2nd Ave. N, Grand Forks, ND 58203, USA

Shannon L. Kesl, Angela M. Poff, Nathan P. Ward, Tina N. Fiorelli, Csilla Ari, Ashley J. Van Putten, Jacob W. Sherwood and Dominic P. D'Agostino
Department of Molecular Pharmacology and Physiology, Morsani College of Medicine, University of South Florida, 12901 Bruce B. Downs Blvd. MDC8, Tampa, FL 33612, USA

Patrick Arnold
Savind Inc, 205 South Main Street, Seymore, IL 61875, USA

Iona Lozano, William Bietiger, Elodie Seyfritz, Claude Peronet, Elisa Maillard, Séverine Sigrist and Stéphanie Dal
UMR DIATHEC, EA 7294, Centre Européen d'Etude du Diabète, Université de Strasbourg, Fédération de Médecine Translationnelle de Strasbourg, Bld René Leriche, 67200 Strasbourg, France

Remmelt Van der Werf
UMR DIATHEC, EA 7294, Centre Européen d'Etude du Diabète, Université de Strasbourg, Fédération de Médecine Translationnelle de Strasbourg, Bld René Leriche, 67200 Strasbourg, France
Equipe de Chimie Analytique des Molécules BioActives, IPHC-LC4, UMR 7178, Faculté de Pharmacie, Ilkirch, France

Michel Pinget and Nathalie Jeandidier
Structure d'Endocrinologie, Diabète, Nutrition et Addictologie, Pôle NUDE, Hôpitaux Universitaires de Strasbourg, (HUS), 67000 Strasbourg, France

Eric Marchioni
Equipe de Chimie Analytique des Molécules BioActives, IPHC-LC4, UMR 7178, Faculté de Pharmacie, Ilkirch, France

Thomas Plötz, Magnus Hartmann, Sigurd Lenzen and Matthias Elsner
Institute of Clinical Biochemistry, Hannover Medical School, 30623 Hannover, Germany

Minjoo Kim
Research Center for Silver Science, Institute of Symbiotic Life-TECH, Yonsei University, Seoul 03722, Republic of Korea

Gayoung Song, Miso Kang and Hye Jin Yoo
National Leading Research Laboratory of Clinical Nutrigenetics/Nutrigenomics, Department of Food and Nutrition, College of Human Ecology, Yonsei University, Seoul 03722, Republic of Korea

Department of Food and Nutrition, Brain Korea 21 PLUS Project, College of Human Ecology, Yonsei University, 50 Yonsei-ro, Seodaemun-gu, Seoul 03722, Republic of Korea

Tae-Sook Jeong
National Research Laboratory of Lipid Metabolism and Atherosclerosis, Korea Research Institute of Bioscience and Biotechnology, Daejeon 34141, Republic of Korea

Sang-Hyun Lee
Department of Family Practice, National Health Insurance Corporation Ilsan Hospital, Goyang 10444, Republic of Korea

Jong Ho Lee
Research Center for Silver Science, Institute of Symbiotic Life-TECH, Yonsei University, Seoul 03722, Republic of Korea
National Leading Research Laboratory of Clinical Nutrigenetics/Nutrigenomics, Department of Food and Nutrition, College of Human Ecology, Yonsei University, Seoul 03722, Republic of Korea
Department of Food and Nutrition, Brain Korea 21 PLUS Project, College of Human Ecology, Yonsei University, 50 Yonsei-ro, Seodaemun-gu, Seoul 03722, Republic of Korea

Wen Guo, Yingyun Gong, Zhenzhen Fu, Jinxiang Fu, Yan Sun, Xianxia Ju, Yina Chang, Wen Wang, Xiaohui Zhu, Beibei Gao, Xiaoyun Liu, Tao Yang and Hongwen Zhou
Department of Endocrinology, the First Affiliated Hospital of Nanjing Medical University, 300 Guangzhou Road, Nanjing 210029, China

Sujoy Ghosh
Pennington Biomedical Research Center, Louisiana State University System, 6400 Perkins Road, Baton Rouge, LA 70808-4124, USA
Duke-NUS Graduate Medical School, Singapore 169857, Singapore

Claudia Kruger, Shawna Wicks, Jacob Simon, William D. Johnson, Randall L. Mynatt, Robert C. Noland and Brenda K. Richards
Pennington Biomedical Research Center, Louisiana State University System, 6400 Perkins Road, Baton Rouge, LA 70808-4124, USA

K. Ganesh Kumar
Pennington Biomedical Research Center, Louisiana State University System, 6400 Perkins Road, Baton Rouge, LA 70808-4124, USA
Present Address: Taconic Biosciences, Inc., Germantown, NY, USA

Nittaya Marungruang, Frida Fåk and Eden Tareke
Food for Health Science Centre, Lund University, Medicon Village, Scheelevägen 2, SE-223 81 Lund, Sweden

David O. Kennedy, Emma J. Stevenson, Philippa A. Jackson, Sarah Dunn, Alexandra Carne, Fiona L. Dodd, Bernadette C. Robertson, Joanne Forster and Crystal F. Haskell-Ramsay
Brain, Performance and Nutrition Research Centre, Northumbria University, Newcastle-upon-Tyne NE1 8ST, UK

Karl Wishart, Gregor Bieri and Luca Barella
Bayer HealthCare - Consumer Care, Peter Merian Strasse 84, P.O. Box 4002, Basel, Switzerland

Ahmed Bakillah
Department of Cell Biology, SUNY Downstate Medical Center, 450 Clarkson Avenue, Brooklyn, NY 11203, USA
Department of Pediatrics, SUNY Downstate Medical Center, 450 Clarkson Avenue, Brooklyn, NY 11203, USA

M. Mahmood Hussain
Department of Cell Biology, SUNY Downstate Medical Center, 450 Clarkson Avenue, Brooklyn, NY 11203, USA

Department of Pediatrics, SUNY Downstate Medical Center, 450 Clarkson Avenue, Brooklyn, NY 11203, USA
VA New York Harbor Healthcare System, Brooklyn, NY 11209, USA

Min-Sup Jung, Yuno Song, Sun-Hee Jang, Wongi Min and Chung-Kil Won
Institute of Animal Medicine, College of Veterinary Medicine, Gyeongsang National University, Jinju 660-701, Korea

Soo-Jung Lee
Department of Foods and Nutrition, Gyeongsang National University, Jinju 660-701, Korea

Hong-Duck Kim
Department of Environmental Health Science, New York Medical College, Valhalla, NY 10595, USA

Tae Hoon Kim
Department of Food Science and Biotechnology, Daegu University, Gyeongsan 38453, Korea

Jae-Hyeon Cho
Institute of Animal Medicine, College of Veterinary Medicine, Gyeongsang National University, Jinju 660-701, Korea
College of Veterinary Medicine, Gyeongsang National University, Jiju Daero 501, Jinju-city, Gyeongsangnamdo 660-701, Korea

Sadako Nakamura and Tsuneyuki Oku
Institute of Food, Nutrition and Health, Jumonji University, 2-1-28, Sugasawa, Niiza, Saitama 352-8510, Japan
Graduate School of Human Health Science, University of Nagasaki Siebold, 1-1-1, Manabino, , Nagayo, Nagasaki 851-2195, Japan

Kenichi Tanabe
Graduate School of Human Health Science, University of Nagasaki Siebold, 1-1-1, Manabino, , Nagayo, Nagasaki 851-2195, Japan
Department of Food Science and Nutrition, Nagoya Women's University, 3-40, Shioji, Mizuho-ku, Nagoya 467-8610, Japan

Shigeki Morita
Graduate School of Human Health Science, University of Nagasaki Siebold, 1-1-1, Manabino, , Nagayo, Nagasaki 851-2195, Japan

Norihisa Hamaguchi
Institute of Food Materials, Nippon Shokuhin Kako Co. Ltd., Tajima, Fuji 417-8530, Japan

Fumio Shimura
Institute of Food, Nutrition and Health, Jumonji University, 2-1-28, Sugasawa, Niiza, Saitama 352-8510, Japan

Christel Björk
Lipid Laboratory, Department of Medicine, Karolinska Institutet, Huddinge, Stockholm, Sweden
Department of Medicine, Karolinska Institutet, Lipid Laboratory, Novum, NVS D4, Hälsovägen 7, 14186 Stockholm, Sweden

Uta Wilhelm, Mikael Rydén, Peter Arner and Jurga Laurencikiene
Lipid Laboratory, Department of Medicine, Karolinska Institutet, Huddinge, Stockholm, Sweden

Susanne Mandrup and Bjørk Ditlev Larsen
Department of Biochemistry and Molecular Biology, University of Southern Denmark, 5230 Odense M, Denmark

Alessandra Bordoni
Department of Agro-Food Sciences and Technologies, University of Bologna, Bologna, Italy

Per Hedén
Department of Plastic Surgery, Akademikliniken, Stockholm, Sweden

Erin D. Giles and Paul S. MacLean
Center for Human Nutrition, University of Colorado Anschutz Medical Campus, Aurora, CO, USA

Division of Endocrinology, Diabetes and Metabolism, School of Medicine, University of Colorado Anschutz Medical Campus, Aurora, CO, USA

Jennifer Hagman
Department of Psychiatry, School of Medicine, University of Colorado Anschutz Medical Campus, Aurora, CO, USA

Zhaoxing Pan
Biostatistics Core, Children's Hospital Colorado Research Institute, Aurora, CO, USA

Janine A. Higgins
Center for Human Nutrition, University of Colorado Anschutz Medical Campus, Aurora, CO, USA
Department of Pediatrics, School of Medicine, University of Colorado Anschutz Medical Campus, Aurora, CO, USA

Kyoko Inagaki-Ohara
Research Institute, National Center for Global Health and Medicine (NCGM), 1-21-1, Toyama Shinjuku, Tokyo 162-0052, Japan
Division of Endocrinology and Metabolism, Department of Developmental Physiology, National Institute for Physiological Sciences (NIPS), 38 Nishigonaka Myodaiji, Okazaki, Aichi 444-8585, Japan
Division of Host Defense, Department of Life Sciences, Faculty of Life and Environmental Sciences, Prefectural University of Hiroshima, 562 Nanatsuka, Shobara, Hiroshima 727-0023, Japan

Shiki Okamoto, Kazuyo Takagi, Kumiko Saito, Lijun Tang and Yasuhiko Minokoshi
Division of Endocrinology and Metabolism, Department of Developmental Physiology, National Institute for Physiological Sciences (NIPS), 38 Nishigonaka Myodaiji, Okazaki, Aichi 444-8585, Japan

Seiya Arita
Division of Host Defense, Department of Life Sciences, Faculty of Life and Environmental Sciences, Prefectural University of Hiroshima, 562 Nanatsuka, Shobara, Hiroshima 727-0023, Japan

Tetsuji Hori and Satoshi Matsumoto
Yakult Central Institute for Microbiological Research, 5-11 Izumi, Kunitachi, Tokyo 186-8650, Japan

Hiroaki Kataoka
Section of Oncopathology and Regenerative Biology, Department of Pathology, Faculty of Medicine, University of Miyazaki, 5200 Kihara, Kiyotake, Miyazaki 889-1692, Japan

Yunqin Chens
Shanghai Institute of Cardiovascular Diseases, Zhongshan Hospital, Fudan University, Shanghai, China
Department of Cell Biology, SUNY Downstate Medical Center, 450 Clarkson Ave, Box 5, Brooklyn, NY 11203, USA

Jibin Dong
School of Pharmacy, Fudan University, Shanghai, China

Xueying Chen, Hui Jiang, Zhiqiang Li, Yunzeng Zou, Haozhu Chen and Junbo Ge
Shanghai Institute of Cardiovascular Diseases, Zhongshan Hospital, Fudan University, Shanghai, China

Ahmed Bakillah, Mahmood Hussain and Xian-Cheng Jiang
Department of Cell Biology, SUNY Downstate Medical Center, 450 Clarkson Ave, Box 5, Brooklyn, NY 11203, USA

Xiaojin Zhang
Obstetrics & Gynecology Hospital, Fudan University, Shanghai, China

Jia Yin,Donghui Liang and Daniel Rader
Southern Medical University, Guangzhou, China

Marina Cuchel
Division of Translational Medicine and Human Genetics, Perelman School of Medicine, University of Pennsylvania, Philadelphia, USA

Milan Holecek and Melita Vodenicarovova
Department of Physiology, Faculty of Medicine in Hradec Kralove, Charles University in Prague, Simkova 870, Hradec Kralove 500 38, Czech Republic

Pavel Siman
Department of Biochemistry, Faculty of Medicine in Hradec Kralove, Charles University Prague, Hradec Kralove, Czech Republic

Roman Kandar
Department of Biological and Biochemical Sciences, Faculty of Chemical Technology, University of Pardubice, Pardubice, Czech Republic

Index